生殖免疫学
第三卷
REPRODUCTIVE IMMUNOLOGY
VOLUME 3

免疫性反复妊娠丢失和反复种植失败

IMMUNOLOGY OF RECURRENT PREGNANCY LOSS
AND IMPLANTATION FAILURE

总主编·［美］GIL MOR

主　编·［美］JOANNE KWAK-KIM

主　译·张稼闻　贺小进　吴　欢

主　审·曹云霞

上海科学技术出版社

图书在版编目（CIP）数据

免疫性反复妊娠丢失和反复种植失败 /（美）吉尔·莫尔（Gil Mor）总主编；（美）乔安妮·夸克-金（Joanne Kwak-Kim）主编；张稼闻，贺小进，吴欢主译. -- 上海：上海科学技术出版社，2025.1. -- ISBN 978-7-5478-6876-8

Ⅰ. R714.21；R339.2

中国国家版本馆CIP数据核字第202435G6A0号

This edition *Immunology of Recurrent Pregnancy Loss and Implantation Failure* by **Joanne Kwak-Kim** is published by arrangement with **Elsevier Inc.** of Suite 800, 230 Park Avenue, New York, NY 10169, USA.

上海市版权局著作权合同登记号　图字：09 - 2022 - 0787 号

基金资助：国家自然科学基金（82471648），上海市自然科学基金（22ZR1450700），大健康研究院健康大数据与群体医学研究所专项资金（JKS2023004），上海申康医院发展中心促进市级医院临床技能和临床创新三年行动计划（SHDC2020CR1046B），松江区科技攻关项目（医药卫生类）。

免疫性反复妊娠丢失和反复种植失败
总主编　[美]GIL MOR
主　编　[美]JOANNE KWAK-KIM
主　译　张稼闻　贺小进　吴　欢
主　审　曹云霞

上海世纪出版（集团）有限公司
上海科学技术出版社　出版、发行
（上海市闵行区号景路159弄A座9F - 10F）
邮政编码201101　www.sstp.cn
浙江新华印刷技术有限公司印刷
开本 889×1194　1/16　印张 17.5
字数：500 千字
2025 年 1 月第 1 版　2025 年 1 月第 1 次印刷
ISBN 978 - 7 - 5478 - 6876 - 8/R · 3132
定价：248.00 元

本书如有缺页、错装或坏损等严重质量问题，请向工厂联系调换

Immunology of Recurrent Pregnancy Loss and Implantation Failure, First Edition
Joanne Kwak-Kim
ISBN: 978-0-323-90805-4
Copyright © 2022 Elsevier Inc. All rights reserved.
Authorized Chinese translation published by Shanghai Scientific & Technical Publishers.

《免疫性反复妊娠丢失和反复种植失败》（第1版）（张稼闻，贺小进，吴欢主译）
ISBN: 978-7-5478-6876-8
Copyright © Elsevier Inc. and Shanghai Scientific & Technical Publishers. All rights reserved.
No part of this publication may be reproduced or transmitted in any form or by any means, electronic or mechanical, including photocopying, recording, or any information storage and retrieval system, without permission in writing from Elsevier Inc. Details on how to seek permission, further information about the Elsevier's permissions policies and arrangements with organizations such as the Copyright Clearance Center and the Copyright Licensing Agency, can be found at our website: www.elsevier.com/permissions.
This book and the individual contributions contained in it are protected under copyright by Elsevier Inc. and Shanghai Scientific & Technical Publishers (other than as may be noted herein).

This edition of Immunology of Recurrent Pregnancy Loss and Implantation Failure is published by Shanghai Scientific & Technical Publishers under arrangement with ELSEVIER INC.
This edition is authorized for sale in China only, excluding Hong Kong, Macao and Taiwan. Unauthorized export of this edition is a violation of the Copyright Act. Violation of this Law is subject to Civil and Criminal Penalties.

本版由 ELSEVIER INC. 授权上海科学技术出版社有限公司在中国大陆地区（不包括香港、澳门以及台湾地区）出版发行。
本版仅限在中国大陆地区（不包括香港、澳门以及台湾地区）出版及标价销售。未经许可之出口，视为违反著作权法，将受民事及刑事法律之制裁。
本书封底贴有 Elsevier 防伪标签，无标签者不得销售。

注 意

本书涉及领域的知识和实践标准在不断变化。新的研究和经验拓展我们的理解，因此须对研究方法、专业实践或医疗方法作出调整。从业者和研究人员必须始终依靠自身经验和知识来评估和使用本书中提到的所有信息、方法、化合物或本书中描述的实验。在使用这些信息或方法时，他们应注意自身和他人的安全，包括注意他们负有专业责任的当事人的安全。在法律允许的最大范围内，爱思唯尔、译文的原文作者、原文编辑及原文内容提供者均不对因产品责任、疏忽或其他人身财产伤害及/或损失承担责任，亦不对由于使用或操作文中提到的方法、产品、说明或思想而导致的人身或财产伤害及/或损失承担责任。

内 容 提 要

本书是全球临床生殖免疫学领域的重要专著,重点聚焦反复妊娠丢失(RPL)和反复种植失败(RIF)的免疫病理学机制,患者的评估、诊断和治疗,主要内容包括:

- 详细阐述了 RPL 和 RIF 的免疫学机制,包括 NK 细胞、T 细胞、B 细胞和肥大细胞等免疫细胞异常,以及抗磷脂综合征、自身免疫性甲状腺病等自身免疫性疾病与 RPL 和 RIF 的关系。
- 探讨了胚胎因素、子宫内膜免疫异常、抗精子抗体等在 RPL 和 RIF 中的作用,并介绍了相关诊断和治疗策略。
- 讨论了神经-免疫-内分泌网络失调在生殖障碍中的作用,包括卵巢免疫病理、多囊卵巢综合征、代谢异常和应激等对生殖功能的影响。

本书汇集了生殖免疫学领域最新研究成果和临床经验,为临床医生和研究人员提供了全面、专业的参考资料,对提高 RPL 和 RIF 的诊治水平具有重要指导意义。

译者名单

主审

曹云霞　安徽医科大学第一附属医院

主译

张稼闻　上海交通大学医学院附属第一人民医院

贺小进　上海交通大学医学院附属第一人民医院

吴　欢　安徽医科大学第一附属医院

译者（按首字汉语拼音排序）

柏明珠　徐州市妇幼保健院

陈佳偰　上海集爱遗传与不育诊疗中心

陈晓悦　同济大学附属妇产科医院

何源莹　上海交通大学医学院附属新华医院

何碧薇　上海交通大学医学院附属国际和平妇幼保健院

胡剑麟　上海交通大学医学院附属第一人民医院

姜　姗　上海交通大学医学院附属第一人民医院

李青先　海军军医大学第二附属医院

李淑元　上海交通大学医学院附属国际和平妇幼保健院

林　慧　复旦大学附属妇产科医院

牛永莉　酒泉市人民医院

齐　家　上海交通大学医学院附属仁济医院

宋　兵　安徽医科大学第一附属医院

王惠惠　上海交通大学医学院附属仁济医院

王清莹　同济大学附属第十人民医院

王炎秋　同济大学附属同济医院

吴　煜　上海交通大学医学院附属第一人民医院

肖　会　安徽医科大学第一附属医院

杨　烨　上海交通大学医学院附属第一人民医院

俞思慧　复旦大学附属中山医院
张箴波　同济大学附属同济医院
张沁怡　上海交通大学医学院附属第一人民医院
张旖旎　上海交通大学医学院附属第一人民医院
周莉娜　上海交通大学医学院附属第一人民医院

编者名单

总主编

Gil Mor
 John M. Malone Jr., MD, Endowed Chair, Scientific Director, C.S. Mott Center for Human Growth and Development, Wayne State University School of Medicine, Detroit MI, USA

主　编

Joanne Kwak-Kim, MD, MPH
 Agnes D. Lattimer MD, Professor, Director, Reproductive Medicine and Immunology, Obstetrics and Gynecology, Clinical Sciences Department, Chicago Medical School, Rosalind Franklin University of Medicine and Science, Vernon Hills, IL, USA

编　者

Maria Socorro L. Agcaoili-De Jesus Division of Allergy and Immunology, Department of Medicine, University of the Philippines College of Medicine, Philippine General Hospital, Manila, Philippines

Lara Theresa C. Alentajan-Aleta Division of Allergy and Immunology, Department of Medicine, University of the Philippines College of Medicine, Philippine General Hospital, Manila, Philippines

Lujain Alsubki Reproductive Medicine and Immunology, Obstetrics and Gynecology, Clinical Sciences Department, Chicago Medical School, Rosalind Franklin University of Medicine and Science, Vernon Hills, IL, United States

Raymond M. Anchan Center for Infertility and Reproductive Surgery, Brigham and Women's Hospital, Harvard Medical School, Boston, MA, United States

Petra Clara Arck Division of Experimental Feto-Maternal Medicine, Department of Obstetrics and Fetal Medicine, University Medical Center Hamburg-Eppendorf, Hamburg, Germany

Shihua Bao Department of Reproductive Immunology, Shanghai First Maternity and Infant Hospital, Tongji University School of Medicine, Shanghai, P.R. China

Ricardo Barini Department of Obstetrics and Gynecology, Campinas University (UNICAMP), Campinas, São Paulo, Brazil

Kenneth Beaman Clinical Immunology Laboratory, Faculty of Microbiology and Immunology, Center for Cancer Biology, Infection and Immunology, The Chicago Medical School, Rosalind Franklin University of Medicine and Science, Chicago, IL, United States

Bonnie L. Bermas Division of Rheumatic Diseases, University of Texas Southwestern Medical Center, Dallas, TX, United States

Elena Borodina Department of Obstetrics, Gynecology and Reproductive Sciences, Saint Petersburg State University, Saint Petersburg, Russia

Laboratory of the Mosaic of Autoimmunity, Saint Petersburg State University, Saint Petersburg, Russia

Tia Brodeur Division of Reproductive Endocrinology and Infertility, Department of Obstetrics and Gynecology and Reproductive Sciences, Larner College of Medicine at the University of Vermont, Burlington, VT, United States

Songchen Cai Shenzhen Key Laboratory for Reproductive Immunology of Peri-implantation, Shenzhen Zhongshan Institute for Reproduction and Genetics, Shenzhen Zhongshan Urology Hospital, Shenzhen, P.R. China

Marcelo Borges Cavalcante Postgraduate Program in Medical Sciences, Universidade de Fortaleza (UNIFOR), Fortaleza, Ceará, Brazil

CONCEPTUS-Reproductive Medicine, Fortaleza, Ceará, Brazil

Yuekun Chen Department of Obstetrics and Gynecology, School of Medicine, Hyogo Medical University, Nishinomiya, Hyogo, Japan

Tiffany Alexis Clinton Department of Obstetrics and Gynecology, Henry Ford Health System, Detroit, MI, United States

Svetlana Dambaeva Clinical Immunology Laboratory, Faculty of Microbiology and Immunology, Center for Cancer Biology, Infection and Immunology, The Chicago Medical School, Rosalind Franklin University of Medicine and Science, Chicago, IL, United States

Nicoletta Di Simone Department of Biomedical Sciences, Humanitas University, Pieve Emanuele, Milan, Italy

IRCCS Humanitas Research Hospital, Rozzano, Milan, Italy

Lianghui Diao Shenzhen Key Laboratory for Reproductive Immunology of Peri-implantation, Shenzhen Zhongshan Institute for Reproduction and Genetics, Shenzhen Zhongshan Urology Hospital, Shenzhen, P.R. China

Kerrilyn R. Diener Clinical and Health Sciences Unit, University of South Australia, Adelaide, SA, Australia

Robinson Research Institute and Adelaide Medical School, The University of Adelaide, Adelaide, SA, Australia

Jinli Ding Reproductive Medicine Center, Renmin Hospital of Wuhan University, Wuhan, Hubei, P.R. China

Mengyang Du Department of Reproductive Immunology, Shanghai First Maternity and Infant Hospital, Tongji University School of Medicine, Shanghai, P.R. China

Joseph Duero Department of Obstetrics, Gynecology and Reproductive Sciences, Yale School of Medicine, New Haven, CT, United States

Lyailya Kh. Dzhemlikhanova Department of Obstetrics, Gynecology and Reproductive Sciences, Saint Petersburg State University, Saint Petersburg, Russia

FSBSI "The Research Institute of Obstetrics, Gynecology and Reproductology named after D.O. Ott," Saint Petersburg, Russia

Navid Esfandiari Division of Reproductive Endocrinology and Infertility, Department of Obstetrics and Gynecology and Reproductive Sciences, Larner College of Medicine at the University of Vermont, Burlington, VT, United States

Xuhui Fang Reproductive Medicine Center, Department of Obstetrics and Gynecology, The First Affiliated Hospital of USTC, Division of Life Sciences and Medicine, University of Science and Technology of China, Hefei, Anhui, P.R. China

Atsushi Fukui Department of Obstetrics and

Gynecology, School of Medicine, Hyogo Medical University, Nishinomiya, Hyogo, Japan

Fukushima Medical Center for Child and Woman, Fukushima Medical University, Fukushima, Japan

Jenny S. George Center for Infertility and Reproductive Surgery, Brigham and Women's Hospital, Harvard Medical School, Boston, MA, United States

Alice Gilman-Sachs Clinical Immunology Laboratory, Faculty of Microbiology and Immunology, Center for Cancer Biology, Infection and Immunology, The Chicago Medical School, Rosalind Franklin University of Medicine and Science, Chicago, IL, United States

Ruth Marian Guzman-Genuino Clinical and Health Sciences Unit, University of South Australia, Adelaide, SA, Australia

Alexander M. Gzgzyan Department of Obstetrics, Gynecology and Reproductive Sciences, Saint Petersburg State University, Saint Petersburg, Russia

FSBSI "The Research Institute of Obstetrics, Gynecology and Reproductology named after D.O. Ott," Saint Petersburg, Russia

Ae Ra Han Cha University, Fertility Center, Daegu, Republic of Korea

Jae Won Han Department of Obstetrics and Gynecology, Konyang University College of Medicine, Daejeon, Republic of Korea

Tetsuro Hanada Deparment of Obstetrics and Gynecology, Shiga University of Medical Science, Otsu, Shiga, Japan

Akiko Hasegawa Department of Obstetrics and Gynecology, School of Medicine, Hyogo Medical University, Nishinomiya, Hyogo, Japan

Gentaro Izumi Department of Obstetrics and Gynecology, Graduate School of Medicine, The University of Tokyo, Tokyo, Japan

Toru Kato Department of Obstetrics and Gynecology, School of Medicine, Hyogo Medical University, Nishinomiya, Hyogo, Japan

Sun Kwon Kim Department of Obstetrics and Gynecology, Division of Maternal-Fetal Medicine, Henry Ford Health System, Detroit, MI, United States

Fuminori Kimura Department of Obstetrics and Gynecology, Nara Medical University, Kashihara, Nara, Japan

Jun Kitazawa Department of Obstetrics and Gynecology, Shiga University of Medical Science, Otsu, Shiga, Japan

Kaori Koga Department of Obstetrics and Gynecology, Graduate School of Medicine, The University of Tokyo, Tokyo, Japan

Keiji Kuroda Division Manager of Implantation Research and Endoscopy, Center for Reproductive Medicine and Implantation Research, Sugiyama Clinic Shinjuku, Tokyo, Japan

Joanne Kwak-Kim Reproductive Medicine and Immunology, Obstetrics and Gynecology, Clinical Sciences Department, Chicago Medical School, Rosalind Franklin University of Medicine and Science, Vernon Hills, IL, United States

Maud Lansiaux Hôpital des Bluets, Centre de PMA, Paris, France

Trespidi Laura Department of Obstetrics and Gynaecology, Fondazione Ca Granda, Ospedale Maggiore Policlinico, Milan, Italy

Nathalie Lédée Hôpital des Bluets, Centre de PMA, Paris, France

MatriceLab Innove, Pépinière Paris-Santé-Cochin, Paris, France

Si won Lee Department of Obstetrics and Gynecology, Mount Sinai Medical Center, Miami Beach, FL, United States

Sung Ki Lee Department of Obstetrics and Gynecology, Konyang University College of

Medicine, Daejeon, Republic of Korea

Meroni Pier Luigi　Istituto Auxologico Italiano, IRCCS, Immunorheumatology Research Laboratory, Milan, Italy

Thanh Luu　Reproductive Medicine and Immunology, Obstetrics and Gynecology, Clinical Sciences Department, Chicago Medical School, Rosalind Franklin University of Medicine and Science, Vernon Hills, IL, United States

Brooke Mills　Division of Rheumatic Diseases, University of Texas Southwestern Medical Center, Dallas, TX, United States

Aina Morimune　Department of Obstetrics and Gynecology, Shiga University of Medical Science, Otsu, Shiga, Japan

Roisin Mortimer　Center for Infertility and Reproductive Surgery, Brigham and Women's Hospital, Harvard Medical School, Boston, MA, United States

Takashi Murakami　Department of Obstetrics and Gynecology, Shiga University of Medical Science, Otsu, Shiga, Japan

Koji Nakagawa　Director, Center for Reproductive Medicine and Implantation Research, Sugiyama Clinic Shinjuku, Tokyo, Japan

Akiko Nakamura　Department of Obstetrics and Gynecology, Shiga University of Medical Science, Otsu, Shiga, Japan

Dariko A. Niauri　Department of Obstetrics, Gynecology and Reproductive Sciences, Saint Petersburg State University, Saint Petersburg, Russia
　Laboratory of the Mosaic of Autoimmunity, Saint Petersburg State University, Saint Petersburg, Russia
　FSBSI "The Research Institute of Obstetrics, Gynecology and Reproductology named after D. O. Ott," Saint Petersburg, Russia

Cherie C. Ocampo-Cervantes　Division of Allergy and Immunology, Department of Medicine, University of the Philippines College of Medicine, Philippine General Hospital, Manila, Philippines

Yutaka Osuga　Department of Obstetrics and Gynecology, Graduate School of Medicine, The University of Tokyo, Tokyo, Japan

Jenifer R. Otadoy-Agustin　Division of Allergy and Immunology, Department of Medicine, University of the Philippines College of Medicine, Philippine General Hospital, Manila, Philippines

Joon Cheol Park　Department of Obstetrics and Gynecology, Keimyung University School of Medicine, Daegu, Republic of Korea

Erra Roberta　Department of Obstetrics and Gynaecology, Fondazione Ca Granda, Ospedale Maggiore Policlinico, Milan, Italy

Shinichiro Saeki　Department of Obstetrics and Gynecology, School of Medicine, Hyogo Medical University, Nishinomiya, Hyogo, Japan

Hiroaki Shibahara　Department of Obstetrics and Gynecology, School of Medicine, Hyogo Medical University, Nishinomiya, Hyogo, Japan

Yehuda Shoenfeld　Laboratory of the Mosaic of Autoimmunity, Saint Petersburg State University, Saint Petersburg, Russia
　Ariel University, Ariel, Israel
　Zabludowicz Center for Autoimmune Diseases; Sheba Medical Center, Tel-Aviv, Israel

Rikikazu Sugiyama　CEO, Center for Reproductive Medicine and Implantation Research, Sugiyama Clinic Shinjuku, Tokyo, Japan

Ryu Takeyama　Department of Obstetrics and Gynecology, School of Medicine, Hyogo Medical University, Nishinomiya, Hyogo, Japan

Reshef Tal　Department of Obstetrics, Gynecology and Reproductive Sciences, Yale School of Medicine, New Haven, CT, United States

Chiara Tersigni　Fondazione Policlinico Universitario

A. Gemelli IRCCS, Dipartimento di Scienze della Salute della Donna e del Bambino e di Sanità Pubblica, Rome, Italy

Kristin Thiele　Division of Experimental Feto-Maternal Medicine, Department of Obstetrics and Fetal Medicine, University Medical Center Hamburg-Eppendorf, Hamburg, Germany

Virginie Vaucoret　Hôpital des Bluets, Centre de PMA, Paris, France

Yu Wakimoto　Department of Obstetrics and Gynecology, School of Medicine, Hyogo Medical University, Nishinomiya, Hyogo, Japan

Ossola Wally　Department of Obstetrics and Gynaecology, Fondazione Ca Granda, Ospedale Maggiore Policlinico, Milan, Italy

Xiao Wang　Department of Reproductive Immunology, Shanghai First Maternity and Infant Hospital, Tongji University School of Medicine, Shanghai, P. R. China

Yanshi Wang　Reproductive Medicine Center, Department of Obstetrics and Gynecology, The First Affiliated Hospital of USTC, Division of Life Sciences and Medicine, University of Science and Technology of China, Hefei, Anhui, P. R. China

Yiqiu Wei　Reproductive Medicine Center, Renmin Hospital of Wuhan University, Wuhan, Hubei, P. R. China

Ronja Wöhrle　Division of Experimental Feto-Maternal Medicine, Department of Obstetrics and Fetal Medicine, University Medical Center Hamburg-Eppendorf, Hamburg, Germany

Katharine Wolf　Clinical Immunology Laboratory, Faculty of Microbiology and Immunology, Center for Cancer Biology, Infection and Immunology, The Chicago Medical School, Rosalind Franklin University of Medicine and Science, Chicago, IL, United States

Li Wu　Reproductive Medicine Center, Department of Obstetrics and Gynecology, The First Affiliated Hospital of USTC, Division of Life Sciences and Medicine, University of Science and Technology of China, Hefei, Anhui, P. R. China

Ayano Yamaya　Department of Obstetrics and Gynecology, School of Medicine, Hyogo Medical University, Nishinomiya, Hyogo, Japan

Tailang Yin　Reproductive Medicine Center, Renmin Hospital of Wuhan University, Wuhan, Hubei, P. R. China

Yong Zeng　Shenzhen Key Laboratory for Reproductive Immunology of Peri-implantation, Shenzhen Zhongshan Institute for Reproduction and Genetics, Shenzhen Zhongshan Urology Hospital, Shenzhen, P. R. China

主编介绍

Joanne Kwak-Kim

医学博士、理学硕士、公共卫生硕士。美国罗莎琳德·富兰克林医科大学芝加哥医学院临床科学系妇产科学/免疫和感染中心教授,美国罗莎琳德·富兰克林大学健康诊所生殖医学和免疫学主任。曾任芝加哥医学院妇产科主任助理和罗莎琳德·富兰克林大学卫生系医学主任。

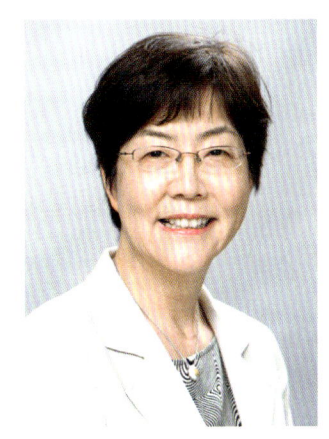

Kwak-Kim 博士在过去的三十年间一直从事临床、研究和教育工作。她对生殖免疫学领域,尤其是反复妊娠丢失和反复种植失败,抱有浓厚的兴趣,这是她研究的重点。她在自然杀伤细胞以及 Th1/Th2 免疫反应方面的研究,特别是针对经历反复妊娠丢失和反复种植失败女性的相关研究,成果显著。她所做的将基础科学研究成果应用于临床的工作,处于该领域的前沿。她在同行评审的杂志和图书中发表了 160 余篇文章。她在《美国生殖免疫学》杂志上编写了两本特刊:《临床生殖免疫学专题》和《临床生殖免疫学》。此外,她还是《子宫内膜基因表达:生殖障碍的新范式》和《生殖免疫学:反复妊娠丢失和反复种植失败》两本书的作者。

Kwak-Kim 博士是《生殖免疫学》杂志的主编,《美国生殖免疫学》杂志的副主编,也是多本同行评审科学期刊的编委会成员。她是一位备受欢迎的讲师,已审阅众多来自各个国家的科学研究。此外,她还为全球的科学机构提供科学咨询服务。

她主要指导医学生、住院医师、博士研究生和博士后研究员。作为培训生导师,她是生殖医学和免疫学领域的坚定支持者。当被问及如何才能成为一名成功的生殖免疫学家时,她指出,需具备创造性思维、乐于倾听和富有同情心——这些品质在 Kwak-Kim 博士超过 30 年的杰出工作中得到了充分体现。

她在美国生殖免疫学会(ASRI)、美国生殖医学会(ASRM)、生殖研究学会和国际生殖免疫学会均有突出贡献。

Kwak-Kim 博士曾多次获奖,包括 2002 年因其在生殖免疫学基础研究或应用研究方面的杰出成就而获得的著名的 J. Christian Herr 奖。2009 年,她获得 ASRI 颁发的杰出服务奖。2011 年,因在研究、教学和临床护理方面的杰出贡献,获得了罗莎琳德·富兰克林医科大学颁发的 Lawrence R. Medoff 奖。在 2015 年第 35 届 ASRI 年会上,Kwak-Kim 博士被授予美国生殖免疫学杂志奖,该奖项表彰在生殖免疫学领域做出杰出贡献的资深研究人员。2017 年,她应邀成为得克萨斯大学举办的第 23 届雷蒙德·O.贝里纪念讲座的演讲人。2018年,她获得了罗莎琳德·富兰克林医科大学芝加哥医学院的"Lattimer教授"职位。Agnes D. Lattimer博士曾克服了令人难以置信的逆境,成为一名受人尊敬、具有影响力的儿科医生,并最终担任库克县医院的医疗主任。为纪念Lattimer博士不懈的服务、勇敢的精神和世代相传的仁慈,该教授职位被命名为"Lattimer教授"。Kwak-Kim博士被认为是"Lattimer教授"的典型代表。2020年,Kwak-Kim还获得了"延世医学大奖",该奖项授予在医学领域做出重大学术贡献的校友。

Kwak-Kim博士曾任ASRI主席,并成功组织和主持了ASRI第21届、22届和38届年会。她担任过国际生殖免疫学会(ISIR)秘书长和财务主管,目前是ISIR的主席。她还是ASRM生殖免疫学特别兴趣小组的主席。2021年,她在美国生殖免疫学会的支持下设立了临床生殖免疫学协会。

Kwak-Kim博士一直担任罗莎琳德·富兰克林大学健康诊所的生殖医学和免疫学主任。该诊所主要治疗种植失败引起的不孕症、免疫因素导致的反复妊娠丢失以及合并同种免疫/自身免疫疾病的妊娠。该诊所在世界范围享有盛誉,为来自美国和其他国家的患者提供服务。她在生殖医学和免疫学领域的专业知识与她对患者的深切同情和全心全意的诊疗相得益彰。她为来自各行各业和世界各地的患者提供帮助,为前来就诊时已经历多次妊娠丢失的女性提供知识和安慰。她的患者常侃侃而谈她是如何改变她们生活的:她们多年的困惑和挫折多亏了她的诊疗才得以结束。作为本领域的先驱,随着生殖免疫学专业的出现,她与她的诊所如今能提供许多治疗方法,这些都是在她数十年的研究和对患者治疗基础上得出的。

中文版序

生殖免疫学是一个充满挑战和机遇的前沿领域。它不仅涉及生殖医学和免疫学，还与内分泌学、遗传学、分子生物学等多个学科密切相关。这种多学科交叉的特性，使得生殖免疫学成为解决复杂生殖问题的关键科学。特别是在反复妊娠丢失（RPL）和反复种植失败（RIF）这两个临床难题上，生殖免疫学为我们提供了全新的视角和方法。

然而，我们必须认识到，尽管生殖免疫学在过去几十年取得了显著进展，但仍有许多未解之谜等待我们去探索。例如，母体免疫系统如何精确调节以接受半同种异体胚胎，却又能维持对病原体的防御能力？胚胎-子宫界面的免疫微环境如何影响胚胎种植和早期妊娠维持？这些问题的答案可能蕴含着解决 RPL 和 RIF 的关键方法和途径。

这本由美国生殖免疫学会专家编写的《免疫性反复妊娠丢失和反复种植失败》全面涵盖了从基础免疫学到临床应用的各个方面，包括 NK 细胞、T 细胞、B 细胞等免疫细胞的作用，自身免疫疾病与生殖障碍的关系，以及新兴的研究热点如子宫内膜免疫病理、代谢异常与生殖免疫等。这些内容不仅反映了当前研究的前沿，也为未来的探索指明了方向。

值得注意的是，生殖免疫学的临床应用仍面临诸多挑战。诊断标准的制定、治疗方案的个体化、疗效评估的客观化等问题，都需要我们进一步研究和探讨。例如，NK 细胞检测在临床中的应用价值、免疫调节治疗的最佳时机和剂量等，都是当前争议较大的问题。这提醒我们，在临床实践中要保持谨慎和批判性思维的态度，避免盲目应用未经充分验证的诊疗方法。

同时，我们也要认识到转化医学在生殖免疫学中的重要性。如何将实验室的发现快速、有效地转化为临床应用，是摆在我们面前的一大挑战。这需要基础研究者和临床医生的紧密合作，也需要建立更加完善的临床研究体系。

此外，随着生物技术的飞速发展，新的研究工具和方法不断涌现，如单细胞测序、多组学分析、人工智能辅助诊断等，这些都为生殖免疫学研究带来了新的机遇。我们应该积极拥抱这些新技术，将其应用于生殖免疫学研究中，以期获得更深入的认识和更有效的诊疗方法。

作为一名长期从事生殖医学研究的实践者，我深感生殖免疫学的魅力和挑战。它不仅涉及人类繁衍这一根本问题，还与多个重大疾病的发生发展密切相关。因此，我们的研究不仅能够帮助那些饱受生育困扰的患者，还可能为其他免疫相关疾病的治疗提供新的思路。

最后，我要特别感谢本书的译者团队。他们的辛勤工作使得这本重要的著作能够以中文版的形式呈现在中国读者面前。这不仅为国内的临床医生和研究人员提供了宝贵的学习资料，也为中国生殖免疫学的发展注入了新的动力。

我相信，本书的出版将极大地促进中国生殖免疫学的发展。它不仅为临床医生提供了宝贵的指导，也为研究者提供了新的思路。让我们携手努力，在这个充满挑战和机遇的领域中不断探索，为揭示生命的奥秘、造福人类健康做出我们的贡献。

曹云霞

国家卫生健康委配子及生殖道异常研究重点实验室主任

中国妇幼健康研究会生殖医学专业委员会主任委员

安徽医科大学妇产科学系主任

2024 年 10 月

中文版前言

生殖免疫学作为生殖医学和免疫学的交叉领域,近年来发展迅速,在解释和治疗诸多生殖健康问题方面发挥着越来越重要的作用。然而,长期以来,国内缺乏系统、全面介绍临床生殖免疫学的专著,尤其是针对反复妊娠丢失(RPL)和反复种植失败(RIF)这两个临床难题的专著。有鉴于此,我们有幸将美国生殖免疫学会专家编著的《免疫性反复妊娠丢失和反复种植失败》一书翻译成中文,以飨国内同道。

本书聚焦临床生殖免疫学,尤其是 RPL 和 RIF 的免疫病理学,以及患者评估、诊断和治疗。全书基于最新的临床和研究数据,系统阐述了影响人类妊娠的自身免疫、细胞免疫和同种免疫疾病,详细讨论了包括抗磷脂综合征、风湿性疾病、自身免疫性甲状腺疾病在内的自身免疫性疾病,以及 T 细胞、B 细胞、NK 细胞和肥大细胞相关的细胞免疫异常。此外,本书还全面总结了可能影响 RPL 和 RIF 的免疫炎症性疾病,如子宫内膜免疫病理、血栓形成状态、卵巢自身免疫、多囊卵巢综合征、子宫内膜异位症等。

本书是目前国际上最新、最全面的临床生殖免疫学专著之一,汇集了该领域最新的研究成果和临床经验。本书不仅深入探讨了 RPL 和 RIF 的免疫学机制,还提供了详细的诊断和治疗指南,具有很强的临床实用性。此外,本书还涵盖生殖免疫学与其他学科的交叉领域,如辅助生殖技术、代谢紊乱和应激反应等,体现了多学科融合的研究趋势。我们将本书翻译出版,旨在为国内生殖医学和免疫学领域的同道提供一本系统全面的参考书。这不仅有助于提高我国临床医生对 RPL 和 RIF 免疫学机制的认识,为患者诊疗提供最新的指导,也将为国内相关领域的科研工作提供宝贵的研究思路和方法。

值得一提的是,近年来我国学者在生殖免疫学领域也取得了显著进展。例如,*JAMA* 杂志陆续发表了乔杰院士和洪天配教授团队开展的甲状腺功能正常的甲状腺自身免疫不同状态妇女接受左旋甲状腺素治疗后的妊娠结局研究(POSTAL 研究)、陈子江院士和孙贇教授团队的全球首个探究强的松治疗反复种植失败有效性的多中心、双盲、随机对照临床研究。这些成果为全球生殖免疫领域的研究提供了中国数据,贡献了中国方案。此外,多位中国专家也参与了原著的编写工作,为本书内容在中国的应用和推广奠定了基础。

在上海科学技术出版社的鼎力支持下,过去一年,来自上海交通大学医学院、复旦大学、同济大学以及安徽医科大学等多家附属医院的中青年骨干医师和研究员,共同完成了本书的翻译工作。在整个翻译过程中，我们始终秉持严谨治学的态度，力求准确传达原著的学术内容，以确保译文既专业准确又通俗易懂。尽管如此，由于译者学识有限，书中难免存在疏漏或不当之处。我们诚挚地希望各位同道不吝赐教，提出宝贵的意见和建议。

让我们携手努力，共同推动中国生殖免疫学领域的蓬勃发展，为提升我国生殖医学水平贡献力量！

张稼闻　贺小进　吴　欢

2024年10月于上海

目 录

第 1 篇
概　述
Introduction

第 1 章　临床生殖免疫学：了解生殖与免疫学的窗口　　　　002
Clinical reproductive immunology: a window to understanding reproduction and immunology

第 2 篇
反复妊娠丢失
Recurrent pregnancy losses

第 2 章　自然杀伤（NK）细胞病理学与生殖障碍：NK 细胞水平、NK 细胞毒性和 KIR/HLA - C　　　　006
Natural killer (NK) cell pathology and reproductive failure: NK cell level, NK cell cytotoxicity, and KIR/HLA-C

第 3 章　辅助性 T 细胞病理学与反复妊娠丢失：Th1/Th2、Treg/Th17 及其他 T 细胞应答　　　　017
T helper cell pathology and recurrent pregnancy losses: Th1/Th2, Treg/Th17, and other T cell responses

第 4 章　B 细胞病理学与反复妊娠丢失　　　　034
B cell pathology and recurrent pregnancy loss

第 5 章　肥大细胞病理学与生殖障碍　　　　044
Mast cell pathology and reproductive failures

第 6 章　人白细胞抗原在反复妊娠丢失发病机制中的作用　　　　058
Role of human leukocyte antigen in the pathogenesis of recurrent pregnancy loss

第 7 章　应激诱导的免疫偏差和生殖障碍　　　　064
Stress-induced immune deviations and reproductive failure

第 8 章　抗磷脂综合征与反复妊娠丢失　　　　075
Antiphospholipid syndrome and recurrent pregnancy losses

第 9 章　抗精子抗体与生殖障碍　　　　085
Antisperm antibodies and reproductive failure

第 10 章　抗甲状腺抗体与生殖功能　　　　093
　　　　　Antithyroid antibodies and reproductive function

第 11 章　胎儿和新生儿同种免疫性血小板减少症与反复妊娠丢失　　　　101
　　　　　Fetal/neonatal alloimmune-mediated thrombocytopenia and recurrent pregnancy loss

第 12 章　感染性和非感染性子宫内膜炎与反复妊娠丢失　　　　109
　　　　　Infections and noninfections endometritis and recurrent pregnancy loss

第 13 章　反复妊娠丢失的血栓病理学　　　　119
　　　　　Thrombophilic pathologies in recurrent pregnancy losses

第 14 章　风湿病与生殖结局　　　　126
　　　　　Rheumatic diseases and reproductive outcomes

第 3 篇

反复种植失败
Repeated implantation failures

第 15 章　生殖免疫学在反复妊娠丢失和反复种植失败中的作用　　　　136
　　　　　The role of reproductive immunology in recurrent pregnancy loss and repeated implantation failure

第 16 章　生殖障碍中的胚胎：免疫学视角　　　　147
　　　　　The embryo in reproductive failure: immunological view

第 17 章　自然杀伤细胞病理学与反复种植失败　　　　158
　　　　　Natural killer cell pathology and repeated implantation failures

第 18 章　辅助性 T 细胞病理学与反复种植失败　　　　167
　　　　　Helper T cell pathology and repeated implantation failures

第 19 章　B 细胞病理学与反复种植失败　　　　175
　　　　　B-cell pathology and repeated implantation failures

第 20 章　子宫内膜病理学和反复种植失败　　　　185
　　　　　Endometrial pathology and repeated implantation failures

第 21 章　易栓症、抗磷脂抗体和抗凝治疗与反复种植失败　　　　193
　　　　　Thrombophilia, antiphospholipid antibodies, and anticoagulation in recurrent implantation failure

第 4 篇

生殖障碍中的神经-免疫-内分泌网络失调
Dysregulated neuroimmune-endocrine network in reproductive failures

第 22 章 卵巢免疫病理学与生殖功能障碍 　　　　　　　　　　　　　　　　　　　204
　　　　　The ovarian immune pathology and reproductive failures

第 23 章 多囊卵巢综合征与生殖障碍 　　　　　　　　　　　　　　　　　　　　　216
　　　　　Polycystic ovarian syndrome and reproductive failure

第 24 章 反复妊娠丢失和反复种植失败女性免疫反应的代谢调控 　　　　　　　　235
　　　　　Metabolic control of immune responses in women with recurrent pregnancy loss and recurrent implantation failure

第 25 章 子宫内膜异位症与生殖障碍 　　　　　　　　　　　　　　　　　　　　　245
　　　　　Endometriosis and reproductive failures

第 26 章 生殖障碍的实验室检查：生殖障碍的免疫学生物标志物 　　　　　　　　250
　　　　　Laboratory approaches for reproductive failure: immunological biomarkers for reproductive failures

第 1 篇

概 述

Introduction

第 1 章

临床生殖免疫学：了解生殖与免疫学的窗口

Clinical reproductive immunology: a window to understanding reproduction and immunology

Joanne Kwak-Kim

Reproductive Medicine and Immunology, Obstetrics and Gynecology, Clinical Sciences Department, Chicago Medical School, Rosalind Franklin University of Medicine and Science, Vernon Hills, IL, United States

生殖免疫学已成为生殖医学的一个活跃领域。尽管已有许多图书和期刊聚焦生殖免疫学的研究工作，但目前还没有对临床生殖免疫学进行系统综述的教科书。本书是生殖免疫学教科书系列的组成部分，内容涉及临床生殖免疫学，特别是基于最新的临床和研究数据，聚焦反复妊娠丢失（recurrent pregnancy losses，RPL）和反复种植失败（repeated implantation failures，RIF）的免疫病理学以及对患者的评估、诊断和治疗。

生殖免疫学概念的临床转化始于 20 世纪 80 年代[1]。William Hunter 通过证明胎儿循环与母体完全隔离，记录了免疫学对人类生殖意义的早期观察[2]。1871 年，Charles Darwin 将女性生育力降低与不良行为联系起来，进而对不孕症进行了免疫学解释[3]。1890 年，Walter Heape 成功将同种异体囊胚移植到代孕母兔体内，是早期免疫学研究的里程碑事件[3]。在 1924 年 Clarence Cook Little 的文献中可找到关于生殖免疫学的最早记载，其中将妊娠的免疫耐受描述为"就个体的遗传独特性而言，雌性哺乳动物必须具有相同的耐受性"[4]。1932 年，Raymond O. Berry 首次成功进行了同种系内胚胎移植，意味着子宫并非免疫豁免部位，胎盘需与母体的免疫相容[5]。1953 年，诺贝尔奖获得者 Peter Medawar 爵士在实验生物学学会的会议上提出"怀孕的母亲是如何将一个作为抗原异物的胎儿在体内养育数周或数月的"这一问题，整合了生殖免疫学的概念[6]。几乎在同一时期，得益于移植生物学的进展，免疫学领域开始将其重点转向免疫生物学[7]。这些变化影响了对移植免疫学感兴趣的生殖科学家，他们于 1981 年成立了美国生殖免疫学会[8]。几年后，Alan E Beer 报道了第一项临床转化研究，并首次报道了淋巴细胞免疫疗法治疗反复妊娠丢失的临床研究[9]。从那时起，针对患有免疫性病因的 RPL 和 RIF 女性的各种免疫疗法的临床试验被陆续报道。

生殖免疫学是研究免疫系统与生殖系统间相互作用的医学领域，其原理被用于认识母胎耐受性，并揭示了一些妇产科疾病，如 Rh 致敏和新生儿早期同种免疫性血小板减少症。20 世纪 80 年代和 90 年代，生殖免疫学概念被应用于研究妊娠丢失、生育力降低和子痫前期的潜在免疫病理学。此外，随着生殖免疫学日益成熟，业已开发了各种治疗方法。然而，在研究成果的临床转化方面，仍存在诸多挑战。

生殖免疫学的临床实践已被公认为妇产科的一个领域。2021 年，在美国生殖免疫学会的支持下设立了临床生殖免疫学协会。虽然注册的临床生殖免疫学家人数还很少，但他们目前正从事生殖免疫学的相关工作。生殖免疫学领域需要实施更多的临床培训计划和编写更多的教材，因此，出版生殖免疫学教科书的时机已经成熟。

本书呈现了妇产科，尤其是与早期妊娠相关的生殖免疫疾病的精髓。本书的内容涵盖了影响人类妊娠的自身免疫、细胞免疫和同种免疫疾病，重点聚焦 RPL 和 RIF，并全面回顾了与其相关的自身免疫疾病，包括抗磷脂综合征、风湿性疾病、自身免疫性甲状腺病、抗精子抗体，以及细胞免疫异常，如 T 细胞、B 细胞、NK 细胞和肥大细胞相关的免疫病理。此外，本书还总结了可能影响 RPL 和 RIF 的免疫炎症性疾病，包括子宫内膜免疫病理、血栓形成状态、卵巢自身免疫、多囊卵巢综合征、子宫内膜异位症、辅助生殖技术、代谢紊乱和应激诱导的免疫异常。

尽管免疫学的发展迅速，临床生殖免疫学仍处于起步阶段。今后需要进一步研究以开发新的生物标志物和治疗靶点。为了实现临床转化，需要进行精心设计的临床试验和系统的数据收集。此外，未来应考虑采用新的疾病命名法和临床报告系统，并建立一个医生网络平台以分享最新的临床知识。随着技术的快速发展和新型生物制剂的问世，临床生殖免疫学正处于一个崭新的阶段。因此，未来需要进行大量的研究，并及时转化生殖免疫学的研究成果。

我希望本书能对临床医生和其他医疗保健提供者在临床生殖免疫学实践中有所帮助。我衷心感谢所有参与并为本书做出贡献的作者，特别是 Na Young Sung 博士，他在本书编写过程中提供了多方面的帮助。最后，我要感谢我的丈夫 Joon Woo Kim 博士，我的孩子 Caroline 和 Michael，他们理解我对这个职业的奉献以及繁忙的工作和日程安排。

参考文献

[1] Beer AE, Quebbeman JF, Ayers JW, Haines RF. Major histocompatibility complex antigens, maternal and paternal immune responses, and chronic habitual abortions in humans. Am J Obstet Gynecol 1981;141(8):987-99. Available from: https://doi.org/10.1016/s0002-9378(16)32690-4.

[2] Shippen Jr W. The hunters. N Engl J Med 1963;268(5):271-2. Available from: https://doi.org/10.1056/nejm196301312680514.

[3] Billingham RE, Beer AE. Reproductive immunology: past, present, and future. Perspect Biol Med 1984;27(2):259-75. Available from: https://doi.org/10.1353/pbm.1984.0042.

[4] Little CC. The genetics of tissue transplantation in mammals. J Cancer Res 1924;8(1):75-95. Available from: https://doi.org/10.1158/jcr.1924.75.

[5] Kwak-Kim J, Sung N, Saab W, Fukui A. Introduction of the special issue, "clinical reproductive immunology.". Am J Reprod immunol (New York, NY: 1989) 2021;85(4):e13415. Available from: https://doi.org/10.1111/aji.13415.

[6] Medawar PB. Some immunological and endocrinological problems raised by the evolution of viviparity in vertebrates. Symp Soc Exp Biol 1953;1953(7):320-37.

[7] Kaufmann SHE. Immunology's coming of age. Review. Front Immunol 2019;10(684). Available from: https://doi.org/10.3389/fimmu.2019.00684.

[8] Officers of The American Society for the. Immunology of reproduction and the international committee for immunology of reproduction. Am J Reprod Immunol 1980;1(1):1. Available from: https://doi.org/10.1111/j.1600-0897.1980.tb00002.x.

[9] Beer AE. 10-New Horizons in the diagnosis, evaluation and therapy of recurrent spontaneous abortion. ClObstet Gynaecol 1986;13(1):115-24. Available from: https://doi.org/10.1016/S0306-3356(21)00158-8.

第 2 篇

反复妊娠丢失

Recurrent pregnancy losses

第 2 章

自然杀伤(NK)细胞病理学与生殖障碍：NK 细胞水平、NK 细胞毒性和 KIR/HLA - C

Natural killer (NK) cell pathology and reproductive failure: NK cell level, NK cell cytotoxicity, and KIR/HLA - C

Svetlana Dambaeva[1], Thanh Luu[2], Lujain Alsubki[2] and Joanne Kwak-Kim[2]

[1] Clinical Immunology Laboratory, Faculty of Microbiology and Immunology, Center for Cancer Biology, Infection and Immunology, The Chicago Medical School, Rosalind Franklin University of Medicine and Science, Chicago, IL, United States
[2] Reproductive Medicine and Immunology, Obstetrics and Gynecology, Clinical Sciences Department, Chicago Medical School, Rosalind Franklin University of Medicine and Science, Vernon Hills, IL, United States

1 引言

早在 20 世纪 20 年代，组织学家就注意到分泌晚期子宫内膜和妊娠早期蜕膜中存在大量颗粒细胞，并认为这些细胞起源于未分化的子宫内膜基质细胞。在 20 世纪 80 年代，研究者们发现它们表达淋巴细胞谱系受体，并进一步鉴定为自然杀伤(NK)细胞[1,2]。免疫组化检测显示，这些子宫内膜的颗粒淋巴细胞具有不寻常的特征——NK 细胞标志物 NKH1(CD56)强染，而对其他 NK 细胞标志物 (CD16)无反应。自从发现子宫内膜 NK(eNK)细胞，eNK 细胞在妊娠中的重要性，在蜕膜化、胚胎植入和胎盘形成中的作用，以及它们的起源，已成为生殖生物学家、妇产科医生和生殖免疫学家感兴趣的话题。

2 自然杀伤细胞的定义

NK 细胞是一种淋巴细胞，在固有免疫中起着至关重要的作用。与 T 淋巴细胞和 B 淋巴细胞不同，它们既不经历体细胞基因重排，也不执行获得性免疫的特异性免疫反应。相反，NK 细胞表达各种受体，使其能够从受病毒感染、处于应激状态或发生恶性转化的细胞中识别出健康细胞。NK 细胞无须事先致敏就能直接破坏肿瘤细胞，这就是它们被命名为自然杀伤细胞的原因。NK 细胞的细胞毒作用机制可以用"缺失自我"的概念来解释。这个概念的基础是，失去自身 HLA Ⅰ 类分子的细胞将被 NK 细胞识别为靶细胞[3]。然而，对 NK 细胞的进一步研究发现，在许多情况下，"缺失自我"并不足以或必须触发 NK 细胞的毒性，还需要通过激活性受体发出额外信号来促进细胞毒性功能[4]。此外，除了细胞毒性作用，NK 细胞还能非常有效地产生细胞因子。NK 细胞的免疫调节能力对于局部和全身免疫反应都很重要[4]。

2.1 自然杀伤细胞的受体

NK 细胞表达多种激活性和抑制性受体。由激活性受体传导的信号受到抑制性受体信号的制约。因此，为了触发细胞毒活性，激活性受体的信号需强于通过抑制性受体接收的信号。

专门识别 HLA Ⅰ 类分子的两大受体家族参与调节 NK 细胞的细胞毒性效应功能。第一类受体在进化上是保守的，包括 C 型凝集素样受体，如 NKG2A、NKG2C 和 NKG2E。它们与 CD94 形成异二聚体复合物。CD94/NKG2A 复合物介导对 NK 细胞的抑制信号，而 CD94/NKC2C 和 CD94/NKG2E 则介导激活信号。这些受体识别非经典的 HLA Ⅰ类分子 HLA-E。与高度多态性的经典 HLA-A、HLA-B、HLA-C 相比，HLA-E 具有有限的多态性，可在抗原结合槽内结合特异的抗原肽。因此，只有来源于其他 HLA Ⅰ类分子的抗原肽才能被 HLA-E 递呈[5]。

NK 细胞表达的 HLA Ⅰ类特异性受体的第二个家族包括了一大类受体，称为杀伤细胞免疫球蛋白样受体（KIR）。KIR 家族与 CD94/NKG2 相似，都包含了激活性和抑制性受体。KIR 由高度多态性的基因编码，构成了位于 19 号染色体上的 KIR 基因座。现已发现了 9 个抑制性受体基因（KIR2DL1、KIR2DL2、KIR2DL3、KIR2DL4、KIR2DL5A、KIR2DL5B、KIR3DL1、KIR3DL2 和 KIR3DL3）和 6 个激活性受体基因（KIR2DS1、KIR2DS2、KIR2ADS3、KIR2DS4、KIR1DS5 和 KIR3DS1）[6]。与 NKG2 相反，KIR 基因座内的基因属于灵长类动物中快速扩增的最新进化基因[7]。人类携带的 KIR 基因数量最多。此外，KIR 基因座上的等位基因含量因个体而异，其中一些 KIR 基因存在或缺失。这些基因的不同组合被称为 KIR 单倍型。单倍型"A"包括一组 6 个抑制性 KIR 和 1 个激活性 KIR。这个单倍型的组成是固定的。KIR 基因座内的所有其他基因组合称为"B"单倍型。具有 2 个"A"单倍型的个体被称为 KIR AA 基因型或"抑制性"KIR 基因型。携带"A"和"B"或两个"B"单倍型的个体被称为 KIR Bx 基因型或"激活性"KIR 基因型。由于 KIR 基因座内基因含量不同，KIR Bx 基因型的特征是 KIR 数量的高度多样性。此外，2 个或多个激活性 KIR 的存在将 KIR Bx 基因型与 KIR AA 基因型区分开来。

KIR 可识别经典的 HLA Ⅰ类分子。HLA Ⅰ类家族中最新进化的成员 HLA-C 是 KIR 的主要配体[8]。根据 KIR 识别的表位，所有作为配体的 HLA-C 分子可分为 C1 或 C2。HLA-C C1 分子是 KIR2DL2 和 KIR2DL3 的配体，HLA-C C2 分子是 KIR2DL1 和 KIR2DS1 的配体。其他 HLA Ⅰ类分子也被认为是 KIR 的配体。HLA-G 被 KIR2DL4 识别。此外，KIR3DL1 识别携带 HLA-B 和 HLA-A 的 Bw4 表位。约 1/3 的 HLA-B 等位基因和少数 HLA-A 等位基因（HLA-A*23、24、32）具有 Bw4 表位[9]。然而，KIR3DL3、KIR2DL5、KIR3DS3 没有明确的配体，只有特定的 HLA Ⅰ类等位基因与 KIR3DL2（HLA-A*03、11）、KIR2DS2（HLA-C*01）、KIR2DS5（一些 HLA-C C2 等位基因）和 KIR3DS1（HLA-B*51）结合[6]。

CD16 是 NK 细胞用来执行固有免疫任务的非 HLA 限制性受体。CD16 是一种低亲和力 Fcγ 受体，能识别被 IgG 调理的细胞，并介导抗体依赖性细胞介导的细胞毒作用（antibody-dependent cellular cytotoxicity，ADCC）[10]。另一个调节 NK 细胞效应功能的受体家族是自然细胞毒性受体（natural cytotoxicity receptors，NCR）。NCR 家族由 3 个受体组成，即 NKp30、NKp44 和 NKp46。它们通过与配体结合主要介导激活信号。与 KIR 和 NKG2 受体不同，NCR 不受 HLA 限制。它们的配体是各种肿瘤或病原体相关分子，包括硫酸乙酰肝素、恶性细胞上的糖胺聚糖、病毒血凝素、巨细胞病毒的蛋白 pp65，以及一些细菌和细菌-真菌配体[11]。

2.2 自然杀伤细胞的细胞因子

NK 细胞产生的主要细胞因子包括 IFN-γ 和 TNF。此外，NK 细胞还分泌白细胞介素（如 IL-6 和 IL-5）、生长因子和血管生成因子（GM-CSF、VEGF），以及各类趋化因子（CXCL8、CCL3、CCL4 等）[12]。其中，一些细胞因子直接影响其他免疫细胞的活性，另一些则对血管生成、血管重塑和组织内稳态很重要。NK 细胞是 IFN-γ 的主要来源，而 IFN-γ 则是免疫反应不可或缺的组成部分，能刺激巨噬细胞和树突状细胞，并对 T 细胞向 Th1 型极化至关重要。TNF 和 IL-6 是急性期反应因子，可引起前列腺素 E2 等炎症介质的表达。趋化因子在招募中性粒细胞和其他白细胞进入组织中发挥积极作用。GM-CSF 是一种调节髓系细胞发育和促进巨噬细胞活化的生长因子。NK 细胞在Ⅰ型 IFN、IL-15 或 IL-18 以及其他细胞因子的刺激下分泌细胞因子。NK 细胞上表达的这些刺激物受体使其能够做出快速反应，产生免疫调节因子。组织环境也会影响 NK 细胞的反应性，缺氧条件可刺激 NK 细胞分泌血管生成因子 VEGF-A[13]。

2.3 自然杀伤细胞的亚群

自 20 世纪 70 年代发现 NK 细胞既不是 T 细胞

也不是 B 细胞以来[14]，研究者们已经清楚认识到 NK 细胞在其驻留、表型和功能特征方面是一个极其多样化的群体[15,16]。NK 细胞约占外周血淋巴细胞的 10%，并且也存在于许多组织中，包括肝脏、肠道、扁桃体和肺。值得注意的是，子宫中 NK 细胞数量最多。

在外周血中，NK 细胞根据其表型可分为两个亚群。外周血 NK(pNK)细胞主要为 CD16 阳性，且 CD56($CD56^{dim}$ pNK 细胞)弱表达。约 10% 的 pNK 细胞的 CD16 呈阴性，并高表达 CD56($CD56^{bright}$ pNK 细胞)。这些亚群之间还存在其他表型差异。例如，$CD56^{bright}$ pNK 细胞的特征是 KIR 低表达，但 NKp46 和 NKG2A 均呈阳性。相反，$CD56^{dim}$ pNK 细胞表达 KIR，而 NKp46 和 NKG2A 的表达变化较大。这两个亚群具有不同的功能。$CD56^{dim}$ pNK 细胞显示出比 $CD56^{bright}$ 细胞更高的细胞毒活性。相比之下，$CD56^{bright}$ pNK 细胞可以快速产生细胞因子和趋化因子，被认为是免疫调节细胞[17]。存在于组织中的 NK 细胞，即组织驻留 NK(trNK)细胞，与上述两种 pNK 细胞亚群不同。它们大多为 CD16 阴性和 $CD56^{dim}$。一般来说，trNK 细胞能够产生细胞因子，但细胞毒性较弱[15]。

子宫 NK(uNK)细胞具有独特的特性。与 $CD56^{bright}$ pNK 细胞或其他 trNK 细胞相似，uNK 缺乏 CD16 表达，不能介导 ADCC。然而，uNK 似乎具有很强的细胞毒活性，因为其充满了含有裂解蛋白酶(颗粒酶)和成孔蛋白(穿孔素)的颗粒。研究表明，与两个 pNK 细胞亚群相比，颗粒酶 A 和 B 及穿孔素在 uNK 细胞中的表达最高[18]。抑制性受体表达的增加可能对于控制这种细胞毒作用的潜在有害触发是必需的。这一发现可能解释了 uNK 细胞的 KIR 高表达。事实上，uNK 细胞比任何其他 NK 细胞亚群具有更高的 KIR 表达[18]。另一种识别 HLA Ⅰ类配体的抑制性受体 CD94/NKG2A 也在 uNK 细胞中高表达[16]。uNK 细胞的免疫调节特性在妊娠支持中起着重要作用，这是由于它们产生的 IFN-γ 对于螺旋动脉重塑至关重要[19]。此外，uNK 细胞分泌趋化因子、生长因子和血管生成因子，促进滋养细胞迁移和胎盘生长[20,21]。在周期性子宫内膜中，uNK 细胞有助于清除衰老的子宫内膜基质细胞。随着每个月经周期孕酮水平的增加，一部分子宫内膜基质细胞会发生急性衰老，这是与种植窗相关的短暂炎症反应的原因[22]。

2.4 自然杀伤细胞的驯化与许可

单个 NK 细胞的功能，包括细胞毒性及细胞因子产生的能力，在其发育过程中通过一个称为"驯化"和"许可"的过程来决定，该过程取决于周围环境中 HLA Ⅰ类分子的表达。为了获得其效应潜能的"许可"，NK 细胞必须接收由连接到相邻细胞上的自身 HLA Ⅰ类分子所触发的抑制信号，没有这种自我识别，NK 细胞就无法获得完整的功能。因此，只有表达识别自身 HLA Ⅰ类分子的抑制性受体的 NK 细胞才能获得完整的功能，而其余 NK 细胞则处于无能状态[23]。此外，基于激活性受体 KIR2DS1 与其 HLA Ⅰ类配体 HLA-C C2 结合的第二种相互作用方式可防止形成有害的自我应答 NK 细胞。这类驯化被称为"解除武装"，它解释了 HLA-C C2 个体表达 KIR2DS1 的 NK 细胞低反应的原因[24,25]。因此，通过识别自身 HLA Ⅰ类分子获得的驯化信号决定了发育中的 NK 细胞的功能。参与 NK 细胞驯化的受体包括 HLA-C 和 HLA-Bw4 结合的 KIR 及 HLA-E 结合的 CD94/NKG2A(表 2.1)。由于高度多态性的 KIR 和 HLA 基因位于不同的染色体上并独立遗传，个体间的受体/配体组合类型存在显著差异。因此，特定 KIR 或其配体的存在/缺失会影响每个个体的 NK 细胞驯化程度。

3 自然杀伤细胞的相关病理

当 NK 细胞异常导致临床免疫缺陷(通常危及生命)或 NK 细胞功能特征对疾病进展有影响时，此类 NK 细胞相关疾病归为原发性缺陷。单纯 NK 细胞免疫缺陷是罕见的[31]。相反，NK 细胞异常通常伴随着其他原发性免疫缺陷，例如严重的联合免疫缺陷——IL2RG 基因缺陷导致 T 细胞缺陷和 NK 细胞缺失。这些原发性 NK 细胞相关疾病的临床表现包括对疱疹病毒的异常易感性，这通常在婴儿期或儿童期变得明显。除了原发性 NK 细胞缺陷外，越来越多的数据正在揭示 NK 细胞的作用，即它们在感染、癌症和自身免疫性疾病中的驯化地位。

作为逃避 T 细胞监视的机制，HLA Ⅰ类分子的表达通常在病毒感染细胞中下调。因此，感染人类免疫缺陷病毒(HIV)的细胞 HLA-B 降低，并成为 KIR3DL1 阳性 NK 细胞的"缺失自我"靶点。在具有对 KIR3DL1 高亲和力的 HLA-Bw4 配体的个

表2.1 在NK细胞发育过程中对其驯化至关重要的受体及配体[23,24,26]

NK细胞受体	基因频率[a]	配体	等位基因频率[b]	驯化模型	NK细胞功能
抑制性受体					
KIR2DL1	95.3	HLA-C C2	0.37	驯化/许可	有功能的
KIR2DL3	86.7	HLA-C C1	0.63	驯化/许可	有功能的
KIR2DL2	52.9	HLA-C C1	0.63	驯化/许可	有功能的
KIR3DL1	94.9	HLA-Bw4	见注释[c]	驯化/许可	有功能的
CD94/NKG2A[d]	100	HLA-E	见注释[e]	驯化/许可	有功能的
激活性受体					
KIR2DS1	41.2	HLA-C C2	0.37	"解除武装"	功能低下

注：[a]北美白种人的KIR基因频率[27]。
[b]北美白种人的等位基因频率。基于单个HLA-C等位基因的报道频率计算HLA-C C1和C2频率[28,29]。
[c]HLA-Bw4包含HLA-B和一些HLA-A等位基因，其特征为血清学上可识别的Bw4表位。
[d]高度保守基因。
[e]HLA-E表达受HLA-B前导肽序列的影响[30]。

体中观察到控制HIV的显著差异，这确保了对KIR3DL1阳性NK细胞的"驯化"。研究发现，缺乏KIR3DL1驯化的NK细胞的个体更易进展为艾滋病[25,32]。

NK细胞的功能活性低下与癌症风险增加相关。在一项研究中，3 625名受试者（40岁及以上）接受了NK细胞毒性测试，11年后的癌症发病率随访调查显示，若受试者具有高度或中等NK细胞毒活性，则癌症发病风险较低[33]。在接受急性髓系白血病（acute myeloid leukemia，AML）治疗的患者中，更高的NK细胞毒活性与更好的长期预后相关[34]。供体来源的NK细胞同种异体反应在用于治疗AML的造血干细胞移植中被认为是有益的[6]。

在自身免疫性疾病，包括原发性胆汁性肝硬化（primary biliary cirrhosis，PBC）、类风湿关节炎（rheumatoid arthritis，RA）、系统性红斑狼疮（systemic lupus erythematosus，SLE）和银屑病的患者中，NK细胞的活性增加或受损[35]。在PBC患者中，NK细胞的数量和细胞毒性增加。SLE和RA患者的pNK细胞计数和细胞毒活性低于正常水平。然而，RA患者的滑膜液中含有大量活化的NK细胞[36]。现已知一些有利于NK细胞活化的KIR/HLA基因型组合与多种自身免疫性疾病的发病风险增加相关，包括激活性受体KIR3DS1和具有Bw4表位Ⅰ-80异构体的HLA-B等位基因（HLA-Bw4-Ⅰ-80），携带这些基因的个体易患RA和银屑病[37,38]。

4 生殖中的自然杀伤细胞

4.1 子宫自然杀伤细胞

胚胎植入时和妊娠早期的子宫内膜中存在大量NK细胞，突显了这些细胞在女性生殖健康中的重要性。前文讨论了uNK细胞和其他NK细胞亚群的特征，强调了它们在血管生成和胎盘生长支持方面的重要作用。子宫内膜样本的CD56免疫组化染色分析显示，特发性反复种植失败（RIF）患者的uNK细胞数量增加[39]。另一项研究表明，RIF患者的子宫内膜样本中uNK细胞计数存在很大差异。与正常生育组相比，在RIF组中可发现$CD56^{dim}$和$CD56^{bright}$细胞[40]。与对照组相比，反复妊娠丢失（RPL）患者的uNK细胞增加[41]和减少[42]均有报道。基因表达分析显示，与对照组相比，不明原因生殖障碍组中NK细胞相关基因的表达谱更广[28]。这意味着uNK细胞群的大小存在很大差异，与正常状态的差异可能是致病的，也可能反映了导致生殖障碍的原因。

4.2 外周血自然杀伤细胞

评估NK细胞的另一个重要方面是其功能特性。检测NK细胞的细胞毒活性、脱颗粒和细胞因子的产生需要活细胞悬液。事实上，与生殖障碍相关的 NK 细胞参数异常可通过外周血检测进行初步观察。研究表明，RIF 患者的 pNK 细胞通常具有比正常对照组更高的细胞毒性[43,44]。外周血淋巴细胞的流式细胞免疫表型分析显示，RPL[45-47] 和 RIF[39] 患者的 pNK 细胞百分比更高，该参数被证明能区分患者组和对照组[46]。此外，在患有 RPL 或不明原因不孕症的女性中，可通过检测 CD69 的表达评估 pNK 细胞活性[48,49]。因此，对 pNK 细胞的频率、活化状态和功能活性进行评估，可揭示 NK 细胞的改变是否可归因于生殖障碍，并指导治疗。

4.3 母体 KIR/胎盘 HLA-C 组合与妊娠风险

胎儿来源的滋养细胞缺乏 HLA-A 和 HLA-B，但高表达 HLA-C。此外，它们还表达非经典的 HLA-G 和 HLA-E。这种 HLA Ⅰ 类分子的表达模式非常适合 NK 细胞在母胎界面的识别。事实上，uNK 细胞的特点是高表达 KIR（其配体为 HLA-C 和 HLA-G 分子）和 CD94/NKG2A（HLA-E），由于 KIR 及其配体家族基因存在高度多态性，多种 KIR/配体组合可能与妊娠疾病相关。研究表明，在母体具有"抑制性"KIR AA 基因型且携带 HLA-C C2C2 基因型胎儿的妊娠中，发生子痫前期的风险很高[50]。这种组合表明 uNK 细胞上的抑制性 KIR2DL1 与胚胎滋养层上的配体 HLA-C2 之间存在高亲和性相互作用。uNK 细胞的强烈抑制可能是导致螺旋动脉重构受损的原因，从而引起子痫前期的发生。在 RPL 患者中发现高频 KIR AA 基因型，且在患者及其伴侣中亦能观察到 HLA-C C2 等位基因的频率增加[51]。在自体新鲜 IVF 周期检测 β-人绒毛膜促性腺激素呈阳性后，对母体 KIR 基因和胚胎 HLA-C 基因进行回顾性队列分析发现，母体 KIR AA 和胎儿 HLA-C C2C2 组合与妊娠丢失风险增加有关[52]。然而，母体 KIR Bx 和胚胎 HLA-C C1C1 组合的风险更大。这意味着 uNK 细胞/滋养细胞的识别和相互作用可能会影响妊娠，其中的一个方面是母体 NK 细胞发挥作用的能力，即其"驯化"状态。

4.4 自然杀伤细胞的驯化（母体 KIR/母体 HLA-C 组合）与妊娠风险

自身 HLA-C、HLA-Bw4、HLA-E 为 NK 细胞提供驯化/许可。这一过程受个体的 KIR 基因型和对驯化/许可具有重要作用的 KIR 存在与否的限制（表 2.1）。研究发现，KIR2DL2/HLA-C C1 识别对于所有表达 KIR2DL2 的 NK 细胞很重要。然而，这种 KIR/配体组合在人群中相对较少，因为 KIR2DL2 存在于大约 53% 的个体中（北美高加索人的数据）[27]。根据 Hardy-Weinberg 平衡，大约 40% 的个体为 HLA-C C1C1（针对北美高加索人测算）[28,29]，相应地，约有 21.2% 的个体预计为 KIR2DL2/HLA-C C1。然而，在 KIR2DL2 阳性的患有 RPL 或不明原因不孕症的女性中，HLA-C C1C1 的频率明显较低（25.9%），只有 13.5% 的女性为 KIR2DL2/HLA-C C1C1[53]。这些数据表明，KIR2DL2/HLA-C1 组合具有保护作用，使携带这些基因的女性妊娠失败的风险较低。另一项研究显示，在 RPL 患者中，KIR2DS1/HLA-C C2C2 组合的频率显著增加，可能引起 NK 细胞的功能低下。该研究队列显示，KIR2DS1/HLA-C C2C2 在 RPL 患者中约占 11.5%，而在对照组人群中的流行率低于 6%[28]。因此，uNK 细胞中功能低下细胞的存在可能与妊娠失败有关，其活性不足以支持胎盘生长。

不能通过识别 HLA-E 的 CD94/NKG2A 受体驯化 NK 细胞也与妊娠疾病有关。HLA-E 的表达受 HLA-B 等位基因衍生结合肽的影响，这些结合肽是 HLA-E 经适当折叠并转运至细胞表面所必需的。然而，HLA-B 等位基因（由前导序列中的苏氨酸，-21T 变体识别）提供了一种无功能肽，导致 HLA-E 表达减少，限制了 NK 细胞的 CD94/NKG2A 驯化[26,30]。一项基于大样本（>160 000 名参与者）的全基因组荟萃分析显示，HLA-B 基因-21T 变体的存在与 7% 的子痫前期相对风险相关[54]。检测母体 HLA-B 等位基因是否不利于 CD94/NKG2A 相关的 NK 细胞驯化也可能与其他妊娠疾病相关。

5 评估

流式细胞术分析是外周血 NK 细胞计数的标准方法。CD56 和 CD16 表达抗体检测可用于获得总 pNK 细胞百分比及两个 pNK 亚群的比例（图 2.1）。对 22 项评估外周血 NK 细胞计数的研究进行的 meta 分析表明，与对照组相比，患有 RPL 的女性 NK 细胞计数显著增加（$P<0.00001$），但与正常生

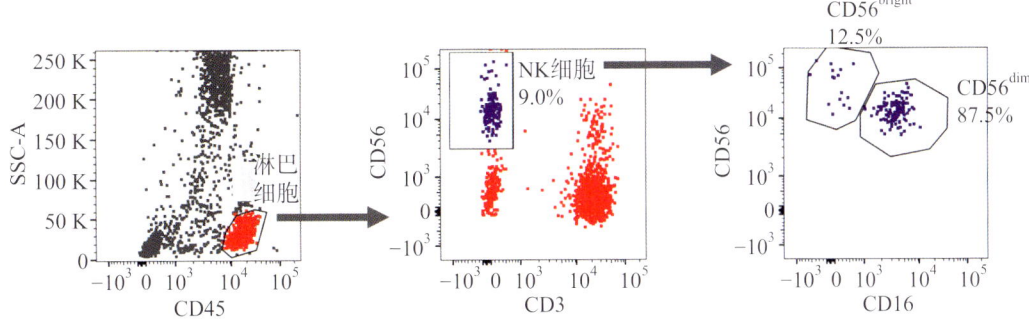

图 2.1 外周血 NK 细胞的流式细胞术分析。

CD45 阳性/侧向散射(SSC)细胞确定为淋巴细胞群。在淋巴细胞中,CD56 阳性且 CD3 阴性细胞为 NK 细胞。在 CD56/CD16 图上可识别 NK 细胞的两个亚群。大多数 pNK 细胞是 $CD56^{dim}$ 和 CD16 阳性,少量 pNK 细胞为 $CD56^{bright}$ 和 CD16 阴性。

育女性相比,不孕女性的 NK 细胞计数并无显著差异[55]。在一项前瞻性队列研究中,RIF 患者的 NK 细胞计数和百分比显著增加,且 $CD56^{dim}$ 和 $CD56^{dim}CD69^+$ 亚群增加[56]。

靶细胞杀伤试验可用于评估 NK 细胞的细胞毒活性。以人红白血病细胞(K562)为靶点的放射性铬(^{51}Cr)释放试验是测定 NK 细胞毒性的金标准。K562 细胞用 ^{51}Cr 标记,并与 NK 细胞以不同的效应物:靶细胞比例孵育。通过测定从 K562 死细胞释放到培养基中的 ^{51}Cr 来确定对靶细胞的杀伤力。这种检测方法的一个改进是使用荧光染料标记 K562 细胞,并利用另一种与死细胞结合的染料,通过流式细胞术测定靶细胞杀伤的百分比(图 2.2)。以 17.8%作为 NK 细胞毒性的阈值,用于区分 RIF 组和对照组,敏感性为 83.2%,特异性为 84%,优势比(OR)为 9.3[57]。在患有 RPL 的女性中,使用 17.7%的截断值,NK 细胞毒性能区分 RPL 组和对照组,敏感性为 78%,特异性为 84%,OR 为 7.2[57]。

用于评估 NK 细胞的其他方法包括 CD69 表达分析和 CD107a 脱颗粒检测。这些标志物反映了 NK 细胞的功能活性。现已知与 K562 细胞共孵育可引起 pNK 细胞活化和 CD69 上调,该现象可通过

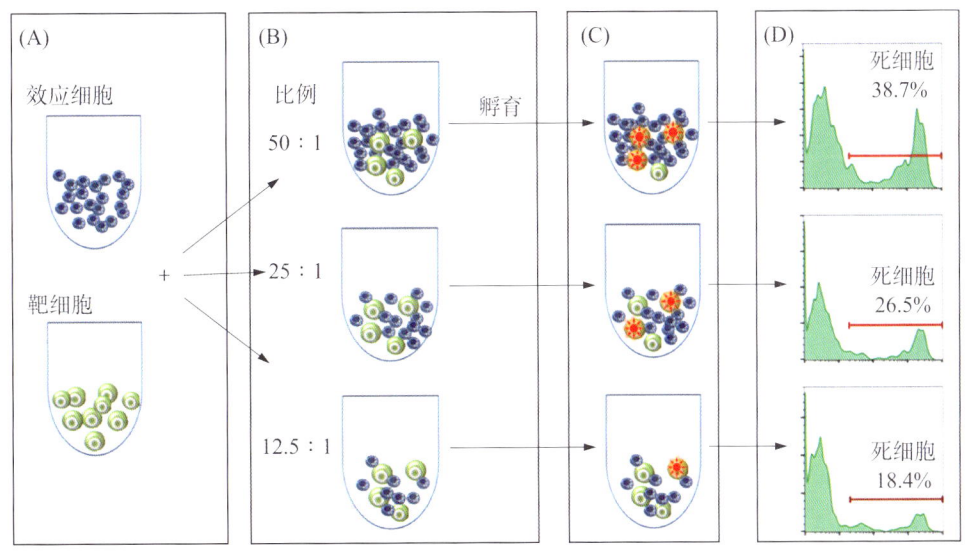

图 2.2 基于流式细胞术的 NK 细胞毒性测定。

(A)效应细胞为外周血单个核细胞,从收集到肝素钠管的静脉血中分离出来。靶细胞为标记 PKH67 绿色荧光染料的 K562 细胞。(B)将效应细胞和靶细胞以指定比例混合并孵育 2 小时。(C)将碘化丙啶(PI)添加到试管中,对被 NK 细胞杀死的靶细胞进行染色。(D)样品通过流式细胞仪检测,其中 K562 细胞通过其绿色荧光进行门控,K562 死细胞则通过 PI 染色进一步鉴定。直方图显示每个效应/靶细胞的 PI 阳性细胞百分比。

流式细胞术进行测定[48,58]。细胞表面检测到 CD107a 表明细胞发生脱颗粒，这是由于 CD107a 通常存在于细胞质颗粒的膜上。同样，将 pNK 细胞与 K562 细胞共孵育刺激，然后用流式细胞术分析 CD107a 的表达。

为了评估子宫内膜活检组织中的 uNK 细胞，可使用 CD56 抗体进行免疫组化染色[59]。通过分子检测分析 mRNA 的表达也可用于评价 uNK 细胞。因此，基于定量 RT-PCR 的子宫内膜免疫表达谱的检测包含了对 CD56 mRNA 的评估[40]。在基于靶向 RNA 测序的蜕膜化评分中，颗粒酶 B 表达可作为 uNK 细胞的标志物[60]。

子宫内膜活检样本采集的时间对 uNK 细胞评估至关重要。在每个月经周期中，uNK 细胞的数量都会发生明显变化，排卵后 7~8 天，uNK 细胞数会迅速增加[59]。

最后，HLA 和 KIR 基因型提供了 KIR 和 HLA 配体可用性的信息。包含对伴侣 HLA-C 的评估有助于预测胚胎 HLA-C 基因型，并可指导判断胚胎移植的潜在风险。

6 生殖结局

在 RPL 患者中，NK 细胞比例和细胞毒性增加。据报道，多种药物可抑制或调节 NK 细胞的毒性和（或）数量，包括强的松、静脉注射免疫球蛋白 G（IVIg）、脂肪乳剂（intralipid）输注等[61-63]。

最新的一项研究表明，免疫因素引起的 RPL 和 RIF 患者（$n=197$）在 IVF/ET 或 FET 周期中，接受个性化免疫调节和抗凝治疗，与基线水平相比，胚胎移植时 NK 细胞水平和细胞毒性显著降低。此外，上述患者的妊娠率、每个胚胎移植周期的活产率（live birth rate，LBR）和每次妊娠的 LBR（分别为 48.2%、39.6% 和 82.1%）显著高于历史对照组（分别为 33%、1.8% 和 5.3%）（$P<0.001$、$P<0.0001$ 和 $P<0.0001$）[64]。

关于 KIR 和 HLA-C 基因型，携带 KIR2DL2pos 和 HLA-C1C1 的女性 NK 细胞毒性显著高于携带 KIR2DL2pos 和 HLA-C2C2 的女性，但 CD56+ NK 细胞水平无差异，体现了 NK 细胞的驯化效果[53]。此外，在 26 例足月分娩的 RPL 患者和 32 例具有产科并发症的患者（包括 22 例早期妊娠丢失、2 例中期妊娠丢失、1 例宫内生长受限、2 例子痫前期和 5 例早产）中，HLA-C、KIR2DL2、KIR AA 和 Bx 基因型频率无差异，表明免疫调节疗法改善了具有 RPL 和 HLA-C 错配的 KIR2DL2pos 女性的妊娠结局[53]。

7 治疗

现已报道了多种 NK 细胞相关生殖障碍的免疫调节疗法，包括强的松、IVIg、脂肪乳剂、粒细胞-巨噬细胞集落刺激因子、TNF 阻断剂、淋巴细胞免疫治疗和羟氯喹。

7.1 皮质类固醇治疗

uNK 细胞表达糖皮质激素受体[65]。在 RPL 患者中，强的松治疗可显著降低 uNK 细胞数量（$P=0.0004$）[66]。此外，强的松治疗可将 Treg/Th17 免疫平衡转化向 Treg 偏移，并改善 RIF 患者的妊娠结局[67]。尽管存在众所周知的副作用，但由于其便捷的给药途径和相对较低的成本，强的松治疗易于应用。在一项针对 160 名不明原因 RPL 患者的随机双盲安慰剂对照研究中，强的松和肝素联合治疗的有效率（70.3%）显著高于肝素和小剂量阿司匹林治疗（9.2%）（$P<0.05$）[68]。该效应可能是由于类固醇对外周血 CD16 NK 细胞浓度的抑制作用[68]。然而，这项研究没有考虑参与者的 NK 细胞评估。在 14 项 IVF 或 ICSI 患者的 RCT 研究中，强的松治疗并未改善活产率（3 项 RTC，OR=1.21）或妊娠率（13 项 RCT，OR=1.16）。然而，对接受 IVF/ICSI（6 项 RCT）的患者进行亚组分析显示，使用糖皮质激素（OR=1.5）的妊娠率显著增加[69]。近期对 4 项 RCT 研究的系统性回顾分析显示，与安慰剂组相比，在 IVF 促排卵期间补充糖皮质激素的临床妊娠率可能会增加，但对活产率几乎没有影响[70]。遗憾的是，这些系统性回顾所包含的 RCT 研究都没有评估参与者是否存在免疫异常，而且糖皮质激素的治疗都是经验性的。因此，低生育力和接受 IVF 或 ICSI 并不是经验性应用糖皮质激素治疗的充分适应证。未来的临床试验应聚焦特定的临床适应证，如 RPL、RIF，以及免疫异常。

7.2 静脉注射免疫球蛋白 G 治疗

研究报道，IVIg 治疗可有效抑制 RPL 和 RIF 患者的 NK 细胞水平和细胞毒性，有利于妊娠结局[61,71,72]。此外，IVIg治疗增加了NK细胞抑制性受体表达，降低激活性受体表达[73]。

在一项对RPL和NK或NKT样细胞扩增患者的观察性研究中，IVIg治疗可将活产率显著提高至96.3%，而在未行IVIg治疗的患者中，活产率仅为30.6%（$P<0.0001$）[74]。在RIF患者中，IVIg组的妊娠率（93.8%）显著高于未治疗组（26.2%）。IVIg组的活产率（80.0%）也显著高于未治疗组（17.0%）[74]。在RPL患者中，接受IVIg治疗的细胞免疫异常（NK细胞水平、细胞毒性或Th1/Th2比值升高）患者的活产率与没有细胞免疫异常且未行治疗的患者相当[75]，表明IVIg对患有细胞免疫异常的RPL具有临床疗效。

Polanski等对接受辅助生殖技术治疗的不孕症患者进行了系统性回顾，这些患者的NK细胞数量和（或）活性升高，该研究报道了不同治疗措施对临床妊娠率的有益影响：强的松的RR为1.63（95% $CI=1.00\sim2.66$），IVIg的RR为3.41（95% $CI=1.90\sim6.11$）。然而，由于存在显著异质性，作者建议谨慎解释上述发现[76]。在最近的一项对197例RPL和（或）RIF的回顾性队列研究中，与历史对照组相比，单用强的松或强的松+IVIg联合抗凝治疗显著提高了IVF周期的妊娠率（48.2% vs 33.0%，$P<0.001$）和活产率（39.6% vs 1.8%，$P<0.001$）[64]。在该项研究中，采用个性化免疫调节治疗，使NK细胞水平、细胞毒性和Th1/Th2细胞比值正常化。总体上看，当免疫标志物得到更好的控制时，免疫调节治疗显著改善了IVF周期的生殖结局。

7.3 其他疗法

其他亦有多种免疫疗法可调节RPL和RIF患者的NK细胞。据报道，淋巴细胞免疫疗法能有效抑制RPL患者的NK细胞水平和细胞毒性[77]。脂肪乳剂可控制外周血NK细胞水平和细胞毒性，改善妊娠结局[78]。在一项50名NKC异常患者接受脂肪乳剂治疗的研究中，2 mL 20%的脂肪乳剂稀释在250 mL生理盐水中，或4 mL 20%的脂肪乳剂稀释在250 mL生理盐水中。1周后的结果显示，78%的患者出现NKC抑制，22%的患者虽出现抑制，但仍高于正常阈值。动物和人体研究均表明，脂肪乳剂治疗能提高胚胎种植率并维持妊娠；在具有异常免疫风险因素的患者中，脂肪乳剂治疗的生殖结局与IVIg相当[79]。然而，近期一项系统性回顾分析表明，脂肪乳剂治疗对IVF/ICSI生殖结局的作用尚不确切[80]。同样，在没有对患者进行NK细胞评估的情况下，只能经验性给予脂肪乳剂治疗。

在一项针对难治性固有免疫性RPL患者的随机对照试验中，与安慰剂组相比，依那西普每周25 mg，起始周期的第1天显著降低TNF-α水平和NK细胞活性（$P<0.05$），并且依那西普治疗组的活产率（89.47%）显著高于安慰剂组（72.04%）（$OR=3.30, 95\% CI=1.49\sim7.32, P=0.01$）。基于该研究，依那西普有望成为难治性固有免疫性RPL的一种治疗策略[81]。

在NK细胞水平或活性异常的患者中，多种免疫疗法可提高胚胎种植率并维持妊娠。然而，仍需在生殖免疫学专家进行全面评估和咨询后，选择潜在药物和免疫调节治疗的候选药物。

8 总结和建议

NK细胞是重要的效应细胞，有助于宿主防御感染和控制恶性肿瘤。此外，NK细胞在母胎界面发挥积极作用，对妊娠支持亦非常重要。NK细胞的活性受到受体/配体识别的严格调控，其中KIR和HLA Ⅰ类分子的相互作用在人类NK细胞中起着关键作用。各类生殖障碍，如RPL或RIF，与外周血或子宫内膜组织样本检测发现的NK细胞异常有关。

- NK细胞是胚胎植入时和妊娠早期子宫内膜中最丰富的免疫细胞。
- NK细胞通过调节血管生成和胎盘生长在母胎界面发挥重要作用。
- 研究报道，RPL患者NK细胞比例和细胞毒性升高。
- 研究报道，多种免疫疗法（包括糖皮质激素、IVIg、淋巴细胞免疫疗法、脂肪乳剂、TNF阻断剂）可抑制/调节NK细胞数量和细胞毒性。
- 未来需要精心设计的临床试验来研究各种免疫疗法的疗效。
- 对于RPL和RIF，免疫治疗应针对免疫异常的患者进行，而非经验性治疗。

参考文献

[1] Bulmer JN, Sunderland CA. Immunohistological characterization of lymphoid cell populations in the early human placental bed. Immunology 1984;52(2):349-57.

[2] Ritson A, Bulmer JN. Endometrial granulocytes in human decidua react with a natural-killer (NK) cell marker, NKH1. Immunology 1987;62(2):329-31.

[3] Karre K, Ljunggren HG, Piontek G, Kiessling R. Selective rejection of H-2-deficient lymphoma variants suggests alternative immune defence strategy. Nature 1986;319(6055):675-8.

[4] Long EO, Kim HS, Liu D, Peterson ME, Rajagopalan S. Controlling natural killer cell responses: integration of signals for activation and inhibition. Annu Rev Immunol 2013;31:227-58.

[5] Braud V, Jones EY, McMichael A. The human major histocompatibility complex class Ib molecule HLA-E binds signal sequence-derived peptides with primary anchor residues at positions 2 and 9. Eur J Immunol 1997;27(5):1164-9.

[6] Pende D, Falco M, Vitale M, et al. Killer Ig-like receptors (KIRs): their role in nk cell modulation and developments leading to their clinical exploitation. Front Immunol 2019;10:1179.

[7] Hao L, Nei M. Rapid expansion of killer cell immunoglobulin-like receptor genes in primates and their coevolution with MHC Class I genes. Gene 2005;347(2):149-59.

[8] Parham P, Norman PJ, Abi-Rached L, Guethlein LA. Human-specific evolution of killer cell immunoglobulin-like receptor recognition of major histocompatibility complex class I molecules. Philos Trans R Soc Lond B Biol Sci 2012;367(1590):800-11.

[9] Gumperz JE, Litwin V, Phillips JH, Lanier LL, Parham P. The Bw4 public epitope of HLA-B molecules confers reactivity with natural killer cell clones that express NKB1, a putative HLA receptor. J Exp Med 1995;181(3):1133-44.

[10] Lanier LL, Le AM, Civin CI, Loken MR, Phillips JH. The relationship of CD16 (Leu-11) and Leu-19 (NKH-1) antigen expression on human peripheral blood NK cells and cytotoxic T lymphocytes. J Immunol 1986;136(12):4480-6.

[11] Barrow AD, Martin CJ, Colonna M. The natural cytotoxicity receptors in health and disease. Front Immunol 2019;10:909.

[12] Fauriat C, Long EO, Ljunggren HG, Bryceson YT. Regulation of human NK-cell cytokine and chemokine production by target cell recognition. Blood. 2010;115(11):2167-76.

[13] Hawke LG, Whitford MKM, Ormiston ML. The production of pro-angiogenic VEGF-A isoforms by hypoxic human NK cells is independent of their TGF-beta-mediated conversion to an ILC1-like phenotype. Front Immunol 2020;11:1903.

[14] Greenberg AH. The origins of the NK cell, or a Canadian in King Ivan's court. Clin Invest Med 1994;17(6):626-31.

[15] Freud AG, Mundy-Bosse BL, Yu J, Caligiuri MA. The broad spectrum of human natural killer cell diversity. Immunity. 2017;47(5):820-33.

[16] Bjorkstrom NK, Ljunggren HG, Michaelsson J. Emerging insights into natural killer cells in human peripheral tissues. Nat Rev Immunol 2016;16(5):310-20.

[17] Cooper MA, Fehniger TA, Turner SC, et al. Human natural killer cells: a unique innate immunoregulatory role for the CD56(bright) subset. Blood. 2001;97(10):3146-51.

[18] Koopman LA, Kopcow HD, Rybalov B, et al. Human decidual natural killer cells are a unique NK cell subset with immunomodulatory potential. J Exp Med 2003;198(8):1201-12.

[19] Ashkar AA, Di Santo JP, Croy BA. Interferon gamma contributes to initiation of uterine vascular modification, decidual integrity, and uterine natural killer cell maturation during normal murine pregnancy. J Exp Med 2000;192(2):259-70.

[20] Lash GE, Schiessl B, Kirkley M, et al. Expression of angiogenic growth factors by uterine natural killer cells during early pregnancy. J Leukoc Biol 2006;80(3):572-80.

[21] Fu B, Zhou Y, Ni X, et al. Natural killer cells promote fetal development through the secretion of growth-promoting factors. Immunity. 2017;47(6):1100-13 e1106.

[22] Brighton PJ, Maruyama Y, Fishwick K, et al. Clearance of senescent decidual cells by uterine natural killer cells in cycling human endometrium. Elife. 2017;6.

[23] Anfossi N, Andre P, Guia S, et al. Human NK cell education by inhibitory receptors for MHC class I. Immunity. 2006;25(2):331-42.

[24] Fauriat C, Ivarsson MA, Ljunggren HG, Malmberg KJ, Michaelsson J. Education of human natural killer cells by activating killer cell immunoglobulin-like receptors. Blood. 2010;115(6):1166-74.

[25] Boudreau JE, Hsu KC. Natural killer cell education and the response to infection and cancer therapy: stay tuned. Trends Immunol 2018;39(3):222-39.

[26] Horowitz A, Djaoud Z, Nemat-Gorgani N, et al. Class I HLA haplotypes form two schools that educate NK cells in different ways. Sci Immunol 2016;1(3).

[27] Hollenbach JA, Meenagh A, Sleator C, et al. Report from the killer immunoglobulin-like receptor (KIR) anthropology component of the 15th International Histocompatibility Workshop: worldwide variation in the KIR loci and further evidence for the co-evolution of KIR and HLA. Tissue Antigens 2010;76(1):9-17.

[28] Dambaeva SV, Lee DH, Sung N, et al. Recurrent pregnancy loss in women with killer cell immunoglobulin-like receptor KIR2DS1 is associated with an increased HLA-C2 allelic frequency. Am J Reprod Immunol 2016;75(2):94-103.

[29] Wang SS, Abdou AM, Morton LM, et al. Human leukocyte antigen class I and II alleles in non-Hodgkin lymphoma etiology. Blood. 2010;115(23):4820-3.

[30] Hallner A, Bernson E, Hussein BA, et al. The HLA-B-21 dimorphism impacts on NK cell education and clinical outcome of immunotherapy in acute myeloid leukemia. Blood 2019;133(13):1479-88.

[31] Orange JS, How I. Manage natural killer cell deficiency. J Clin Immunol 2020;40(1):13-23.

[32] Boudreau JE, Mulrooney TJ, Le Luduec JB, Barker E, Hsu KC. KIR3DL1 and HLA-B density and binding calibrate nk education and response to HIV. J Immunol 2016;196(8):3398-410.

[33] Imai K, Matsuyama S, Miyake S, Suga K, Nakachi K. Natural cytotoxic activity of peripheral-blood lymphocytes and cancer incidence: an 11-year follow-up study of a general

population. Lancet. 2000;356(9244):1795-9.

[34] Carlsten M, Jaras M. Natural killer cells in myeloid malignancies: immune surveillance, NK cell dysfunction, and pharmacological opportunities to bolster the endogenous NK cells. Front Immunol 2019;10:2357.

[35] Fogel LA, Yokoyama WM, French AR. Natural killer cells in human autoimmune disorders. Arthritis Res Ther 2013;15(4):216.

[36] Dalbeth N, Callan MF. A subset of natural killer cells is greatly expanded within inflamed joints. Arthritis Rheum 2002;46(7):1763-72.

[37] Yen JH, Moore BE, Nakajima T, et al. Major histocompatibility complex class I-recognizing receptors are disease risk genes in rheumatoid arthritis. J Exp Med 2001;193(10):1159-67.

[38] Nelson GW, Martin MP, Gladman D, Wade J, Trowsdale J, Carrington M. Cutting edge: heterozygote advantage in autoimmune disease: hierarchy of protection/susceptibility conferred by HLA and killer Ig-like receptor combinations in psoriatic arthritis. J Immunol 2004;173(7):4273-6.

[39] Santillan I, Lozano I, Illan J, et al. Where and when should natural killer cells be tested in women with repeated implantation failure? J Reprod Immunol 2015;108:142-8.

[40] Ledee N, Petitbarat M, Prat-Ellenberg L, et al. Endometrial immune profiling: a method to design personalized care in assisted reproductive medicine. Front Immunol 2020;11:1032.

[41] El-Azzamy H, Dambaeva SV, Katukurundage D, et al. Dysregulated uterine natural killer cells and vascular remodeling in women with recurrent pregnancy losses. Am J Reprod Immunol 2018;80(4):e13024.

[42] Lucas ES, Vrljicak P, Muter J, et al. Recurrent pregnancy loss is associated with a pro-senescent decidual response during the peri-implantation window. Commun Biol 2020;3(1):37.

[43] Fukui A, Fujii S, Yamaguchi E, Kimura H, Sato S, Saito Y. Natural killer cell subpopulations and cytotoxicity for infertile patients undergoing in vitro fertilization. Am J Reprod Immunol 1999;41(6):413-22.

[44] Coulam CB, Roussev RG. Correlation of NK cell activation and inhibition markers with NK cytoxicity among women experiencing immunologic implantation failure after in vitro fertilization and embryo transfer. J Assist Reprod Genet 2003;20(2):58-62.

[45] Kwak JY, Beaman KD, Gilman-Sachs A, Ruiz JE, Schewitz D, Beer AE. Up-regulated expression of CD56+, CD56+/CD16+, and CD19+ cells in peripheral blood lymphocytes in pregnant women with recurrent pregnancy losses. Am J Reprod Immunol 1995;34(2):93-9.

[46] King K, Smith S, Chapman M, Sacks G. Detailed analysis of peripheral blood natural killer (NK) cells in women with recurrent miscarriage. Hum Reprod 2010;25(1):52-8.

[47] Kuon RJ, Vomstein K, Weber M, et al. The "killer cell story" in recurrent miscarriage: Association between activated peripheral lymphocytes and uterine natural killer cells. J Reprod Immunol 2017;119:9-14.

[48] Ntrivalas EI, Kwak-Kim JY, Gilman-Sachs A, et al. Status of peripheral blood natural killer cells in women with recurrent spontaneous abortions and infertility of unknown aetiology. Hum Reprod 2001;16(5):855-61.

[49] Thum MY, Bhaskaran S, Abdalla HI, et al. An increase in the absolute count of CD56dimCD16+CD69+ NK cells in the peripheral blood is associated with a poorer IVF treatment and pregnancy outcome. Hum Reprod 2004;19(10):2395-400.

[50] Hiby SE, Walker JJ, O'Shaughnessy KM, et al. Combinations of maternal KIR and fetal HLA-C genes influence the risk of preeclampsia and reproductive success. J Exp Med 2004;200(8):957-65.

[51] Hiby SE, Regan L, Lo W, Farrell L, Carrington M, Moffett A. Association of maternal killer-cell immunoglobulin-like receptors and parental HLA-C genotypes with recurrent miscarriage. Hum Reprod 2008;23(4):972-6.

[52] Morin SJ, Treff NR, Tao X, et al. Combination of uterine natural killer cell immunoglobulin receptor haplotype and trophoblastic HLA-C ligand influences the risk of pregnancy loss: a retrospective cohort analysis of direct embryo genotyping data from euploid transfers. Fertil Steril 2017;107(3):677-83 e672.

[53] Yang X, Yang E, Wang WJ, et al. Decreased HLA-C1 alleles in couples of KIR2DL2 positive women with recurrent pregnancy loss. J Reprod Immunol 2020;142:103186.

[54] Shreeve N, Depierreux D, Hawkes D, et al. The CD94/NKG2A inhibitory receptor educates uterine NK cells to optimize pregnancy outcomes in humans and mice. Immunity 2021;54(6):1231-44 e1234.

[55] Seshadri S, Sunkara SK. Natural killer cells in female infertility and recurrent miscarriage: a systematic review and meta-analysis. Hum Reprod Update 2014;20(3):429-38.

[56] Sacks G, Yang Y, Gowen E, Smith S, Fay L, Chapman M. Detailed analysis of peripheral blood natural killer cells in women with repeated IVF failure. Am J Reprod Immunol 2012;67(5):434-42.

[57] Salazar MD, Wang W, Skariah A, et al. Post-hoc evaluation of peripheral blood natural killer cell cytotoxicity in predicting the risk of recurrent pregnancy losses and repeated implantation failures. J Reprod Immunol 2022.

[58] Dons'koi BV, Chernyshov VP, Osypchuk DV. Measurement of NK activity in whole blood by the CD69 up-regulation after co-incubation with K562, comparison with NK cytotoxicity assays and CD107a degranulation assay. J Immunol Meth 2011;372(1-2):187-95.

[59] Russell P, Sacks G, Tremellen K, Gee A. The distribution of immune cells and macrophages in the endometrium of women with recurrent reproductive failure. III: further observations and reference ranges. Pathology 2013;45(4):393-401.

[60] Dambaeva S, Bilal M, Schneiderman S, et al. Decidualization score identifies an endometrial dysregulation in samples from women with recurrent pregnancy losses and unexplained infertility. F S Rep 2021;2(1):95-103.

[61] Ruiz JE, Kwak JY, Baum L, et al. Effect of intravenous immunoglobulin G on natural killer cell cytotoxicity in vitro in women with recurrent spontaneous abortion. J Reprod Immunol 1996;31(1-2):125-41.

[62] Nair MP, Schwartz SA. Immunomodulatory effects of corticosteroids on natural killer and antibody-dependent cellular cytotoxic activities of human lymphocytes. J Immunol 1984;132(6):2876-82.

[63] Austin Taylor M, Bennett M, Kumar V, Schatzle JD. Functional defects of NK cells treated with chloroquine mimic the lytic defects observed in perforin-deficient mice. J Immunol 2000;165(9):5048-53.

[64] Sung N, Khan SA, Yiu ME, et al. Reproductive outcomes of women with recurrent pregnancy losses and repeated implantation failures are significantly improved with

[64] immunomodulatory treatment. J Reprod Immunol 2021；148：103369.
[65] Henderson TA, Saunders PT, Moffett-King A, Groome NP, Critchley HO. Steroid receptor expression in uterine natural killer cells. J Clin Endocrinol Metab 2003；88(1)：440-9.
[66] Quenby S, Kalumbi C, Bates M, Farquharson R, Vince G. Prednisolone reduces preconceptual endometrial natural killer cells in women with recurrent miscarriage. Fertil Steril 2005；84(4)：980-4.
[67] Huang Q, Wu H, Li M, Yang Y, Fu X. Prednisone improves pregnancy outcome in repeated implantation failure by enhance regulatory T cells bias. J Reprod Immunol 2021；143：103245.
[68] Gomaa MF, Elkholy AG, El-Said MM, Abdel-Salam NE. Combined oral prednisolone and heparin vs heparin: the effect on peripheral NK cells and clinical outcome in patients with unexplained recurrent miscarriage. A double-blind placebo randomized controlled trial. Arch Gynecol Obstet 2014；290(4)：757-62.
[69] Boomsma CM, Keay SD, Macklon NS. Peri-implantation glucocorticoid administration for assisted reproductive technology cycles. Cochrane Database Syst Rev 2012；6 CD005996.
[70] Kalampokas T, Pandian Z, Keay SD, Bhattacharya S. Glucocorticoid supplementation during ovarian stimulation for IVF or ICSI. Cochrane Database Syst Rev 2017；3 CD004752.
[71] Kwak JY, Kwak FM, Ainbinder SW, Ruiz AM, Beer AE. Elevated peripheral blood natural killer cells are effectively downregulated by immunoglobulin G infusion in women with recurrent spontaneous abortions. Am J Reprod Immunol 1996；35(4)：363-9.
[72] Ruiz JE, Kwak JY, Baum L, et al. Intravenous immunoglobulin inhibits natural killer cell activity in vivo in women with recurrent spontaneous abortion. Am J Reprod Immunol 1996；35(4)：370-5.
[73] Ahmadi M, Ghaebi M, Abdolmohammadi-Vahid S, et al. NK cell frequency and cytotoxicity in correlation to pregnancy outcome and response to IVIG therapy among women with recurrent pregnancy loss. J Cell Physiol 2019；234(6)：9428-37.
[74] Ramos-Medina R, Garcia-Segovia A, Gil J, et al. Experience in IVIg therapy for selected women with recurrent reproductive failure and NK cell expansion. Am J Reprod Immunol 2014；71(5)：458-66.
[75] Lee SK, Kim JY, Han AR, et al. Intravenous immunoglobulin g improves pregnancy outcome in women with recurrent pregnancy losses with cellular immune abnormalities. Am J Reprod Immunol 2016；75(1)：59-68.
[76] Polanski LT, Barbosa MA, Martins WP, et al. Interventions to improve reproductive outcomes in women with elevated natural killer cells undergoing assisted reproduction techniques: a systematic review of literature. Hum Reprod 2014；29(1)：65-75.
[77] Kwak JY, Gilman-Sachs A, Moretti M, Beaman KD, Beer AE. Natural killer cell cytotoxicity and paternal lymphocyte immunization in women with recurrent spontaneous abortions. Am J Reprod Immunol 1998；40(5)：352-8.
[78] Roussev RG, Acacio B, Ng SC, Coulam CB. Duration of intralipid's suppressive effect on NK cell's functional activity. Am J Reprod Immunol 2008；60(3)：258-63.
[79] Coulam CB, Acacio B. Does immunotherapy for treatment of reproductive failure enhance live births? Am J Reprod Immunol 2012；67(4)：296-304.
[80] Zhou P, Wu H, Lin X, Wang S, Zhang S. The effect of intralipid on pregnancy outcomes in women with previous implantation failure in in vitro fertilization/intracytoplasmic sperm injection cycles: a systematic review and meta-analysis. Eur J Obstet Gynecol Reprod Biol 2020；252：187-92.
[81] Fu J, Li L, Qi L, Zhao L. A randomized controlled trial of etanercept in the treatment of refractory recurrent spontaneous abortion with innate immune disorders. Taiwan J Obstet Gynecol 2019；58(5)：621-5.

第 3 章

辅助性 T 细胞病理学与反复妊娠丢失，Th1/Th2、Treg/Th17 及其他 T 细胞应答

T helper cell pathology and recurrent pregnancy losses: Th1/Th2, Treg/Th17, and other T cell responses

Joon Cheol Park [1], Jae Won Han [2] and Sung Ki Lee [2]

[1] Department of Obstetrics and Gynecology, Keimyung University School of Medicine, Daegu, Republic of Korea
[2] Department of Obstetrics and Gynecology, Konyang University College of Medicine, Daejeon, Republic of Korea

1 反复妊娠丢失的免疫学视角

1986 年，Mosmann 等[1]首次提出 T 辅助细胞 1（Th1）和 Th2 的概念。随后，Wegmann 等[2]采用 Th1/Th2 模式来解释妊娠期母体对胎儿同种抗原的耐受性。10 余年前，Th1/Th2 模式进一步扩展到 Th1/Th2/Th17/调节性 T（Treg）细胞模式[3]。从那时起，其他 Th 细胞亚群，包括 Th9、Th22、滤泡辅助性 T 细胞（Tfh）和记忆细胞被陆续引入。此外，免疫检查点分子在调节免疫效应中的作用亦受到广泛研究。反复妊娠丢失（RPL）的免疫病理学是生殖免疫学领域的热点之一，其深深植根于 T 细胞病理学。本章将全面回顾 RPL 相关 Th 细胞免疫的最新进展。

2 反复妊娠丢失的定义

最近，RPL 被重新定义为两次或两次以上的妊娠丢失[4,5]。这一新定义现已受到许多临床医生和研究人员的欢迎。妊娠丢失或流产可定义为胎儿在达到具有存活能力之前的自然死亡，通常是在妊娠 24 周之前[6]。然而，对于妊娠的定义还没有达成共识。美国生殖医学会（American Society of Reproductive Medicine，ASRM）认为，妊娠是指通过超声或组织病理检查确定的临床妊娠[5]。而欧洲人类生殖与胚胎学会（European Society of Human Reproduction and Embryology，ESHRE）将妊娠定义为通过尿液和血清 β-人绒毛膜促性腺激素（hCG）试验确定的临床和生化妊娠[6]。

3 患病率

很难估计 RPL 的确切患病率。许多文献报道，在妊娠 20 周前，有 1%~2% 的夫妇出现 3 次或 3 次以上的连续临床妊娠丢失[4,6,7]。如果将生化妊娠也包括在内，患病率将增加到 2%~3%[8]。最近，一项针对 18~42 岁瑞典女性的流行病学研究表明，当 RPL 定义为妊娠 22 周前连续 3 次或以上的妊娠丢失时，RPL 的患病率在 2003 年至 2012 年间增加了 74%[9]。免疫、炎症和环境因素被认为是 RPL 增加的可能原因[9]。然而，还需进一步探索 RPL 迅速增加的原因。

尽管 RPL 有多种原因，但细胞免疫异常仍是最重要的病因之一。根据我们先前对 RPL 非妊娠女性外周血（peripheral blood，PB）NK 细胞水平、NK 细胞毒性和分泌 Th1/Th2 细胞因子的 Th 细胞比值的研究，细胞免疫异常占所有 RPL 的 64%，占特发性 RPL 的 76%[10]。此外，分泌 Th1/Th2 细胞因子的 Th 细胞比值异常相对常见，在所有 RPL 组中占

34.7%，在不明原因组中占38.1%。

4 正常妊娠和反复妊娠丢失的免疫调节

4.1 月经周期中的T细胞

外周血和子宫中的淋巴细胞随月经周期波动。与卵泡期相比，黄体期循环CD3$^+$和CD4$^+$T细胞比例显著降低[11]。然而，CD8$^+$T细胞比例在月经周期中无显著变化。因此，黄体期Th/Tc比值低于卵泡期。与T细胞相比，排卵后CD3$^-$CD56$^+$NK细胞的比例显著增加。在CD4$^+$T细胞中，肿瘤坏死因子(TNF)-α、干扰素(IFN)-γ和IL-10的产生，以及Th1/Th2比值，不随月经周期的变化而波动[11]。

在非妊娠子宫内膜中，与增殖期相比，分泌期T细胞的比例降低(1.4% vs 0.8%)[12]。CD8$^+$T细胞在所有CD3$^+$细胞中的百分比从增殖期的63%显著降低到黄体期的54.2%。另一方面，由于CD4$^+$T细胞略有增加，CD4$^+$/CD8$^+$T细胞比值从增殖期的1.9增加到黄体期的4.2。这种变化可能是由于分泌晚期子宫内膜NK细胞增加所致。

外周血Foxp3$^+$Treg细胞的比例在卵泡期随着血清雌激素浓度的增加而提高[13]，子宫内膜Foxp3$^+$细胞则在整个增殖期逐渐增加[14]。非妊娠女性外周血中的Th17占Th细胞的一小部分，约为1.4%[15]。然而，目前尚不清楚Th17是否同Treg细胞一样随月经周期波动[16]。

4.2 人类妊娠中的T细胞

子宫内膜通过白细胞的流入为胚胎种植做好准备[17]。在月经周期中，NK细胞和巨噬细胞的密度随增殖期到分泌期而增加[18]。在妊娠早期，T细胞占蜕膜免疫细胞的比例仅为10%～20%，但随着妊娠的进展，该比例增加至44%[19]。然而，CD4$^+$和CD8$^+$T细胞的数量在妊娠期间没有变化[19]。在妊娠早期的蜕膜CD3$^+$T细胞中，CD4$^+$T细胞占30%～45%，CD8$^+$T细胞占45%～75%，Treg细胞占5%[20]。近期的单细胞转录组测序分析亦证实了妊娠早期蜕膜中CD8$^+$T细胞多于CD4$^+$T细胞[21]。在比较三个不同妊娠阶段外周血Th细胞的细胞因子产生情况时发现，IL-4$^+$Th细胞的绝对计数在妊娠早期最高[22]。Th细胞的TNF-α/IL-10比值在妊娠晚期显著增加[22]。然而，也有研究报道，与非妊娠女性相比，妊娠晚期外周血CD4$^+$IFN-γ$^+$Th1和CD4$^+$IL-10$^+$Th2细胞的百分比没有差异[23]。尽管如此，蜕膜中Th2细胞因子产生的增加，表明Th2偏移不是Th细胞的固有特征，而是受微环境的调节[20]。

外周血中的CD4$^+$CD25$^+$Foxp3$^+$抑制性Treg细胞从妊娠开始便逐渐增加，在妊娠中期达到峰值，直至产后才逐渐减少[24]。与非妊娠时外周血单个核细胞(peripheral blood mononuclear cells，PBMC)和月经血相比，足月蜕膜中Treg细胞的比例增加[17]。值得注意的是，足月蜕膜Treg细胞的高比例主要是由于分化的Treg增加，而非幼稚Treg。在同一项研究中，非妊娠子宫内膜和足月蜕膜中Th1、Th2和Th17细胞的分布相似。同样，非妊娠期、妊娠早期、中期和晚期的循环Th17细胞也没有差异[15,16]。另一项研究表明，与非妊娠期相比，妊娠晚期外周血Th17细胞减少[23]。总的来说，蜕膜具有独特的免疫环境以适应潜在的妊娠。

4.3 妊娠期间的三个免疫学阶段

过去，组织炎症被认为对妊娠有害，抗炎或Th2优势型维持了健康妊娠。然而，既往20年的研究表明，正常妊娠需要在妊娠早期发生局部组织炎症，于是产生了一个新的概念[25]。对于成功的妊娠，母体免疫系统必须适应妊娠的每个阶段。Gil等[25]将妊娠期母体的免疫适应描述为三个阶段。

4.3.1 胚胎种植和胎盘形成：促炎期

胚胎种植和早期胎盘形成的过程与组织损伤及修复的过程非常相似。在植入部位，子宫内膜基质细胞和局部免疫细胞产生多种炎性介质，包括白细胞介素-6(IL-6)、IL-8、IL-15、粒细胞-巨噬细胞集落刺激因子(GM-CSF)、CXC趋化因子配体1(CXCL1)、CC趋化因子配体4(CCL4)、骨桥蛋白和肿瘤坏死因子(TNF)[25]。植入期子宫内膜的这种促炎环境增加了黏附分子的表达、重组和亲和力，并去除了黏蛋白层。这些过程对子宫内膜容受性和早期胎盘形成至关重要。子宫树突状细胞(dendritic cells，DC)也通过调节组织重塑和血管生成在子宫内膜容受性中发挥作用[26]。子宫DC不会迁移至淋巴结，促进了对父系抗原的耐受性[27]。

4.3.2 胎儿生长：抗炎期

胚胎种植和胎盘形成后的胎儿生长阶段处于Th2型环境。这一阶段从妊娠13周持续至妊娠27周。子宫内抗炎微环境在此阶段由M2巨噬细胞、蜕膜NK(dNK)细胞和Treg细胞建立[25]。M2巨噬细胞对于组织更新和凋亡滋养细胞的吞噬至关重要，防止父系抗原释放[25]。此外，具有低细胞毒性的dNK细胞通过与巨噬细胞相互作用诱导Treg细胞[28]。在妊娠早期，Treg细胞在母胎界面系统性扩增和积聚，保护胎儿细胞免受排斥，并通过其抗炎和抗凋亡能力调节Th17介导的炎症[25]。

4.3.3　分娩：促炎转换

当胎儿完成发育后，子宫中的抗炎环境转换为促炎环境。促炎核因子-κB(NF-κB)信号通路在子宫收缩和分娩中起着关键作用。TLR4通过连接胎儿的肺表面活性物质相关蛋白A和内源性损伤相关分子模式(DAMP)，如高迁移率族蛋白1(HMGB1)，诱导NF-κB活化[25]。在此过程中，免疫细胞侵入子宫肌层，引起子宫收缩和分娩。

综上，在胚胎植入阶段需要Th1优势型，在胎盘发育后的妊娠阶段，Th1优势转换为Th2免疫。然后，当分娩开始时，Th2免疫被重新转换为Th1免疫，为分娩和产后做准备。

4.4　妊娠期父系和胎儿抗原的特异性耐受

1953年，Peter Medawar爵士为母体如何在其子宫中支持半异体胎儿生长9个月的"免疫学悖论"提出了三个假设，包括：①胎盘将胎儿与母体从解剖学上分离。②胎儿抗原不成熟。③妊娠期间母体免疫系统的免疫惰性[29]。上述假设已经演变为妊娠期间母胎界面免疫耐受的概念。然而，最新研究表明，母体免疫系统对胎儿抗原表现出特异性反应，提示同时存在对胎儿的攻击性和免疫耐受性。

针对父系抗原的特异性免疫首先是由母体接触精液引起的。此外，在妊娠期间，会持续接触胎儿细胞和胎儿细胞衍生物质。即使在分娩后，胎儿细胞仍可通过微嵌合继续挑战母体系统[20,30]。由此产生了父系和胎儿抗原特异性记忆T细胞。尽管记忆T细胞的发育可能对妊娠有害，但微妙的记忆T细胞平衡有助于成功妊娠[30]。

精液诱导的Treg细胞不仅为胚胎植入子宫内膜做准备，亦能减轻子宫炎症，但与胎盘抗原暴露无关[31]。胎儿抗原由抗原递呈细胞(APC)——树突状细胞间接递呈给CD4$^+$T细胞。人类蜕膜T细胞识别错配的胎儿HLA-C，并在蜕膜中诱导CD4$^+$CD25^{dim}T细胞活化和功能性CD4$^+$CD25^{bright}Treg细胞增殖[32]。然而，HLA-C匹配或HLA-A、B、Dr或DQ不匹配的妊娠没有表现出这种反应，表明母体T细胞识别胎儿HLA-C抗原。此外，在动物模型中已报道了胎儿抗原特异性效应T细胞的存在。然而，受免疫调节机制控制的效应T细胞在妊娠结束时变得更加强大。

4.5　损害生殖的基础免疫病理学

显然，过度的全身和局部炎症环境对妊娠有害。现已对Th1和Th2免疫失衡，以及Th17和Treg细胞失调进行了深入研究(图3.1)。

4.5.1　反复妊娠丢失中Th1免疫强于Th2免疫

Th1细胞

活化的Th1细胞产生IL-2、TNF-α和IFN-γ，是宿主防御的主要效应物[33]。受控的Th1优势状态似乎有利于植入期间的绒毛外滋养细胞(extravillous trophoblasts，EVT)侵袭[33]。TNF-α调节滋养细胞的过度侵袭[34]，同时促进子痫前期蜕膜中MMP9的表达[35]。IFN-γ在早期胎盘形成中发挥作用，如血管重塑的启动[36]、EVT凋亡和EVT侵袭的调节[33]。然而，在人类妊娠期，过度Th1免疫会导致不良生殖结局。与行人工流产的女性相比，胎儿核型正常的流产患者蜕膜中IFN-γ$^+$Th1细胞增加得更多[37]。与正常妊娠女性相比，在RPL患者的蜕膜和外周血中观察到Th1占优势[38]。在比较PBMC产生的细胞因子时，RPL流产患者上清液中的IL-2、TNF-α和IFN-γ浓度高于正常早孕女性。同样，在RPL和反复植入失败(RIF)患者中亦发现全身性Th1偏移[22,39,40]。众所周知，一些自身免疫性疾病与Th1和Th17免疫相关，如系统性红斑狼疮、多发性硬化、硬皮病、抗磷脂综合征和桥本甲状腺炎[33]。鉴于许多RPL患者也有上述自身免疫状况，与自身免疫疾病相关的Th1免疫增强可能导致流产。

Th2细胞

Th2细胞负责不依赖于吞噬细胞的宿主防御细胞外病原体，并产生IL-4、IL-5、IL-10和IL-13[20]。据报道，在小鼠和人类健康妊娠中存在局部Th2环境[20,41]。Th2细胞在妊娠期由子宫DC诱导[42]，并被滋养层表达的父系抗原激活[20]。在LPS诱导的大鼠流产模型中，IL-10或TNF-α受体抑制剂(依那西普)可预防妊娠丢失[43]。与正常妊娠女性相比，不明原因RPL患者蜕膜T细胞的LIF、IL-4和IL-10分泌降低[44]。在比较PBMC产生

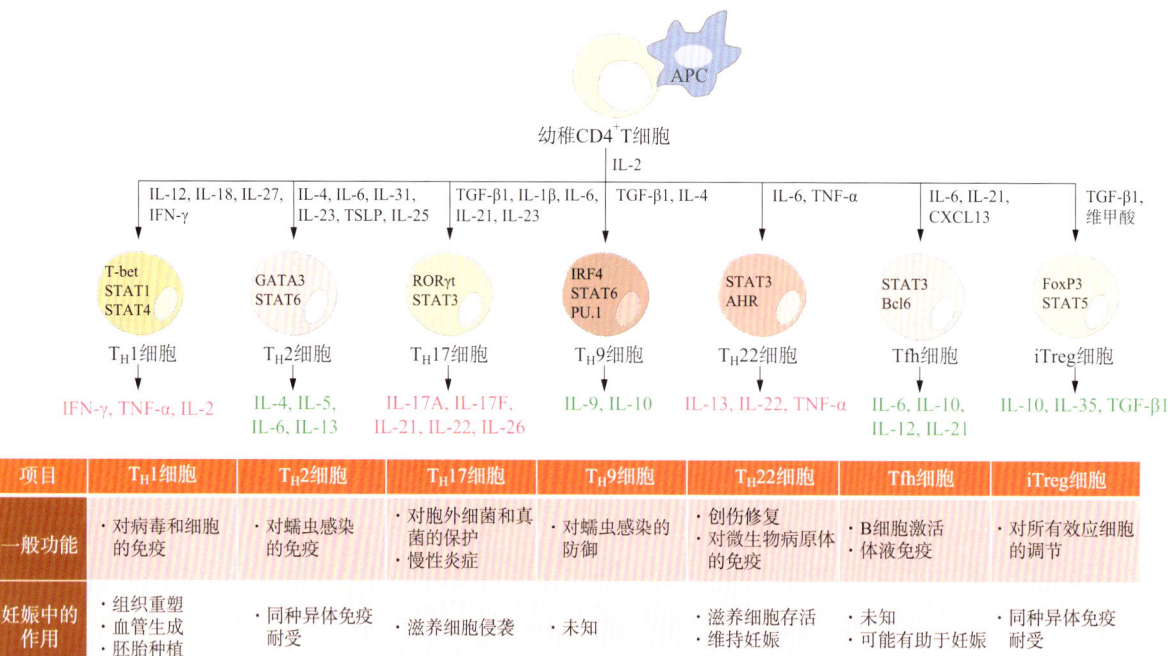

图 3.1 人类 CD4⁺ T 细胞亚群及其在妊娠中的作用。

幼稚 CD4⁺ T 细胞受抗原递呈细胞刺激发育为活化 CD4⁺ T 细胞。CD4⁺ T 细胞根据其被激活的条件分化为 CD4⁺ T 细胞的不同亚群。图中,细胞内显示每个亚群对应的转录因子。此外,主要由 T 细胞亚群分泌的细胞因子以红色和绿色标识。红色代表促炎细胞因子,绿色代表具有调节功能的细胞因子。图中还标注了每个亚群在妊娠中的功能和作用。

的细胞因子时,RPL 流产患者的 IL-6 和 IL-10 水平均低于正常早孕女性[38]。

反复妊娠丢失中的 Th1 和 Th2 失衡

Th1 免疫应答在器官移植排斥反应中起着关键作用,Th2 免疫则有助于免疫耐受。基于此,妊娠期 Th1 和 Th2 平衡的概念可简单理解为:对胎儿过度的 Th1 反应会导致不良妊娠结局,而 Th2 反应则能抵消 Th1 反应,有利于成功妊娠[20]。与对照组 CBA/J × BALB/c 小鼠相比,流产模型 CBA/J × DBA/2 小鼠的 TNF-α、IFN-γ 和 IL-2 表达增加。流产模型小鼠注射重组 IL-10 后,高胚胎吸收率被逆转[45]。

与正常生育组相比,非妊娠 RPL 女性外周血中 TNF-α⁺Th/IL-10⁺Th、TNF-α⁺Th/IL-4⁺Th 和 TNF-γ⁺Th/IL-4⁺Th 细胞比例增高[39,40]。一项研究表明,与正常早孕女性相比,流产的 RPL 患者中各种组合的 Th1/Th2 细胞因子比例持续增加[38]。在另一项比较 PBMC 产生细胞因子的研究中,与正常妊娠女性在早期妊娠结束时相比,RPL 患者流产时 Th1/Th2 细胞因子比例显著增加[46]。在培养蜕膜 T 细胞时发现,与接受人工流产的女性相比,流产的特发性 RPL 患者中 IL-4 和 IL-10 产生减少[44]。在这项研究中,与正常孕妇相比,RPL 患者蜕膜 Th 细胞的白血病抑制因子(LIF)和巨噬细胞集落刺激因子(M-CSF)产生亦受损,流产患者蜕膜 T 细胞的 IL-2 和 IFN-γ 表达较高,IL-4 和 IL-10 表达较低[47]。此外,Th1 细胞因子的产生与共刺激分子(如 CD86 和 CD28)的表达呈正相关[47]。蜕膜 IL-2 和 IFN-γ 的分泌与母胎界面的 CD86 和 CD28 表达呈正相关,与 CTLA4 表达呈负相关[47]。

4.5.2 反复妊娠丢失中 Treg 和 Th17 细胞失调

Foxp3⁺ Treg 细胞

Sasaki 等[48]于 2004 年首次报道了 Treg 细胞在自然流产中的作用。他们发现,与正常妊娠相比,流产组外周血和蜕膜中 CD4⁺ CD25^bright T 细胞减少。此后,多项研究证实了 RPL 女性体内全身和局部的 Foxp3⁺ Treg 细胞数量和抑制性功能降低[13,16,49]。外周血 Treg 细胞水平在月经周期的增殖晚期达到峰值,并与血清雌二醇水平呈正相关[13]。相反,RPL 女性的外周血 Treg 细胞没有这种变化[13]。

Th17 细胞

Th17 细胞在对抗细胞外细菌和真菌方面发挥作用,并通过分泌 IL-17A、IL-17F、IL-21、

IL-22和IL-26引起慢性炎症、同种异体移植排斥反应和某些自身免疫性疾病[20,40]。在人类妊娠中,蜕膜基质细胞从外周血向蜕膜募集Th17细胞[50]。在妊娠早期,蜕膜Th17细胞通过分泌IL-17促进滋养细胞的增殖与侵袭,并抑制其调亡[50]。这一发现表明,Th17细胞在早期胎盘形成中是必需的。在一项比较外周血和蜕膜Th17细胞的研究中,蜕膜Th17细胞在淋巴细胞中的百分比高于外周血Th17细胞[15]。由于IL-17能诱导中性粒细胞募集,随着蜕膜Th17细胞增多,蜕膜的中性粒细胞浸润可能也会增加。与正常生育组相比,非妊娠和妊娠RPL女性的外周血Th17细胞增多,而外周血Treg细胞减少[40,51]。与正常妊娠女性相比,特发性RPL患者流产物蜕膜中的Th17细胞增多,Treg细胞减少[51]。这些研究提示,Th17和Treg细胞失调可能是导致RPL的一个关键免疫机制。

此外,对非妊娠RPL女性的Th亚群和Treg细胞间的相关性分析表明,外周血Th17细胞比例与TNF-α$^+$ Th细胞及TNF-α$^+$CD4$^+$/IL-10$^+$CD4$^+$ T细胞和TNF-γ$^+$CD4$^+$/IL-10$^+$CD4$^+$ T细胞比值呈正相关[40]。此外,Th17/Foxp3$^+$ Treg细胞比值也与TNF-α$^+$ Th细胞、IFN-γ$^+$ Th细胞和Th1/Th2细胞比值呈正相关。这些结果表明Th1和Th17都参与了RPL的免疫病理学。

4.5.3 生殖中的其他Th细胞

Th9细胞

分泌IL-9的Th细胞,称为Th9细胞,可能在过敏性炎症、自身免疫性疾病、肿瘤免疫和寄生虫感染中发挥作用[52,53]。在小鼠模型中,Th9细胞控制子宫的局部炎症,而IL-6能诱导蜕膜Th9细胞减少,从而加速分娩[54]。然而,Th9细胞在人类妊娠中的作用尚不明确。

Th22细胞

IL-22由Th22、Th17、γδT、NKT和固有淋巴细胞产生,在肠、肺、肝、肾、胸腺、胰腺、皮肤和胎盘等多种组织中均已发现[55]。IL-22在组织再生中发挥作用,并调节屏障表面的宿主防御。在生殖过程中,IL-22可能参与促进滋养细胞存活并维持妊娠。流产患者胎盘绒毛中IL-22R1的表达低于正常妊娠女性,表明IL-22/IL-22R信号传导不足与流产存在关联[56]。Th22细胞具有显著的可塑性,可分化为Th1或Th2细胞。目前尚不明确外周血Th22细胞或蜕膜IL-22的产生是否在RPL中增加。然而,RPL患者的蜕膜IL-22$^+$IL-17$^+$IL-4$^+$ Th细胞少于正常妊娠女性。Th22细胞的作用仍有待进一步研究。

滤泡辅助性T细胞

滤泡辅助性T(Tfh)细胞在B细胞活化、抗体类别转换和生发中心形成中起着关键作用[57]。在一项小鼠研究中发现,CXCR5$^+$ Tfh细胞在妊娠中期的子宫中积聚并达到峰值,并在妊娠晚期的胎盘中增加[33]。PDL1阻断引起的胚胎再吸收与Tfh细胞积聚相关,表明Tfh的过度积聚可能不利于妊娠。此外,妊娠晚期女性的外周血Tfh细胞比例显著高于非妊娠女性[58]。外周血雌激素水平(而非孕酮)与CXCR3$^+$ Tfh细胞呈正相关[58]。总的来说,妊娠期高雌激素水平可能导致Tfh细胞比例增加,激活B细胞并促进体液免疫。因此,充足的Tfh细胞可能有助于成功妊娠。Tfh细胞在RPL中的作用仍需进一步研究加以阐明。

4.5.4 新型调节性T细胞

除了Foxp3$^+$ Treg细胞,其他具有调节功能的新T细胞亚群亦被发现。CD4$^+$HLA-G$^+$CD25$^-$Foxp3$^-$ Treg细胞可通过膜结合型HLA-G1表达及分泌IL-10和可溶性HLA-G5,以细胞接触依赖和非依赖的方式抑制T细胞增殖[59]。CD4$^+$和CD8$^+$ T细胞可通过HLA-G1的细胞间转移(即胞啃作用)从APC获得调节功能[60]。与非妊娠女性相比,正常妊娠女性外周血中的CD4$^+$HLA-G$^+$ Treg细胞增加,并且蜕膜中的这些细胞在正常妊娠时较子痫前期时更多[61]。

有趣的是,Th1细胞能选择性杀死APC,但不杀死T细胞和B细胞[62]。然而,CD4$^+$CD25$^-$FoxP3$^-$ T调节细胞,即Th3细胞,同时产生IL-10和IL-4,并通过产生TGF-β和IL-10抑制免疫细胞。尽管在蜕膜中发现了Th3细胞,但其在妊娠中的作用仍有待探索。相反,1型调节性T(Tr1)细胞通过产生IL-10和TGF-β并利用KIR受体或胞外酶以细胞间接触的方式抑制其他免疫细胞[59]。在外周血和许多组织(包括人类蜕膜)中发现了Tr1细胞。Tr1细胞由EVT通过HLA-G直接诱导,并高表达PD-1。然而,最近的一项质谱研究未能证实人类蜕膜中存在Tr1细胞[63]。因此,仍需进一步研究。

4.5.5 生殖中的记忆T细胞

动物和人类的免疫系统对父系和胎儿抗原表现

出特异性免疫反应。一些由父系抗原激活的母体免疫细胞可作为记忆细胞存活很长时间。这些细胞在随后的妊娠中对胎儿抗原表现出更快的反应和增殖，并在妊娠结局中发挥积极作用。迄今，尚未引入代表记忆T细胞的可靠标志物；然而，CD45RO⁺表达或CD45RA⁻表达被广泛用作表型标记[30]。主要的两个记忆T细胞亚群是效应记忆（EM）和中央记忆（CM）细胞（图3.2A）。一些产科并发症（如子痫前期、妊娠糖尿病和早产）患者外周血中总记忆T细胞的比例高于正常妊娠[30]。

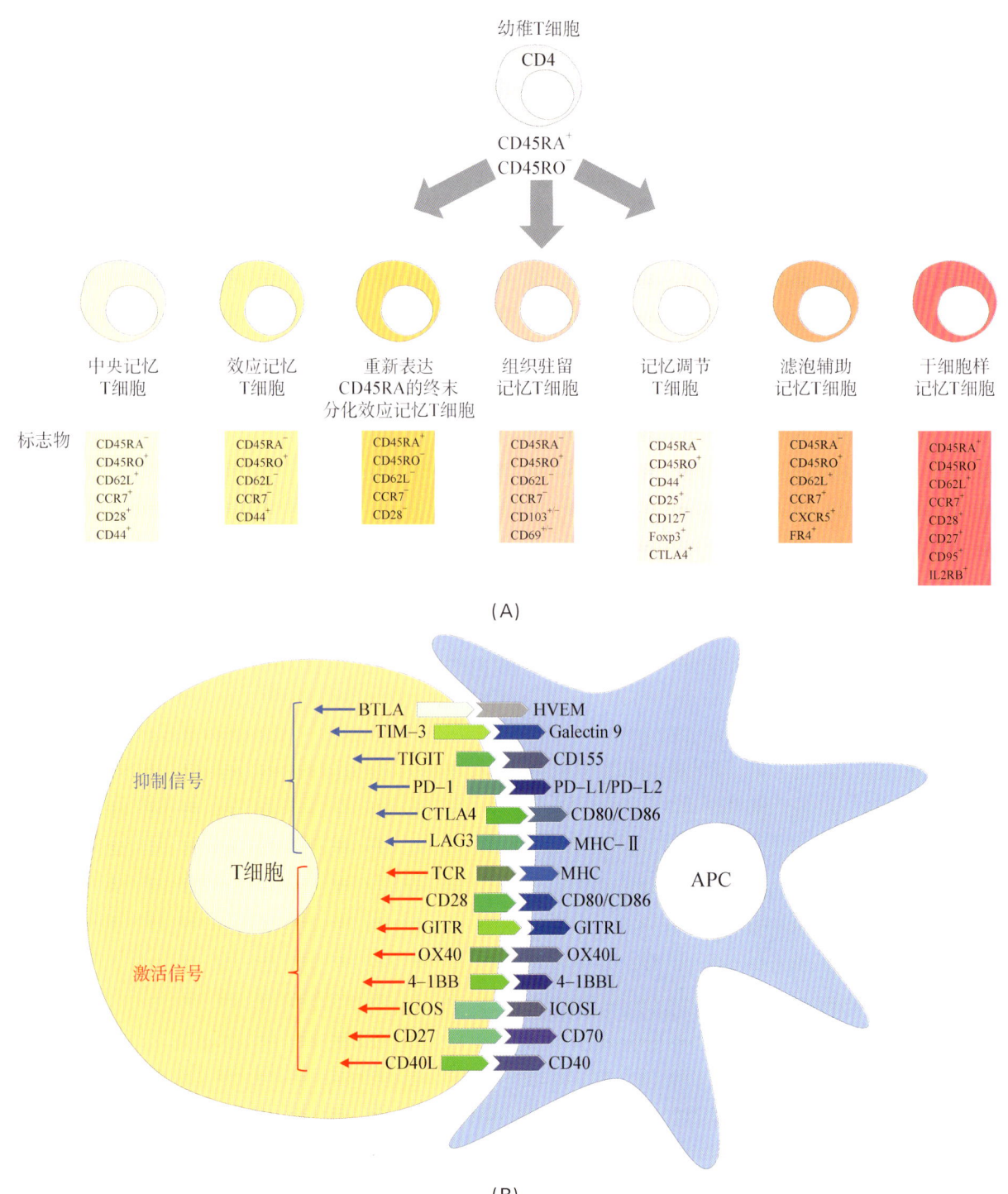

图3.2 人类记忆CD4⁺T细胞亚群通过免疫检查点分子与抗原递呈细胞（APC）相互作用。

(A)人类记忆CD4⁺T细胞亚群。活化CD4⁺T细胞亚群起效应器作用，但其中一部分也发育为记忆细胞。图中标记了每种记忆CD4⁺细胞的表型。(B)T细胞通过免疫检查点分子接受APC的抑制信号和激活信号。图中的蓝色箭头表示T细胞的抑制信号，红色箭头表示激活信号。

CD4$^+$效应记忆T细胞(T_{EM})

Th亚群如Th1、Th2和Th17细胞可分化为CD4$^+$ T_{EM}细胞。CD4$^+$ T_{EM}细胞的特征是缺乏淋巴结归巢受体CCR7和CD62L（L-选择素），并迁移至外周非淋巴组织[64]。与非妊娠状态相比，外周血CD4$^+$ T_{EM}细胞在妊娠期增加，表达更多的CD69和PD-1。不仅在妊娠期间，外周血中的CD4$^+$ T_{EM}细胞水平在分娩后的数年里仍高于未曾妊娠的女性[65]。

CD4$^+$ T_{EM}细胞可能参与胎儿母体免疫环境的调节。蜕膜CD4$^+$ T_{EM}细胞上的免疫检查点受体，如PD-1、T细胞免疫球蛋白和黏蛋白结构域分子-3（Tim-3）、CTLA-4和淋巴细胞激活基因3（LAG3）的表达高于外周血CD4$^+$ T_{EM}细胞[30]。人类蜕膜中的大多数CD4$^+$ T_{EM}细胞表达PD-1和Tim-3，并表现出Th2表型，产生IL-4[66]。此外，流产患者蜕膜CD4$^+$ T_{EM}细胞上PD-1和Tim-3共表达显著低于正常妊娠[66]。在小鼠中，阻断Tim-3和PD-1通路能增加胚胎再吸收率。总的来说，蜕膜CD4$^+$ T_{EM}细胞可能在母胎界面具有调节功能，并防止流产[66]。然而，RPL女性血液和子宫内膜中CD3$^+$CD69$^+$ T_{EM}细胞的频率显著高于正常生育女性[67]。因此，需要进一步研究以阐明CD4$^+$ T_{EM}细胞在生殖中的作用。

CD4$^+$重新表达CD45RA的终末分化效应记忆T细胞（T_{EMRA}）

CD4$^+$ T_{EMRA}细胞是一种独特的CD4$^+$ T_{EM}亚群，在抗原刺激后重新表达CD45RA，并参与了对登革热病毒和巨细胞病毒感染的保护性免疫[68]。然而，此类CD4$^+$ T_{EMRA}细胞在生殖中的作用很少被研究。

CD4$^+$中央记忆T细胞（T_{CM}）

CD4$^+$ T_{CM}细胞表达淋巴结归巢受体，如CCR7和CD62L[22]。与正常妊娠和正常生育女性的非妊娠对照组相比，子痫前期和非妊娠RPL患者血液中的CD4$^+$ T_{CM}细胞显著增加[30]。

CD4$^+$调节记忆T细胞（记忆Treg）

长期存活的记忆Treg细胞亚群在抗原暴露后持续存在[54]。记忆Treg细胞尚无明确的标志物，目前通过Foxp3$^+$、CD25$^+$、CD127$^-$、CD45RO$^+$和CD45RA$^-$的组合来鉴定[30]。有趣的是，记忆Treg细胞在子痫前期和妊娠期糖尿病中增加[30]，然而它们的作用并未在高危妊娠中得到充分评估。

CD4$^+$滤泡辅助记忆T细胞（T_{FHM}）

T_{FHM}细胞以表达CXCR5、CD62L、CCR7和叶酸受体4为特征，产生IL-10和IL-21，并可根据PD-1、CCR8、诱导性T细胞共刺激受体（ICOS）的表达区分不同亚群[30]。在小鼠中，T_{FHM}细胞在妊娠晚期的子宫和胎盘中增加，阻断PD-L1（抑制PD-1效应）诱导胚胎再吸收和CD4$^+$ T_{FHM}积聚，表明T_{FHM}可能参与胎儿母体耐受[30]。与择期终止妊娠的正常孕妇相比，流产患者蜕膜中PD-1$^+$CCR7$^+$和PD-1$^+$ICOS$^+$细胞更多，而外周血中没有显著差异[69]。

CD4$^+$组织驻留记忆T细胞（T_{RM}）

由于没有确切的分子标志物，对CD4$^+$ T_{RM}细胞的研究具有挑战性[30]。迄今尚无CD4$^+$ T_{RM}细胞与生殖的相关研究发表。

CD4$^+$干细胞样记忆T细胞（T_{SCM}）

CD4$^+$ T_{SCM}细胞表达CD45RA$^+$、CCR7$^+$、CD62L$^+$、CD28$^+$、CD27$^+$、CXCR3$^+$、CD95$^+$和IL2RB$^+$[30]。CD4$^+$ T_{SCM}细胞亦尚未在妊娠期进行研究。

4.5.6 Th细胞上的免疫检查点分子与生殖

免疫检查点分子是携带共刺激或共抑制信号的免疫系统的调节分子（图3.2B）。目前研究最多的分子是抑制性免疫检查点分子，如CTLA-4、PD-1、Tim-3、TIGIT和LAG-3[70]。CTLA-4、Tim-3和PD-1是维持母胎界面免疫耐受的关键分子。

细胞毒性T淋巴细胞相关抗原4（CTLA-4）

在人类妊娠中，CTLA-4存在于蜕膜Treg细胞。CTLA-4、CD80和CD86的配体在蜕膜APC上表达，如树突状细胞和巨噬细胞[71]。由于蜕膜CTLA-4的表达与蜕膜Th2免疫呈正相关，与Th1呈负相关，因此CTLA-4可能涉及子宫内的免疫调节[71]。CTLA-4在流产中的作用存在争议。与正常妊娠相比，流产患者的CTLA-4$^+$蜕膜淋巴细胞显著减少。然而，另一项研究表明，蜕膜中CTLA-4$^+$Treg细胞/Treg细胞的比例在正常妊娠和流产之间没有差异[48]。

Tim-3

Tim-3最初被鉴定为Th1特异性细胞表面分子，在蜕膜基质细胞和免疫细胞上表达，如NK、巨噬细胞、CD8$^+$T、Th1、Th2、Th17、Treg、γδT和NKT细胞。Tim-3通过Galectin-9转导凋亡信号下调 Th1 应答[72]。Tim-3 能结合两种配体,磷脂酰丝氨酸(PtdSer)和 Galectin-9。PtdSer 暴露于凋亡细胞的表面。APC 上的 Tim-3 与 PtdSer 连接诱导凋亡细胞的吞噬作用,有助于维持对自身抗原的耐受[72]。Galectin-9 由 Treg、T、B 和肥大细胞、子宫内膜上皮细胞、滋养细胞和胃肠道上皮细胞分泌。Tim-3-Gal-9 通路诱导 Th1 和 Th17 的凋亡、Treg 的增殖和抗凋亡、dNK 的转化,以及对巨噬细胞、树突状细胞和 CD8⁺ T 细胞的调节功能[72]。在小鼠中,阻断 Tim-3 导致胚胎再吸收率增加,产仔数减少[70]。在 RPL 患者中,蜕膜 CD4⁺ T 细胞上的 CTLA-4 和 Tim-3 共同表达显著低于正常早期妊娠[73]。一项对接受胚胎移植的不孕患者的研究发现,与成功妊娠组相比,妊娠失败组的种植期 Tim-3⁺PD-1⁺CD4⁺ T 细胞和 Tim-3⁺PD-1⁺CD8⁺ T 细胞的比例降低[74]。

程序性细胞死亡蛋白1(PD-1)

PD-1 是一种跨膜受体,通过与其配体 PD-L1 和 PD-L2 结合产生有效的抑制信号[71]。PD-1 在 T、B、NK、树突状细胞和巨噬细胞上表达。PD-L1 也在胎盘、心脏和脾脏等一些组织中表达[71]。在小鼠流产模型中,阻断 PD-1 导致流产率增加,但阻断 CTLA-4 不影响妊娠结局[75]。在外周血淋巴细胞的流式细胞分析中,PD-L1 在 Th1、Th17 和 Treg 细胞中的表达比 PD-1 在 RPL 和对照组中的表达更普遍[76]。然而,非妊娠 RPL 女性的 PD-1⁺Th1、PD-1⁺Th17 和 PD-L1⁺Th17 细胞明显低于正常生育对照组[76]。在人类妊娠中,蜕膜淋巴细胞 PD-1 的表达在正常妊娠和 RPL 之间没有差异,但 RPL 患者蜕膜 PD-L1 mRNA 的表达明显低于正常妊娠女性[77]。多项研究证实,子痫前期患者 PD-1⁺Treg 细胞增加。近期的一项研究表明,蜕膜 PD-1^{high}CD8⁺ 细胞比例在流产和正常早期妊娠之间没有差异;但与正常妊娠晚期相比,蜕膜 PD-1^{high}CD8⁺ 细胞比例在子痫前期中降低[78]。

5 诊断方法

5.1 实验室技术

5.1.1 流式细胞术

流式细胞分析是计数子宫内膜/蜕膜/血液中淋巴细胞及其亚群(包括 T 细胞、B 细胞和 NK 细胞)的最常用评估方法。在临床实践中,外周血 Th1/Th2 细胞因子比例在多个方面具有优势:①静脉血比子宫内膜组织更易获得和处理。②由于在妊娠早期,循环免疫细胞被迅速招募到分泌期子宫内膜和蜕膜中,外周血免疫细胞似乎反映了子宫内膜免疫细胞。许多研究证实,基于外周血免疫检测的免疫治疗可改善生殖障碍患者的临床结局。子宫内膜和蜕膜 T 细胞免疫也可通过流式细胞术测定。

Th1/Th2 细胞比例的检测步骤如下[39]:从 10~15 mL 外周血或子宫内膜中分离 PBMC,并用佛波酯(PMA)和离子霉素激活。使用含布雷非德菌素A(BFA)的蛋白转运抑制剂来抑制细胞因子分泌,并添加细胞表面抗原(如 CD3、CD4 或 CD8)的特异性荧光素偶联单克隆抗体。破膜进行细胞内染色,并用 TNF-α、IFN-γ、IL-4 或 IL-10 荧光素偶联单克隆抗体对细胞进行染色。用流式细胞仪对细胞进行检测分析[11,39]。

然而,全球只有少数实验室具有 Th 细胞亚群的临界值,并将其应用于临床实践。Winger 等[79] 报道,与未经免疫治疗的患者相比,IVIg 免疫治疗提高了具有较高外周血 Th1/Th2 比值或 NK 细胞水平(TNF-α/IL-10>30.6,IFN-γ/IL-10>20.5,NK 细胞水平>12%)患者的活产率(LBR)。Lee 等[10] 也确定了分泌细胞因子的 CD4 细胞临界值:CD4⁺ T 细胞中 TNF-α>70.1%,分泌 TNF-β/IL-10 的 Th 细胞比例>36.2。在临床实践中,医生可以制定自己的 Th 细胞免疫临界值或采用已报道的参考值。

5.1.2 聚合酶链反应和酶联免疫吸附试验

转录因子和各种细胞因子的基因表达可以通过聚合酶链反应(PCR)在外周血和(或)子宫内膜/蜕膜组织中测定。此外,也可通过商业化酶联免疫吸附试验(ELISA)试剂盒检测外周血中的各种细胞因子以评估 T 细胞免疫。

5.2 候选人群的评估

对于需进行 Th 细胞亚群评估的候选人群尚无普遍共识。然而,在评估 T 细胞免疫时,应考虑两次或两次以上流产的 RPL 女性,尤其是具有以下一种或多种因素:①存在亚临床自身免疫,如抗磷脂抗体、抗核抗体、抗 DNA 抗体和抗甲状腺抗体。②既往或活动性自身免疫性和(或)风湿性疾病病史。③既往或活动性 NK 细胞病理改变。④母胎同种异体免疫疾病。⑤特发性 RPL(表 3.1)。

表 3.1 在正常妊娠和反复妊娠丢失中比较外周血和子宫内膜/蜕膜的辅助 T 细胞免疫

Th 亚群	月经周期(分泌期 vs 卵泡期)		正常妊娠		反复妊娠丢失(RPL)			
					非妊娠 (RPL vs 对照组)		妊娠 (RPL vs 对照组)	
	外周血	内膜	外周血	蜕膜	外周血	内膜	外周血	蜕膜
Th1	→	?	↓(妊娠早期)	↓	→	↑	↑→	↑
Th2	→	?	↑(妊娠早期)	→	?	↓	↓	
Th1/Th2	→	?	↑(妊娠晚期)	?	↑	?	↑	?
Th17	?	?	→	↑	↑	?	→↑	↑
Treg	↓(卵泡后期峰值)	↓(增殖期较高)	↑(妊娠中期峰值)	↑	↓	↓	↓	↓
Th17/Treg	?	?	?	?	↑	?	?	?
Th9	?	?	?	?	?	?	?	?
Th22	?	?	?	?	?	?	?	↓
Tfh	?	?	?	?	?	?	?	?
CD4$^+$ T$_{EM}$	?	?	?	?	?	?	?	↓
CD4$^+$ T$_{EMRA}$	?	?	?	?	?	?	?	?
CD4$^+$ T$_{CM}$	?	?	?	?	?	?	↑	?
记忆 Treg	?	?	?	?	?	?	?	?
CD4$^+$ T$_{FHM}$	?	?	?	?	?	?	↑	↑
CD4$^+$ T$_{RM}$	?	?	?	?	?	?	?	?
CD4$^+$ T$_{SCM}$	?	?	?	?	?	?	?	?

注:?,未知;↑,升高;↓,降低;→,无变化。

6 治疗与生殖结局

当前,RPL 患者 T 细胞免疫异常的治疗方案包括皮质类固醇、静脉注射免疫球蛋白(IVIg)、他克莫司、环孢素、TNF-α 抑制剂和维生素 D(表 3.2)[80]。

6.1 皮质类固醇

糖皮质激素影响早期妊娠的几个关键环节,包括母体免疫反应、胚胎附着/植入、滋养细胞生长和侵袭,以及胎儿及胎盘发育[87]。由于皮质类固醇对高 Th1/Th2 或 Treg/Th17 及 NK 细胞的细胞毒性具有免疫抑制作用,现已被用于治疗患有 RPL 的女性[88]。

在一项对不明原因 RPL 女性进行的随机对照试验中,与安慰剂组(9.7%)相比,在肝素和低剂量阿司匹林治疗时添加强的松(20 mg/d)显著提高了妊娠成功率(70.3%),这可能是由于皮质类固醇对外周 CD16$^+$ NK 细胞浓度和 Th1 细胞免疫的抑制作用[81]。关于 Th1/Th2 比值失调,目前对糖皮质激素作用的研究有限。皮质类固醇能恢复正常 Th1 和 Th2 细胞因子间的平衡,如降低 IFN-γ 和提高 IL-4。皮质类固醇的抗炎作用部分是由于通过抑制 IL-2 的产生从而发挥对 T 细胞增殖的抑制作用。皮质类固醇以药效相关和剂量依赖的方式调节 T 细胞的细胞因子产生。越有效的皮质类固醇,对 T 细胞产 IFN-γ 和 IL4 的抑制作用越强。然而,低浓度和药效较弱的皮质类固醇(如地塞米松),可增强 IL-4 的产生[89,90]。Sasaki 等[91] 报道了 RPL 和 Th1/Th2 比值升高的女性在强的松治疗后成功活产。强的松治疗后 Th1/Th2 比值随时间延长而降低。

表 3.2 治疗异常 T 细胞免疫的免疫调节药物

药物	机制	剂量/周期	妊娠结局	副作用
皮质类固醇	↓Th1/Th2	强的松每天 5~20 mg	活产率:强的松+肝素+低分子肝素组 70.3% vs 安慰剂组 9.7%[81]	早产、胎儿宫内生长迟缓、子痫前期、绒毛膜羊膜炎
IVIg	↓Th1/Th2 ↓Th17/Treg	400 mg/kg 每 3~4 周	活产率:IVIg 组 87.5% vs 对照组 41.6%[82] 活产率:IVIg 组 47.5% vs 对照组 21.8%[83]	头痛、发热、恶心、过敏、急性肾功能衰竭
他克莫司	↓Th1/Th2 ↓细胞毒 T 细胞	每天 1~3 mg	活产率:他克莫司组 60.0% vs 对照组 0.0%[84]	没有与产科和围产期并发症相关的报道
环孢素	↓Th1 频率,T-bet mRNA 表达,IFN-γ 和 TNFα; ↑Th2 频率,GATA 结合蛋白 mRNA 表达,IL-10	50 mg 口服,每天 3 次,6 个月	活产率:环孢素组 81.5% vs 对照组 42.1%[85]	—
TNF-α 抑制剂	↓TNF-α	阿达木单抗 40 mg 皮下注射,每 1~2 周一次,直至通过超声检查确认胎儿心跳	活产率:阿达木单抗+IVIg+肝素组 71.0% vs IVIg+肝素组 54%[86]	机会性感染、淋巴瘤、神经后遗症

在患有免疫障碍的女性中,妊娠中、晚期暴露于糖皮质激素可能会导致产科并发症,包括胎儿宫内生长受限、早产、子痫前期、绒毛膜羊膜炎,以及与产前和产后行为改变相关的对胎儿大脑发育的影响[87]。相反,最近的研究表明,用类固醇治疗早产儿不会增加神经发育迟缓的风险[92]。对糖皮质激素在早期妊娠中的影响研究较少,大多数可用证据来自接受辅助生殖技术患者的妊娠率[87]。皮质类固醇的不良反应似乎是剂量依赖的,在较低剂量应用强的松时发生率较低。暴露于大剂量强的松(≥每天 10 mg/kg)与早产相关,而较低剂量(≤每天 10 mg/kg)则与早产无关[93]。在患有肠易激综合征的女性中,口服皮质类固醇 140 天以内不会增加早产的风险,而口服超过 140 天则会增加早产风险。然而,妊娠早、中期服用大剂量皮质类固醇与 SLE 患者的早产增加相关[94]。由此可见,皮质类固醇的副作用似乎与妊娠期间的剂量和暴露时间有关。在妊娠早期,RPL 患者的低剂量暴露可能不会增加早产风险。由于滋养细胞浸润和胎盘生长受损,RPL 本身与早产风险有关。此类研究受局限于各种混杂因素难以区分。最近,德国/奥地利/瑞士的妇产科协会指南建议,皮质类固醇仅用于既往有自身免疫性疾病患者的治疗。正如 ESHRE 指南所指出的,妊娠期间存在使用皮质类固醇与重大不良事件相关的可能性[4,95]。然而,值得注意的是,在有限的时间内接受低至中等剂量强的松治疗的 RPL 患者并未出现产科并发症[93]。严格挑选皮质类固醇治疗患者,如使用外周血 Th1/Th2 细胞比例和连续随访 T 细胞免疫,可能会增加 RPL 患者的妊娠成功率,且不增加产科并发症。

6.2 静脉注射免疫球蛋白

IVIg 具有抑制和中和自身抗体、减弱 NK 细胞的细胞毒性、抑制补体结合、调节细胞因子产生和扩增调节性 T 淋巴细胞的多种免疫调节作用[96]。一些病例对照研究与探索 IVIg 对 RPL 患者疗效的随机对照试验显示了相互矛盾的结果。在一项 Cochrane 系统回顾和荟萃分析中,包括 8 项对不明原因 RPL 患者进行的随机对照试验,IVIg 与安慰剂相比没有增加活产率($OR = 0.98$, 95% $CI = 0.61 \sim 1.58$)[97]。与原发性 RPL 相比,免疫紊乱可能在继发性 RPL 中发挥更为重要的作用。Egerup 等[98]的荟萃分析显示,继发性 RPL 患者更有可能从 IVIg 中获得潜在的益处。然而,另一项 RCT 研究未显示继发性 RPL 患者经 IVIg 治疗后活产率增加[99]。最新的荟萃分析显示,与对照组相比,IVIg 治疗的患者活产率增加($RR=1.20$,$95\% CI=1.0\sim1.37$,固定效应法 $P=0.004$)[100]。由于研究人群存在显著异质性,研究主要报道了随机效应模型的统计结果($RR=1.17$,$95\% CI=0.95\sim1.44$,$P=0.14$)。然而,值得注意的是,当干预效应分布模式因研究较少而不对称时,随机效应模型对干预效应的分布宽度估计较差,而固定效应模型受影响较小[101]。IVIg 似乎在特定的亚群中起作用。亚组分析显示,妊娠前 IVIg 治疗显著增加活产率($RR=1.69$,$95\% CI=1.33\sim2.14$,$P<0.0001$),而 IVIg 对二次流产者的治疗效果处于临界($RR=1.24$,$95\% CI=0.96\sim1.59$,$P=0.06$)[101]。最近,Won 等[102]进行了一项荟萃分析,以评估基于异常 NK 细胞水平和(或)活性而特别选择的患者的免疫治疗效果。非 RCT 的 IVIg 研究(312 例干预,245 例对照)显示,IVIg 治疗组的活产数增加($RR=2.57$,$95\% CI=1.79\sim3.69$,$P<0.05$)。

IVIg 显示出对 RPL 中 Th1/Th2 和 Th17/Treg 细胞比例的显著调节作用。Yamada 等[103]报道,IVIg 治疗(20 g/d,持续 5 天)调节了外周血细胞因子水平并降低了 Th1/Th2 细胞比例。每 4 周静脉注射 400 mg/kg 免疫球蛋白,也显著降低了 Th1 淋巴细胞、转录因子表达和细胞因子水平,同时显著增加了 Th2 淋巴细胞参数[82]。通过向 Th2 反应的转换,IVIg 治疗组的活产率(87.5%)显著高于未治疗组(41.6%)[82]。Lee 等[104]还报道了在患有 RPL 和异常细胞免疫(数量、NK 细胞的细胞毒性或 Th1/Th2 比值增加)的女性中,每 3 周给予一次 400 mg/kg 免疫球蛋白,活产率为 84.7%(94/111)。

Kim 等[105]报道,IVIg 治疗调节了 RPL 妊娠患者体内 Th17 和 $Foxp3^+$ Treg 细胞的失衡。IVIg 下调最高四分位数(Q4)中的 Th17 细胞($P=0.001$),上调较低四分位数(Q1 和 Q2)中的 $CD4^+Foxp3^+$ T 细胞(分别为 $P=0.025$ 和 $P=0.029$)。76% 的 RPL 患者(28/37)在 IVIg 治疗后获得成功的妊娠结局。首次 IVIg 治疗时免疫异常的 RPL 患者的妊娠成功率(80.6%)高于无免疫异常的妇女(50%)。据推测,IVIg 介导的对 Th17 和 Treg 细胞失调的免疫调节也与早期妊娠期间细胞免疫异常的 RPL 患者的成功妊娠结局有关[105]。Ahmadi 等[83]证实,在 RIF 患者中,IVIg 治疗显著增加了 Treg 细胞相关参数,如 Treg 比例、Foxp3 表达和细胞因子 mRNA 水平(IL-10 和 TGF-β)。RIF 患者经 IVIg 治疗后的活产率为 47.5%,显著高于对照组(21.8%)[83]。

RPL 患者通常耐受 IVIg,不良反应(包括头痛、发热和恶心)发生率低于 5%[96]。严重且罕见的并发症,如过敏反应和急性肾衰竭,与 IgA 缺乏和使用含糖稳定剂的 IVIg 溶液有关[106,107]。因此,IVIg 输注前应检查血清 IgA 和肌酐水平[108]。如今,大多数 IVIg 制剂不使用含糖稳定剂。假定产前接触药物会导致胎儿免疫的表观遗传变化,研究调查了宫内暴露于 IVIg 的儿童自身免疫和过敏性疾病的患病率。然而,未观察到所调查疾病的患病率差异。到目前为止,这一领域在过去 30 年中,没有任何报道表明母体在妊娠前和妊娠期间接受 IVIg 治疗对婴儿有明显的副作用[108,109]。

6.3 他克莫司

他克莫司用于器官移植的受者及患有类风湿关节炎和系统性红斑狼疮等自身免疫性疾病的患者,即使是在妊娠期或哺乳期。他克莫司抑制淋巴细胞增殖、细胞毒性 T 细胞生成、IL-2 受体表达和细胞因子(如 IL-2 和 IFN-γ)的产生[110]。他克莫司被用于 RIF 和妊娠丢失患者,并显示出 Th1/Th2 细胞比例升高(≥ 10.3);他克莫司组的活产率显著高于对照组(60.0% vs 0%)[84]。

FDA 将他克莫司归类为妊娠 C 类药物。此外,他克莫司对新生儿 Th 细胞或其他免疫细胞的药物作用是无法预计的,因为其半衰期为 7.9 ± 5.2 小时。在多份女性移植受者的报告和最近一份 RIF 患者的报告中,他克莫司对母亲和胎儿/婴儿的安全性得到了充分证明[111,112]。美国国家移植妊娠登记处的数据显示,活产婴儿先天畸形的发生率与普通人群相似,并且移植受者后代的 20 年长期随访观察为此提供了保证[113]。Nakagawa 等[111]的一份报道显示,妊娠前和妊娠期他克莫司治疗(1~4 mg/d)与产科和围产期并发症无关。

6.4 其他免疫抑制剂

环孢素是一种广泛应用于器官移植和自身免疫疾病的免疫抑制剂。一些研究表明,低剂量的环孢素可诱导母胎免疫耐受,同时增强滋养细胞侵袭[114]。据报道,环孢素治疗通过降低 Th1 细胞数量、T-bet mRNA 表达、IFN-γ 和 TNF-α 水平,并增加 Th2 细胞数量、GATA 结合蛋白 mRNA 表达和 IL-10 水平,使 RPL 患者的 Th1/Th2 比值显著降低($P<0.0001$)[85]。尽管研究规模较小($n=38$),但接受环孢素治疗的 RPL 患者的活产率明显高于对照组[85,114]。

西罗莫司(rapamune)是一种 mTOR 抑制剂,通过抑制 IL-2 激活的 T 细胞增殖,有效防止同种异体移植排斥[115]。此外,西罗莫司促进 $CD4^+$ $CD25^+$ $FoxP3^+$ Treg 细胞的产生,同时抑制人和动物模型外周组织中 Th17 细胞的分化。与对照组(21.2%)相比,接受西罗莫司治疗的 RIF 患者的活产率(48.8%)显著增加($P<0.0001$)[115]。关于西罗莫司对妊娠和儿童相关影响的数据有限。西罗莫司归类为妊娠 C 类药物,产前暴露的婴儿未发现明显异常[116,117]。

6.5 TNF-α 抑制剂

TNF-α 抑制剂,如英夫利昔单抗(remicade)、阿达木单抗(humira)和依那西普(enbrel),用于减轻类风湿关节炎、炎症性肠病(克罗恩病)和强直性脊柱炎的炎性反应。已知 Th1 细胞因子,包括 IFN-γ、TNF-α 和 IL-2,会增加妊娠丢失。特别是在 Th1/Th2 升高的女性中,TNF-α 抑制剂与 IVIg 联合使用显示出活产率的显著提高。对于 RPL 患者,TNF-α 抑制剂、IVIg 和肝素的三重组合疗法与单独使用肝素或 IVIg 联合肝素相比,活产率得到改善(单用肝素 19%;肝素+IVIg 54%;肝素+IVIg+阿达木单抗 71%,$P=0.0026$)[86]。

TNF-α 抑制剂是一种相对安全的药物,但仍可能会导致一些严重的不良事件,如结核分枝杆菌再激活、机会性感染、淋巴瘤、神经后遗症如脱髓鞘疾病[118]。此外,TNF-α 抑制剂可用于植入期和妊娠期,也适用于母乳喂养。然而,医生应意识到这些药物在妊娠期间的潜在胚胎-胎儿毒性风险,尽管发生率很低[119]。

6.6 维生素 D

在 RPL 和维生素 D 缺乏的女性中,自身和细胞免疫异常的风险增加。在 T 细胞培养时添加维生素 D,TNF-α/IL-10 和 INF-γ/IL-10 表达的 $CD3^+$/$CD4^+$ 细胞比例显著降低。在 NK 细胞培养时添加维生素 D 可抑制 Ⅰ 型细胞因子(如 IFN-γ 和 TNF-α)的分泌,并增加 Ⅱ 型细胞因子(如 IL-10)[120]。维生素 D 通过 Th2 和 NK2 转换促进形成更优的妊娠环境。此外,维生素 D_3 还能使 RPL 患者外周血中的 Th17 细胞数和 Th17/Treg 比值降低[121]。

7 总结和建议

- 母体的免疫系统能差异性适应妊娠的各个阶段,包括胚胎种植、胎儿发育、分娩和产后。
- 循环血和母胎界面中 Th 细胞失调引起的过度促炎环境对妊娠有害。
- 妊娠期 Th1 免疫显著强于 Th2 免疫,形成不利于胚胎植入的环境,导致流产和 RIF。
- 现已研究了 Th 细胞的各亚群及其在生殖障碍中的作用。Th17 细胞/Treg 细胞失衡也会促进 RPL 的发生发展。
- 对于有两次或两次以上流产和其他危险因素(如亚临床自身免疫异常、活动性自身免疫性疾病、NK 细胞病理改变和特发性 RPL)的 RPL 患者,可考虑行 Th 细胞亚群分析。
- 免疫调节剂(如皮质类固醇、IVIg、他克莫司和 TNF 抑制剂)可调节 RPL 和 T 细胞免疫异常患者的免疫失衡,并改善妊娠结局。
- 对 RPL 和免疫异常(如 NK 细胞水平和细胞毒性增加、Th1/Th2 细胞比例增加、自身免疫异常和特发性 RPL)患者在孕前进行免疫调节治疗更为有效。

参考文献

[1] Mosmann TR, Cherwinski H, Bond MW, Giedlin MA, Coffman RL. Two types of murine helper T cell clone. I. Definition according to profiles of lymphokine activities and secreted proteins. Comparative study. J Immunol 1986;136(7):2348-57 Apr 1.

[2] Wegmann TG, Lin H, Guilbert L, Mosmann TR. Bidirectional cytokine interactions in the maternal-fetal relationship: is successful pregnancy a TH2 phenomenon? Immunol Today 1993;14(7):353-6. Available from: https://doi.org/10.1016/0167-5699(93)90235-D Jul.

[3] Saito S, Nakashima A, Shima T, Ito M. Th1/Th2/Th17 and regulatory T-cell paradigm in pregnancy. Am J Reprod

Immunol 2010;63(6):601-10. Available from: https://doi.org/10.1111/j.1600-0897.2010.00852.x Jun.

[4] EGGo RPL, Bender Atik R, Christiansen OB, et al. ESHRE guideline: recurrent pregnancy loss. Hum Reprod Open 2018;2018(2):hoy004. Available from: https://doi.org/10.1093/hropen/hoy004.

[5] Practice Committee of American Society for Reproductive M. Definitions of infertility and recurrent pregnancy loss: a committee opinion. Fertil Steril 2013;99(1):63. Available from: https://doi.org/10.1016/j.fertnstert.2012.09.023 Jan.

[6] Group EEPGD. Recurrent pregnancy loss. https://www.eshre.eu/Guidelines-and-Legal/Guidelines/Recurrent-pregnancy-loss/.

[7] van Dijk MM, Kolte AM, Limpens J, et al. Recurrent pregnancy loss: diagnostic workup after two or three pregnancy losses? A systematic review of the literature and meta-analysis. Hum Reprod Update 15 2020;26(3):356-67. Available from: https://doi.org/10.1093/humupd/dmz048 Apr.

[8] Larsen EC, Christiansen OB, Kolte AM, Macklon N. New insights into mechanisms behind miscarriage. BMC Med 2013;11:154. Available from: https://doi.org/10.1186/1741-7015-11-154 Jun 26.

[9] Rasmark Roepke E, Matthiesen L, Rylance R, Christiansen OB. Is the incidence of recurrent pregnancy loss increasing? A retrospective register-based study in Sweden. Acta Obstet Gynecol Scand 2017;96(11):1365-72. Available from: https://doi.org/10.1111/aogs.13210 Nov.

[10] Lee SK, Na BJ, Kim JY, et al. Determination of clinical cellular immune markers in women with recurrent pregnancy loss. Am J Reprod Immunol 2013;70(5):398-411. Available from: https://doi.org/10.1111/aji.12137 Nov.

[11] Lee S, Kim J, Jang B, et al. Fluctuation of peripheral blood T, B, and NK cells during a menstrual cycle of normal healthy women. J Immunol 2010;185(1):756-62. Available from: https://doi.org/10.4049/jimmunol.0904192 Jul 1.

[12] Flynn L, Byrne B, Carton J, Kelehan P, Orsquo;Herlihy C, Orsquo;Farrelly C. Menstrual cycle dependent fluctuations in NK and T-lymphocyte subsets from nonpregnant human endometrium. Am J Reprod Immunol 2000;43(4):209-17. Available from: https://doi.org/10.1111/j.8755-8920.2000.430405.x Apr.

[13] Arruvito L, Sanz M, Banham AH, Fainboim L. Expansion of CD4+ CD25+ and FOXP3+ regulatory T cells during the follicular phase of the menstrual cycle: implications for human reproduction. J Immunol 2007;178(4):2572-8 Feb 15.

[14] Berbic M, Hey-Cunningham AJ, Ng C, et al. The role of Foxp3+ regulatory T-cells in endometriosis: a potential controlling mechanism for a complex, chronic immunological condition. Hum Reprod 2010;25(4):900-7. Available from: https://doi.org/10.1093/humrep/deq020 doi:deq020 [pii].

[15] Nakashima A, Ito M, Yoneda S, Shiozaki A, Hidaka T, Saito S. Circulating and decidual Th17 cell levels in healthy pregnancy. Am J Reprod Immunol 2010;63(2):104-9. Available from: https://doi.org/10.1111/j.1600-0897.2009.00771.x doi:AJI771 [pii].

[16] Lee SK, Kim JY, Lee M, Gilman-Sachs A, Kwak-Kim J. Th17 and regulatory T cells in women with recurrent pregnancy loss. Am J Reprod Immunol 2012;67(4):311-18. Available from: https://doi.org/10.1111/j.1600-0897.2012.01116.x Apr.

[17] Feyaerts D, Benner M, van Cranenbroek B, van der Heijden OWH, Joosten I, van der Molen RG. Human uterine lymphocytes acquire a more experienced and tolerogenic phenotype during pregnancy. Sci Rep 2017;7(1):2884. Available from: https://doi.org/10.1038/s41598-017-03191-0 Jun 6.

[18] Lee SK, Kim CJ, Kim DJ, Kang JH. Immune cells in the female reproductive tract. Immune Netw 2015;15(1):16-26. Available from: https://doi.org/10.4110/in.2015.15.1.16 Feb.

[19] Williams PJ, Searle RF, Robson SC, Innes BA, Bulmer JN. Decidual leucocyte populations in early to late gestation normal human pregnancy. J Reprod Immunol 2009;82(1):24-31. Available from: https://doi.org/10.1016/j.jri.2009.08.001 Oct.

[20] Piccinni MP, Lombardelli L, Logiodice F, Kullolli O, Romagnani S, Le Bouteiller P. T helper cell mediated-tolerance towards fetal allograft in successful pregnancy. Clin Mol Allergy 2015;13(1):9. Available from: https://doi.org/10.1186/s12948-015-0015-y.

[21] Vento-Tormo R, Efremova M, Botting RA, et al. Single-cell reconstruction of the early maternal-fetal interface in humans. Nature 2018;563(7731):347-53. Available from: https://doi.org/10.1038/s41586-018-0698-6 Nov.

[22] Ng SC, Gilman-Sachs A, Thaker P, Beaman KD, Beer AE, Kwak-Kim J. Expression of intracellular Th1 and Th2 cytokines in women with recurrent spontaneous abortion, implantation failures after IVF/ET or normal pregnancy. Am J Reprod Immunol 2002;48(2):77-86. Available from: https://doi.org/10.1034/j.1600-0897.2002.01105.x Aug.

[23] Santner-Nanan B, Peek MJ, Khanam R, et al. Systemic increase in the ratio between Foxp3+ and IL-17-producing CD4+ T cells in healthy pregnancy but not in preeclampsia. J Immunol 2009;183(11):7023-30. Available from: https://doi.org/10.4049/jimmunol.0901154 doi:jimmunol.0901154 [pii].

[24] Somerset DA, Zheng Y, Kilby MD, Sansom DM, Drayson MT. Normal human pregnancy is associated with an elevation in the immune suppressive CD25+ CD4+ regulatory T-cell subset. Research support, Non-U.S. Govrsquo;t. Immunology 2004;112(1):38-43. Available from: https://doi.org/10.1111/j.1365-2567.2004.01869.x May.

[25] Mor G, Aldo P, Alvero AB. The unique immunological and microbial aspects of pregnancy. Nat Rev Immunol 2017;17(8):469-82. Available from: https://doi.org/10.1038/nri.2017.64 Aug.

[26] Plaks V, Birnberg T, Berkutzki T, et al. Uterine DCs are crucial for decidua formation during embryo implantation in mice. J Clin Invest 2008;118(12):3954-65. Available from: https://doi.org/10.1172/jci36682 Dec.

[27] Morelli AE, Thomson AW. Tolerogenic dendritic cells and the quest for transplant tolerance. Nat Rev Immunol 2007;7(8):610-21. Available from: https://doi.org/10.1038/nri2132 Aug.

[28] Vacca P, Cantoni C, Vitale M, et al. Crosstalk between decidual NK and CD14+ myelomonocytic cells results in induction of Tregs and immunosuppression. Proc Natl Acad Sci U S A 2010;107(26):11918-23. Available from: https://doi.org/10.1073/pnas.1001749107 Jun 29.

[29] Billington WD. The immunological problem of pregnancy: 50 years with the hope of progress. A tribute to Peter Medawar. J Reprod Immunol 2003;60(1):1-11. Available from:

https://doi.org/10.1016/s0165-0378(03)00083-4 Oct.

[30] Kieffer TEC, Laskewitz A, Scherjon SA, Faas MM, Prins JR. Memory T cells in pregnancy. Front Immunol 2019;10:625. Available from: https://doi.org/10.3389/fimmu.2019.00625.

[31] Robertson SA, Prins JR, Sharkey DJ, Moldenhauer LM. Seminal fluid and the generation of regulatory T cells for embryo implantation. Am J Reprod Immunol 2013;69(4):315-30. Available from: https://doi.org/10.1111/aji.12107 Apr.

[32] Tilburgs T, Scherjon SA, van der Mast BJ, et al. Fetal-maternal HLA-C mismatch is associated with decidual T cell activation and induction of functional T regulatory cells. J Reprod Immunol 2009;82(2):148-57. Available from: https://doi.org/10.1016/j.jri.2009.05.003 Nov.

[33] Wang W, Sung N, Gilman-Sachs A, Kwak-Kim JT. Helper (Th) cell profiles in pregnancy and recurrent pregnancy losses: Th1/Th2/Th9/Th17/Th22/Tfh cells. Front Immunol 2020;11:2025. Available from: https://doi.org/10.3389/fimmu.2020.02025.

[34] Todt JC, Yang Y, Lei J, et al. Effects of tumor necrosis factor-alpha on human trophoblast cell adhesion and motility. Am J Reprod Immunol 1996;36(2):65-71. Available from: https://doi.org/10.1111/j.1600-0897.1996.tb00141.x Aug.

[35] Lockwood CJ, Oner C, Uz YH, et al. Matrix metalloproteinase 9 (MMP9) expression in preeclamptic decidua and MMP9 induction by tumor necrosis factor alpha and interleukin 1 beta in human first trimester decidual cells. Biol Reprod 2008;78(6):1064-72. Available from: https://doi.org/10.1095/biolreprod.107.063743 Jun.

[36] Ashkar AA, Di Santo JP, Croy BA. Interferon gamma contributes to initiation of uterine vascular modification, decidual integrity, and uterine natural killer cell maturation during normal murine pregnancy. J Exp Med 2000;192(2):259-70. Available from: https://doi.org/10.1084/jem.192.2.259 Jul 17.

[37] Ebina Y, Shimada S, Deguchi M, Maesawa Y, Iijima N, Yamada H. Divergence of helper, cytotoxic, and regulatory T cells in the decidua from miscarriage. Am J Reprod Immunol 2016;76(3):199-204. Available from: https://doi.org/10.1111/aji.12546 Sep.

[38] Makhseed M, Raghupathy R, Azizieh F, Omu A, Al-Shamali E, Ashkanani L. Th1 and Th2 cytokine profiles in recurrent aborters with successful pregnancy and with subsequent abortions. Hum Reprod 2001;16(10):2219-26 Oct.

[39] Kwak-Kim JY, Chung-Bang HS, Ng SC, et al. Increased T helper 1 cytokine responses by circulating T cells are present in women with recurrent pregnancy losses and in infertile women with multiple implantation failures after IVF. Hum Reprod 2003;18(4):767-73 Apr.

[40] Lee SK, Kim JY, Hur SE, et al. An imbalance in interleukin-17-producing T and Foxp3+ regulatory T cells in women with idiopathic recurrent pregnancy loss. Hum Reprod 2011;26(11):2964-71. Available from: https://doi.org/10.1093/humrep/der301 Nov.

[41] Lin H, Mosmann TR, Guilbert L, Tuntipopipat S, Wegmann TG. Synthesis of T helper 2-type cytokines at the maternal-fetal interface. J Immunol 1993;151(9):4562-73 Nov 1.

[42] Fallon PG, Jolin HE, Smith P, et al. IL-4 induces characteristic Th2 responses even in the combined absence of IL-5, IL-9, and IL-13. Immunity 2002;17(1):7-17. Available from: https://doi.org/10.1016/s1074-7613(02) 00332-1 Jul.

[43] Renaud SJ, Cotechini T, Quirt JS, Macdonald-Goodfellow SK, Othman M, Graham CH. Spontaneous pregnancy loss mediated by abnormal maternal inflammation in rats is linked to deficient uteroplacental perfusion. J Immunol 2011;186(3):1799-808. Available from: https://doi.org/10.4049/jimmunol.1002679 Feb 1.

[44] Piccinni MP, Beloni L, Livi C, Maggi E, Scarselli G, Romagnani S. Defective production of both leukemia inhibitory factor and type 2 T-helper cytokines by decidual T cells in unexplained recurrent abortions. Nat Med 1998;4(9):1020-4. Available from: https://doi.org/10.1038/2006 Sep.

[45] Chaouat G, Assal Meliani A, Martal J, et al. IL-10 prevents naturally occurring fetal loss in the CBA x DBA/2 mating combination, and local defect in IL-10 production in this abortion-prone combination is corrected by in vivo injection of IFN-tau. J Immunol 1995;154(9):4261-8 May 1.

[46] Raghupathy R, Makhseed M, Azizieh F, Omu A, Gupta M, Farhat R. Cytokine production by maternal lymphocytes during normal human pregnancy and in unexplained recurrent spontaneous abortion. Hum Reprod 2000;15(3):713-18 Mar.

[47] Jin LP, Fan DX, Zhang T, Guo PF, Li DJ. The co-stimulatory signal upregulation is associated with Th1 bias at the maternal-fetal interface in human miscarriage. Am J Reprod Immunol 2011;66(4):270-8. Available from: https://doi.org/10.1111/j.1600-0897.2011.00997.x Oct.

[48] Sasaki Y, Sakai M, Miyazaki S, Higuma S, Shiozaki A, Saito S. Decidual and peripheral blood CD4+CD25+ regulatory T cells in early pregnancy subjects and spontaneous abortion cases. Mol Hum Reprod 2004;10(5):347-53. Available from: https://doi.org/10.1093/molehr/gah044 May.

[49] Mei S, Tan J, Chen H, Chen Y, Zhang J. Changes of CD4+CD25high regulatory T cells and FOXP3 expression in unexplained recurrent spontaneous abortion patients. Fertil Steril 2010;94(6):2244-7. Available from: https://doi.org/10.1016/j.fertnstert.2009.11.020 doi:S0015-0282(09)04049-7 [pii].

[50] Wu HX, Jin LP, Xu B, Liang SS, Li DJ. Decidual stromal cells recruit Th17 cells into decidua to promote proliferation and invasion of human trophoblast cells by secreting IL-17. Cell Mol Immunol 2014;11(3):253-62. Available from: https://doi.org/10.1038/cmi.2013.67 May.

[51] Wang WJ, Hao CF, Yi L, et al. Increased prevalence of T helper 17 (Th17) cells in peripheral blood and decidua in unexplained recurrent spontaneous abortion patients. J Reprod Immunol 2010;84(2):164-70. Available from: https://doi.org/10.1016/j.jri.2009.12.003 doi:S0165-0378(10)00009-4 [pii].

[52] Kaplan MH. Th9 cells: differentiation and disease. Immunol Rev 2013;252(1):104-15. Available from: https://doi.org/10.1111/imr.12028 Mar.

[53] Licona-Limon P, Henao-Mejia J, Temann AU, et al. Th9 cells drive host immunity against gastrointestinal worm infection. Immunity 2013;39(4):744-57. Available from: https://doi.org/10.1016/j.immuni.2013.07.020 Oct 17.

[54] Gomez-Lopez N, Olson DM, Robertson SA. Interleukin-6 controls uterine Th9 cells and CD8(+) T regulatory cells to accelerate parturition in mice. Immunol Cell Biol 2016;94(1):79-89. Available from: https://doi.org/10.1038/icb.2015.63 Jan.

[55] Dudakov JA, Hanash AM, van den Brink MR. Interleukin-22: immunobiology and pathology. Annu Rev Immunol 2015; 33: 747 - 85. Available from: https://doi.org/10.1146/annurev-immunol-032414-112123.

[56] Wang Y, Xu B, Li MQ, Li DJ, Jin LP. IL - 22 secreted by decidual stromal cells and NK cells promotes the survival of human trophoblasts. Int J Clin Exp Pathol 2013;6(9):1781 - 90.

[57] Jogdand GM, Mohanty S, Devadas S. Regulators of Tfh cell differentiation. Front Immunol 2016;7:520. Available from: https://doi.org/10.3389/fimmu.2016.00520.

[58] Monteiro C, Kasahara TM, Castro JR, et al. Pregnancy favors the expansion of circulating functional follicular helper T cells. J Reprod Immunol 2017;121:1 - 10. Available from: https://doi.org/10.1016/j.jri.2017.04.007 Jun.

[59] Krop J, Heidt S, Claas FHJ, Eikmans M. Regulatory T cells in pregnancy: it is not all about FoxP3. Front Immunol 2020; 11:1182. Available from: https://doi.org/10.3389/fimmu.2020.01182.

[60] LeMaoult J, Caumartin J, Daouya M, et al. Immune regulation by pretenders: cell-to-cell transfers of HLA-G make effector T cells act as regulatory cells. Blood 2007;109 (5):2040 - 8. Available from: https://doi.org/10.1182/blood-2006-05-024547 Mar 1.

[61] Hsu P, Santner-Nanan B, Joung S, Peek MJ, Nanan R. Expansion of CD4(＋) HLA-G(＋) T cell in human pregnancy is impaired in preeclampsia. Am J Reprod Immunol 2014;71(3):217 - 28. Available from: https://doi.org/10.1111/aji.12195 Mar.

[62] Magnani CF, Alberigo G, Bacchetta R, et al. Killing of myeloid APCs via HLA class I, CD2 and CD226 defines a novel mechanism of suppression by human Tr1 cells. Eur J Immunol 2011;41(6):1652 - 62. Available from: https://doi.org/10.1002/eji.201041120 Jun.

[63] van der Zwan A, van Unen V, Beyrend G, et al. Visualizing dynamic changes at the maternal-fetal interface throughout human pregnancy by mass cytometry. Front Immunol 2020; 11: 571300. Available from: https://doi.org/10.3389/fimmu.2020.571300.

[64] Reinhardt RL, Khoruts A, Merica R, Zell T, Jenkins MK. Visualizing the generation of memory CD4 T cells in the whole body. Nature 2001; 410 (6824): 101 - 5. Available from: https://doi.org/10.1038/35065111 Mar 1.

[65] Kieffer TE, Faas MM, Scherjon SA, Prins JR. Pregnancy persistently affects memory T cell populations. J Reprod Immunol 2017;119:1 - 8. Available from: https://doi.org/10.1016/j.jri.2016.11.004 Feb.

[66] Wang S, Zhu X, Xu Y, et al. Programmed cell death-1 (PD - 1) and T-cell immunoglobulin mucin-3 (Tim-3) regulate CD4＋ T cells to induce Type 2 helper T cell (Th2) bias at the maternal-fetal interface. Hum Reprod 2016;31(4):700 - 11. Available from: https://doi.org/10.1093/humrep/dew019 Apr.

[67] Ramhorst R, Garcia V, Agriello E, et al. Intracellular expression of CD69 in endometrial and peripheral T cells represents a useful marker in women with recurrent miscarriage: modulation after allogeneic leukocyte immunotherapy. Am J Reprod Immunol 2003; 49 (3): 149 - 58. Available from: https://doi.org/10.1034/j.1600-0897.2003.00021.x Mar.

[68] Tian Y, Babor M, Lane J, et al. Unique phenotypes and clonal expansions of human CD4 effector memory T cells re-expressing CD45RA. Nat Commun 2017; 8 (1): 1473. Available from: https://doi.org/10.1038/s41467-017-01728-5 Nov 13.

[69] Luan X, Kang X, Li W, Dong Q. An investigation of the relationship between recurrent spontaneous abortion and memory T follicular helper cells. Am J Reprod Immunol 2017. Available from: https://doi.org/10.1111/aji.12714 Jun 21.

[70] Zhang YH, Sun HX. Immune checkpoint molecules in pregnancy: focus on regulatory T cells. Eur J Immunol 2020; 50(2):160 - 9. Available from: https://doi.org/10.1002/eji.201948382 Feb.

[71] Miko E, Meggyes M, Doba K, Barakonyi A, Szereday L. Immune checkpoint molecules in reproductive immunology. Front Immunol 2019; 10: 846. Available from: https://doi.org/10.3389/fimmu.2019.00846.

[72] Hu XH, Tang MX, Mor G, Liao AH. Tim-3: expression on immune cells and roles at the maternal-fetal interface. J Reprod Immunol 2016;118:92 - 9. Available from: https://doi.org/10.1016/j.jri.2016.10.113 Nov.

[73] Wang S, Chen C, Li M, et al. Blockade of CTLA - 4 and Tim - 3 pathways induces fetal loss with altered cytokine profiles by decidual CD4(＋)T cells. Cell Death Dis 2019;10(1):15. Available from: https://doi.org/10.1038/s41419-018-1251-0 Jan 8.

[74] Zhang T, Zhu W, Zhao Y, et al. Early transient suppression of immune checkpoint proteins T-cell immunoglobulin mucin-3 and programmed cell death-1 in peripheral blood lymphocytes after blastocyst transfer is associated with successful implantation. Fertil Steril 2020;114(2):426 - 35. Available from: https://doi.org/10.1016/j.fertnstert.2019.12.022 Aug.

[75] Wafula PO, Teles A, Schumacher A, et al. PD - 1 but not CTLA - 4 blockage abrogates the protective effect of regulatory T cells in a pregnancy murine model. Research support, non-U.S. Govrsquo;t. Am J Reprod Immunol 2009; 62(5):283 - 92. Available from: https://doi.org/10.1111/j.1600-0897.2009.00737.x Nov.

[76] Wang WJ, Salazar Garcia MD, Deutsch G, et al. PD - 1 and PD - L1 expression on T-cell subsets in women with unexplained recurrent pregnancy losses. Am J Reprod Immunol 2020;83(5):e13230. Available from: https://doi.org/10.1111/aji.13230 May.

[77] Li G, Lu C, Gao J, et al. Association between PD - 1/PD - L1 and T regulate cells in early recurrent miscarriage. Int J Clin Exp Pathol 2015;8(6):6512 - 18.

[78] Morita K, Tsuda S, Kobayashi E, et al. Analysis of TCR repertoire and PD - 1 expression in decidual and peripheral CD8(＋) T cells reveals distinct immune mechanisms in miscarriage and preeclampsia. Front Immunol 2020;11:1082. Available from: https://doi.org/10.3389/fimmu.2020.01082.

[79] Winger EE, Reed JL, Ashoush S, El-Toukhy T, Ahuja S, Taranissi M. Elevated preconception CD56＋ 16＋ and/or Th1:Th2 levels predict benefit from IVIG therapy in subfertile women undergoing IVF. Am J Reprod Immunol 2011;66(5):394 - 403. Available from: https://doi.org/10.1111/j.1600-0897.2011.01018.x Nov.

[80] Vomstein K, Feil K, Strobel L, et al. Immunological risk factors in recurrent pregnancy loss: guidelines vs current state of the art. J Clin Med 2021;10(4). Available from: https://doi.org/10.3390/jcm10040869 Feb 20.

[81] Gomaa MF, Elkholy AG, El-Said MM, Abdel-Salam NE. Combined oral prednisolone and heparin vs heparin: the

effect on peripheral NK cells and clinical outcome in patients with unexplained recurrent miscarriage. A double-blind placebo randomized controlled trial. Arch Gynecol Obstet 2014;290(4):757 – 62. Available from: https://doi.org/10.1007/s00404-014-3262-0 Oct.

[82] Ahmadi M, Abdolmohammadi-Vahid S, Ghaebi M, et al. Effect of Intravenous immunoglobulin on Th1 and Th2 lymphocytes and improvement of pregnancy outcome in recurrent pregnancy loss (RPL). Biomed Pharmacother 2017; 92:1095 – 102. Available from: https://doi.org/10.1016/j.biopha.2017.06.001 Aug.

[83] Ahmadi M, Abdolmohammadi-Vahid S, Ghaebi M, et al. Regulatory T cells improve pregnancy rate in RIF patients after additional IVIG treatment. Syst Biol Reprod Med 2017; 63(6):350 – 9. Available from: https://doi.org/10.1080/19396368.2017.1390007 Dec.

[84] Nakagawa K, Kwak-Kim J, Ota K, et al. Immunosuppression with tacrolimus improved reproductive outcome of women with repeated implantation failure and elevated peripheral blood TH1/TH2 cell ratios. Am J Reprod Immunol 2015;73 (4):353 – 61. Available from: https://doi.org/10.1111/aji.12338 Apr.

[85] Azizi R, Ahmadi M, Danaii S, et al. Cyclosporine A improves pregnancy outcomes in women with recurrent pregnancy loss and elevated Th1/Th2 ratio. J Cell Physiol 2019;234(10):19039 – 47. Available from: https://doi.org/10.1002/jcp.28543 Aug.

[86] Winger EE, Reed JL. Treatment with tumor necrosis factor inhibitors and intravenous immunoglobulin improves live birth rates in women with recurrent spontaneous abortion. Am J Reprod Immunol 2008;60(1):8 – 16 Jul.

[87] Michael AE, Papageorghiou AT. Potential significance of physiological and pharmacological glucocorticoids in early pregnancy. Hum Reprod Update 2008;14(5):497 – 517. Available from: https://doi.org/10.1093/humupd/dmn021 Sep-Oct.

[88] Kemp MW, Newnham JP, Challis JG, Jobe AH, Stock SJ. The clinical use of corticosteroids in pregnancy. Hum Reprod Update 2016;22(2):240 – 59. Available from: https://doi.org/10.1093/humupd/dmv047 Mar-Apr.

[89] Snijdewint FG, Kapsenberg ML, Wauben-Penris PJ, Bos JD. Corticosteroids class-dependently inhibit in vitro Th1- and Th2-type cytokine production. Immunopharmacology 1995;29 (2):93 – 101. Available from: https://doi.org/10.1016/0162-3109(94)00048-k Mar.

[90] Milburn HJ, Poulter LW, Dilmec A, Cochrane GM, Kemeny DM. Corticosteroids restore the balance between locally produced Th1 and Th2 cytokines and immunoglobulin isotypes to normal in sarcoid lung. Clin Exp Immunol 1997;108(1): 105 – 13. Available from: https://doi.org/10.1046/j.1365-2249.1997.d01-979.x Apr.

[91] Sasaki A, Kuroda K, Hisano M, Ozawa N, Sago H, Yamaguchi K. Successful treatment for a recurrent pregnancy loss woman with high Th1/Th2 ratio using medium-dose corticosteroids. J Obstet Gynaecol 2017;37(5):685 – 7. Available from: https://doi.org/10.1080/01443615.2017.1285873 Jul.

[92] Harmon HM, Jensen EA, Tan S, et al. Timing of postnatal steroids for bronchopulmonary dysplasia: association with pulmonary and neurodevelopmental outcomes. J Perinatol 2020;40(4):616 – 27. Available from: https://doi.org/10.1038/s41372-020-0594-4 Apr.

[93] Palmsten K, Bandoli G, Vazquez-Benitez G, et al. Oral corticosteroid use during pregnancy and risk of preterm birth. Rheumatol (Oxf) 2020;59(6):1262 – 71. Available from: https://doi.org/10.1093/rheumatology/kez405 Jun 1.

[94] Palmsten K, Bandoli G, Watkins J, Vazquez-Benitez G, Gilmer TP, Chambers CD. Oral corticosteroids and risk of preterm Birth in the California medicaid program. J Allergy Clin Immunol Pract 2021;9(1):375 – 84. Available from: https://doi.org/10.1016/j.jaip.2020.07.047 e5.

[95] Toth B, Wurfel W, Bohlmann M, et al. Recurrent miscarriage: diagnostic and therapeutic procedures. guideline of the DGGG, OEGGG and SGGG (S2k-Level, AWMF registry number 015/050). Geburtshilfe Frauenheilkd 2018; 78(4):364 – 81. Available from: https://doi.org/10.1055/a-0586-4568 Apr.

[96] Schwab I, Nimmerjahn F. Intravenous immunoglobulin therapy: how does IgG modulate the immune system? Nat Rev Immunol 2013;13(3):176 – 89. Available from: https://doi.org/10.1038/nri3401 Mar.

[97] Wong LF, Porter TF, Scott JR. Immunotherapy for recurrent miscarriage. Cochrane Database Syst Rev 2014; 10:CD000112. Available from: https://doi.org/10.1002/14651858.CD000112.pub3 Oct 21.

[98] Egerup P, Lindschou J, Gluud C, Christiansen OB. ImmuRe MIPDSG. the effects of intravenous immunoglobulins in women with recurrent miscarriages: a systematic review of randomised trials with meta-analyses and trial sequential analyses including individual patient data. PLoS One 2015;10 (10):e0141588. Available from: https://doi.org/10.1371/journal.pone.0141588.

[99] Christiansen OB, Larsen EC, Egerup P, Lunoee L, Egestad L, Nielsen HS. Intravenous immunoglobulin treatment for secondary recurrent miscarriage: a randomised, double-blind, placebo-controlled trial. BJOG. 2015;122(4):500 – 8. Available from: https://doi.org/10.1111/1471-0528.13192 Mar.

[100] Christiansen OB, Kolte AM, Krog MC, Nielsen HS, Egerup P. Treatment with intravenous immunoglobulin in patients with recurrent pregnancy loss: An update. J Reprod Immunol 2019;133:37 – 42. Available from: https://doi.org/10.1016/j.jri.2019.06.001 Jun.

[101] Saab W, Seshadri S, Huang C, Alsubki L, Sung N, Kwak-Kim J. A systemic review of intravenous immunoglobulin G treatment in women with recurrent implantation failures and recurrent pregnancy losses. Am J Reprod Immunol 2021;85 (4):e13395. Available from: https://doi.org/10.1111/aji.13395 Apr.

[102] Woon EV, Day A, Bracewell-Milnes T, Male V, Johnson M. Immunotherapy to improve pregnancy outcome in women with abnormal natural killer cell levels/activity and recurrent miscarriage or implantation failure: a systematic review and meta-analysis. J Reprod Immunol 2020;142: 103189. Available from: https://doi.org/10.1016/j.jri.2020.103189 Nov.

[103] Yamada H, Morikawa M, Furuta I, et al. Intravenous immunoglobulin treatment in women with recurrent abortions: increased cytokine levels and reduced Th1/Th2 lymphocyte ratio in peripheral blood. Am J Reprod Immunol 2003;49(2):84 – 9 Feb.

[104] Lee SK, Kim JY, Han AR, et al. Intravenous immunoglobulin G improves pregnancy outcome in women

[105] Kim DJ, Lee SK, Kim JY, et al. Intravenous immunoglobulin G modulates peripheral blood Th17 and Foxp3(+) regulatory T cells in pregnant women with recurrent pregnancy loss. Am J Reprod Immunol 2014; 71(5): 441 – 50. Available from: https://doi.org/10.1111/aji.12208 May.

[106] Rachid R, Bonilla FA. The role of anti-IgA antibodies in causing adverse reactions to gamma globulin infusion in immunodeficient patients: a comprehensive review of the literature. J Allergy Clin Immunol 2012; 129(3): 628 – 34. Available from: https://doi.org/10.1016/j.jaci.2011.06.047 Mar.

[107] Zhang R, Szerlip HM. Reemergence of sucrose nephropathy: acute renal failure caused by high-dose intravenous immune globulin therapy. South Med J 2000; 93(9): 901 – 4 Sep.

[108] Han AR, Lee SK. Immune modulation of i.v. immunoglobulin in women with reproductive failure. Reprod Med Biol 2018; 17(2): 115 – 24. Available from: https://doi.org/10.1002/rmb2.12078 Apr.

[109] Triggianese P, Lattavo G, Chimenti MS, et al. Reproductive outcomes 20 years after the intravenous immunoglobulin treatment in women with recurrent pregnancy losses. Am J Reprod Immunol 2020; 83(4): e13224. Available from: https://doi.org/10.1111/aji.13224 Apr.

[110] Kino T, Hatanaka H, Miyata S, et al. FK – 506, a novel immunosuppressant isolated from a Streptomyces. II. Immunosuppressive effect of FK – 506 in vitro. J Antibiot (Tokyo) 1987; 40(9): 1256 – 65. Available from: https://doi.org/10.7164/antibiotics.40.1256 Sep.

[111] Nakagawa K, Kwak-Kim J, Hisano M, et al. Obstetric and perinatal outcome of the women with repeated implantation failures or recurrent pregnancy losses who received pre- and post-conception tacrolimus treatment. Am J Reprod Immunol 2019; 82(2): e13142. Available from: https://doi.org/10.1111/aji.13142 Aug.

[112] Nakagawa K, Kwak-Kim J, Kuroda K, Sugiyama R, Yamaguchi K. Immunosuppressive treatment using tacrolimus promotes pregnancy outcome in infertile women with repeated implantation failures. Am J Reprod Immunol 2017; 78(3). Available from: https://doi.org/10.1111/aji.12682 Sep.

[113] Coscia LA, Constantinescu S, Moritz MJ, et al. Report from the national transplantation pregnancy registry (NTPR): outcomes of pregnancy after transplantation. Clin Transpl 2010; 65 – 85.

[114] Ling Y, Huang Y, Chen C, Mao J, Zhang H. Low dose Cyclosporin A treatment increases live birth rate of unexplained recurrent abortion — initial cohort study. Clin Exp Obstet Gynecol 2017; 44(2): 230 – 5.

[115] Ahmadi M, Abdolmohamadi-Vahid S, Ghaebi M, et al. Sirolimus as a new drug to treat RIF patients with elevated Th17/Treg ratio: a double-blind, phase II randomized clinical trial. Int Immunopharmacol 2019; 74: 105730. Available from: https://doi.org/10.1016/j.intimp.2019.105730 Sep.

[116] Perez-Garcia LF, Dolhain R, Vorstenbosch S, et al. The effect of paternal exposure to immunosuppressive drugs on sexual function, reproductive hormones, fertility, pregnancy and offspring outcomes: a systematic review. Hum Reprod Update 2020; 26(6): 961 – 1001. Available from: https://doi.org/10.1093/humupd/dmaa022 Nov 1.

[117] Shen L, Xu W, Gao J, et al. Pregnancy after the diagnosis of lymphangioleiomyomatosis (LAM). Orphanet J Rare Dis 2021; 16(1): 133. Available from: https://doi.org/10.1186/s13023-021-01776-7 Mar 17.

[118] Steeland S, Libert C, Vandenbroucke RE. A new venue of TNF targeting. Int J Mol Sci 2018; 19(5). Available from: https://doi.org/10.3390/ijms19051442 May 11.

[119] Alijotas-Reig J, Esteve-Valverde E, Ferrer-Oliveras R, Llurba E, Gris JM. Tumor necrosis factor-alpha and pregnancy: focus on biologics. an updated and comprehensive review. Clin Rev Allergy Immunol 2017; 53(1): 40 – 53. Available from: https://doi.org/10.1007/s12016-016-8596-x Aug.

[120] Ota K, Dambaeva S, Han AR, Beaman K, Gilman-Sachs A, Kwak-Kim J. Vitamin D deficiency may be a risk factor for recurrent pregnancy losses by increasing cellular immunity and autoimmunity. Hum Reprod 2014; 29(2): 208 – 19. Available from: https://doi.org/10.1093/humrep/det424 Feb.

[121] Rafiee M, Gharagozloo M, Ghahiri A, et al. Altered Th17/Treg ratio in recurrent miscarriage after treatment with paternal lymphocytes and vitamin D3: a double-blind placebo-controlled study. Iran J Immunol. 2015; 12(4): 252 – 262. doi:IJIv12i4A3.

第 4 章

B 细胞病理学与反复妊娠丢失
B cell pathology and recurrent pregnancy loss

Ruth Marian Guzman-Genino[1] and Kerrilyn R. Diener[1,2]

[1] Clinical and Health Sciences Unit, University of South Australia, Adelaide, SA, Australia
[2] Robinson Research Institute and Adelaide Medical School, The University of Adelaide, Adelaide, SA, Australia

1 引言

一次成功的妊娠需要母体免疫系统执行不同的功能：必须对半异体胚胎具有免疫耐受性，同时保持对外来病原体的有效免疫。免疫功能异常可能导致妊娠障碍，如反复妊娠丢失（RPL）、子痫前期和免疫性不孕。因此，确定和了解各类免疫细胞、子宫内膜细胞和胎儿细胞的功能及其复杂的相互作用关系，对于开发有效治疗病理妊娠的方法至关重要。

B 细胞因其具有产生病原体特异性抗体的能力，在经典体液免疫中起着核心作用。抗体的产生在妊娠期间非常重要，这是由于针对父系抗原的保护性抗体的产生使母体免疫系统能够对生长中的胎儿保持耐受性。研究证实，B 细胞在妊娠期发挥关键的调节作用，并在增殖、亚型转换、抗体产生、细胞因子分泌和免疫细胞调节等多方面发生变化[1,2]。

越来越多的研究发现，异常的 B 细胞亚群与不孕症和不良产科结局相关。在小鼠中，成熟 B 细胞的缺乏与产仔数减少、胚胎尺寸减小和产前感染的易感性增加有关[3]。患有 RPL 和子痫前期女性的免疫图谱显示，记忆 B 细胞的诱导和功能发生了改变[4,5]。因此，B 细胞亚群的发育和功能变化被认为是妊娠期间发生免疫改变的主要因素[2]。

免疫系统内的失衡常被认为是导致不良生殖结局的原因，尤其是在特发性的病例中。免疫失调的指标包括：淋巴细胞数量、表型和功能异常（如细胞因子失调）、抗磷脂（aPL）抗体或其他自身抗体的存在，以及不平衡的辅助性 T 细胞（Th）1 和 Th2 比例[6]。免疫适应不足会导致植入失败，而次优免疫适应则会增加病理妊娠的风险，包括早期 RPL、宫内生长受限（intrauterine growth restriction，IUGR）、子痫前期和早产。

目前，针对由免疫适应不足或次优免疫适应导致的妊娠丢失的治疗选择，是通过静脉免疫球蛋白（IVIg）疗法和淋巴细胞免疫疗法（LIT）等一般免疫治疗方式来调节女性的免疫系统。然而，近期的综述和荟萃分析发现，免疫治疗并不能改善所有特发性 RPL 患者的妊娠结局，这表明，只有明确免疫异常与治疗之间的关联，才能有效开展治疗[6,7]。

与 RPL 相关的 B 细胞病理学是生殖免疫学中一个相对较少被研究的领域。信息的缺乏意味着很少有针对 B 细胞作为 RPL 病因的特异性疗法。本章介绍了 B 细胞在 RPL 和其他免疫相关妊娠并发症中的作用，并讨论了针对 B 细胞的潜在治疗方法。

2 妊娠期 B 细胞的功能

2.1 体液免疫

B 细胞的功能主要与体液免疫有关，B 细胞被认为在妊娠期通过产生抗体发挥作用。早期研究表明，母体血清中的免疫球蛋白（Ig）G 在人滋养层抗原体外模型中阻止了母体效应 T 细胞对异体滋养层组织的细胞毒性作用[8]。妊娠小鼠子宫引流淋巴结中 IgG 和 IgM 分泌细胞数量的增加进一步支持了抗体在维持同种异体胚胎中发挥抑制作用的观点[9]。近期的小鼠和临床研究强化了这一概念。妊娠小鼠血清样本中的 IgM 和 IgA 水平显著高于非妊娠对照组；与年龄匹配的非妊娠女性相比，健康孕妇血清中天然 IgM、IgA、IgG3 和 IgG4 的产生增加[10-12]。在一项关于妊娠期记忆 B 细胞亚群的研究中，记忆 B 细胞标志物 CD27 的表达水平直接影响了 Ig 同种型的产生：CD27 表达上调与 IgG 和 IgA 产生增加相关[13]。这些结果表明，B 细胞活化和抗体产生是实现健康妊娠的必要步骤。

2.2 不对称抗体和自身抗体

不对称抗体是 IgG 抗体的一个亚群，仅在分子的一个 Fab 区携带碳水化合物残基，使其功能单一，无法触发免疫效应器功能，如补体固定、吞噬和细胞毒性[14]。研究表明，健康孕妇血清中的不对称抗体（大多数具有父系抗原特异性）水平高于非妊娠女性，而经历反复自然流产的女性血清不对称抗体比例明显降低[15-17]。因此，不对称抗体被认为在妊娠期间具有保护性，称为"保护性母体抗体"，尽管支持这种现象的机制尚不清楚。

自身抗体与不良妊娠结局相关。多种 aPL（如狼疮抗凝血因子、抗心磷脂和抗 β-2 糖蛋白 I）与 RPL 和不孕症有关，而甲状腺抗原（如甲状腺球蛋白和甲状腺过氧化物酶）、核抗原、抗层粘连蛋白、抗凝血酶原和抗酿酒酵母抗体也与妊娠并发症有关[18]。近期的研究集中于 aPL 和激动性自身抗体对血管紧张素 Ⅱ Ⅰ 型受体（AT1-AA）的影响[19-21]。高水平血清 aPL 可发生在自身免疫性疾病——抗磷脂综合征（antiphospholipid syndrome，APS）中。在妊娠期，APS 会导致不良生殖结局，如胎儿丢失和严重子痫前期[19,22,23]。AT1-AA 自身抗体在子痫前期的发病和病理过程中起着重要作用。这些激动性自身抗体模拟 AT1-AA 的天然配体，诱导下游产生抗血管生成因子，如可溶性 fms 样酪氨酸激酶 1（s-Flt1）和内皮素，导致子痫前期症状的发作，并引起胎盘异常和胚胎缺陷[24,25]。

2.3 B 淋巴细胞减少症

妊娠期间，B 细胞亚群的数量、分布和功能可能会发生波动。最早的研究描述了妊娠期间 B 细胞数量的普遍减少以及 B 细胞对内分泌激素（如雌激素和人绒毛膜生长素）的条件性反应[26,27]。异基因妊娠小鼠模型显示，在妊娠后半期，前 B 细胞、祖 B 细胞、骨髓未成熟 B 细胞和脾脏滤泡 B 细胞的数量显著减少[10,11,28]。临床研究也证实了 B 细胞在妊娠时存在普遍减少，低风险孕妇的外周血 CD19$^+$ B 细胞在妊娠中、晚期及分娩当天明显低于非妊娠女性[29-32]。其他研究确定了发生淋巴细胞减少症的特定 B 细胞亚群，包括 IgD$^+$CD38^{hi} 过渡 B 细胞、CD24^{hi}CD38^{hi} 过渡 B 细胞、IgD$^+$CD38$^-$ 非转换记忆 B 细胞、IgD$^-$CD38$^-$ 静息记忆 B 细胞、IgD$^-$CD38^{hi} 浆细胞和 CD5$^+$ B 细胞[12,31,33,34]。除了较低水平外，还有证据表明人类妊娠期间 B 细胞功能亦受到抑制[35]。相比之下，多项实验小鼠研究发现，一些 B 细胞亚群在妊娠期间扩增，这些细胞包括脾脏边缘区 B 细胞、腹膜 B1 和 B2 细胞、子宫引流淋巴结和子宫内的 B 细胞以及蜕膜中的 B 细胞[11,28,36,37]。此外，在妊娠晚期，循环 IgD$^+$CD38$^+$ 幼稚 B 细胞的百分比增加[31]。

循环 B 细胞的减少可能是由于生长胎盘中 B 淋巴细胞生成减少或 B 细胞重新分布所致[10,27,36]。对妊娠早期胎盘免疫浸润的组织学检测表明，正常妊娠蜕膜中存在 B 细胞，并且在发生葡萄胎的蜕膜组织中显著增加[38]。胎盘绒毛间血液富含趋化因子配体 CCL20，吸引表达趋化因子受体 CCR6 的成熟/幼稚 B 细胞[39]。研究发现，胎盘组织中的 B 细胞可能通过产生孕酮诱导阻断因子 1（PIBF1）以保护足月妊娠[29,39,40]。

B 细胞分布的变化与 RPL 和不孕症有关。与对照组相比，RPL 患者的子宫内膜 CD20$^+$ B 细胞数量显著增加[41,42]。同样，有 RPL 和产科并发症病史的患者外周血 CD19$^+$ B 细胞增多，CD27$^+$IgD$^-$ 和 CD27$^+$IgD$^+$ 记忆 B 细胞减少[43]。然而，另一项研究发现，RPL 患者外周血 CD19$^+$IL-10$^+$ B 细胞减少，白细胞介素（IL）-10 和程序性死亡配体 1（PD-L1）基因的 mRNA 表达水平降低[44,45]。B 细胞与妊娠病理之间的关系仍有待进一步研究。

2.4 调节性 B 细胞

表现为免疫抑制功能的 B 细胞亚群称为调节性 B 细胞（Breg）[1]。在小鼠妊娠中，Breg 包括 IL-10$^+$ B 细胞、CD5$^+$CD1d$^+$ B 细胞、CD80$^+$CD86$^+$ B 细胞、CD80$^+$CD86$^+$CD27$^+$IL-10$^+$ B 细胞、IL-35$^+$ B 细胞以及孕酮免疫调节结合因子 1 阳性（PIBF1$^+$）绒毛膜蜕膜 B 细胞。在人类妊娠中，鉴定出的 Breg 包括 IL-10$^+$ B 细胞、CD24^{hi}CD27$^+$ B 细胞、CD24^{hi}CD38^{hi} 过渡 B 细胞、CD 27$^+$IgM$^+$ 记忆

B细胞、CD38^{hi}CD27^{hi}浆细胞、边缘区B细胞和IL-35$^+$B细胞。B细胞产生IL-10和转化生长因子-β(TGF-β)的能力仍是不同物种间Bregs的统一特征。其他标志物,如IL-35和PIBF1,亦在妊娠期促进B细胞的调节能力[40,46-49]。

妊娠会引起正常小鼠脾脏边缘区B细胞群的扩张,而具有妊娠并发症的小鼠不会出现这种现象。在成功的妊娠中,边缘区B细胞产生较高水平的IgM和IgA,这有助于或提示细胞免疫应答从Th1向Th2转化。在小鼠胚胎植入期,子宫组织中产生IL-10的B细胞表现出调节特性,共刺激分子CD80和CD86表达水平显著上调[28]。同样,脾脏B细胞在此期间也上调了共刺激分子的表达[50-52],这可能允许局部和全身B细胞控制调节性T细胞群和细胞因子的产生,为成功的胚胎植入做准备。

研究发现,在妊娠小鼠的子宫引流淋巴结、脾脏以及妊娠女性外周血中的Bregs具有产生和响应IL-35的能力,并有助于建立母体免疫耐受性和维持健康妊娠[47,49]。在小鼠模型中,由于妊娠晚期IL-33介导的B细胞产生PIBF1可预防早产,并且通过治疗性应用IL-33可增强该疗效[40]。绒毛膜蜕膜B细胞亦被归为Bregs。此外,绒毛膜蜕膜B细胞表达的活化记忆B细胞和浆细胞相关分子(如CD11c、CD27、CD38、CD70、CD80、CD86、CD95、CD138和B细胞成熟抗原)水平升高,表明其存在更高的激活状态、类别转换,以及记忆和浆细胞样分化[40]。

Bregs也被证明在小鼠胚胎植入期间发挥功能。脾脏B细胞中Toll样受体9和CD86(Breg相关标志物)在受精后3.5天上调,而在受精后2.5～8.5天,子宫B细胞扩增,B细胞表型改变[28,50]。子宫B细胞能有效抑制同源CD4$^+$效应T细胞的增殖和活化[28],并且妊娠早期的滋养细胞驯化可能促成了B细胞表型的改变[46]。与健康对照组相比,在反复种植失败的患者中发现外周血B细胞IL-10 mRNA水平较低,体外再刺激时IL-10分泌水平显著降低[45],提示B细胞的IL-10生成受损可能是反复种植失败的关键机制。这些研究表明,Bregs在妊娠早期支持胚胎植入。

3 与生殖相关的免疫病理学

3.1 妊娠期B细胞免疫失调

妊娠早期,功能正常的母体免疫细胞间的相互协调作用对于成功、健康、足月妊娠所需的生理变化至关重要。免疫失调,包括病理B细胞,被认为是不明原因RPL的潜在病因。母体免疫耐受的特征是诱导调节性T细胞和抗炎性Th2。如果没有这些条件,异常的母体同种异体免疫反应可能会导致妊娠丢失。

B细胞亚群的免疫改变可能与不明原因RPL的发病机制有关。例如,与健康女性相比,RPL患者B-1 CD19$^+$ CD5$^+$淋巴细胞的百分比明显提高[53]。此外,B细胞上的CD83表达受局部调节,并在小鼠妊娠障碍中差异表达[54]。因此,B细胞数量和功能的失调可能与APS、种植失败、IUGR、子痫前期和早产的发生有关(图4.1)。

3.2 抗磷脂综合征

APS是一种体液性自身免疫性疾病,其特征是存在针对膜磷脂的aPL。APS的临床特征与高凝状态有关,可能通过血栓形成和内皮功能受损引起产科并发症[21,55]。

由于APS是一种自身抗体介导的疾病,B细胞被认为在其发病机制中起着关键的作用;然而,很少有研究涉及B细胞失调与aPL产生克隆的特性。在B细胞分化和B细胞耐受检查点期间,B细胞稳态的受损可能会改变B细胞池和产生自身抗体的细胞。在产科APS患者中,B细胞激活和分化异常与浆细胞分化偏差有关,导致记忆B细胞减少[4,56]。血栓并发症患者中,记忆B细胞的减少及随后循环幼稚细胞的增加与血清C4浓度降低以及IgG抗心磷脂和抗β-2糖蛋白Ⅰ抗体的增加有关[4]。一项对11名血栓性原发APS患者淋巴细胞亚群分析的研究支持了这一发现:B1细胞、过渡B细胞(CD24$^+$ CD38$^+$)和幼稚B细胞(CD27$^-$ IgD$^+$)比例增加,记忆B细胞(CD27$^+$ IgD$^+$和CD27$^+$ IgD$^-$)减少[57]。然而,近期的一篇论文报道了相互矛盾的发现:与健康对照组相比,血栓性和产科APS患者幼稚B细胞的比例较低[56]。

迄今,关于幼稚B细胞在APS发病机制中的作用仍有争议。近期的研究表明,APS患者在B细胞稳态方面存在异常,表现为总的记忆B细胞、转换前记忆B细胞和转换后记忆B细胞以及分泌IL-10的Bregs减少[58]。此外,CD20$^-$ B细胞是aPL的主要来源,而CD20$^+$ B细胞则部分有助于抗心磷脂抗体的产生[58]。另一种尚未被充分研究的可能导致B

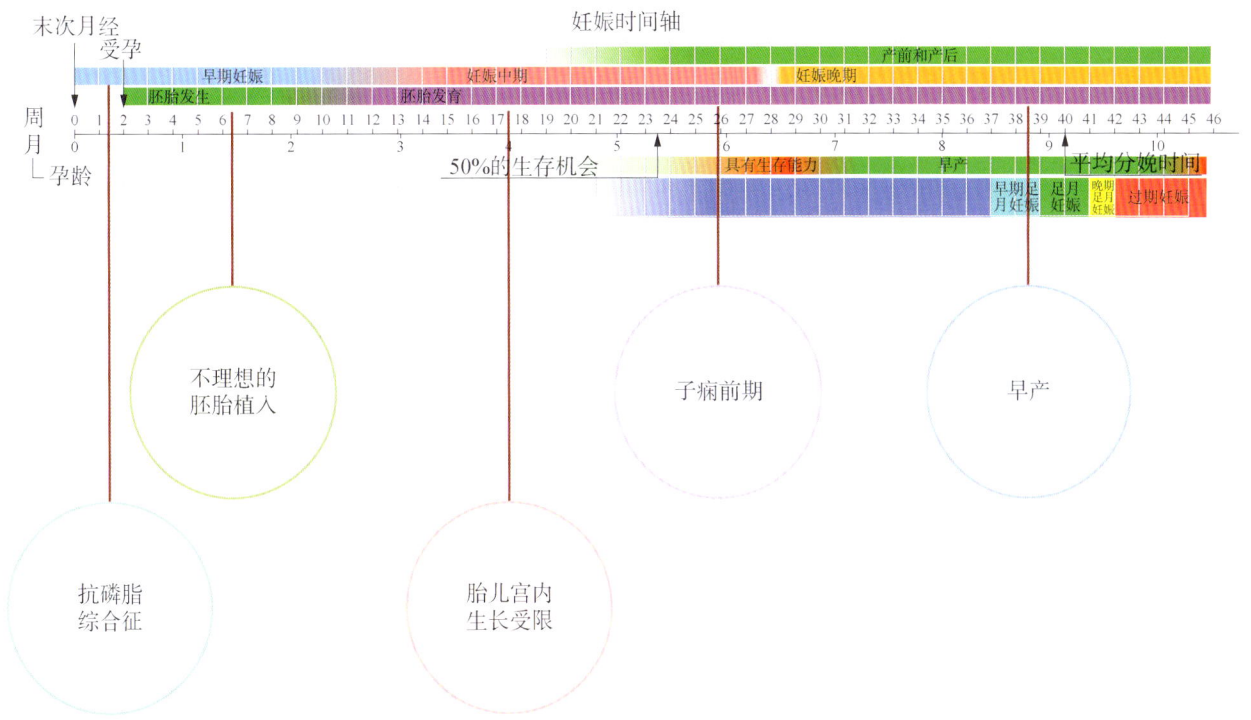

图 4.1 B 细胞失调对妊娠的潜在影响。
来源：由 BioRender.com 创建，改编自 Mikael Häggström 2014 年的医学图谱。

细胞存活和分化失调的可溶性介质是肿瘤坏死因子（TNF）家族（BAFF）的 B 细胞激活因子。在 APS 中，原发性或继发性产科 APS 患者的可溶性 BAFF 水平升高，并与较高的血栓事件风险相关[59]。BAFF 有望在未来作为产科 APS 患者的生物标志物或治疗靶点。

3.3 胚胎种植失败

胚胎种植失败会导致妊娠丢失。潜在的原因可能与配子/胚胎的问题或子宫内膜环境不佳有关。在后一种情况下，假设囊胚完好无损且完全具有植入能力，母胎界面免疫成分的募集、诱导或激活受损就可能导致种植失败[60]。胚胎植入时的免疫网络是复杂的，对其仍知之甚少；然而，B 细胞可能在妊娠早期发挥作用。在小鼠模型中，子宫 B 细胞的比例在胚胎种植期增加，B 细胞在体外表现出比 T 细胞更高的分泌 IL-10 和调节能力[28]。同样，腹腔内分泌 IL-10 的 Bregs 比例在妊娠早期逐渐增加，在妊娠中期下降[61]。

尽管很少有研究检测妊娠早期 B 细胞的功能，但 B 细胞仍被发现有助于胚胎成功植入。最新的报道显示，蜕膜 B 细胞在妊娠早期和中期增加，尤其是 $CD24^{hi}CD27^+$ B 细胞和 $CD24^{hi}CD38^{hi}$ B 细胞。与外周血 B 细胞相比，蜕膜 B 细胞具有更高的分泌 IL-10 的能力[36]。此外，有研究观察到蜕膜 B 细胞与 T 细胞存在共定位，可能调控调节性 T 细胞的诱导和维持，并抑制幼稚 T 细胞向 Th1 或 Th17 细胞发育[36]。一项体外研究表明，B 细胞在滋养细胞存在时产生了调节表型，并对 T 细胞介导的有害炎症提供免疫保护[46]。这些发现支持一种新观点，即 B 细胞与促进最佳植入的条件密切相关，B 细胞稳态的改变或紊乱可能会导致自然流产。事实上，对妊娠期 Breg 功能的临床研究表明，妊娠开始时 $CD24^{hi}CD27^+$ B 细胞水平不足与自然流产相关[48]，而过继转移分泌 IL-10 的 Breg 则可恢复易流产小鼠的妊娠耐受性[62]。

3.4 胎儿宫内生长受限

IUGR 定义为胎儿未能达到其遗传生长潜能，与围产期死亡率和发病率增加有关。IUGR 是母体、胎盘、胎儿或遗传因素，或这些因素共同导致的结果。IUGR 的主要原因是胎盘功能不全，占所有妊娠的 5%～10%[63]。由于胎盘功能不全发生时，蜕膜的细胞免疫限制了滋养细胞的侵袭，从而减弱了胎盘的微循环和新陈代谢，胚胎移植的部分排斥可能是 IUGR 的免疫学病因。近期的一项研究发现，免疫系统的严重异常会导致孕妇出现适应障碍，包括胎盘功能不全[63]。然而,IUGR 与母胎界面免疫网络紊乱之间的关联和机制尚不清楚。

一些评估 IUGR 患者淋巴细胞亚群的研究表明,B 细胞失调与出生体重呈显著负相关[64,65]。IUGR 患者外周血胞浆 IgM、IgG 和 IgA 阳性的淋巴样细胞数明显增加,B 细胞的绝对数和百分比也更高。功能上,扩增的 B 细胞亚群可能与 IUGR 患者的抗体产生增加和淋巴系统慢性激活有关[64,66]。一项针对 IUGR 患者的队列研究发现,脐带血中 B 淋巴细胞的百分比和数量与婴儿出生时的体重、身长和头围呈正相关[65]。外周血细胞因子谱的比较显示,与健康孕妇相比,IUGR 患者的促炎细胞因子 IL-8、IL-6、IL-12 和 TNF 水平增加。与 IUGR 患者相比,同时患有 IUGR 和胎盘功能不全的女性 IL-10 更低[67-69]。由于包括 B 细胞在内的多种免疫细胞能分泌上述细胞因子,目前尚不清楚 B 细胞是如何影响这些结果的。然而,这些发现都表明 B 细胞参与了 IUGR 的病理生理学。

3.5 子痫前期

子痫前期的特征是血压升高、肾功能降低、宫内发育迟缓、慢性免疫激活和多器官功能障碍,始于妊娠后半期。子痫前期使孕妇及其胎儿面临很大的卒中、早产和死亡风险。与 IUGR 一样,该疾病归因于胎盘血管重塑不足和胎盘循环不良,导致胎盘缺氧和缺血[70]。有关 B 细胞在高血压中的作用的证据有限;然而,B 细胞通过其记忆免疫反应和自身抗体的产生与子痫前期密切相关。一项研究观察到 B 细胞数量和功能的失调:与正常对照组相比,循环记忆 B 细胞($CD27^+CD38^-$ 和 $CD27^+CD38^+$)的百分比和 B 细胞的增殖水平在子痫前期患者中增加[71]。此外,子痫前期胎盘的 B1 B 淋巴细胞($CD5^+$)标志物染色呈阳性,该 B 细胞亚群表现出更强的产生 AT1-AA 特异性 IgG 自身抗体的能力[72]。胎盘低灌注压(RUPP)大鼠模型进一步支持了 B 细胞在胎盘缺血引起的高血压病理生理中的作用。过继性转移患者来源的 AT1-AA 可诱导妊娠大鼠的子痫前期,而使用非特异性 CD20 抗体利妥昔单抗耗尽循环 B 细胞则能缓解子痫前期[25,73]。

3.6 早产

早产是指在妊娠 37 周之前发生的分娩。早产是一种复杂的现象,是新生儿死亡的主要原因,并使存活的新生儿易患上远期疾病[74]。宫内和全身感染以及随之而来的炎症是早产最常见的病理生理机制。

在分娩前和足月分娩开始时,底蜕膜和壁蜕膜中均有 B 细胞,而 B 细胞仅在底蜕膜中扩增[75]。小鼠妊娠羊水中发现的 B 细胞表型及功能特征显示存在大量自发产生 IgM 的 B1 B 细胞[76]。在自发性早产患者的壁蜕膜中,总 B 细胞比例显著增加,而在足月分娩中没有观察到这种变化[40,77]。胎盘及绒毛膜的早产标本也显示分泌自身抗体和多反应性抗体的 B1 细胞具有更高的数量和活化[40]。

最近的研究突出了 B 细胞在分娩过程中的调节作用。在脂多糖(LPS)诱导的小鼠早产模型中,B 细胞缺乏促进子宫炎症,并增加了早产和新生儿死亡的发生率[3,40]。在足月和自发性早产中,人绒毛膜间质中的 B 细胞表现出较高的活性、类别转换、记忆性及浆细胞样分化的表型和功能特征。然而,蜕膜 B 细胞在早产中功能发生了改变(即异常扩增、活化增强和抗体产生增多)[40]。LPS 诱导的小鼠早产模型显示,IL-33 介导的蜕膜 B 细胞产生 PIBF1 可保护足月妊娠,而这一机制在早产中存在缺陷[40,78]。

LPS 诱导的小鼠早产模型亦证明了 IL-10 在足月妊娠中的重要作用[79]。分泌 IL-10 的 Bregs 已成为维持健康妊娠的关键因素,因为最近的一项研究表明,过继转移分泌 IL-10 的 Bregs 可减少胎儿丢失并恢复体内免疫平衡[3]。

4 反复妊娠丢失

RPL 发生在 1%~3% 的女性中[6]。原发性 RPL 定义为与同一性伴侣连续两次或两次以上临床妊娠丢失,且之前未曾有过活产,而继发性 RPL 定义为在一次或多次活产后连续发生的妊娠丢失[80,81]。妊娠丢失的原因包括:胎儿染色体异常、父母染色体缺陷、感染、内分泌失调或子宫异常[6,80,82]。超过一半的 RPL 病例是特发性的,尽管其可能的原因是免疫失调引起的母体耐受性缺乏或启动不当[6,7,80]。由于对 RPL 的免疫学病因研究有限,且缺乏标准化的诊断流程,很难评估病理 B 细胞导致 RPL 的患病率。

5 诊断

不同免疫细胞亚群间复杂的相互协作是成功妊

娠所必需的，并在很大程度上成为了 RPL 的潜在病因。目前，对于异常妊娠同种免疫反应的检测，或评估特发性 RPL 的方法尚无共识。因此，RPL 通常以排除性诊断来确定。

RPL 的最低诊断标准包括完整的病史、手术史、遗传史、家族史和体格检查。排除遗传性病因后，通过子宫输卵管造影、超声子宫造影或宫腔镜检查，并检测 IgG 和 IgM 抗心磷脂抗体、狼疮抗凝物和自身抗体以评估免疫相关指标。此外，还可通过使用生物标志物或临床分析以进行免疫学检测，如免疫细胞分析、人类白细胞抗原分型、淋巴细胞毒交叉试验和混合淋巴细胞培养反应。这些检测是确定 RPL 免疫学诊断的基础[7]。

可预测妊娠丢失的 B 细胞病理指标包括低水平的 IL-10+ B 细胞和循环 CD5+ B 细胞数增多[48,72]。然而，这些指标目前仅限于验证以研究为目的的妊娠结局预测，尚未被临床用于孕前预测妊娠丢失风险。

6 治疗

基于在移植前输血以减少器官移植排斥反应的证据，一些研究人员尝试对特发性 RPL 进行多种免疫治疗。母体免疫调节最常用的方法是在受孕前父源白细胞输血及妊娠期 IVIg 被动免疫[82]。其他干预措施包括第三方淋巴细胞免疫（LIT）和父系抗原脱敏，尽管这些方法尚未被证明对 RPL 有效[6,82]（图 4.2）。

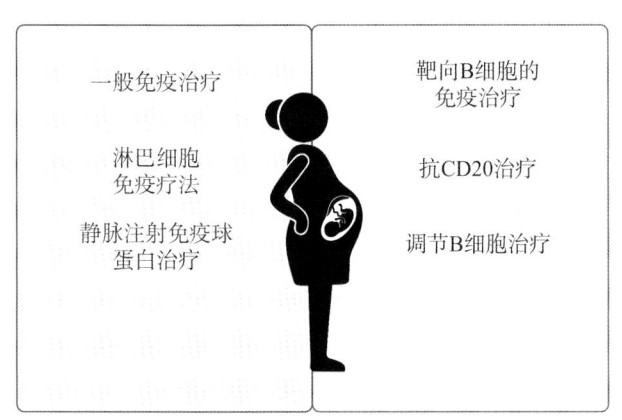

图 4.2　免疫相关反复妊娠丢失的免疫治疗方案。
来源：BioRender.com。

6.1 淋巴细胞免疫治疗

特发性 RPL 患者可考虑使用淋巴细胞免疫。LIT 是基于使准母亲适应外来细胞以提高父源细胞免疫耐受性的理论而开发的。对于 RPL，LIT 治疗包括从供体中提取淋巴细胞并将其注射到准母亲体内。LIT 通过几种潜在机制诱导母体免疫系统的变化以维持妊娠：抗父源淋巴细胞毒性抗体、PIBF、抗独特型抗体和混合淋巴细胞反应阻断抗体的表达，降低 Th1/Th2，以及改变细胞因子的产生模式[83]。

关于 LIT 的有效性和安全性尚无共识。一些 RPL 的临床研究表明，LIT 的有效率为 38%~70%；然而，2006 年的一项 Cochrane 系统综述发现，免疫治疗对不明原因的 RPL 没有任何益处[6,82-84]。此外，父源淋巴细胞应用部位的反应可能持续 15 天，但 LIT 并未增加自身免疫并发症的风险[84]。因此，仍需更多的研究以建立 LIT 临床应用的共识。

6.2　静脉注射免疫球蛋白治疗

在临床实践中发现患有 RPL 的女性存在免疫异常后，可通过多种免疫调节疗法以维持母胎界面的免疫平衡。基于 IgG 抗体的各种免疫调节作用，提出应用 IVIg 进行免疫抑制治疗。免疫调节作用包括：阻断抗体介导的免疫损伤、阻断 T 细胞受体、抑制自然杀伤细胞活性、抑制 Th1 细胞因子分泌、阻断 Fc 受体、补体失活、下调 B 细胞反应性和增强抑制性 T 细胞功能[85,86]。

据报道，IVIg 治疗的副作用包括头痛、皮疹和 APS 易血栓形成，但无明显先天性畸形风险。对自然妊娠期间使用了 IVIg 的患者进行的 20 年随访显示，母亲的血栓状态或新的自身免疫性疾病的发生没有变化，子痫前期和早产的发生率也较低，这可能是由于 IVIg 改善了胎盘形成[87]。

多项关于 IVIg 对 RPL 患者治疗效果的研究得出了相互矛盾的结果。虽然有一些研究表明，IVIg 可显著改善 RPL 患者的妊娠结局，但其他研究发现 IVIg 并没有明显的治疗效果[6,82,85,86]。因此，IVIg 尚未纳入 RPL 的临床治疗指南。随着 IVIg 在免疫性 RPL 中的作用机制越来越清楚，这一点在未来可能会发生变化。

6.3　B 细胞靶向治疗

靶向 B 细胞的免疫疗法仍处于实验阶段。然而，基于抗 CD20 抗体疗法（利妥昔单抗）在癌症患者中的应用，其已在由自身抗体介导的疾病中进行了试验。APS 患者受益于利妥昔单抗治疗,一些患者表现出 aPL 滴度降低或正常化,临床指标显著降低,如血小板减少[88]。但目前尚不清楚这种变化如何转化为成功妊娠。

现已提出基于 B 细胞调节能力的治疗方法用于病理性妊娠,特别是已知免疫来源的病理情况,以建立和维持支持胚胎植入所需的免疫改变。例如,从女性身上获得的 B 细胞可以扩增为 Breg 亚群,重新输注以激活维持妊娠所需的适当免疫改变。

这些治疗仍处于实验阶段,这一事实凸显了需要更为深入理解 B 细胞介导的病理生理学机制的必要性。全面了解决定健康妊娠的细胞间复杂的相互作用网络,对于开发和测试新一代疗法至关重要。

7　总结和建议

调节 B 细胞分布和功能以改善妊娠结局的靶向疗法尚处于研究的初始阶段。理论上,通过单克隆抗 CD20 抗体以耗竭 B 细胞,或使用 B 细胞细胞因子特异性炎症介质可抑制有害的炎症反应;然而,这些疗法仍有待改进,以避免限制有助于妊娠健康的特定 B 细胞亚群的功能。

因此,为了推进治疗病理妊娠的不同类型免疫疗法,建议:

- 拓展旨在破解母体耐受诱导机制的研究。
- 同时利用临床样本进行评估,以确定所提出机制的有效性。
- 确定进一步的免疫参数对不明原因不孕和 RPL 进行检测。
- 扩大对其他病理妊娠中免疫细胞亚群和功能的评估。
- 继续探索适用于早期妊娠的新治疗方案,以设置或纠正异常的免疫适应。

参考文献

[1] Guzman-Genuino RM, Diener KR. Regulatory B cells in pregnancy: lessons from autoimmunity, graft tolerance, and cancer. Front Immunol 2017;8:172.

[2] Guzman-Genuino RM, Hayball JD, Diener KR. Regulatory B cells: dark horse in pregnancy immunotherapy? J Mol Biol 2021;433(1):166596.

[3] Busse M, Campe KJ, Nowak D, et al. IL-10 producing B cells rescue mouse fetuses from inflammation-driven fetal death and are able to modulate T cell immune responses. Sci Rep 2019;9(1):9335.

[4] Carbone J, Gallego A, Lanio N, et al. Quantitative abnormalities of peripheral blood distinct T, B, and natural killer cell subsets and clinical findings in obstetric antiphospholipid syndrome. J Rheumatol 2009;36(6):1217-25.

[5] Zeng B, Kwak-Kim J, Liu Y, Liao AH. Treg cells are negatively correlated with increased memory B cells in preeclampsia while maintaining suppressive function on autologous B-cell proliferation. Am J Reprod Immunol 2013;70(6):454-63.

[6] Achilli C, Duran-Retamal M, Saab W, Serhal P, Seshadri S. The role of immunotherapy in in vitro fertilization and recurrent pregnancy loss: a systematic review and meta-analysis. Fertil Steril 2018;110(6):1089-100.

[7] Beaman KD, Ntrivalas E, Mallers TM, Jaiswal MK, Kwak-Kim J, Gilman-Sachs A. Immune etiology of recurrent pregnancy loss and its diagnosis. Am J Reprod Immunol 2012;67(4):319-25.

[8] Taylor PV, Hancock KW. Antigenicity of trophoblast and possible antigen-masking effects during pregnancy. Immunology. 1975;28(5):973-82.

[9] Carter J, Dresser DW. Pregnancy induces an increase in the number of immunoglobulin-secreting cells. Immunology. 1983;49(3):481-90.

[10] Muzzio DO, Soldati R, Ehrhardt J, et al. B cell development undergoes profound modifications and adaptations during pregnancy in mice. Biol Reprod 2014;91(5):115.

[11] Muzzio DO, Ziegler KB, Ehrhardt J, Zygmunt M, Jensen F. Marginal zone B cells emerge as a critical component of pregnancy wellbeing. Reproduction. 2016;151(1):29-37.

[12] Ziegler KB, Muzzio DO, Matzner F, et al. Human pregnancy is accompanied by modifications in B cell development and immunoglobulin profile. J Reprod Immunol 2018;129:40-7.

[13] Grimsholm O, Piano Mortari E, Davydov AN, et al. The interplay between CD27(dull) and CD27(bright) B cells ensures the flexibility, stability, and resilience of human B cell memory. Cell Rep 2020;30(9):2963-77 e2966.

[14] Margni RA, Paz CB, Cordal ME. Immunochemical behavior of sheep non-precipitating antibodies isolated by immunoadsorption. Immunochemistry. 1976;13(3):209-14.

[15] Barrientos G, Fuchs D, Schrocksnadel K, et al. Low levels of serum asymmetric antibodies as a marker of threatened pregnancy. J Reprod Immunol 2009;79(2):201-10.

[16] Malan Borel I, Gentile T, Angelucci J, et al. IgG asymmetric molecules with antipaternal activity isolated from sera and placenta of pregnant human. J Reprod Immunol 1991;20(2):129-40.

[17] Zenclussen AC, Gentile T, Kortebani G, Mazzolli A, Margni R. Asymmetric antibodies and pregnancy. Am J Reprod Immunol 2001;45(5):289-94.

[18] Carp HJ, Meroni PL, Shoenfeld Y. Autoantibodies as predictors of pregnancy complications. Rheumatol (Oxf) 2008;47(Suppl 3):iii6-8.

[19] Di Prima FA, Valenti O, Hyseni E, et al. Antiphospholipid

[19] syndrome during pregnancy: the state of the art. J Prenat Med 2011;5(2):41-53.

[20] Herse F, LaMarca B. Angiotensin II type 1 receptor autoantibody (AT1-AA)-mediated pregnancy hypertension. Am J Reprod Immunol 2013;69(4):413-18.

[21] Salmon JE, Girardi G. Antiphospholipid antibodies and pregnancy loss: a disorder of inflammation. J Reprod Immunol 2008;77(1):51-6.

[22] Heilmann L, Schorsch M, Hahn T, Fareed J. Antiphospholipid syndrome and preeclampsia. Semin Thromb Hemost 2011;37(2):141-5.

[23] Vinatier D, Dufour P, Cosson M, Houpeau JL. Antiphospholipid syndrome and recurrent miscarriages. Eur J Obstet Gynecol Reprod Biol 2001;96(1):37-50.

[24] Robinson CJ, Johnson DD, Chang EY, Armstrong DM, Wang W. Evaluation of placenta growth factor and soluble Fms-like tyrosine kinase 1 receptor levels in mild and severe preeclampsia. Am J Obstet Gynecol 2006;195(1):255-9.

[25] Zhou CC, Zhang Y, Irani RA, et al. Angiotensin receptor agonistic autoantibodies induce preeclampsia in pregnant mice. Nat Med 2008;14(8):855-62.

[26] Christiansen JS, Andersen AR, Osther K, Peitersen B, Bach-Mortensen N, Lebech PE. The relationship between pregnancy, HCS and B lymphocytes. Acta Pathol Microbiol Scand C 1976;84(4):313-18.

[27] Medina KL, Smithson G, Kincade PW. Suppression of B lymphopoiesis during normal pregnancy. J Exp Med 1993;178(5):1507-15.

[28] Guzman-Genuino RM, Eldi P, Garcia-Valtanen P, Hayball JD, Diener KR. Uterine B cells exhibit regulatory properties during the peri-implantation stage of murine pregnancy. Front Immunol 2019;10:2899.

[29] de Carvalho Schettini JA, Gomes TV, Junior C, Heraclio SA, Coelho I, Torres LC. Evaluation of immunological parameters in pregnant women: low levels of B and NK cells. Rev Bras Ginecol Obstet 2019;41(4):213-19.

[30] Kraus TA, Engel SM, Sperling RS, et al. Characterizing the pregnancy immune phenotype: results of the viral immunity and pregnancy (VIP) study. J Clin Immunol 2012;32(2):300-11.

[31] Lima J, Martins C, Leandro MJ, et al. Characterization of B cells in healthy pregnant women from late pregnancy to post-partum: a prospective observational study. BMC Pregnancy Childbirth 2016;16(1):139.

[32] Mahmoud F, Abul H, Omu A, Al-Rayes S, Haines D, Whaley K. Pregnancy-associated changes in peripheral blood lymphocyte subpopulations in normal Kuwaiti women. Gynecol Obstet Invest 2001;52(4):232-6.

[33] Bhat NM, Mithal A, Bieber MM, Herzenberg LA, Teng NN. Human CD5+ B lymphocytes (B-1 cells) decrease in peripheral blood during pregnancy. J Reprod Immunol 1995;28(1):53-60.

[34] Watanabe M, Iwatani Y, Kaneda T, et al. Changes in T, B, and NK lymphocyte subsets during and after normal pregnancy. Am J Reprod Immunol 1997;37(5):368-77.

[35] Birkeland SA, Kristoffersen K. Lymphocyte transformation with mitogens and antigens during normal human pregnancy: a longitudinal study. Scand J Immunol 1980;11(3):321-5.

[36] Benner M, Feyaerts D, Garcia CC, et al. Clusters of tolerogenic B cells feature in the dynamic immunological landscape of the pregnant uterus. Cell Rep 2020;32(13):108204.

[37] Carter J, Newport A, Keeler KD, Dresser DW. FACS analysis of changes in T and B lymphocyte populations in the blood, spleen and lymph nodes of pregnant mice. Immunology. 1983;48(4):791-7.

[38] Hussein MR, Abd-Elwahed AR, Abodeif ES, Abdulwahed SR. Decidual immune cell infiltrate in hydatidiform mole. Cancer Invest 2009;27(1):60-6.

[39] Solders M, Lundell AC, Gorchs L, Gidlof S, Tiblad E, Kaipe H. Mature naive B cells are retained in the placental intervillous blood and positively associate with specific chemokines in full-term healthy pregnancy. Am J Reprod Immunol 2019;82(3):e13154.

[40] Huang B, Faucette AN, Pawlitz MD, et al. Interleukin-33-induced expression of PIBF1 by decidual B cells protects against preterm labor. Nat Med 2017;23(1):128-35.

[41] Harrity C, Bereir MM, Walsh DJ, Marron KD. Moving from peripheral blood to local uterine immunophenotype analysis in patients with poor reproductive history: pilot study of a novel technique. Ir J Med Sci 2019;188(3):893-901.

[42] Marron K, Walsh D, Harrity C. Detailed endometrial immune assessment of both normal and adverse reproductive outcome populations. J Assist Reprod Genet 2019;36(2):199-210.

[43] Sung N, Byeon HJ, Garcia MDS, et al. Deficiency in memory B cell compartment in a patient with infertility and recurrent pregnancy losses. J Reprod Immunol 2016;118:70-5.

[44] Danaii S, Ghorbani F, Ahmadi M, et al. IL-10-producing B cells play important role in the pathogenesis of recurrent pregnancy loss. Int Immunopharmacol 2020;87:106806.

[45] Koushaeian L, Ghorbani F, Ahmadi M, et al. The role of IL-10-producing B cells in repeated implantation failure patients with cellular immune abnormalities. Immunol Lett 2019;214:16-22.

[46] Guzman-Genuino RM, Dimova T, You Y, et al. Trophoblasts promote induction of a regulatory phenotype in B cells that can protect against detrimental T cell-mediated inflammation. Am J Reprod Immunol 2019;82(6):e13187.

[47] Liu J, Chen X, Hao S, et al. Human chorionic gonadotropin and IL-35 contribute to the maintenance of peripheral immune tolerance during pregnancy through mediating the generation of IL-10(+) or IL-35(+) Breg cells. Exp Cell Res 2019;383(2):111513.

[48] Rolle L, Memarzadeh Tehran M, Morell-Garcia A, et al. Cutting edge: IL-10-producing regulatory B cells in early human pregnancy. Am J Reprod Immunol 2013;70(6):448-53.

[49] Slawek A, Lorek D, Kedzierska AE, Chelmonska-Soyta A. Regulatory B cells with IL-35 and IL-10 expression in a normal and abortion-prone murine pregnancy model. Am J Reprod Immunol 2020;83(3):e13217.

[50] Lorek D, Kedzierska AE, Slawek A, Chelmonska-Soyta A. Expression of Toll-like receptors and costimulatory molecules in splenic B cells in a normal and abortion-prone murine pregnancy model. Am J Reprod Immunol 2019;82(2):e13148.

[51] Maj T, Slawek A, Chelmonska-Soyta A. CD80 and CD86 co-stimulatory molecules differentially regulate OT-II CD4(+) T lymphocyte proliferation and cytokine response in cocultures with antigen-presenting cells derived from pregnant and pseudopregnant mice. Mediators Inflamm 2014;2014:769239.

[52] Slawek A, Maj T, Chelmonska-Soyta A. CD40, CD80, and CD86 co-stimulatory molecules are differentially expressed on murine splenic antigen-presenting cells during the pre-implantation period of pregnancy, and they modulate regulatory T-cell abundance, peripheral cytokine response, and pregnancy outcome. Am J Reprod Immunol 2013;70(2):116-26.

[53] Darmochwal-Kolarz D, Leszczynska-Gorzelak B, Rolinski J, Oleszczuk J. The immunophenotype of patients with recurrent pregnancy loss. Eur J Obstet Gynecol Reprod Biol 2002;103(1):53-7.

[54] Einenkel R, Packhauser KRH, Ehrhardt J, Tungler A, Zygmunt M, Muzzio DO. CD83 is locally regulated and differentially expressed in disturbed murine pregnancy. Reproduction. 2019;158(4):323-33.

[55] Satta R, Biondi G. Antiphospholipid syndrome and pregnancy. G Ital Dermatol Venereol 2019;154(3):277-85.

[56] Alvarez-Rodriguez L, Riancho-Zarrabeitia L, Calvo-Alen J, Lopez-Hoyos M, Martinez-Taboada V. Peripheral B-cell subset distribution in primary antiphospholipid syndrome. Int J Mol Sci 2018;19:2.

[57] Simonin L, Pasquier E, Leroyer C, et al. Lymphocyte disturbances in primary antiphospholipid syndrome and application to venous thromboembolism follow-up. Clin Rev Allergy Immunol 2017;53(1):14-27.

[58] Hisada R, Kato M, Sugawara E, et al. Circulating plasmablasts contribute to antiphospholipid antibody production, associated with type I interferon upregulation. J Thromb Haemost 2019;17(7):1134-43.

[59] Li XY, Duan HJ, Liu XY, Deng XL. Change of serum B-cell activating factor level in patients with positive antiphospholipid antibodies and previous adverse pregnancy outcomes and its significance. Chin Med J (Engl) 2020;133(19):2287-94.

[60] Mor G, Cardenas I, Abrahams V, Guller S. Inflammation and pregnancy: the role of the immune system at the implantation site. Ann N Y Acad Sci 2011;1221:80-7.

[61] Schumacher A, Ehrentraut S, Scharm M, et al. Plasma cell alloantigen 1 and IL-10 secretion define two distinct peritoneal B1a B cell subsets with opposite functions, PC1(high) cells being protective and PC1(low) cells harmful for the growing fetus. Front Immunol 2018;9:1045.

[62] Jensen F, Muzzio D, Soldati R, Fest S, Zenclussen AC. Regulatory B10 cells restore pregnancy tolerance in a mouse model. Biol Reprod 2013;89(4):90.

[63] Bekmukhambetov Y, Mamyrbayev A, Dzharkenov T, et al. Metabolic and immunologic aspects of fetoplacental insufficiency. Am J Reprod Immunol 2016;76(4):299-306.

[64] Bartha JL, Comino-Delgado R. Lymphocyte subpopulations in intrauterine growth retardation in women with or without previous pregnancies. Eur J Obstet Gynecol Reprod Biol 1999;82(1):23-7.

[65] Xiong F, Tong Y, You Y, et al. Prospective cohort study about the lymphocyte subpopulations' change and impact on the pregnancy outcome in fetal growth restriction. J Matern Fetal Neonatal Med 2012;25(12):2773-7.

[66] Selvaggi L, Lucivero G, Iannone A, et al. Analysis of mononuclear cell subsets in pregnancies with intrauterine growth retardation. Evidence of chronic B-lymphocyte activation. J Perinat Med 1983;11(4):213-17.

[67] Al-Azemi M, Raghupathy R, Azizieh F. Pro-inflammatory and anti-inflammatory cytokine profiles in fetal growth restriction. Clin Exp Obstet Gynecol 2017;44(1):98-103.

[68] Bartha JL, Romero-Carmona R, Comino-Delgado R. Inflammatory cytokines in intrauterine growth retardation. Acta Obstet Gynecol Scand 2003;82(12):1099-102.

[69] Raghupathy R, Al-Azemi M, Azizieh F. Intrauterine growth restriction: cytokine profiles of trophoblast antigen-stimulated maternal lymphocytes. Clin Dev Immunol 2012;2012:734865.

[70] LaMarca B, Cornelius D, Wallace K. Elucidating immune mechanisms causing hypertension during pregnancy. Physiol (Bethesda) 2013;28(4):225-33.

[71] Liao AH, Liu LP, Ding WP, Zhang L. Functional changes of human peripheral B-lymphocytes in preeclampsia. Am J Reprod Immunol 2009;61(5):313-21.

[72] Jensen F, Wallukat G, Herse F, et al. CD19+ CD5+ cells as indicators of preeclampsia. Hypertension. 2012;59(4):861-8.

[73] Laule CF, Odean EJ, Wing CR, et al. Role of B1 and B2 lymphocytes in placental ischemia-induced hypertension. Am J Physiol Heart Circ Physiol 2019;317(4):H732-42.

[74] Quinn JA, Munoz FM, Gonik B, et al. Preterm birth: case definition & guidelines for data collection, analysis, and presentation of immunisation safety data. Vaccine. 2016;34(49):6047-56.

[75] Rinaldi SF, Makieva S, Saunders PT, Rossi AG, Norman JE. Immune cell and transcriptomic analysis of the human decidua in term and preterm parturition. Mol Hum Reprod 2017;23(10):708-24.

[76] Bommer I, Juriol L, Muzzio D, et al. Characterization of murine amniotic fluid B cells in normal pregnancy and in preterm birth. Reproduction. 2019;158(4):369-76.

[77] Leng Y, Romero R, Xu Y, et al. Are B cells altered in the decidua of women with preterm or term labor? Am J Reprod Immunol 2019;81(5):e13102.

[78] Valeff N, Juriol L, Quadrana F, et al. Expression of IL-33 receptor is significantly up-regulated in B cells during pregnancy and in the acute phase of preterm birth in mice. Front Immunol 2020;11:446.

[79] Robertson SA, Skinner RJ, Care AS. Essential role for IL-10 in resistance to lipopolysaccharide-induced preterm labor in mice. J Immunol 2006;177(7):4888-96.

[80] Zarnani AH. Recurrent pregnancy loss through the lens of immunology. J Reprod Infertil 2015;16(2):59-60.

[81] Pillarisetty LS, Gupta N. Recurrent Pregnancy Loss. Treasure Island (FL): StatPearls; 2021.

[82] Wong LF, Porter TF, Scott JR. Immunotherapy for recurrent miscarriage. Cochrane Database Syst Rev 2014;10:CD000112.

[83] Hajipour H, Nejabati HR, Latifi Z, et al. Lymphocytes immunotherapy for preserving pregnancy: mechanisms and challenges. Am J Reprod Immunol 2018;80(3):e12853.

[84] Cavalcante MB, Sarno M, Araujo Junior E, Da Silva Costa F, Barini R. Lymphocyte immunotherapy in the treatment of recurrent miscarriage: systematic review and meta-analysis. Arch Gynecol Obstet 2017;295(2):511-18.

[85] Palmeira P, Quinello C, Silveira-Lessa AL, Zago CA, Carneiro-Sampaio M. IgG placental transfer in healthy and pathological pregnancies. Clin Dev Immunol 2012;2012:985646.

[86] Sung N, Han AR, Park CW, et al. Intravenous immunoglobulin G in women with reproductive failure: The Korean Society for reproductive immunology practice

guidelines. Clin Exp Reprod Med 2017;44(1):1-7.

[87] Woon EV, Day A, Bracewell-Milnes T, Male V, Johnson M. Immunotherapy to improve pregnancy outcome in women with abnormal natural killer cell levels/activity and recurrent miscarriage or implantation failure: a systematic review and meta-analysis. J Reprod Immunol 2020;142:103189.

[88] Dieudonne Y, Guffroy A, Poindron V, et al. B cells in primary antiphospholipid syndrome: review and remaining challenges. Autoimmun Rev 2021;20(5):102798.

第 5 章

肥大细胞病理学与生殖障碍
Mast cell pathology and reproductive failures

Maria Socorro L. Agcaoili De Jesus[1], Lara Theresa C. Alentajan-Aleta[1], Cherie C. Ocampo-Cervantes[1], Jenifer R. Otadoy-Agustin[1] and Joanne Kwak-Kim[2]

[1] Division of Allergy and Immunology, Department of Medicine, University of the Philippines College of Medicine, Philippine General Hospital, Manila, Philippines

[2] Reproductive Medicine and Immunology, Obstetrics and Gynecology, Clinical Sciences Department, Chicago Medical School, Rosalind Franklin University of Medicine and Science, Vernon Hills, IL, United States

1 引言

肥大细胞（mast cell，MC）长期以来一直被认为与过敏性疾病有关。然而，肥大细胞不仅是过敏性疾病的关键细胞介质，还可调节机体的生理和病理过程，包括生殖。肥大细胞在男性和女性生殖道中的广泛分布凸显了其在免疫反应中的积极作用，且对生育能力及妊娠的建立和维持具有积极和消极的影响。肥大细胞的激活导致脱颗粒，释放各种预合成的和（或）新合成的炎症介质。在本章中，将深入探讨肥大细胞及其颗粒的功能、在生殖道中的分布和在生殖过程中的作用。此外，还将探讨由异常肥大细胞密度和病理引起的生殖和产科疾病以及妊娠结局。

2 肥大细胞生物学

肥大细胞是多功能组织驻留细胞，主要驻留在黏膜和上皮组织中，是固有免疫系统的一部分，也是机体的第一道防线。Paul Ehrlich 于 1878 年首次发现肥大细胞，由于其分泌颗粒的特征性异染，最初被命名为"mastzellen"[1]。德语中的"mast"一词表示"增肥"或"哺乳"功能，这是基于它的颗粒具有营养功能。约 60 年后，肥大细胞与组胺之间的联系被建立起来。从那时起，肥大细胞就与过敏性疾病和寄生虫感染紧密相连[2]。

然而，肥大细胞存在于所有种类的脊椎动物中，并且肥大细胞在脊椎动物中的组胺储备及其作为炎症介质的功能大约在 2.76 亿年前的原始爬行动物中便已建立。这表明，肥大细胞介导了生命的基本功能，而不仅仅代表免疫系统的退化残余。此外，迄今尚未发现肥大细胞缺陷的人类，表明肥大细胞具有重要的生物学作用[3]。

2.1 肥大细胞的起源

肥大细胞来源于称为共同髓系祖细胞（common myeloid progenitor，CMP）的多能造血骨髓干细胞，以未分化的 CD34 受体、酪氨酸激酶 Kit 阳性（CD117$^+$）单核细胞释放到全身循环[4]。它是唯一在未成熟状态下离开骨髓的免疫细胞，在成熟之前进入结缔组织和黏膜衬里。肥大细胞的数量和分布存在种间差异。人、猴、大鼠、小鼠和鱼的肥大细胞数量众多，而兔的肥大细胞数量很少。肥大细胞主要存在于皮肤的真皮和皮下组织。在消化系统的网膜、肠和舌中有大量肥大细胞。然而，由于肝脏、脾脏和肾上腺缺乏结缔组织，这些器官中的肥大细胞很少。近期有研究表明，肥大细胞在子宫肌层中大量存在，但在子宫内膜中很少，且局限于基底层[5]。正常增生期和分泌期子宫内膜中的肥大细胞数量似乎没有明显差异；然而，在月经前期，子宫内膜肥大细胞显著减少[5]。据推测，肥大细胞几乎只存在于子宫内膜基底层，加之其细胞质颗粒在月经周期结束时排出，可能与月经前螺旋动脉发生缺血性痉挛的月经机制有关。功能层中肥大细胞的相对缺乏可能有助于子宫内膜对囊胚植入的免疫耐受。

2.2 肥大细胞的分化和发育

肥大细胞由释放到外周循环中的多能造血干细胞发育而来。这些细胞迁移到组织中并增殖，在局部细胞因子、组织基质和常驻细胞（如成纤维细胞）的影响下成熟。干细胞因子（SCF）和 c-kit 之间的相互作用及随后的信号传导对肥大细胞的生长和发育至关重要。

促进肥大细胞发育的细胞因子已被研究。在含血清和无血清的培养基中添加 SCF、IL-3、IL-4、IL-5 或 IL-6 能以剂量依赖的方式延长肥大细胞的存活时间[6]。SCF 和 IL-6 是必需的生长因子，从培养基中去除会导致肥大细胞凋亡。多种辅助因子可根据肥大细胞的来源和成熟程度增强或抑制 SCF 的作用。神经生长因子、IL-3、IL-6、IL-9 和 IL-10 可增强 SCF 依赖的肥大细胞生长和（或）存活[7,8]。粒细胞-巨噬细胞集落刺激因子（GM-CSF）、维甲酸和转化生长因子-β（TGF-β）则能抑制肥大细胞的生长和分化[8]。

2.3 肥大细胞的活化

由于肥大细胞与过敏性疾病密切相关，目前研究最为深入的肥大细胞活化机制是无害过敏原通过 IgE 与肥大细胞表面高亲和力 IgE 受体 FcεRI 交联所介导的机制。然而，在生理环境下，其他受体（如 KIT 或 CD117、Toll 样受体和 TNF-α 受体）也可能显著影响肥大细胞释放介质[6]。肥大细胞活化的其他途径包括蛋白酶（如类胰蛋白酶）、神经肽（特别是皮肤肥大细胞）、污染物、职业化学制剂、细胞间接触和高渗压。

组织损伤或识别病原体可激活固有免疫反应。由于肥大细胞的分布以及其处于异物进入人体的关键位置，它们已成为人体的第一道防线。据报道，肥大细胞由多种病原体激活，如寄生虫、细菌和病毒等[6]。

2.4 肥大细胞的类型

据报道，肥大细胞存在形态、生化和功能特征的变异，这种现象被称为肥大细胞的异质性。肥大细胞的超微结构、受体表达、介质含量、免疫和非免疫激活以及药理反应性使其具有异质性。不同物种间、不同器官间甚至在同一器官内的肥大细胞也可能不相同。导致这种异质性的因素是多样化的，包括与组织基质和常驻细胞（如成纤维细胞）的相互作用。尽管可能是祖细胞在发育早期就决定了特定表型，但蛋白酶表达的显著可塑性亦很明显。根据蛋白酶含量，人类肥大细胞分为两组：一组仅含类胰蛋白酶（MC_T），另一组同时含有类胰蛋白酶、糜蛋白酶、羧肽酶 A 和组织蛋白酶 G（MC_{TC}）。MC_T 表型通常出现在黏膜表面，如鼻和下呼吸道上皮。MC_{TC} 表型则存于结缔组织（如健康皮肤）中。肥大细胞的异质性也延伸到其细胞因子含量。IL-4 和 IL-13 主要存在于 MC_{TC} 中，而 IL-5 和 IL-6 几乎只存在于 MC_T 中，提示这些表型具有独特的功能[9]。

2.5 肥大细胞脱颗粒

作为人体速发型超敏反应的主要效应细胞，肥大细胞已被证明在暴露后几分钟内便对刺激产生反应。经 FcεRI 激活，预合成和新合成的介质被分泌，该过程也称为脱颗粒。主要的预合成介质包括组胺、类胰蛋白酶[10]、糜蛋白酶和肝素[9]。除了储存的颗粒衍生介质外，在 IgE 依赖性激活后，肥大细胞还能释放新合成的花生四烯酸、白三烯 C4 和 D4、前列腺素 D2 和血小板活化因子的代谢物。这些颗粒能以非 IgE 介导的方式释放，作为对病毒、寄生虫和细菌的固有免疫反应的一部分。研究还发现肥大细胞颗粒富含锌——一种有效的 caspase 抑制剂和 NF-κB 核易位调节剂，并与肥大细胞在机体稳态中的作用相关[11]。

一旦肥大细胞被激活，在抗原结合后的几秒钟内便开始脱颗粒[12]。颗粒内容物包括组胺、丝氨酸酯酶和蛋白酶（如糜蛋白酶和类胰蛋白酶）[13]。组胺和肝素作为毒性介质，有助于清除寄生物感染，增加血管通透性，引起平滑肌收缩以排出寄生物，并促进抗凝。胰蛋白酶、糜蛋白酶、组织蛋白酶 G 和羧肽酶是纤维化过程中的重要介质，有助于炎症后的组织重塑[13]。胰蛋白酶不仅对成纤维细胞有促增殖作用，还能作为这些细胞的趋化剂，并能诱导成纤维细胞中的胶原合成。肥大细胞在激活后合成的细胞因子、趋化因子和脂质介质有助于维持促炎状态，根据不同的炎症部位，促炎状态可能发挥有益或有害作用。

3 肥大细胞在生殖系统中的作用

3.1 男性生殖道

肥大细胞在男性生殖器官中起着重要作用[14]。含类胰蛋白酶和糜蛋白酶的 MC_{TC} 肥大细胞及含类胰蛋白酶的 MC_T 肥大细胞仅在人类睾丸和附睾中发现，而 MC_{TC} 是人类睾丸中的主要种群。肥大细胞的数量在生命的不同发育阶段有所不同，在婴儿期的睾丸和附睾中略有增加，随后在儿童期减少，在青春期再次增加[15]。成年后，睾丸结缔组织中的肥大细胞逐渐减少。健康男性睾丸的平均肥大细胞约为 $(4.8±3.1)×10^6\ \mu m$[16]。

肥大细胞存在于睾丸生精小管固有层、附睾和输出小管。其中大多数位于间质室，小部分靠近生精小管或在固有层[16]。附睾和前列腺中也有肥大细胞。在附睾中，肥大细胞均匀分布在头部、体部和尾部，其数量随生命的不同阶段而发生改变。在可生育男性的精液中亦发现肥大细胞[17,18]。

3.2 女性生殖系统

肥大细胞在女性生殖道发挥诸多功能。例如，在排卵、胚胎种植、妊娠早期的组织重塑、蜕膜化、胎盘形成、胎儿发育和分娩中都具有重要作用。

3.2.1 排卵

与绝经后卵巢相比，在功能正常卵巢和多囊卵巢的皮质和髓质中，胰蛋白酶阳性肥大细胞的数量多于糜蛋白酶阳性肥大细胞。在正常卵巢中，神经纤维密度适中的区域含有大量肥大细胞。随着多囊卵巢中神经纤维密度的增加，肥大细胞的数量减少，而在绝经后卵巢中则未发现肥大细胞。肥大细胞数量的减少与神经纤维密度的增加表明神经-免疫通信发生了变化[19]。

3.2.2 胚胎种植和妊娠早期的组织重塑

肥大细胞表达雌激素和孕激素受体，这些激素可诱导肥大细胞进入子宫[20]。人类子宫肥大细胞的数量和结构随着月经周期的变化而变化，表明这种变化是激素依赖的。在增生期和分泌期子宫内膜中，肥大细胞的数量保持不变，但在月经周期的经前阶段减少[5]。在非妊娠子宫中，类胰蛋白酶-糜蛋白酶阳性肥大细胞占优势，而在妊娠子宫肌层中，类蛋白酶阳性肥大细胞占主导[21]。含有糜蛋白酶的肥大细胞通常存在于妊娠子宫肌层、胎盘和脐带的血管周围[22]。

肥大细胞产生组胺，可能参与囊胚的植入。然而，在小鼠的研究中发现，囊胚植入甚至发生在肥大细胞缺乏的情况下[23]，这表明其他细胞（如内皮细胞或蜕膜细胞）可能是组胺的来源[24]。活化的肥大细胞释放预合成和新合成的介质，如类胰蛋白酶、糜蛋白酶、组胺和 TGF-β，这些介质可能参与囊胚植入。在植入过程中，子宫内膜组织分泌诱导型一氧化氮合酶，产生一氧化氮。一氧化氮在子宫内膜的功能（如子宫内膜容受性、胚胎种植和月经）中起着至关重要的作用。肥大细胞分泌 IL-8 和弹性蛋白酶，前者触发中性粒细胞迁移至基质，后者则分解Ⅲ型胶原，在基质中产生空隙。与透明质酸的相互作用促进基质细胞中的水分滞留，导致在植入过程中可观察到水肿发生[25]。

3.2.3 蜕膜和胎盘

子宫内膜上皮和蜕膜细胞在囊胚附着子宫内膜及滋养细胞侵入蜕膜期间分泌趋化因子。趋化因子（如 CX3CL1、CCL14 和 CCL4）在子宫内膜细胞和基质成纤维细胞中大量表达，而相应的受体（CX3R1、CCR1、CCR2 和 CCR5）则在滋养细胞中表达[26]。趋化因子的分泌促进了滋养细胞迁移，体现了其在母胎界面交互中的重要性[27]。

在子宫内膜中，肥大细胞围绕子宫内膜腺体和螺旋动脉，表达类胰蛋白酶、糜蛋白酶和羧肽酶 A3。此外，子宫内膜肥大细胞还分泌 CCL8，促进子宫内膜上皮和基质细胞的迁移。据报道，CCL8 及其受体 CCR1 在卵巢子宫内膜样病灶和异位子宫内膜中过度表达，引起子宫内膜异位症[28]。深度浸润性子宫内膜异位症患者的病灶活检显示神经纤维周围有大量活化和脱颗粒的肥大细胞。肥大细胞与神经细胞的密切关系表明肥大细胞在子宫内膜异位症疼痛和痛觉过敏的发展中起着关键作用[29]。

3.2.4 胎儿和母体免疫应答的调节

蜕膜肥大细胞分泌血管内皮生长因子-A（VEGF-A）和精氨酸酶-1，促进血管生成[30]。小鼠研究表明，位于蜕膜中的肥大细胞分泌 IL-9，有助于母胎界面的 Treg 依赖性同种异体免疫耐受[31]。近期研究表明，蜕膜中的肥大细胞亦表达杀伤细胞 Ig 样受体（KIR）2DL4，可作为滋养细胞表达的 HLA-G 的受体。NK 细胞上 HLA-G 与 KIR2DL4 的相互作用抑制 NK 细胞的细胞毒活性，进一步支持母体免疫耐受[32]。

肥大细胞通过对螺旋动脉重塑的影响在胎盘形成中发挥作用。对肥大细胞缺陷小鼠胎盘部位的检查显示，胎盘体积减小，螺旋动脉重塑受损[33]。胎盘肥大细胞来源的组胺也参与胎盘发育的不同步骤。组胺通过组胺 1 型受体增强人类细胞滋养层细胞的侵袭[34]。组胺还能增加滋养细胞 αvβ3 整合素的表达[35]，并通过与 H1 受体的相互作用影响细胞滋养层细胞的凋亡活性[36]。

3.2.5 胎儿发育和分娩

当暴露于变应原和组胺时，非妊娠和妊娠子宫组织会产生强烈的子宫肌层收缩。由于妊娠子宫中含有大量的肥大细胞，表明肥大细胞参与了妊娠期间的子宫收缩[21]。子宫肌层组织的伸展以适应生长中的胎儿，释放诸如 SCF 和其他趋化因子等介质，将肥大细胞吸引到子宫肌层。趋化因子如 CXCL‐1、CXCL‐2、CXCL‐3、CXCL‐5 和 CXCL‐8 在足月分娩期间的子宫内膜、子宫颈和胎膜中占主导地位。这些趋化因子的受体 CXCR‐1 和 CXCR‐2 存在于中性粒细胞和肥大细胞中，促使它们募集到子宫[37]。

4 生殖中肥大细胞相关免疫病理学

4.1 男性不育

4.1.1 肥大细胞相关男性不育

据报道，患有特发性少精症、弱精症或无精症的不育男性精液中肥大细胞密度增加。睾丸细针穿刺抽吸活检涂片的定量分析显示肥大细胞显著增加。在特发性男性不育症患者中仅呈现 Sertoli 细胞和增多的肥大细胞（平均值为 19.5 个肥大细胞/20 个视野）。H&E 染色显示，肥大细胞呈圆形或椭圆形，含有大量紫色颗粒。这一发现与正常精子发生的病例（0.66 个肥大细胞/20 个视野；$P<0.001$）相比具有显著性差异。同样，晚期精子发育成熟阻滞病例的肥大细胞数（8 个肥大细胞/20 个视野；$P<0.01$）也显著高于正常精子发生。在早期精子发育成熟阻滞病例中，肥大细胞/20 个视野的平均数为 3.5；然而，由于病例数较少，该研究未行统计学分析[38]。

4.1.2 患病率

特发性弱精子症的男性精液样本中有 64.5% 存在肥大细胞，弱精子症和阴囊精索静脉曲张的男性精液标本中有 68.8% 存在肥大细胞。相比之下，正常生育对照组的精液样本仅 34.8% 存在肥大细胞[18]。

4.1.3 免疫病理学

肥大细胞已被证明会影响男性的生育能力。免疫组化研究表明，大多数男性生育障碍与大量睾丸肥大细胞有关。肥大细胞在炎症过程及可能导致器官功能障碍的纤维化中起着至关重要的作用。肥大细胞导致不育的病理生理机制如下[39,40]：①肥大细胞来源的类胰蛋白酶和组胺诱导纤维化，影响正常的精子发生。②类胰蛋白酶和糜蛋白酶诱导成纤维细胞的促有丝分裂作用，导致睾丸纤维化和胶原沉积。③管壁增厚破坏生精小管与间质之间的液体交换。④肥大细胞来源的基质金属蛋白酶（尤其是 MMP‐9）诱导纤维化。⑤核心蛋白聚糖干扰包括表皮生长因子（EGF）在内的生长因子信号转导。肥大细胞来源的类胰蛋白酶可诱导睾丸管周细胞产生核心蛋白聚糖，后者调节胶原纤维形成，并能与 TGF‐β 和血小板衍生生长因子（PDGF）结合[41]。⑥肥大细胞来源的糜蛋白酶生成血管紧张素 II，作用于管周细胞分泌促炎因子。

与正常生育对照组相比，特发性弱精症和精索静脉曲张相关的弱精症患者精液中肥大细胞显著增加[18,42]。此外，梗阻性无精症患者的肥大细胞计数和 MC_{TC}/总 MC 增加。在精索静脉曲张患者中，与对照组相比，每个生精小管的平均 MC_{TC} 显著增加[43]。精液中肥大细胞增加与精子浓度、前向精子活力和总精子数呈负相关，可能是精索静脉曲张引起不育的潜在病理生理机制[17]。精液中肥大细胞来源的介质（如类胰蛋白酶）通过激活丝裂原激活的蛋白激酶途径降低精子活力[14,44]。单侧中重度精索静脉曲张患者的精液中肥大细胞显著增加[45]，在精索静脉曲张相关不育患者中也发现了精液氧化应激[46]。精索静脉曲张程度决定了精液质量，随着精索静脉曲张严重程度升高，精液活性氧（ROS）水平增加，精液浓度降低。精液中产生的 ROS 可刺激肥大细胞脱颗粒，随后释放介质（如类胰蛋白酶和组胺）。ROS 与精子的异常形态相关，影响精子活力、DNA 完整性并加速凋亡。

4.1.4 评估和候选标志物

检测不育男性的精液中是否存在肥大细胞，可将精液滴于载玻片上进行风干固定，用 1% 甲苯胺蓝‐派若宁染色，并用油浸物镜进行评估[18]。亦可使用检测 c‐kit（CD117）表达的流式细胞术进行评估[47]。

患有以下任何情况的不育男性可能需要进行肥大细胞评估：精索静脉曲张相关的、特发性弱精子症[18]，非梗阻性无精子症[48]，吸烟[18]及年龄超过40岁[18]。

4.1.5 治疗方案

用抗蛋白酶激活受体2（抗PAR-2）抗血清和抗胰蛋白酶抗体进行预处理，或用人输卵管液（HTFM）冲洗都可逆转胰蛋白酶对精子活性的负面影响[40,49]。

如前所述，鉴于肥大细胞在男性不育中的作用，可选择使用肥大细胞稳定剂和抗组胺药。每12小时口服1 mg酮替芬（ketotifen）可显著提高不育[50,51]且无精索静脉曲张[52]男性患者的妊娠率、精子计数和活力。每日300 mg曲尼司特（tranilast）亦可提高妊娠率、精子计数和活力[53,54]。在抗组胺药中，每日10 mg依巴斯汀（ebastine）有助于提高妊娠率和精子质量[55]，而非索非那定（fexofenadine）则未显示出益处[56]。这三种药物的常见副作用主要为轻度嗜睡。表5.1总结了在少精子症和弱精子症患者中使用酮替芬、曲尼司特、依巴斯汀和非索非那定的各项研究。

表5.1 男性不育中肥大细胞稳定剂和抗组胺药的研究概述

作者	人群	研究类型	干预措施	结局
Schill[52]	17位特发性少精子症患者，精子<20×10⁶/mL；22位特发性弱精子症患者	前瞻性队列研究	酮替芬1 mg/片×2片/日×3个月	少精子症：提高精子数量和总精子产量；治疗1年后妊娠率为9%；弱精子症：前向运动精子和活动精子总数增加；治疗1年后妊娠率为20%
Azadi[50]	103位接受精索静脉曲张手术的不育男性；酮替芬组：$n=51$；对照组：$n=52$	随机对照研究	精索静脉曲张术后每12小时服用1 mg酮替芬	术后9个月的妊娠率：酮替芬：41.17%；对照组：21.15%、$P<0.05$；3个月后精子数量、精蛋白含量和DNA完整性显著改善
Zaazaa[51]	120位精索静脉曲张的不育男性	前瞻性队列研究	第1组：精索静脉曲张手术；第2组：酮替芬1 mg×每日2次×3个月；第3组：精索静脉曲张手术+酮替芬1 mg×每日2次×3个月	与单纯精索静脉曲张手术或酮替芬相比，精索静脉曲张术后+酮替芬显著改善了精子DNA碎片指数
Yamamoto[54]	50位严重少精子症患者，精子<5×10⁶/mL	安慰剂对照、单盲研究	曲尼司特300 mg/d×3个月	妊娠率曲尼司特组：28.6%；安慰剂组：0%；$P<0.05$；曲尼司特组的精子密度、精子活力和总活动精子数显著高于对照组
Hibi[53]	17位严重少精子症患者，精子<10×10⁶/mL	前瞻性队列研究	曲尼司特300 mg/d，≥12周	41.1%的患者精子数量增加，妊娠率18%
Matsuki[55]	15位特发性少精子症患者	前瞻性队列研究	依巴斯汀10 mg/d×3个月	66.7%的患者精子质量明显改善，6个月内妊娠率为20%
Cayan[56]	16位特发性无精子症或少精子症患者	前瞻性队列研究	非索非那定180 mg/d×4~9个月	无获益

然而据报道,抗组胺药对男性生殖功能有潜在的不良影响,因为这些药物可能影响睾丸稳态,降低精子活力,并减弱人类性行为和阴茎勃起[57]。

4.2 子宫内膜异位症

4.2.1 肥大细胞与子宫内膜异位症

子宫内膜异位症是育龄期女性常见的雌激素依赖性炎性疾病。其特征是子宫内膜组织在子宫外植入,导致盆腔瘢痕、疼痛和不孕[58]。近期研究表明,肥大细胞通过其介质直接抑制精子运动,并在子宫内膜异位症和不孕中发挥作用。肥大细胞相关的子宫内膜异位症可表现为子宫内膜异位症患者的宫颈刷和宫颈涂片中肥大细胞的数量增加。

Sugamata等[59]比较了有或无子宫内膜异位症的患者的子宫内膜异位病灶、在位子宫内膜和正常子宫浆膜间脱颗粒肥大细胞的形态和数量(表5.2)。在子宫内膜异位病灶的区域,观察到肥大细胞出现了脱颗粒及分散的颗粒。在有或无子宫内膜异位症的患者的在位子宫内膜和正常子宫浆膜标本中,脱颗粒肥大细胞罕见。Matsuzaki等[60]研究了腹膜子宫内膜异位病灶的肥大细胞密度。在腹膜子宫内膜异位病灶中可检测到肥大细胞,黑色病变基质中的肥大细胞密度明显高于红色病变(表5.3)。此外,子宫内膜异位症患者的腹膜红色病变和在位子宫内膜之间的肥大细胞密度存在显著差异。在腹膜子宫内膜异位症中,肥大细胞存在显著的不均匀分布。

表5.2 肥大细胞群形态和数量的比较[59]

病灶	合并子宫内膜异位症(mean±1 S.D.)	不合并子宫内膜异位症(mean±1 S.D.)
异位子宫内膜病灶	颗粒:0.69±0.72 脱颗粒:10.97±3.71 总计:11.66±4.07 肥大细胞出现脱颗粒可观察到分散的颗粒	—
在位子宫内膜	颗粒:0.82±0.97 脱颗粒:0.18±0.40 总计:1.00±1.19	颗粒:0.95±0.96 脱颗粒:0.47±0.73 总计:1.42±1.37
腹腔镜手术采集的正常浆膜标本	颗粒:0.54±0.63 脱颗粒:0.16±0.37 总计:0.70±0.86	颗粒:0.52±0.65 脱颗粒:0.16±0.42 总计:0.68±0.84

表5.3 腹膜子宫内膜异位症的肥大细胞密度[60]

项目	黑色病变	红色病变	P
肥大细胞密度	15.6%±4.9%	3.1%±1.5%	0.0002
每0.13 mm²基质的肥大细胞数	0~12	0~26	—

4.2.2 患病率

截至本书撰写,尚无关于子宫内膜异位症患者肥大细胞数量增加的患病率数据。然而,Tsuji等[61]的研究表明,与没有痛经的患者相比,所有痛经患者的宫颈刷和宫颈涂片中的肥大细胞数量均增加。

4.2.3 免疫病理学

在正常子宫内膜的月经过程中,肥大细胞促进组织脱落,并吸引其他免疫效应物进入组织参与这一过程。然而,在子宫内膜异位症患者的在位子宫内膜中,肥大细胞于整个周期内波动,表明肥大细胞的调节或功能异常[58],尽管存在相互矛盾的研究报道[58-60]。子宫内膜异位症病灶中肥大细胞数量增加,通过释放促炎因子加剧炎症,从而增加其他免疫效应物对病灶的浸润[58]。现已证实在子宫内膜异位症患者中存在肥大细胞及其主要介质类胰蛋白酶,腹腔液中的肥大细胞与精子相互作用导致肥大细胞脱颗粒,可直接调节精子功能[62]。相反,肥大细胞可能在子宫内膜异位症的发展中发挥作用。在子宫内膜异位症的发展过程中,业已证明了子宫内膜细胞与肥大细胞间通过CCL8/CCR1发生交互对话[28]。

4.2.4 评估

出现子宫内膜异位症症状的患者,如痛经和性交困难,可能是需评估的对象。

痛经患者和子宫内膜异位症患者的宫颈刷和宫颈涂片可使用亚甲基蓝染色检测肥大细胞。痛经组和对照组的肥大细胞数量存在显著差异(痛经组中位数35,四分位数范围17~58;对照组中位数2,四分位数范围0~6)[61]。亦可检测腹腔液中是否存在肥大细胞[62]和IL-25水平[63]。

4.2.5 治疗方案

在子宫内膜异位症的动物模型中,靶向肥大细胞的抑制剂,如扎鲁司特(zafirlukast)、色氨酸钠、JAK2抑制剂tyrphostin和超微粉化棕榈酰乙醇胺显示了良好的结果。酮替芬(ketotifen)通过调节肥大细胞活性显著抑制痛觉过敏,减少大鼠子宫内膜异位病灶的有害信号所致的外周敏化[64]。一些小型临床试验（4～30位参与者）表明，棕榈酰乙醇胺、白藜芦醇苷和左炔诺孕酮宫内系统在减少肥大细胞数量及痛经、性交困难和盆腔疼痛等方面具有良好效果[65]。

4.3 反复妊娠丢失

4.3.1 肥大细胞与反复妊娠丢失

据报道，有妊娠丢失史的患者子宫内膜各层存在肥大细胞积聚[40]。此外，反复妊娠丢失患者的黄体中期子宫内膜肥大细胞增加。Derbala等[66]认为，根据子宫内膜基因表达测序，可将肥大细胞相关的反复妊娠丢失定义为连续两次或两次以上妊娠丢失，且子宫内膜组织SCF>0.0418、类胰蛋白酶>0.0035、基质金属蛋白酶（MMP2）>0.1534及硫酸乙酰肝素>0.0121。然而，该结论尚未得到其他研究的证实。

4.3.2 患病率

迄今为止，没有关于反复妊娠丢失患者肥大细胞病理改变的患病率数据。

4.3.3 免疫病理学

尽管肥大细胞通过释放组胺在胚胎种植过程的组织重塑中发挥积极作用，但据推测，肥大细胞在妊娠后期具有消极影响，其激活的增加与早产相关[33]。小鼠肥大细胞缺乏与严重的胚胎植入受损有关，可通过全身或局部过继骨髓来源的肥大细胞予以纠正[67]。肥大细胞还与螺旋动脉重塑受损导致的血流减少有关，引起宫内生长受限[68]。此外，易流产小鼠的子宫中肥大细胞数量不足，过继转移Tregs可通过增强螺旋动脉重塑和胎盘发育以防止妊娠丢失[69]。

肥大细胞存在于子宫内膜的不同组织层。在反复妊娠丢失患者的子宫内膜中，肥大细胞计数和各种介质（如SCF、类胰蛋白酶、硫酸乙酰肝素和MMP-2）的mRNA表达与正常生育对照组相比显著增加。在黄体中期，即种植窗，肥大细胞计数和活性增加[66]。此外，在对妊娠早期流产的患者研究中发现，其宫颈中存在胶原蛋白骨架组织紊乱、反应性成纤维细胞，且肥大细胞数量增加。这表明，流产患者的宫颈内发生了炎症样反应[70]。

压力能触发促肾上腺皮质激素释放激素（CRH）的分泌，激活下丘脑-垂体-肾上腺轴，可能引起自然流产。除了下丘脑外，CRH及其类似物尿皮质素（Ucn）亦在大脑外局部分泌，并可激活肥大细胞，导致炎症。Ucn、类胰蛋白酶（肥大细胞分泌的介质）和IL-8在至少两次自然流产患者的妊娠组织中显著高于仅一次自然流产和选择性流产的患者。因此，反复妊娠丢失患者的高应激水平引起的CRH和Ucn分泌增加可能会激活子宫肥大细胞，分泌促流产的类胰蛋白酶和IL-8[71]。

由问卷评估的感知压力评分与蜕膜基底层中含类胰蛋白酶的肥大细胞（MC_T）及分泌TNF-α的$CD8^+$T细胞的数量呈正相关[72]。除了炎性细胞因子的分泌，肥大细胞中类胰蛋白酶的释放可能对妊娠造成额外的危害。胰蛋白酶裂解蛋白酶激活受体2（PAR-2）并诱导广泛炎症。表达PAR-2的初级脊髓传入神经元含有促炎性神经肽P物质。胰蛋白酶促使神经元刺激这些神经肽的释放，从而介导炎症水肿。这些机制有助于应激触发肥大细胞在流产患者子宫蜕膜中的促炎效应[73]。

4.3.4 评估

经超声或生化检测证实有两次或两次以上临床妊娠丢失的患者，初筛时未发现病因，如染色体异常、解剖缺陷、内分泌失调、自身免疫性疾病和伴有静脉血栓栓塞个人或家族史的易栓症（遗传或获得性），可考虑评估肥大细胞相关的反复妊娠丢失（基于Derbala等[66]的研究）。然而，尚无关于临床应用的特定检测方法的报道。

根据Derbala等[66]的研究，在排卵后5～7天或黄体中期进行子宫内膜活检以评估子宫内膜的肥大细胞。可使用c-kit单克隆抗体和肥大细胞类胰蛋白酶抗体对连续切片进行染色以检测肥大细胞的表面（c-kit）和活化（类胰蛋白酶）标志物。需注意免疫染色强度分级和每平方毫米阳性细胞的数量。该方法基于Derbala的反复妊娠丢失与正常生育对照组之间的对比研究。

4.3.5 治疗方案

目前尚无临床试验报告，需进一步研究。

4.4 肥大细胞与体外受精-胚胎移植失败

组胺是肥大细胞释放的一种介质，可能在体外受精-胚胎移植（ET）及冷冻胚胎移植周期的种植失败中发挥作用。过量的组胺可能会增强Th1反应，并在胚胎种植前抑制Th2反应，导致免疫排斥和种植失败[40]。然而，关于辅助生殖技术中肥大细胞与种植失败之间关系的研究仍十分有限。

4.5 肥大细胞活化疾病

4.5.1 定义

肥大细胞活化疾病(mast cell activation disease, MCAD)是一组以病理性肥大细胞在任何或所有器官和组织中积聚和(或)可变肥大细胞介质异常释放为特征的疾病。MCAD 包括肥大细胞增多症、肥大细胞活化综合征(mast cell activation syndrome, MCAS)和肥大细胞白血病(mast cell leukemia, MCL)。

肥大细胞增多症是一种罕见的疾病,其特征是肥大细胞在器官中克隆性增殖和积聚。在皮肤肥大细胞增多症(cutaneous mastocytosis, CM)中,肥大细胞的皮肤积聚增加,且仅限于皮肤。皮肤外组织受累则引起系统性肥大细胞增多症(systemic matocytosis, SM),这是由于应激、感染、药物等多种刺激引起的肥大细胞介质释放所致。MCAS 亦是一种罕见的疾病,定义为肥大细胞活化引起的急性和(或)慢性症状,在基线或急性发作期间,肥大细胞介质增加,而无肥大细胞增生[74]。患者不仅有过敏反应,还有其他炎性和(或)过敏性合并症,且有肥大细胞活化的实验室证据,但没有其他明确的诊断(如肥大细胞增多症),可诊断为 MCAS。MCL 是一种侵袭性肥大细胞肿瘤,定义为骨髓涂片中的肥大细胞数量增加(>20%)且存在循环肥大细胞。据报道,肥大细胞增多症可累及生殖道,特别是子宫和宫颈[75,76]。

4.5.2 患病率

关于 MCAD 患病率的数据很少。SM 和 MCL 都是罕见的疾病。肥大细胞增多症的确切发病率和患病率因其罕见而无具体数据。在西欧人群中,发病率为(5~10)/1 000 000,患病率为(5~13)/1 000 000[77,78]。CM 比 SM 的数量约为 10∶1。在其所有类型中,估计患病率为 1/10 000,而成年后女性略占优势。相比之下,MCAS 似乎更为常见。目前仅有 MCAS 的初步数据。有证据表明 MCAS 可能是各种临床表现的潜在原因。因此,MCAS 的患病率可能在个位数百分比范围内。MCAS 中亦可观察到女性略占优势(3∶1)。

欧洲肥大细胞增多症网络追踪了 23 位肥大细胞增多症患者,记录到了 5 次自然流产和 4 次早产,其中一次是 26 周时发生子痫前期,导致新生儿死亡[79]。

4.5.3 免疫病理学

肥大细胞疾病(如 MCAS)患者可表现为子宫内膜异位症、不孕和流产等生殖功能障碍。这些最有可能是由于肥大细胞释放的炎性和(或)纤维化介质所致[66,80]。

约 20% 的肥大细胞增多症孕妇报告了疾病相关症状恶化,30% 的孕妇在妊娠早期出现临床症状改善,另外 50% 的孕妇没有出现肥大细胞介质相关的症状。当 T 辅助因子 1(Th1)介导的促炎环境占主导时,在妊娠早期或晚期亦观察到症状恶化[81]。妊娠和分娩期间的许多生理变化也会触发多种应激源,这些应激源会加重肥大细胞增多症的症状。反过来,组胺水平升高可能引起子宫收缩,导致肥大细胞增多症患者早产,增加其他产科并发症的风险。据报道,肥大细胞增多症患者出现了自然流产、早产、新生儿死亡以及因过敏反应导致胎儿死亡的罕见病例[79,82,83]。另有一例患有肥大细胞增多症的患者分娩的新生儿发生 CM[79]。

4.5.4 评估

具有流产、不孕症和子宫内膜异位症病史,并伴随肥大细胞活化相关体征和症状的患者,如反复不明原因的过敏反应、潮红、骨质疏松、溃疡性肠胃疾病、慢性腹部疼挛、特发性性交困难、功能失调性子宫出血、生殖道炎症或多系统炎症/过敏/生长问题,需筛查 MCAD。

由于 MCAD 倾向于影响免疫系统,包括诱导自身免疫,MCAD 患者发生特发性流产应立即进行抗磷脂抗体综合征(MCAS 源性抗磷脂抗体综合征)检测[84]。尽管肥大细胞含有肝素,但 MCAD 诱导的凝血功能紊乱可能会刺激胎盘微血栓,妨碍胎盘形成,扰乱胚胎血供,导致流产[78]。如表 5.4 和表 5.5 所示,肥大细胞增多症的诊断和分类基于世界卫生组织制定的标准。

表 5.4 世界卫生组织的肥大细胞增多症临床分型[85,86]

(1) 皮肤肥大细胞增多症(CM):
A. 色素性荨麻疹(UP)/斑丘疹型皮肤肥大细胞增多症(MPCM);
B. 弥漫性皮肤肥大细胞增多症;
C. 皮肤孤立性肥大细胞瘤

(2) 惰性系统性肥大细胞增多症(ISM)
-符合系统性肥大细胞增多症(SM)的标准[a]。没有"C"项所见[a]。
没有相关血液肿瘤的证据。
-分离的骨髓肥大细胞增多症[b]。
符合 ISM 标准,但骨髓受累,无皮肤受累,肥大细胞负荷一般较低

(续表)

(3) 冒烟型系统性肥大细胞增多症(SSM)
符合 ISM 标准,有 2 项或 2 项以上"B"项所见,但没有"C"项所见[1],肥大细胞负荷一般较高

(4) 系统性肥大细胞增多症伴相关造血肿瘤(SM-AHN)
-符合 SM 标准,符合世界卫生组织分类中独特类型的AHN 标准

(5) 侵袭性系统性肥大细胞增多症(ASM)
-符合 SM 标准,有 1 项或 1 项以上"C"项所见[a]。没有MCL 证据

(6) 肥大细胞白血病(MCL)
-符合 SM 标准,骨髓活检显示不典型的未成熟肥大细胞弥漫性浸润,通常是致密的。
骨髓穿刺涂片显示≥20%的肥大细胞。在经典病例中,肥大细胞占外周血白细胞≥10%。非白血病 MCL(<10%循环肥大细胞)

(7) 肥大细胞肉瘤(MCS)
-没有 SM 证据,呈局部破坏性生长模式。细胞形态高度不典型

注:[a] SM 的诊断标准及"B"项和"C"项的定义见表 5.5。
[b] 暂定类别。

表 5.5 世界卫生组织的系统性肥大细胞增多症诊断标准[85,86]

确诊 SM 需符合主要标准和 1 个次要标准,或至少 3 个次要标准

主要标准
在骨髓和(或)其他皮肤外器官的切片中检测到多灶性、密集的肥大细胞浸润(呈集簇状存在的肥大细胞≥15 个)

次要标准
(1) 在骨髓或其他皮肤外器官的活检切片中,>25%的浸润肥大细胞呈梭形或形态不典型,或骨髓穿刺涂片所有肥大细胞中>25%为未成熟或不典型。
(2) 骨髓、血液或其他皮肤外器官中 KIT 基因 816 位密码子的活化位点突变。
(3) 骨髓、血液或其他皮肤外器官中的肥大细胞除表达正常肥大细胞标志物外,还表达 CD25 和(或)CD2[a]。
(4) 血清总类胰蛋白酶持续>20 ng/mL(除非合并相关的髓系肿瘤,此时该参数无效)

"B"项所见
(1) 骨髓活检显示肥大细胞高负荷:肥大细胞(局灶性、紧密聚集)浸润>30%,和(或)血清总类胰蛋白酶>200 ng/mL。
(2) 非肥大细胞系中出现发育异常或骨髓增生征象,但诊断相关血液肿瘤(AHN)的条件不足,血细胞计数正常或仅轻度异常。
(3) 肝脏肿大,无肝功能损害,可触摸的脾肿大,无脾功能亢进,和(或)触诊或影像学发现淋巴结肿大

(续表)

"C"项所见
(1) 肿瘤性肥大细胞浸润引起的骨髓功能障碍,表现为一系或多系细胞减少[ANC<$1.0×10^9$/L,Hgb<10 g/dL,和(或)血小板计数<$100×10^9$/L]。
(2) 可触及的肝肿大伴肝功能损害,腹水和(或)门静脉高压。
(3) 骨骼受累,大的溶骨性病变,伴或不伴病理性骨折(骨质疏松导致的病理性骨折不属于"C"项所见)。
(4) 可触及脾肿大伴脾功能亢进。
(5) 胃肠道肥大细胞浸润导致的吸收不良和体重减轻

注:[a] 肥大细胞的 CD25 是流式细胞术和免疫组化检测的更敏感的标志物。
ANC,中性粒细胞计数;Hgb,血红蛋白;ng,纳克;mL,毫升;L,升;dL,分升。

4.5.5 治疗方案

MCAD 的治疗包括识别触发因素、避免和控制肥大细胞介质的产生及活性。阻断介质增多可能会有所帮助。可以考虑使用强效或慢作用免疫抑制剂。H1 抗组胺药、色甘酸钠、奥马珠单抗(omalizumab)、类固醇、白三烯受体拮抗剂以及干扰素 α2b 等细胞减量疗法可减少 MCAD 相关并发症[82,87]。

综合报道显示组胺 H1 和 H2 受体阻滞剂在妊娠期是安全的[84],但尚无对妊娠期 MCAD 人群进行药物安全性研究。糖皮质激素有助于控制疾病加重,但慢性毒性限制了它们的使用。抗 IgE 单克隆抗体奥马珠单抗在多个病例报道中显示对 MCAD 安全有效[88]。对于肥大细胞增多症临床症状严重的患者,需服用细胞减量药物,其中包括干扰素-α(IFN-α)和克拉屈滨(cladribine),通常与糖皮质激素联合使用[89-91]。在 5 位慢性特发性性交困难、功能失调性子宫出血和生殖器感染的MCAS 患者中报道了肥大细胞靶向治疗的成功案例[92]。

妊娠期肥大细胞增多症患者通常需要继续服用药物,包括抗组胺药。然而,由于胎儿安全性问题,药物剂量通常会减少。而这种药物减量,有时再加上不规律的药物摄入,可能导致肥大细胞增多症的症状恶化。未经诊断和治疗不当的肥大细胞增多症可导致严重的妊娠并发症,包括胎儿死亡[93]。

接受剖宫产的肥大细胞增多症患者是一个特别的挑战。由于麻醉存在诱发过敏反应的风险,分娩期间可能会发生危及生命的并发症。因此,在分娩

和产后,应始终提供紧急药物,如肾上腺素、抗组胺药和糖皮质激素。

除了上述个性化的治疗外,成人 SM 的治疗也是以症状为导向。表 5.6 列出了各类治疗方案[86]。

表 5.6 系统性肥大细胞增多症的治疗方案

惰性/冒烟型系统性肥大细胞增多症	侵袭性系统性肥大细胞增多症	系统性肥大细胞增多症伴相关造血肿瘤
避免触发肥大细胞脱颗粒(如阿司匹林、镇静剂、酒精、麻醉剂); 肥大细胞脱颗粒症状(症状负荷的评估,治疗方案包括肾上腺素、皮质类固醇、组胺 H1/H2 阻断剂、色甘酸钠、白三烯抑制剂、外用药物、阿司匹林、酮替芬、奥马珠单抗,严重/难治性病例中考虑肥大细胞的细胞减量疗法); 骨质疏松症/骨质减少(骨密度评估、钙和维生素 D 补充、双磷酸盐、地舒单抗、干扰素-α、椎体成形术/后凸成形术); 围手术期管理(参考专业文献,咨询麻醉和外科团队,审查先前的麻醉记录,使用"更安全"的药物)	临床试验(高效、选择性 KIT 突变激酶抑制剂,如阿伐替尼); midostaurin 或 cladribine(若需快速去除肥大细胞,首选 cladribin,而 midostaulin 在移植后起维持作用); 伊马替尼(FIP1L1-PGFRA 或 KITD816V 阴性的嗜酸性粒细胞增多症); 干扰素-α(聚乙二醇化形式可能耐受性更好,伴或不伴强的松); 异基因干细胞移植(难治性/复发性疾病)	整合临床、组织学和分子数据,以评估哪些疾病(即 SM 或 AHN)需立即治疗; 对于侵袭性 AHN(具有低负荷或偶然发现的 SM)(对于 AML 或低风险 CMML,按标准方案治疗 AHN,如 AML,同种异体干细胞移植,并管理 SM 的症状); 对于 SM 引起的器官病(惰性 AHN)(对于侵袭性 SM,惰性 AHN 如 PV 或 ET,观察或按标准方案治疗); 疾病进展(重新评估疾病进展的主要构成——SM vs AHN,适当的挽救治疗,包括同种异体干细胞移植,分子评估以指导靶向治疗)

5 总结和建议

- 肥大细胞除了在过敏性疾病中发挥功能外,在生殖方面也具有重要作用。
- 肥大细胞释放预合成和新合成的介质参与诸多生理过程,如男性生殖道的类固醇生成和精子生成,以及女性生殖道的排卵、胚胎种植、蜕膜化、胎盘形成、胎儿发育和分娩。
- 男性睾丸和精液中肥大细胞数量增加、肥大细胞释放的类胰蛋白酶水平升高与男性不育和精子运动障碍有关。
- 肥大细胞稳定剂和抗组胺药的使用已成为男性生育障碍的潜在治疗选择。
- 肥大细胞在胚胎种植过程中具有积极作用,肥大细胞缺乏与严重的胚胎种植和螺旋动脉重塑受损相关,可导致宫内生长受限。
- 肥大细胞活性增加与早产有关。
- 在反复妊娠丢失患者中观察到肥大细胞计数升高及各种肥大细胞炎症介质 mRNA 表达增加。
- 组胺水平过高可能会导致体外受精(in vitro fertilization,IVF)失败。
- 肥大细胞疾病患者(如肥大细胞增多症、MCAS)可能有生殖障碍的临床表现,如子宫内膜异位症、不孕、早产和自然流产。
- H1 抗组胺药、色甘酸钠、奥马珠单抗、类固醇、白三烯受体拮抗剂和细胞减量疗法可减少肥大细胞障碍患者的妊娠并发症。

参考文献

[1] Beaven MA. Our perception of the mast cell from Paul Ehrlich to now. Eur J Immunol 2009;39(1):11-25. Available from: https://ncbi.nlm.nih.gov/pubmed/19130582 Accessed April 21,2021.

[2] Yong L. The mast cell: origin, morphology, distribution, and function. Exp Toxicol Pathol 1997;49(6):409-24. Available from: https://doi.org/10.1016/s0940-2993(97)80129-7.

[3] Abraham St S, John A. Mast cell-orchestrated immunity to pathogens. Nat Rev Immunol 2010;10(6):440-52. Available from: https://doi.org/10.1038/nri2782.

[4] Dahlin JS, Hallgren J. Mast cell progenitors: origin, development and migration to tissues. Molecular Immunology. Mol Immunol 2015;63(1):9-17. Available from: https://sciencedirect.com/science/article/pii/s0161589014000340 Accessed April 24,2021.

[5] Sivridis E, Giatromanolaki A, Agnantis E, Anastasiadis P. Mast cell distribution and density in the normaluterus Ð metachromatic staining using lectins. Eur J Obstet Gynecol Reprod Biol 2001;98:109-13. Available from: https://doi.org/10.1016/s0301-2115(00)00564-9.

[6] Gilfillan A. M., Tkaczyk C. Integrated signalling pathways

[7] Razin E, Ihle J, Seldin D, Menchia-Huerta J. Interleukin 3: a differentiation and growth factor for the mouse mast cell that contains chondroitin sulfate E proteoglycan. J Immunol 1984; 132(3): 1479-86. Available from: http://www.jimmunol.org/cgi/pmidlookup?view=long&pmid=6198393 Accessed April 24, 2021.

[8] Abbas AK, Lichtman AH, Pillai S. Cellular and Molecular Immunology. Elsevier; 2011.

[9] Bradding PA. Biology of mast cells and their mediators. Middleton's Allergy Principles and Practice. 9th (ed.) Edinburgh London New York Oxford Philadelphia St Louis Sydney: Elsevier; 2020. p.215-35.

[10] Hogan AD, Schwartz L. B. Markers of mast cell degranulation. Methods. 13(1):45-52. https://doi.org/10.1006/meth.1997.0494.

[11] Ho LH, Ruffin RE, Murgia C, Li L, Krilis SA, Zalewski PD. Labile zinc and zinc transporter ZnT4 in mast cell granules: role in regulation of caspase activation and NF-kappaB translocation. J Immunol 2004; 172(12): 7750-68. Available from: https://doi.org/10.4049/jimmunol.172.12.7750.

[12] Murphy K. M. In: Janeway's Immunobiology. https://books.google.com/?id=WDMmAgAAQBAJ&dq=janeway+immunobiology.

[13] Duan L., Mukherjee E. Janeway's immunobiology. 9th (ed.). Yale Journal of Biology and Medicine; 2016. http://europepmc.org/articles/pmc5045153 [accessed 25.04.21].

[14] Haidl G, Duan Y, Chen S, Kohn F, Schuppe H, Allam JP. The role of mast cells in male infertility. Exp Rev Clin Immunol 2011;7(5): 627-34. Available from: https://doi.org/10.1586/eci.11.57.

[15] Nistal M, Santamaria L, Paniagua R. Mast cells in the human testis and epididymis from birth to adulthood. Acta Anat 1984;119:155-60.

[16] Jezek D, Banek L, Hittmair A, Pezerovic-Panijan R, Goluza T, Schulze W. Mast cells in testicular biopsies of infertile men with 'mixed atrophy' of seminiferous tubules. Andrologia. 1999;31:2013-210.

[17] Cincik M, Sezen SC. The mast cells in semen: their effects on sperm motility. Arch Androl 2003;49(4):307-11.

[18] El-Karasky A, Mostafa T, Shaeer O, Bahgat D, Samir N. Seminal mast cells in infertile asthenozoospermic males. Andrologia. 2007;39(6):244-7.

[19] Heider U, Pedal I, Spanel-Borowski K. Increase in nerve fibers and loss of mast cells in polycystic and postmenopausal ovaries. Fertil Steril 2001;75(6):1141-7. Available from: https://doi.org/10.1016/S0015-0282(01)01805-2.

[20] Jensen F, Woudwyk M, Teles A, et al. Estradiol and progesterone regulate the migration of mast cells from the periphery to the uterus and induce their maturation and degranulation. PLoS ONE 2010; 5(12). Available from: https://doi.org/10.1371/journal.pone.0014409.

[21] Garfield RE, Irani AM, Schwartz LB, Bytautiene E, Romero R. Structural and functional comparison of mast cells in the pregnant vs nonpregnant human uterus. Am J Obstet Gynecol 2006;194(1): 261-7. Available from: https://doi.org/10.1016/j.ajog.2005.05.011.

[22] Mitani R, Maeda K, Fukui R, et al. Production of human mast cell chymase in human myometrium and placenta in cases of normal pregnancy and preeclampsia. Eur J Obstet Gynecol Reprod Biol 2002; 101(12): 155-60. Available from: https://doi.org/10.1016/S0301-2115(01)00546-2.

[23] Robinson-White A, Beaven MA. Presence of histamine and histamine-metabolizing enzyme in rat and guinea-pig microvascular endothelial cells. J Pharmacol Exp Ther 1982; 223(2):440-5.

[24] Schrey MP, Hare AL, Ilson SL, Walters MP. Decidual histamine release and amplification of prostaglandin F2α production by histamine in interleukin-1 β-primed decidual cells: potential interactive role for inflammatory mediators in uterine function at term. J Clin Endocrinol Metab 1995; 80(2): 648-53. Available from: https://doi.org/10.1210/jcem.80.2.7531717.

[25] Okada Y., Asahina T., Kobayashi T., Goto J., Terao T. Studies on the mechanism of edematous changes at the endometrial stroma for implantation. Semin Thromb Hemost. 27(2):67-68. https://doi.org/10.1055/s-2001-14063.

[26] Hannan NJ, Jones RL, White CA, Salamonsen LA. The chemokines, CX3CL1, CCL14, and CCL4, promote human trophoblast migration at the feto-maternal interface. Biol Reprod 2006;74(5):896-904. Available from: https://doi.org/10.1095/biolreprod.105.045518.

[27] Red-Horse K, Drake PM, Fisher SJ. Human pregnancy: the role of chemokine networks at the fetal-maternal interface. Expert Rev Mol Med 2004; 6(11): 1-14. Available from: https://doi.org/10.1017/S1462399404007720.

[28] Li T, Wang J, Guo X, et al. Possible involvement of crosstalk between endometrial cells and mast cells in the development of endometriosis via CCL8/CCR1. Biomed Pharmacother 2020; 129(110476). Available from: https://doi.org/10.1016/j.biopha.2020.110476.

[29] Anaf V, Chapron C, El Nakadi I, De Moor V, Simonart T, Noël J-C. Pain, mast cells, and nerves in peritoneal, ovarian, and deep infiltrating endometriosis. Fertil Steril 2006;86(5): 1336-43. Available from: https://doi.org/10.1016/j.fertnstert.2006.03.057.

[30] Amsalem H, Kwan M, Hazan A, et al. Identification of a novel neutrophil population: proangiogenic granulocytes in second-trimester human decidua. J Immunol 2014; 193(6): 3070-9. Available from: https://doi.org/10.4049/jimmunol.1303117.

[31] Popovic M, Teles A, Stancic O, Volk HD, Zenclussen AC. Mast-cell-associated genes Thp1, Mcpt1 and Mcpt5 are up-regulated after Treg-induced tolerance at the fetal-maternal interface: new role for mast cells in tolerance? J Reprod Immunol 2007;75(1):A16. Available from: https://doi.org/10.1016/j.jri.2007.06.043.

[32] Ueshima C, Kataoka TR, Hirata M, et al. Possible involvement of human mast cells in the establishment of pregnancy via killer cell Ig-like receptor 2DL4. Am J Pathol 2018;188(6): 1497-508. Available from: https://doi.org/10.1016/j.ajpath.2018.02.012.

[33] Woidacki K, Jensen F, Zenclussen AC. Mast cells as novel mediators of reproductive processes. Front Immunol 2013;4 (FRB): 29. Available from: https://doi.org/10.3389/fimmu.2013.00029.

[34] Liu Z, Kilburn B, Leach R, Romero R, Paria B, Armant DR. Histamine enhances cytotrophoblast invasion by inducing intracellular calcium transients through the histamine type-1 receptor. Mol Reprod Dev 2004; 68: 345-53. Available from: https://doi.org/10.1002/mrd.20082.

[35] Szewczyk G, Pyzlak M, Smierta W, Klimkiewicz J,

[35] Szukiewicz D. Histamine stimulates av-b3 integrin expression of the human trophoblast through the H1 receptor. Inflamm Res 2006;55:79-80.

[36] Pyzlak M, Szewczyk G, Szukiewicz D. Histamine influence on apoptosis in trophoblast cell cultures. Inflamm Res 2010;59:213-15. Available from: https://doi.org/10.1007/s00011-009-0133-4.

[37] Bollopragada S, Youssef R, Jordan F, Greer I, Norman J, Nelson S. Term labor is associated with a core inflammatory response in human fetal membranes, myometrium, and cervix. Am J Obstet Gynecol 2009;200(1):104.e1-104.e11. Available from: https://doi.org/10.1016/j.ajog.2008.08.032.

[38] Dey P, Ray R. Quantitative analysis of mast cells in testicular aspiration cytology smears in azoospermic males. Diagn Cytopathol 1993;9(6):685-6. Available from: https://doi.org/10.1002/dc.2840090617.

[39] Albrecht M, Ramsch R, Kohn F, Schwarzer J, Mayerhofer A. Isolation and cultivation of human testicular peritubular cells: a new model for the investigation of fibrotic processes in the human testis and male infertility. J Clin Endocrinol Metab 2006;91(5):1956-69. Available from: https://doi.org/10.1210/jc.2005-2169.

[40] Elich Ali Komi D, Shafaghat F, Haidl G. Significance of mast cells in spermatogenesis, implantation, pregnancy, and abortion: cross talk and molecular mechanisms. Am J Reprod Immunol N Y N 1989 2020;83(5):e13228. Available from: https://doi.org/10.1111/aji.13228.

[41] Adam M, Schwarzer J, Kohn F, Strauss L, Poutanen M, Mayerhofer A. Mast cell tryptase stimulates production of decorin by human testicular peritubular cells: possible role of decorin in male infertility by interfering with growth factor signaling. Hum Reprod Oxf Engl 2011;26(10):2613-25. Available from: https://doi.org/10.1093/humrep/der245.

[42] Agrawal S, Alvin J. Mast cells and idiopathic male infertility. Int J Fertil 1987;32:283-6.

[43] Yamanaka K, Fujisawa M, Tanaka H, Okada H, Arakawa S, Kamidono S. Significance of human testicular mast cells and their subtypes in male infertility. Hum Reprod 2000;15:1543-7. Available from: https://doi.org/10.1093/humrep/15.7.1543.

[44] Weidinger S, Mayerhofer A, Kunz L. Tryptase inhibits motility of human spermatozoa mainly by activation of the mitogen-activated protein kinase pathway. Hum Reprod 2005;20:456-61. Available from: https://doi.org/10.1093/humrep/deh618.

[45] Mostafa R, Abol-Magd R, Younis S, Dessouki O, Azab M, Mostafa T. Assessment of seminal mast cells in infertile men with varicocele after surgical repair. Andrologia. 2017;49(3):e12625. Available from: https://doi.org/10.1111/and.13756.

[46] Mostafa T, Rashed L, Nabil N, Osman I, Mostafa R, Farag M. Seminal miRNA relationship with apoptotic markers and oxidative stress in infertile men with varicocele. Biomed Res Int 2016;2016. Available from: https://doi.org/10.1155/2016/4302754.

[47] Allam J-P, Langer M, Fathy A, et al. Mast cells in the seminal plasma of infertile men as detected by flow cytometry. Andrologia. 2009;41(1):1-6. Available from: https://doi.org/10.1111/j.1439-0272.2008.00879.x.

[48] Abdel-Hamid AAM, Atef H, Zalata KR, Abdel-Latif A. Correlation between testicular mast cell count and spermatogenic epithelium in non-obstructive azoospermia. Int J Exp Pathol 2018;99(1):22-8. Available from: https://doi.org/10.1111/iep.12261.

[49] Weidinger S, Mayerhofer A, Frungieri MB, Meineke V, Ring J, Kohn FM. Mast cell-sperm interaction: evidence for tryptase and proteinase-activated receptors in the regulation of sperm motility. Hum Reprod Oxf Engl 2003;18(12):2519-24. Available from: https://doi.org/10.1093/humrep/deg476.

[50] Azadi L, Abbasi H, Deemeh MR, et al. Zaditen (Ketotifen), as mast cell blocker, improves sperm quality, chromatin integrity and pregnancy rate after varicocelectomy. Int J Androl 2011;34(5 Pt 1):446-52. Available from: https://doi.org/10.1111/j.1365-2605.2010.01112.x.

[51] Zaazaa A, Adel A, Fahmy I, Elkhiat Y, Awaad AA, Mostafa T. Effect of varicocelectomy and/or mast cells stabilizer on sperm DNA fragmentation in infertile patients with varicocele. Andrology 2018;6(1):146-50. Available from: https://doi.org/10.1111/andr.12445.

[52] Schill WB, Schneider J, Ring J. The use of ketotifen, a mast cell blocker, for treatment of oligo- and asthenozoospermia. Andrologia. 1986;18(6):570-3. Available from: https://doi.org/10.1111/j.1439-0272.1986.tb01831.x.

[53] Hibi H, Kato K, Mitsui K, et al. The treatment with tranilast, a mast cell blocker, for idiopathic oligozoospermia. Arch Androl 2001;47(2):107-11. Available from: https://doi.org/10.1080/014850101316901307.

[54] Yamamoto M, Hibi H, Miyake K. New treatment of idiopathic severe oligozoospermia with mast cell blocker: results of a single-blind study. Fertil Steril 1995;64(6):1221-3. Available from: https://doi.org/10.1016/s0015-0282(16)57992-8.

[55] Matsuki S, Sasagawa I, Suzuki Y. The use of ebastine, a mast cell blocker, for treatment of oligozoospermia. Arch Androl 2000;44(2):129-32. Available from: https://doi.org/10.1080/014850100262290.

[56] Cayan S, Apa DD, Akbay E. Effect of fexofenadine, a mast cell blocker, in infertile men with significantly increased testicular mast cells. Asian J Androl 2002;4(4):291-4.

[57] Mondillo C, Varela ML, Abiuso AMB, Vázquez R. Potential negative effects of anti-histamines on male reproductive function. Reprod Camb Engl 2018;155(5):R221-7. Available from: https://doi.org/10.1530/REP-17-0685.

[58] Vallvé-Juanico J, Houshdaran S, Giudice LC. The endometrial immune environment of women with endometriosis. Hum Reprod Update 2019;25(5):564-91. Available from: https://doi.org/10.1093/humupd/dmz018.

[59] Sugamata M, Ihara T, Uchiide I. Increase of activated mast cells in human endometriosis. Am J Reprod Immunol 2005;53(3):120-5. Available from: https://doi.org/10.1111/j.1600-0897.2005.00254.x.

[60] Matsuzaki S, Canis M, Darcha C, Fukaya T, Yajima A, Bruhat MA. Increased mast cell density in peritoneal endometriosis compared with eutopic endometrium with endometriosis. Am J Reprod Immunol 1998;40(4):291-4. Available from: https://doi.org/10.1111/j.1600-0897.1998.tb00420.x.

[61] Tsuji S, Tsuji K, Otsuka H, Murakami T. Increased mast cells in endocervical smears of women with dysmenorrhea. CytoJournal. 2018;15:27. Available from: https://doi.org/10.4103/cytojournal.cytojournal_54_17.

[62] Borelli V, Martinelli M, Luppi S, et al. Mast cells in peritoneal fluid from women with endometriosis and their

[62] possible role in modulating sperm function. Front Physiol 2019;10:1543. Available from: https://doi.org/10.3389/fphys.2019.01543.

[63] Bungum HF, Nygaard U, Vestergaard C, Martensen PM, Knudsen UB. Increased IL-25 levels in the peritoneal fluid of patients with endometriosis. J Reprod Immunol 2016;114:6-9. Available from: https://doi.org/10.1016/j.jri.2016.01.003.

[64] Zhu T-H, Zou G, Ding S-J, et al. Mast cell stabilizer ketotifen reduces hyperalgesia in a rodent model of surgically induced endometriosis. J Pain Res 2019;12:1359-69. Available from: https://doi.org/10.2147/JPR.S195909.

[65] Binda MM, Donnez J, Dolmans M-M. Targeting mast cells: a new way to treat endometriosis. Expert Opin Ther Targets 2017;21(1):67-75. Available from: https://doi.org/10.1080/14728222.2017.1260548.

[66] Derbala Y, Elazzamy H, Bilal M, et al. Mast cell-induced immunopathology in recurrent pregnancy losses. Am J Reprod Immunol N Y N 1989 2019;82(1):e13128. Available from: https://doi.org/10.1111/aji.13128.

[67] Woidacki K, Popovic M, Metz M, et al. Mast cells rescue implantation defects caused by c-kit deficiency. Cell Death Dis 2013;4:e462. Available from: https://doi.org/10.1038/cddis.2012.214.

[68] Meyer N, Schüler T, Zenclussen AC. Simultaneous ablation of uterine natural killer cells and uterine mast cells in mice leads to poor vascularization and abnormal doppler measurements that compromise fetal well-being. Front Immunol 2017;8:1913. Available from: https://doi.org/10.3389/fimmu.2017.01913.

[69] Woidacki K, Meyer N, Schumacher A, Goldschmidt A, Maurer M, Zenclussen AC. Transfer of regulatory T cells into abortion-prone mice promotes the expansion of uterine mast cells and normalizes early pregnancy angiogenesis. Sci Rep 2015;5:13938. Available from: https://doi.org/10.1038/srep13938.

[70] Radulovic NV, Ekerhovd E, Abrahamsson G, Norström A. Cervical tissue changes in women with miscarriage: a morphological and biochemical investigation. Acta Obstet Gynecol Scand 2010;89(1):54-64. Available from: https://doi.org/10.3109/00016340903390737.

[71] Madhappan B, Kempuraj D, Christodoulou S, et al. High levels of intrauterine corticotropin-releasing hormone, urocortin, tryptase, and interleukin-8 in spontaneous abortions. Endocrinology. 2003;144(6):2285-90. Available from: https://doi.org/10.1210/en.2003-0063.

[72] Arck PC, Rose M, Hertwig K, Hagen E, Hildebrandt M, Klapp BF. Stress and immune mediators in miscarriage. Hum Reprod Oxf Engl 2001;16(7):1505-11. Available from: https://doi.org/10.1093/humrep/16.7.1505.

[73] Arck PC. Stress and pregnancy loss: role of immune mediators, hormones and neurotransmitters. Am J Reprod Immunol 2001;46(2):117-23. Available from: https://doi.org/10.1111/j.8755-8920.2001.460201.x.

[74] Castells M, Butterfield J. Mast cell activation syndrome and mastocytosis: initial treatment options and long-term management. J Allergy Clin Immunol Pract 2019;7(4):1097-106. Available from: https://doi.org/10.1016/j.jaip.2019.02.002.

[75] Jia Q, Fang K, Liu Y. Rare lesion in the uterine cervix with irregular vaginal bleeding. Am J Obstet Gynecol 2019;220(6):598-9. Available from: https://doi.org/10.1016/j.ajog.2018.11.1104.

[76] Zhao D, Zhang L, Li W, Duan M, Zhuang J, Zhou D. Well-differentiated systemic mastocytosis with KIT K5091 mutation and uterus infiltration in an Asian woman with good response to imatinib. Chin Med J Engl 2019;132(16):2002-3. Available from: https://doi.org/10.1097/CM9.0000000000000355.

[77] Brockow K. Epidemiology, prognosis, and risk factors in mastocytosis. Immunol Allergy Clin North Am 2014;34(2):283-95. Available from: https://doi.org/10.1016/j.iac.2014.01.003.

[78] Cohen S, Skovbo S, Vestergaard H, Kristensen T, Moller M, Bindslev-Jensen C. Epidemiology of systemic mastocytosis in denmark. Br J Haematol 2014;166:521-8. Available from: https://doi.org/10.1111/bjh.12916.

[79] Ciach K, Niedoszytko M, Abacjew-Chmylko A, et al. Pregnancy and delivery in patients with mastocytosis treated at the polish center of the european competence network on mastocytosis (ECNM). PLoS ONE 2016;11(1):e0146924. Available from: https://doi.org/10.1371/journal.pone.0146924.

[80] Murray DB, editor. Mast Cells: Phenotypic Features, Biological Functions and Role in Immunity. New York: Nova Biomedical; 2013.

[81] Woidacki K, Zenclussen AC, Siebenhaar F. Mast cell-mediated and associated disorders in pregnancy: a risky game with an uncertain outcome? Fronti Immunol 2014;5(231). Available from: https://doi.org/10.3389/fimmu.2014.00231.

[82] Watson KD, Arendt KW, Watson WJ, Volcheck GW. Systemic mastocytosis complicating pregnancy. Obstet Gynecol 2012;119:486-9. Available from: https://doi.org/10.1097/AOG.0b013e318242d3c5.

[83] Matito A, Álvarez-Twose I, Morgado JM, Sánchez-Muñoz L, Orfao A, Escribano L. Clinical impact of pregnancy in mastocytosis: a study of the Spanish network on mastocytosis (REMA) in 45 cases. Int Arch Allergy Immunol 2011;156(1):104-11. Available from: https://doi.org/10.1159/000321954.

[84] Afrin L, Butterfield J, Raithel M, Molderings G. Often seen, rarely recognized: mast cell activation disease-a guide to diagnosis and therapeutic options. Ann Med 2016;48(3):190-201. Available from: https://doi.org/10.3109/07853890.2016.1161231.

[85] Horny HP, Metcalfe DD, Akin C. WHO Classification of Tumors of Hematopoietic and Lymphoid Tissues. Lyon, France: International Agency for Research and Cancer (IARC); 2017.

[86] Pardanani A. Systemic mastocytosis in adults: 2019 update on diagnosis, risk stratification and management. Am J Hematol 2019;94(3):363-77. Available from: https://doi.org/10.1002/ajh.25371.

[87] Lei D, Akin C, Kovalszki A. Management of mastocytosis in pregnancy: a review. J Allergy Clin Immunol Pract 2017;5(5):1217-23. Available from: https://doi.org/10.1016/j.jaip.2017.05.021.

[88] Molderings G, Raithel M, Kratz F, Azemar M, Haenisch B, Harzer S. Omalizumab treatment of systemic mast cell activation disease: experiences from four cases. Intern Med 2011;50:1-5. Available from: https://doi.org/10.2169/internalmedicine.50.4640.

[89] Lim K, Tefferi A, Lasho T, Finke C, Patnaik M, Butterfield J. Systemic mastocytosis in 342 consecutive adults: survival

studies and prognostic factors. Blood. 2009;113:5727-36. Available from: https://doi.org/10.1182/blood-2009-02-205237.

[90] Valent P, Sperr W, Akin C. How I treat patients with advance systemic mastocytosis. Blood. 2010;116:5812-17. Available from: https://doi.org/10.1182/blood-2010-08-292144.

[91] Butterfield J. Interferon treatment for hypereosinophilic syndromes and systemic mastocytosis. Acta Haematol 2005;114:26-40. Available from: https://doi.org/10.1159/000085560.

[92] Afrin L, Dempsey T, Rosenthal L, Dorff S. Successful mast-cell-targeted treatment of chronic dyspareunia, vaginitis, and dysfunctional uterine bleeding. J Obstet Gynaecol. https://www.tandfonline.com/action/showCitFormats?doi=10.1080/01443615.2018.1550475

[93] Watson K, Arendt K, Watson W, Volcheck G. Systemic mastocytosis complicating pregnancy. Obstetr Gynecol. 119(2Pt2):486-910. Available from: https://doi.org/10.1097/AOG.0b013e318242d3c5.

第 6 章

人白细胞抗原在反复妊娠丢失发病机制中的作用

Role of human leukocyte antigen in the pathogenesis of recurrent pregnancy loss

Chiara Tersigni[1] and Nicoletta Di Simone[2,3]

[1] Fondazione Policlinico Universitario A. Gemelli IRCCS, Dipartimento di Scienze della Salute della Donna e del Bambino e di Sanità Pubblica, Rome, Italy
[2] Department of Biomedical Sciences, Humanitas University, Pieve Emanuele, Milan, Italy
[3] IRCCS Humanitas Research Hospital, Rozzano, Milan, Italy

1 引言

人类妊娠可被视为自然界中完美的同种异体移植。这种现象是由胎盘而不是胎儿造成的。这一非同寻常的器官采用了一种从母体免疫系统逃逸的复杂策略，其主要机制可归纳为三个方面：①母体与胎儿间的解剖分离。②人类白细胞抗原（HLA）分子表达的改变。③抑制母体细胞介导的免疫。胎盘组织中的 HLA 转录抑制阻止了经典的 T 细胞对胎儿抗原的应答。有趣的是，完全表达 HLA 分子的胎儿体细胞在解剖学上被胎盘滋养层屏障与母体组织隔开，从而阻止了胎儿抗原与母体 T 细胞的直接接触。作为对胎儿的额外保护机制，母体细胞免疫经历了低反应性转变。在本章中，我们主要讨论正常妊娠胎盘中 HLA 表达的生理改变，以及 HLA 分子的异常表达在反复妊娠丢失（RPL）发生中的潜在作用。

2 RPL 和人白细胞抗原研究

妊娠丢失是指在胎儿存活之前的妊娠自然终止，包括从受孕到妊娠 20~23 周的所有丢失[1]。在所有临床确认的妊娠中，15%~20% 发生了这种情况。欧洲人类生殖与胚胎学学会（ESHRE）和美国生殖医学会（ASRM）的指南将 RPL 定义为两次或两次以上临床确认的妊娠失败。RPL 是一种病因多样化的产科综合征，在育龄期女性中的患病率为 3%~5%[1,2]。表 6.1 总结了 RPL 的主要病因。然而，仍有约 40% 的 RPL 病例被诊断为不明原因，无法找到确切的病因。据报道，在这些不明原因的病例中，母胎界面 HLA 分子的表达和（或）功能失调发挥了一定作用[3-12]。

表 6.1 RPL 的主要原因及患病率

主要原因	患病率
不明原因（包括非 APS 血栓形成）	40%~50%
自身免疫	20%
内分泌因素	17%~20%
解剖学因素	10%~15%
遗传因素	2%~5%

3 人白细胞抗原 I 类和 II 类分子

HLA 系统是编码主要组织相容性复合体（MHC）蛋白或 HLA 分子的人类基因复合体，是介导细胞与免疫系统之间相互作用的细胞表面蛋白[13]。HLA I 类（A、B 和 C）分子（Ⅰa）由糖基化重链和轻链 β2-微球蛋白组成。重链具有 3 个胞外结构域（α1、α2 和 α3），1 个跨膜区域和 1 个胞质内结构域。α1 和 α2 结构域的氨基酸序列决定了 HLA I 类分子的抗原特异性（图 6.1A）。I 类 HLA 分子在所有有核真核细胞的细胞表面表达。它们也存在于血小板上,但不存在于红细胞上。它们的作用是保护健康的"自我"细胞免受免疫细胞的识别。根据"缺失自我"假说,HLA Ⅰ类分子的缺失或表达改变可使靶细胞易受自然杀伤(NK)细胞攻击[13]。此外,HLA Ⅰa 类分子的另一个功能是将受损或感染细胞中的蛋白质片段展示给细胞毒性 T 细胞,从而触发免疫系统对非自身抗原的即时反应[14]。

HLA Ⅱ类分子(DP、DM、DO、DQ 和 DR)是由 2 个非共价糖基化多肽链组成的异源二聚体:α 和 β (图 6.1B)。α 链和 β 链是跨膜多肽,具有相同的整体结构。由 2 个结构域(α1 和 α2,或 β1 和 β2)组成的细胞外部分锚定在膜上。Ⅱ类分子的多态性发生在第 1 个氨基末端 β1 结构域中。HLA Ⅱ类分子在专业抗原递呈细胞(APC)上构成性表达,如树突状细胞、单核吞噬细胞和 B 细胞。Ⅱ类肽提供的抗原来自细胞外,通过吞噬作用加载到 HLA Ⅱ类分子上。这些抗原刺激辅助 T 细胞的增殖,进而引发 B 细胞分泌抗原特异性抗体[13]。T 细胞的激活需要 2 个信号。第 1 个信号是抗原特异性的,通过 T 细胞受体(TCR)提供,它与 APC 膜上的肽-HLA Ⅱ类分子相互作用。第 2 个信号,即共刺激信号,是抗原非特异性的,由 APC 膜上表达的共刺激分子(即 CD80 和 CD86)和 T 细胞(即 CD28)之间的相互作用提供。

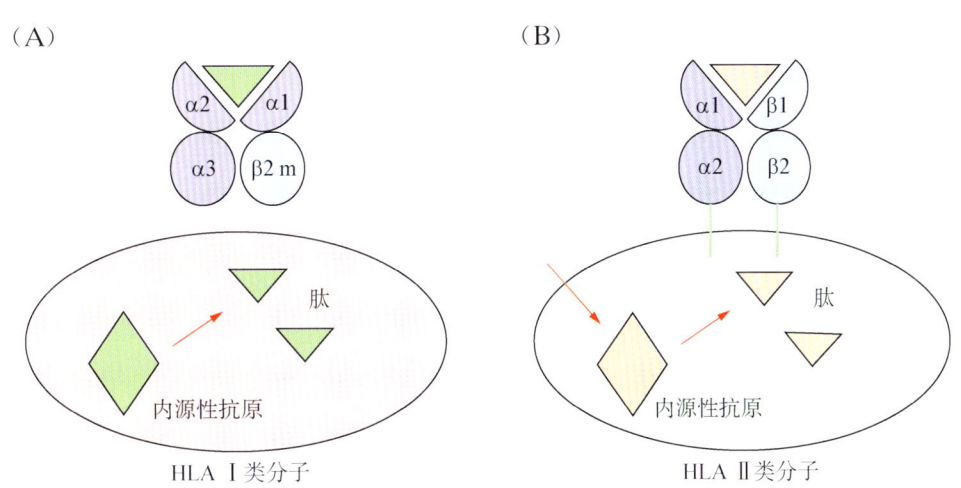

图 6.1 人类细胞中人白细胞抗原Ⅰ(A)和Ⅱ(B)类分子的分子结构。
β2 m:β2 微球蛋白。

3.1 人白细胞抗原Ⅰ、Ⅱ类分子在胎盘中的表达

在人类中,严格控制绒毛膜和绒毛外滋养层(EVT)中 HLA Ⅰ类和Ⅱ类的表达对于成功的妊娠结局至关重要[15]。合体滋养层细胞不表达任何 HLA Ⅰ类或Ⅱ类分子[16]。因此,在理论上,T 细胞无法识别并结合到主要的胎盘屏障上。EVT 表达非经典的 HLA Ⅰ类分子,如 HLA-G 和 HLA-E,以及经典的 HLA Ⅰ类分子 HLA-C,但不表达 HLA Ⅱ类分子[17,18]。经典的Ⅰ类 HLA-A 和 HLA-B 的缺乏,以及 EVT 中普遍缺乏 HLA-Ⅱ类分子表达,阻碍了母体 T 细胞对父源性 HLA 抗原的同种免疫应答。此外,仅表达经典的 HLA-C 和非典型的Ⅰ类抗原(Ⅰb)(如 HLA-G 和 HLA-E 分子),被认为可以保护 EVT 免受蜕膜自然杀伤(dNK)和 T 细胞的免疫攻击[19]。在胚胎植入和胎盘早期发育过程中,EVT 侵入母体蜕膜,其中母体白细胞由 dNK 细胞(80%)、巨噬细胞(10%)和 T 细胞(10%)组成[20]。因此,与母体其他免疫细胞相比,NK 在妊娠前半期母体蜕膜中相对丰富。母体免疫适应妊娠的一个中心机制是 dNK 通过失去细胞毒活性和获得免疫调节特性而表现出耐受性表型。dNK 的低细胞毒性是通过特定的受体表达谱实现的。它们表达杀伤细胞免疫球蛋白样受体(KIR),该受体在其他配体中识别多态性 HLA-C,表达可识别 HLA-E 的自然杀伤细胞群 2 受体(NKG2),以及表达识别 HLA-G 的免疫球蛋白类转录物 2 受体(ILT-2)(图 6.2)[21]。

EVT 细胞表面的 HLA-C 表达在调节母体 NK 细胞和 T 细胞中起着核心作用,并影响妊娠结局。一般来说,它调节对病毒抗原、同种异体和自身抗原的细胞免疫应答[20]。NK 细胞特异性识别两组 HLA-C 同种异型,HLA-C1 和 HLA-C2。它们

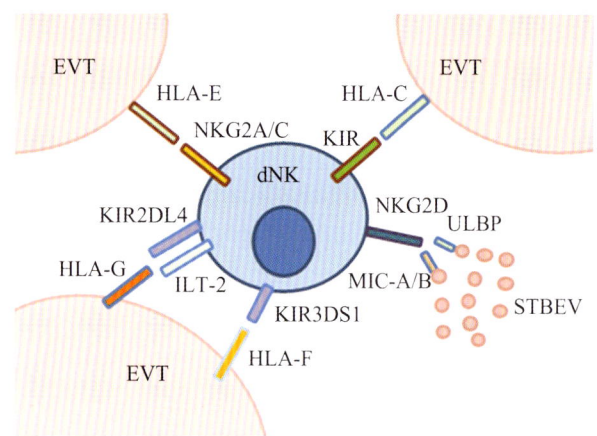

图 6.2 介导蜕膜自然杀伤(dNK)细胞、由绒毛外滋养层(EVT)表达的非经典人白细胞抗原Ⅰ类分子和由合体滋养层细胞衍生的细胞外囊泡携带的可溶性免疫调节受体之间相互作用的主要受体。

NKG2,自然杀伤细胞2型受体;KIR,杀伤细胞免疫球蛋白样受体;ILT-2,免疫球蛋白样转录物2受体;MIC,MHCⅠ类链相关蛋白;ULBP,UL-16结合蛋白。

在 HLA-C 重链 80 位氨基酸上有所不同：HLA-C1 为天冬酰胺,而 HLA-C2 为赖氨酸[20]。KIR 的表达谱赋予 dNK 细胞特异性识别 EVT 上的 HLA 同种异型的能力。HLA-C1 与抑制性 KIR2DL2/3 受体连接,HLA-C2 与抑制性 KIR2DL1 或激活性 KIR2DS1 受体连接[17,20,22]。因此,dNK 细胞与 EVT 的相互作用在每次妊娠时均有不同,并且由母体 KIR 单体型、母体和胎儿 HLA-C 同种型以及 NK 细胞共同决定。

最后,除了 HLA-C-KIR 在母体-滋养层界面的相互作用外,滋养层还存在另一种抑制 dNK 细胞毒性的机制。特别是,已知 NK 细胞的细胞毒性通常由 NK 细胞受体 NKG2D 与其配体,即 MHC Ⅰ类链相关(MIC)蛋白 A 和 B 以及 UL-16 结合蛋白(ULBP)的相互作用诱导。这种受体-配体相互作用激活穿孔素介导的细胞毒性途径,清除受损和(或)感染的细胞。有趣的是,MIC 和 ULBP 在人胎盘中组成型表达,这些蛋白质在妊娠期间通过合体滋养层细胞衍生的胞外囊泡以可溶性形式释放[22]。胎盘来源的可溶性 MIC 和 ULBP 下调 NKG2D 受体,并间接下调 NKG2D 介导的对外周血单核细胞、纯化的 NK 细胞、CD8$^+$ 细胞和 γδT 细胞的细胞毒性(图 6.2)[23,24]。

此外,母体蜕膜 CD8$^+$ 细胞直接识别父源的同种异体 HLA-C 分子。这种免疫相互作用是妊娠期间胎儿免疫耐受发展的关键过程。有趣的是,蜕膜 CD8$^+$ 细胞高表达共抑制分子,如细胞毒性 T 淋巴细胞相关蛋白-4(CTLA4),程序性细胞死亡 1(PD1)和淋巴细胞激活基因-3(LAG3),而低表达细胞溶解分子。这种子宫微环境的作用是抑制 CD8$^+$ 效应 T 细胞活性,并维持胎盘耐受[25]。然而,已有研究表明,蜕膜 CD8$^+$ T 细胞保留了对促炎事件反应的能力,因为在体外刺激时,它们能产生干扰素-γ、肿瘤坏死因子-α、穿孔素和颗粒酶 B[25]。另外,母体调节性 T 细胞(Treg)在建立对侵入 EVT 的免疫耐受和防止对胎盘抗原的炎症反应方面发挥着关键作用[19,26]。事实上,Tregs 在人类蜕膜中高表达[16]。非同寻常的是,幼稚的 CD4$^+$ T 细胞与 EVT 在体外共培养时,通过分化为 CD4$^+$ FOXP3$^+$ Tregs,直接增加 T 细胞的比例[27,28]。有趣的是,一些研究者提出 Treg 分化可能发生在母体 T 细胞特异性识别胎儿 HLA-C 后[20],但确切的机制仍有待进一步研究。总之,HLA-C 分子在调节细胞介导的母体对胎儿耐受的主要参与者(即 NK 细胞、CD8$^+$ 细胞和 Treg 细胞)的活性中起着核心作用。

相较于经典的 HLA-C,HLA Ⅰa 和 Ⅰb 类分子具有不同的多态性,表达不同数量的等位基因。HLA-Ⅰa 类分子具有高度多态性,大量的等位基因编码多种功能蛋白,而 HLA Ⅰb 类分子具有低度多态性,少量等位基因编码少量蛋白。与 HLA Ⅰa 分子类似,HLA Ⅰb 分子也可结合由蛋白酶体驱动的胞浆蛋白降解产生的肽,并将其递呈给特定的 CD8$^+$ T 细胞亚群[19]。这些分子的主要功能是调节生理和病理条件下的免疫应答[29]。HLA-G 具有有限的多态性并形成一个同型二聚体,可与由所有蜕膜 APC 表达的抑制性受体 LILRB1、由 NK 细胞表达的 KIR2DL4[30]及在 T 淋巴细胞、NK 细胞和内皮细胞[31]中表达的 CD160 高亲和力结合。这些相互作用使免疫应答偏向耐受性而不是免疫原性应答。特别是在与这些受体相互作用后,HLA-G 能够：①抑制 T 细胞增殖和细胞毒性[32],诱导调节性 T 细胞的扩增[33]。②抑制 B 细胞的分化、增殖和细胞因子产生[34]。③抑制外周血和子宫 NK 细胞的增殖和细胞毒性[35]。④通过下调 T、B 和 NK 细胞表面趋化因子受体的表达来抑制不同 T、B 和 NK 细胞群的趋化性[36]。⑤抑制中性粒细胞的吞噬作用和活性氧的产生[37]。母体和胎儿之间这种非同寻常的选择性免疫相互作用的益处在于只有当 HLA-G$^+$ EVT 和子宫 APC 之间有直接接触时才会发生,从而使母体其他部位的 APC 能够正常运作[20]。最后,NK-EVT 相互作用涉及 HLA-E 与 NKG2A/C 以及 HLA-F 与 KIR3DS1 的相互作用,可能导致脱颗粒以及释放穿孔素(PRF)和颗粒酶(GZM)(图 6.2),引发免疫调节作用[20],这些仍是有待研究的问题。有趣的是,来源于妊娠组织的间充质基质细胞(特别是来源于脐带血的间充质基质细胞)免疫原性较差,这与其细胞表面 HLA-G 和 HLA-E 的共表达有关[38]。同样,诱导多能干细胞(iPSC)表达低水平的经典 HLA Ⅰ 类分子,但表达高水平的 HLA-G 和 HLA-E,能够避免 HLA 限制性细胞毒性 T 细胞的识别,这些 T 细胞在与 iPSC 共培养时会进入无应答状态[39]。

3.2 RPL 中人白细胞抗原分子的异常表达

HLA 分子在母胎界面的表达和(或)功能异常已被认为是不明原因 RPL 的潜在发病机制。HLA-G 是 RPL 中研究最多的 HLA 分子。从 RPL 患者中收集的流产组织显示了 HLA-G 的表达降低[3,4]。同样,在 RPL 患者的底蜕膜中发现 HLA-G 表达降低[5]。另一方面,与无不良妊娠结局的女性相比,既往有 RPL 病史的足月胎盘中 HLA-G 的表达增高[6]。JEG-3 细胞的体外研究表明,过表达 miR-133a 可能通过减少 HLA-G 的转录而降低 HLA-G 表达,可能是不明原因 RPL 的发病机制之一[3]。有趣的是,研究表明,地塞米松和氢化可的松均可上调 RPL 患者滋养细胞中 HLA-G 的表达[7]。因此,糖皮质激素可能具有潜在调节体外 HLA-G 表达的作用,应进一步确认其在 RPL 中的治疗适应证。

胎儿 HLA-C 分子的正确表达对于成功妊娠结局的重要性已被间接证明,RPL 患者在妊娠早期的血清抗 HLA-C 抗体水平高于正常妊娠女性。这提示抗 HLA-C 抗体可能参与不明原因 RPL 发病机制的假设[8]。

一些研究还分析了 HLA 基因图谱和多态性与 RPL 的高风险相关。特别是,在蛋白质水平上发现了 15 个多态性和 2 个无效等位基因与 RPL 相关。大多数研究集中在无效等位基因 G*01:05 N[9-11]。这一等位基因的发现引起了人们对胎儿 G*01:05N 的纯合性是否可能为 RPL 夫妇致病因素的猜想,尽管一些研究未能证实这一理论[40-44]。因此,需要进一步的研究以确定 HLA-G 多态性在 RPL 发病机制中的确切作用。

尽管目前还没有研究表明 HLA Ⅱ 类分子在 RPL 患者子宫内膜/滋养细胞中的表达,但一些队列研究分析了 HLA 单倍型的表达。在有过 4 次或更多次妊娠丢失的患者中:DRB1*0101、DQA1*0101、DQB1*0501;DRB1*0102、DQA1*0101、DQB1*0501;DRB1*0103、DQA1*0101、DQB1*0501;或 DRB1*0301、DQA1*0501、DQB1*0201,单体频率高于对照组[45]。在一项印度的队列研究中发现,DQB1*03:03:02 等位基因与 RPL 相关[46]。在最近一项黎巴嫩的病例对照研究中发现,单倍型 DPB1*04:01:01-DQB1*02:01:01-DRB1*07:01:01 与 RPL 相关[47]。尽管研究结果各不相同,但这些研究表明 HLA 在决定妊娠结局中起着关键作用,凸显了 RPL 的免疫学特征。

研究发现,HLA-Dr 分子在子痫前期患者的合体滋养层中异常表达[12],证实母体免疫系统对胎盘父源抗原的免疫耐受性降低,可能是子痫前期发病机制中滋养细胞侵袭下降和胎盘发育迟缓的原因。然而,据作者所知,目前尚无关于自然流产女性滋养细胞组织中 HLA Ⅱ 类分子异常表达的研究。

4 评估辅助生殖中的人白细胞抗原

已有研究提出将检测卵泡液中可溶性 HLA-G 作为在体外人工受精时选择卵母细胞的方法[48]。多项研究指出,早期胚胎中 HLA-G 抗原的表达可能是种植率提高的标志[49-51]。事实上,HLA-G 阳性胚胎来源的囊泡在胚胎培养分泌体中含量高,并被子宫内膜上皮细胞和基质细胞吸收,提示绒毛外交换是母胎界面的一种交互方式。需要进一步的研究来验证卵泡液和(或)胚胎中 HLA-G 表达水平对成功妊娠的预测价值。

5 治疗

目前尚无可用的药物用于治疗 HLA 抗原异常表达引起的 RPL 或其他妊娠并发症(子痫前期或早产)。体外研究表明,糖皮质激素可以上调 RPL 患者滋养细胞的 HLA-G 表达[7]。需要进一步的研究来验证在患有 RPL 和 HLA 抗原异常表达的女性中应用糖皮质激素的临床效果。

6 结论

HLA-Ⅰb类分子在EVT中的适当表达和功能，以及滋养层组织中HLA-Ⅱ类分子的完全抑制，是胚胎种植和胎盘形成的关键免疫机制。多项研究表明，HLAⅠ类和Ⅱ类分子的遗传多态性与RPL之间存在关联。已在RPL患者的滋养层组织和蜕膜中发现HLA-G的表达降低。然而，除HLA-G或HLAⅡ类分子外的其他HLAⅠb类分子在母胎界面异常表达的研究仍十分有限。因此，这是一个基本上未被探索的领域，需要进一步的研究。

7 总结和建议

- 绒毛外滋养层表达HLAⅠb类（HLA-C，HLA-E，HLA-F，HLA-G）分子。
- 合体滋养层细胞不表达HLAⅠb类分子。
- 在正常妊娠中，滋养细胞不表达HLAⅡ类分子。
- 在RPL患者中，HLA-G的表达减少。
- HLAⅠ类和Ⅱ类分子的遗传多态性与RPL有关。

参考文献

[1] Bender Atik, R. et al. ESHRE guideline: recurrent pregnancy loss. An in-depth evaluation of the evidence base that underpins the use of diagnostic tests and treatments in the contemporary management of recurrent pregnancy loss. Hum. Reprod. Open 2018, hoy004(2018).

[2] Practice Committee of the American Society for Reproductive Medicine. Evaluation and treatment of recurrent pregnancy loss: a committee opinion. Fertil Steril 2012;98:1103-11.

[3] Wang X, Li B, Wang J, Lei J, Liu C, Ma Y, et al. Evidence That miR-133a Causes Recurrent Spontaneous Abortion by Reducing HLA-G Expression. Reprod Biomed Online 2012;25:415-24.

[4] Mosaferi E, Alizadeh Gharamaleki N, Farzadi L, Majidi J, Babaloo Z, Kazemi T, et al. The study of HLA-G gene and protein expression in patients with recurrent miscarriage. Adv Pharm Bull 2019;9(1):70-5.

[5] Papamitsou T, Toskas A, Papadopoulou K, Sioga A, Lakis S, Chatzistamatiou M, et al. Immunohistochemical study of immunological markers: HLAG, CD16, CD25, CD56 and CD68 in placenta tissues in recurrent pregnancy loss. Histol Histopathol 2014;29(8):1047-55.

[6] Craenmehr MHC, Nederlof I, Cao M, Drabbels JJM, Spruyt-Gerritse MJ, Anholts JDH, et al. Increased HLA-G expression in term placenta of women with a history of recurrent miscarriage despite their genetic predisposition to decreased HLA-G levels. Int J Mol Sci 2019;20:625.

[7] Akhter A, Faridi RM, Das V, Pandey A, Naik S, Agrawal S. In vitro up-regulation of HLA-G using dexamethasone and hydrocortisone in first-trimester trophoblast cells of women experiencing recurrent miscarriage. Tissue Antigens 2012;80(2):126-35.

[8] Meuleman T, van Beelen E, Kaaja RJ, van Lith JM, Claas FH, Bloemenkamp KW. HLA-C antibodies in women with recurrent miscarriage suggests that antibody mediated rejection is one of the mechanisms leading to recurrent miscarriage. J Reprod Immunol 2016;116:28-34.

[9] Pfeiffer KA, Fimmers R, Engels G, van der Ven H, van der Ven K. Implantation and pregnancy: The HLA-G genotype is potentially associated with idiopathic recurrent spontaneous abortion. Mol Hum Reprod 2001;7:373-8.

[10] Aldrich CL, Stephenson MD, Karrison T, Odem RR, Branch DW, Scott JR, et al. HLA-G genotypes and pregnancy outcome in couples with unexplained recurrent miscarriage. Mol Hum Reprod 2001;7:1167-72.

[11] Hviid TV, Hylenius S, Hoegh AM, Kruse C, Christiansen OB. HLA-G polymorphisms in couples with recurrent spontaneous abortions. Tissue Antigens 2002;60:122-32.

[12] Tersigni C, Redman CW, Dragovic R, Tannetta D, Scambia G, Di Simone N, et al. HLA-DR is aberrantly expressed at feto-maternal interface in pre-eclampsia. J Reprod Immunol 2018;129:48-52.

[13] Rock KL, Reits E, Neefjes J. Present yourself! By MHC class I and MHC class II molecules. Trends Immunol 2016;37:724-37.

[14] Blees A, Januliene D, Hofmann T, Koller N, Schmidt C, Trowitzsch S, et al. Structure of the human MHC-I peptide-loading complex. Nature 2017;551:525-8.

[15] Moffett A, Chazara O, Colucci F. Maternal allo-recognition of the fetus. Fertil Steril 2017;107:1269-72.

[16] Apps R, Murphy SP, Fernando R, Gardner L, Ahad T, Moffett A. Human leucocyte antigen (HLA) expression of primary trophoblast cells and placental cell lines, determined using single antigen beads to characterize allotype specificities of anti-HLA antibodies. Immunology 2009;127:26-39.

[17] Parham P, Norman PJ, Abi-Rached L, Hilton HG, Guethlein LA. Review: immunogenetics of human placentation. Placenta 2012;33:71-80.

[18] Burton G, Jauniaux E. What is the placenta? Am J Obstet Gynecol 2015;213:6-8.

[19] Datema G, Van Meir CA, Kanhai HH, Van Den Elsen PJ. Pre-term birth and severe pre-eclampsia are not associated with altered expression of HLA on human trophoblasts. Am J Reprod Immunol 2003;49:193-201.

[20] Papúchová H, Meissner TB, Li Q, Strominger JL, Tilburgs T. The dual role of HLA-C in tolerance and immunity at the maternal-fetal interface. Front Immunol 2019;10:2730.

[21] Olmos-Ortiz A, Flores-Espinosa P, Mancilla-Herrera I, Vega-Sánchez R, Díaz L, Zaga-Clavellina V. Innate immune cells and toll-like receptor-dependent responses at the maternal-fetal interface. Int J Mol Sci 2019;20:3654.

[22] Sharkey AM, Gardner L, Hiby S, Farrell L, Apps R, Masters L, et al. Killer Ig-like receptor expression in uterine NK cells is biased toward recognition of HLA-C and alters with gestational age. J Immunol 2008;181:39-46.

[23] Mincheva-Nilsson L, Nagaeva O, Chen T, Stendahl U, Antsiferova J, Mogren I, et al. Placenta-derived soluble MHC class I chain-related molecules down-regulate NKG2D receptor on peripheral blood mononuclear cells during human pregnancy: a possible novel immune escape mechanism for fetal survival. J Immunol 2006;176:3585-92.

[24] Hedlund M, Stenqvist AC, Nagaeva O, Kjellberg L, Wulff M, Baranov V, et al. Human placenta expresses and secretes NKG2D ligands via exosomes that down-modulate the cognate receptor expression: evidence for immunosuppressive function. J Immunol 2009;183:340-51.

[25] Van der Zwan A, Bi K, Norwitz ER, Crespo AC, Claas FHJ, Strominger JL, et al. Mixed signature of activation and dysfunction allows human decidual CD8(+) T cells to provide both tolerance and immunity. Proc Natl Acad Sci USA 2018; 115:385-90.

[26] Tilburgs T, Roelen DL, van der Mast BJ, van Schip JJ, Kleijburg C, de Groot-Swings GM, et al. Differential distribution of CD4+ CD25bright and CD8+ CD28− T-cells in decidua and maternal blood during human pregnancy. Placenta 2006;27:47-53.

[27] Tilburgs T, Crespo ÂC, van der Zwan A, Rybalov B, Raj T, Stranger B, et al. Human HLAG+ extravillous trophoblasts: immune-activating cells that interact with decidual leukocytes. Proc Natl Acad Sci USA 2015;112:7219-24.

[28] Svensson-Arvelund J, Mehta RB, Lindau R, Mirrasekhian E, Rodriguez-Martinez H, Berg G, et al. The human fetal placenta promotes tolerance against the semi-allogeneic fetus by inducing regulatory T cells and homeostatic M2 macrophages. J Immunol 2015;194:1534-44.

[29] Reeves E, James E. Tumour and placenta establishment: the importance of antigen processing and presentation. Placenta 2017;56:34-9.

[30] Persson G, Jørgensen N, Nilsson LL, Andersen LHJ, Hviid TVF. A role for both HLA-F and HLA-G in reproduction and during pregnancy? Hum Immunol 2020;81:127-33.

[31] Le Page ME, Goodridge JP, John E, Christiansen FT, Witt CS. Killer Ig-like receptor 2DL4 does not mediate NK cell IFN-γ responses to soluble HLA-G preparations. J Immunol 2014;192:732-40.

[32] Pistoia V, Morandi F, Wang X, Ferrone S. Soluble HLAG: are they clinically relevant? Seminars in Cancer Biology, Volume 17. Cambridge, MA, USA: Academic Press; 2007. p.469-79.

[33] Fournel S, Aguerre-Girr M, Huc X, Lenfant F, Alam A, Toubert A, Le Bouteiller P. Cutting edge: soluble HLA-G1 triggers CD95/CD95 ligand-mediated apoptosis in activated CD8+ cells by interacting with CD8. J Immunol 2000;164: 6100-4.

[34] Naji A, Menier C, Morandi F, Agaugué S, Maki G, Ferretti E, et al. Binding of HLA-G to ITIM-bearing Ig-like transcript 2 receptor suppresses B cell Responses. J Immunol 2014;192: 1536-46.

[35] Morandi F, Rizzo R, Fainardi E, Rouas-Freiss N, Pistoia V. Recent advances in our understanding of HLA-G biology: lessons from a wide spectrum of human diseases. J Immunol Res 2016;4326495.

[36] Morandi F, Rouas-Freiss N, Pistoia V. The emerging role of soluble HLA-G in the control of chemotaxis. Cytokine Growth Factor Rev 2014;25:327-35.

[37] Baudhuin J, Migraine J, Faivre V, Loumagne L, Lukaszewicz AC, Payen D, et al. Exocytosis acts as a modulator of the ILT4-mediated inhibition of neutrophil functions. Proc Natl Acad Sci USA 2013;110:17957-62.

[38] Stubbendorff M, Deuse T, Hua X, Phan TT, Bieback K, Atkinson K, et al. Immunological properties of extraembryonic human mesenchymal stromal cells derived from gestational tissue. Stem Cell Dev 2013;22:2619-29.

[39] Kim EM, Manzar G, Zavazava N. Human iPS cell-derived hematopoietic prog-enitor cells induce T-cell anergy in in vitro-generated alloreactive CD8(+) T cells. Blood 2013; 121:5167-75.

[40] Penzes M, Rajczy K, Gyodi E, Reti M, Feher E, Petranyi G. HLA-G gene polymorphism in the normal population and in recurrent spontaneous abortion in Hungary. Transpl Proc 1999;31:1832-3.

[41] Yamashita T, Fujii T, Tokunaga K, Tadokoro K, Hamai Y, Miki A, et al. Analysis of human leukocyte antigen-G polymorphism including intron 4 in Japanese couples with habitual abortion. Am J Reprod Immunol 1999;41:159-63.

[42] Yan WH, Fan LA, Yang JQ, Xu LD, Ge Y, Yao FJ. HLA-G polymorphism in a Chinese Han population with recurrent spontaneous abortion. Int J Immunogenet 2006;33:55-8.

[43] Yan WH, Lin A, Chen XJ, Dai MZ, Gan LH, Zhou MY, et al. Association of the maternal 14-bp insertion polymorphism in the HLA-G gene in women with recurrent spontaneous abortions. Tissue Antigens 2006;68:521-3.

[44] Abbas A, Tripathi P, Naik S, Agrawal S. Analysis of human leukocyte antigen (HLA)-G polymorphism in normal women and in women with recurrent spontaneous abortions. Eur J Immunogenet 2004;31:275-8.

[45] Christiansen OB, Rasmussen KL, Jersild C, Grunnet N. HLA class II alleles confer susceptibility to recurrent fetal losses in Danish women. Tissue Antigens 1994;44(4):225-33.

[46] Aruna M, Nagaraja T, Andal Bhaskar S, Tarakeswari S, Reddy AG, Thangaraj K, et al. Novel alleles of HLA-DQ and -DR loci show association with recurrent miscarriages among South Indian women. Hum Reprod 2011;26(4):765-74.

[47] Aimagambetova G, Hajjej A, Malalla ZH, Finan RR, Sarray S, Almawi WY. Maternal HLA-DR, HLA-DQ, and HLA-DP loci are linked with altered risk of recurrent pregnancy loss in Lebanese women: a case-control study. Am J Reprod Immunol 2019;82(4):e13173.

[48] Rizzo R, Fuzzi B, Stignani M, Criscuoli L, Melchiorri L, Dabizzi S, et al. Soluble HLA-G molecules in follicular fluid: a tool for oocyte selection in IVF? J Reprod Immunol 2007;74 (1-2):133-42.

[49] Desai N, Filipovits J, Goldfarb J. Secretion of soluble HLA-G by day 3 human embryos associated with higher pregnancy and implantation rates: assay of culture media using a new ELISA kit. Reprod Biomed Online 2006;13(2):272-7.

[50] Sher G, Keskintepe L, Fisch JD, Acacio BA, Ahlering P, Batzofin J, et al. Soluble human leukocyte antigen G expression in phase I culture media at 46 hours after fertilization predicts pregnancy and implantation from day 3 embryo transfer. Fertil Steril 2005;83(5):1410-13.

[51] Díaz RR, Zamora RB, Sánchez RV, Pérez JG, Bethencourt JCA. Embryo sHLA-G secretion is related to pregnancy rate. Zygote 2019;27(2):78-81.

第 7 章

应激诱导的免疫偏差和生殖障碍
Stress-induced immune deviations and reproductive failure

Ronja Wöhrle, Petra Clara Arck and Kristin Thiele

Division of Experimental Feto-Maternal Medicine, Department of Obstetrics and Fetal Medicine, University Medical Center Hamburg-Eppendorf, Hamburg, Germany

1 正常妊娠的免疫内分泌适应

60多年前,Peter Medawar 爵士发现,来自非亲属个体的器官排斥反应是基于免疫学原理。这很快使人们关注到妊娠亦是一个免疫学之谜,因为胎儿表现出与母体不同的父系抗原,但不会发生排斥反应。Medawar 提出了三种机制来解释这个谜团:①胎盘的解剖分离。②胎儿抗原的不成熟阻止了母体免疫反应。③母体免疫系统的免疫惰性[1]。这些尝试性的解释开启了大量研究工作,并奠定了生殖免疫学基础。如今,人们普遍认为,母体对妊娠的免疫适应是固有免疫系统和适应性免疫系统中激素与各种免疫细胞相互作用的一个非常复杂的精细调节过程,以促进并维持胎儿的生长和发育[2,3]。

母体对妊娠的免疫适应发生在受精开始及正常妊娠进展直至足月的过程中,包括子宫内膜的周期性更新,即反复形成的一种免疫能力,以接受胚胎植入[4]。受精后,受精卵不断分裂并发育成囊胚。其外层为滋养层,可分为绒毛滋养层和绒毛外滋养层(EVT)。前者既不表达主要组织相容性复合体(MHC)Ⅰ类分子,也不表达Ⅱ类分子,防止母体免疫应答,而后者则表达多态性人白细胞抗原(HLA)-C分子和非多态性 HLA-E、HLA-G 和 HLA-F[5]。通过 HLA-C,EVT 细胞可调控子宫自然杀伤(uNK)细胞、CD8⁺ T 效应细胞和 CD4⁺ T 细胞[6,7]。随后,免疫细胞聚集在分化的滋养细胞周围,以促炎细胞因子和趋化因子反应为特征,白细胞介素(IL)-6、IL-15、肿瘤坏死因子(TNF)、CXCL10、CXCL8、CCL2 的存在则反映了这一现象[8]。炎症被认为是胎儿滋养细胞分化和侵入蜕膜所必需的[9]。

在炎症激增后不久,迫切需要一种耐受性的环境以确保胎儿的耐受性。与先前对免疫系统持续抑制的假设不同,这种对胎儿的免疫耐受是通过免疫细胞向母胎界面的主动募集而获得的[9]。这些免疫细胞具有不同的表型,其效应功能受到限制。简单来说,NK 细胞、巨噬细胞和树突状细胞(DC)表现出耐受性,不同于它们在外周的表型。NK 细胞的细胞毒性较小,巨噬细胞仍不成熟。两者都具有抗炎作用,对蜕膜和血管重塑非常重要[10,11]。DC 的积聚数量高于外周,表现出不成熟的耐受性特征[12]。此外,这些固有免疫细胞有助于 CD4⁺ T 细胞亚群的变化。辅助性 T 细胞(Th)1/Th2-和 Th17/调节性 T 细胞(Treg)平衡向抗炎 T 细胞类型转变。因此,表现为 Th2 和 Treg 细胞在蜕膜中积聚,而不是 Th1 和 Th17 表型[13]。在这段长时间的耐受之后,分娩开始,意味着妊娠期炎症的再一次激增。母体对妊娠免疫适应的所有表现和功能变化均由激素介导,如人绒毛膜促性腺激素(hCG)、孕激素、糖皮质激素和雌激素[14],它们对不同免疫细胞群的影响见表7.1。

上述母体对妊娠复杂而精细的免疫适应极易受药物、感染、营养和应激感知的干扰。后者是本章的重点。

表 7.1 妊娠激素及其对免疫系统的影响

激素	对免疫系统的影响	对适应性免疫的影响
hCG	• 诱导子宫 NK 细胞[15] • 单核细胞产生具有趋化性的 IL-8[16] • 促进巨噬细胞向 M2 表型转变[17] • 诱导耐受性 DC[18]	• 抑制 Th1 细胞[19] • Treg[17] 和 Breg[20] 增加 • Th17 募集到蜕膜[17]
孕酮	• 诱导耐受性 DC[21] • 促进巨噬细胞向 M2 表型转变[22] • NK 细胞:细胞凋亡,细胞毒性降低[23]	• Th2 细胞聚集[24] • Tregs 增加[25] • Th1 细胞[24] 和 Th17 细胞[26] 的抑制 • 低细胞毒性 CD8$^+$ T 细胞[27]
雌激素	• 促进 M2 表型[28] • DC 成熟[21]	• 高浓度促进 Th2 细胞[29] 和 Treg 细胞[30] • 低浓度促进 Th1 细胞[29]
糖皮质激素	• 未成熟 DC[31] • 抗炎巨噬细胞[32] • 子宫 NK 降低[33]	• 取代 Th1 向 Th2 转变[34,35] • 诱导 Tregs[36]

1.1 母体对妊娠免疫适应的独特免疫学特征

1.1.1 固有免疫

在妊娠早期,NK 细胞占免疫细胞的大多数。与外周 NK 细胞相比,子宫 NK 细胞的特点是 CD56^{bright}CD16^{dim} 表达,细胞因子产量更高,细胞毒性更小。它们通过细胞因子、趋化因子和血管生成生长因子的分泌促进血管和蜕膜基质重塑。此外,子宫 NK 细胞能促进 CD4$^+$ Treg 细胞的诱导,同时通过分泌 IFN-γ 抑制 Th17 细胞,分泌 Galectin-1 促进 Th2 转换和活化细胞毒性 T 细胞的凋亡[10,37-40]。

单核细胞,尤其是中间型单核细胞(CD14^{high}CD16^{intermediate}),在妊娠期间增多,导致 TNF-α 产生增加,而吞噬作用减弱。它们优先分化为支持滋养细胞侵袭、螺旋动脉形成和重塑的免疫抑制性 M2 巨噬细胞表型[11,41]。

蜕膜中的 DC 显著高于外周血,其特征是炎性细胞因子(如 IL-12)产生降低,抗原递呈受到抑制,共刺激信号减少。相反,这些未成熟的耐受性 DC 表达 Galectin-1,分泌 IL-10,促进 CD4$^+$ Treg 的扩增并向 Th2 转化[12,39,42]。

1.1.2 适应性免疫

辅助性 T 细胞(Th)1 及其相关细胞因子 IFN-γ、IL-2、IL-12、IL-18 可对病原体产生适当的免疫应答,它们在妊娠期间下调,有利于向 Th2 细胞转化,后者通过经典的细胞因子 IL-4、IL-5、IL-10 和 IL-13 介导体液免疫反应,以促进容受性和抗炎反应[43]。

调节性 T(Treg)细胞是建立和维持胎儿耐受的主要参与者,表达 CD4、CD25 和 Foxp3,并通过分泌 IL-10、前列腺素 E2(PGE2)和 TGF-β 支持耐受性微环境。Th17 细胞则具有促炎性,其特点是分泌 IL-17,促进滋养细胞的侵袭。然而,它们在蜕膜中的普遍存在受到 NK 细胞调节而减少[13,37,43-45]。

γδT 细胞是血液和蜕膜中含量较少的一个细胞群,在妊娠期间出现扩增。它们表现出低细胞毒性,其分泌的 IL-10 和 TGF-β 促进耐受性环境的形成[46]。

调节性 B(Breg)细胞在妊娠期间增加,分泌 IL-10,从而抑制 T 细胞产生 TNF-α。此外,有研究表明 Bregs 能使 DC 停滞在未成熟状态,从而促进 CD4$^+$ Treg 扩增[20,47]。

2 母体应激感知

应激通常被理解为是一种心理压力,描述了能够引起困扰、愤怒和焦虑,并损害个人心理和身体健康的事件或环境。此外,应激具有多面性,由于个人感知,不同的文化、社会和环境背景及应激源的多样性,很难对其进行普适性的定义与衡量[48,49]。然而,描述应激的不同方式包括以下几个方面。

2.1 应激源

应激源具高度异质性,是能被个体感受并产生压力的事件或状况、人或环境。通常分为内部应激源和外部应激源,两者均可以是积极的(eustress)或是消极的(distress)。内部应激源是个人童年时期性格及成长方式的结果,包括高标准与自我期望、完美主义、未实现的愿望和低负荷能力。根据应对的效率,这些条件可能是激励性的,也可能是过度的。外部应激源则是各种环境因素(如噪声、严寒或酷暑)、医疗干预或疼痛、财务问题、失去家人或好友,导致具有各种症状的高压力。妊娠期间,孕妇面临着一种全新的情况,往往与不确定性和焦虑有关。这种"妊娠期特有压力"的存在是科学界公认的,具体包括对母亲和孩子的健康担忧、对分娩的恐惧以及即将成为父母[49,50]。此外,改变个人生活的事件,如搬迁、离婚、失业,或可怕的环境灾难,如地震,都可能对孕妇的健康和婴儿的发育产生负面影响(图 7.1)[51-53]。

2.2 应激强度

对母亲心理和生理健康的影响强度很大程度上取决于应对策略和现有的社会支持,如伴侣或其他家庭成员(图 7.1)[54]。此外,对应激事件的感知受到个体间差异的影响[48]。妊娠稳态可能受主要和次要应激源的干扰,产前应激的严重程度可从轻度日常困扰,到中度生活事件变化,直至严重创伤[55]。对压力的感知进一步取决于妊娠的不同时间段。有研究表明,如果在妊娠早期经历同样的应激源,则会感觉更为严重,这表明随着妊娠的进展,应激源的影响会减小[52,56]。

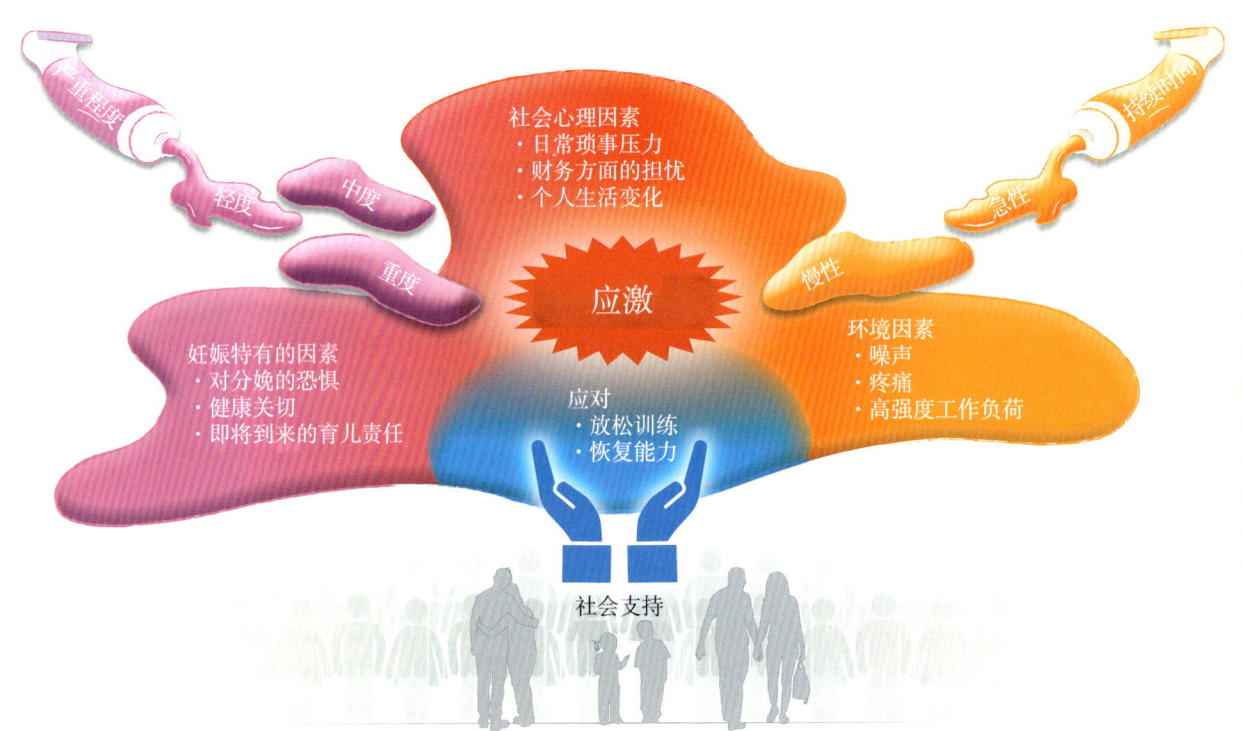

图 7.1 妊娠期间的应激感知:应激源可能是高度异质的,包括各种环境因素、心理压力和妊娠期特有的问题。产前应激对健康的影响取决于应激源的严重程度、持续时间、现有的应对策略和社会支持。

2.3 应激源的严重程度

应激源的严重程度及其对母亲和胎儿健康的影响在很大程度上取决于暴露时间的长短[57]。因此,可区分为急性应激和慢性应激。急性应激通常是由我们日常生活中的特定情况引起的,而慢性应激则为长时间内反复暴露于相同或不同的应激源。两者均可释放压力荷尔蒙(如皮质醇)。然而,在急性应激时,这种释放可能有助于提高人们对特定情况的认识或解决相应的问题。相反,慢性应激所引起的皮质醇持续释放可能会对各种身体功能产生负面影响,例如心血管系统。特别是当两者相结合时更易产生问题。在自然流产的女性中,不仅是急性应激本身,慢性应激史可能是急性应激源导致妊娠事件的关键因素[58]。

3 应激的流行病学

由于没有明确的定义,也没有诊断标志,因此很难确定应激的流行程度。此外,应激及其被感知和处理的方式是相当主观的。据报道,100 名孕妇中有 84 人面临各种形式的产前应激,大部分是轻至中度的[59]。另外,几乎每100 名孕妇中就有11 人可能受到抑郁和焦虑等慢性应激的影响[60]。有报道称,产前普遍存在感知应激的风险,尤其是有一个或多个孩子的女性[61]。根据国家儿童健康与人类发展研究所的胎儿生长研究报告,妊娠期间的应激会逐渐降低,尤其是初产妇,这是因为焦虑主要发生在妊娠早期[61]。此外,在年轻女性、初产妇和计划外妊娠或社会经济地位较低的女性中,妊娠期特有的应激被越来越多地观察到[50]。然而,这种妊娠期特有应激在临近分娩的晚期妊娠时再次增加。

4 神经-内分泌-免疫失衡与妊娠

妊娠期应激相关病理的早期研究已于20世纪开展,例如,应激暴露后胎儿出生体重减轻[48]。因此,妊娠进展受损与近期不良生活事件相关[62]。目前,产前应激对妊娠结局的各种已知影响包括早期胚胎种植失败、反复流产、早产以及胎儿免疫和认知发育缺陷[49,62]。

生理应激反应由自主神经系统和下丘脑-垂体-肾上腺(HPA)轴控制。为了快速适应应激,交感肾上腺髓质轴通过将能量分配给所需的身体系统,诱导肾上腺素从肾上腺释放到血液中,从而激活"战斗或逃跑"反应。之后,副交感神经系统恢复机体的稳态。HPA轴由慢性应激暴露激活,调节肾上腺皮质醇的释放,其基本的先决条件是下丘脑释放促肾上腺皮质激素释放激素(CRH),从而触发垂体释放促肾上腺皮质激素[55]。应激反应的典型表现为心率、血压和呼吸频率增加,葡萄糖和脂肪从临时储存场所释放,以促进大脑、肌肉和心脏的能量供应。因此,慢性应激对心血管、免疫和代谢系统存在影响[55,63]。

胎儿抗原的耐受性在很大程度上依赖于精细调节的内分泌和免疫适应过程,而这些过程会被产前应激感知所破坏,导致各种妊娠并发症,如自然流产或早产。例如,血清孕酮水平的降低,孕酮诱导的阻断因子减少,导致母体免疫系统进入炎症性Th1状态[64]。此外,hCG分泌也受应激的抑制,进一步影响了孕酮的合成。更为重要的是,孕激素、雌激素和糖皮质激素都由孕烯醇酮转化而来,且存在竞争关系。由于HPA轴的激活需要皮质醇产生增加,同时损害了孕酮和雌激素的分泌,导致激素平衡发生改变(图7.2)。因此,过量的糖皮质激素能控制重要的妊娠保护激素的产生,并破坏它们的抑制能力[65]。有趣的是,尽管80%~90%的糖皮质激素被胎盘酶11β-羟基类固醇脱氢酶2型灭活,但这种糖皮质激素的溢出也存在于胎儿体内[66]。除糖皮质激素外,

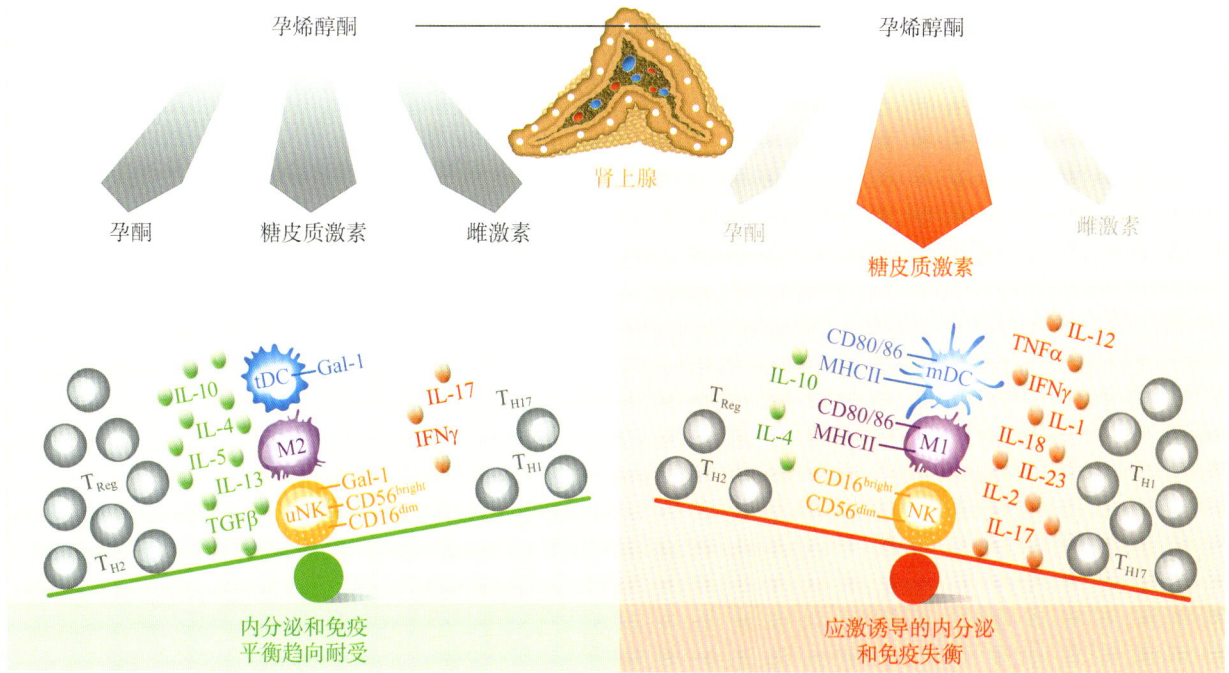

图7.2 妊娠期的内分泌与免疫平衡及应激引起的失衡。

在正常妊娠过程中,激素平衡有利于具有耐受表型的固有免疫细胞,包括表达半乳糖凝集素-1(Gal-1)的耐受性树突状细胞(tDCs)、2型巨噬细胞(M2)和以CD56^{bright}、CD16^{dim}和Gal-1表达为特征的子宫自然杀伤细胞(uNK)。这支持了向抗炎T细胞类型、辅助T细胞(Th)2、调节T细胞(Treg)及其相关的细胞因子,如白细胞介素(IL)-4、IL-5、IL-10、IL-13和转化生长因子-β(TGF-β)的转变。相反,应激引起的对皮质醇需求的增加导致了对肾上腺产生的孕烯醇酮的竞争,损害了孕酮和雌激素的产生。因此,共刺激分子MHCII和CD80/86上调,诱导树突状细胞(mDC)和巨噬细胞(M1)成熟,支持Th1和Th17细胞形成促炎环境,包括促炎细胞因子IL-1、IL-2、IL-12、IL-18、IL-23、肿瘤坏死因子-α(TNF-α)和干扰素-γ(IFN-γ)的分泌。

CRH 在妊娠期间增加，不仅在下丘脑产生，亦由胎盘产生。如参考文献[67]所述，其作为宫缩诱导剂，一旦过度表达，会导致早产。此外，较高水平的 CRH 与流产相关[68]。

这种应激诱导的妊娠激素失衡破坏了免疫细胞和细胞因子环境[69]。因此，尽管糖皮质激素具有免疫抑制和抗炎作用，但由于应激感知，过量的糖皮质激素会对孕酮、雌激素和 hCG 水平产生负面影响。一般来说，母胎界面的白细胞减少，以应对影响固有免疫和适应性免疫的应激[70]。只有 NK 细胞，尤其是 $CD56^{dim}CD16^+CD69^+$ NK 细胞，在子宫内膜和血液中增加，导致 $CD56^{bright}/CD56^{dim}$ 比例降低，这与细胞毒性增加引起的反复妊娠丢失和不孕相关[71-73]。然而，其他研究没有发现蜕膜中 NK 细胞数量存在差异，仅提示 $CD56^{bright}$ dNK 细胞下调[74]。

产前应激可进一步诱导树突状细胞成熟，表现为子宫引流淋巴结和皮肤中的树突状细胞 CD11c、MHC Ⅱ 和 ICAM-1 表达上调[75,76]。成熟状态的树突状细胞增加与自然流产相关。

应激时，$CD4^+$ T 细胞的组成发生比例和表型的改变。因此，Th1 免疫在母胎界面得到促进，而 Th2 细胞受损[69]，包括分泌促炎细胞因子（如 TNF-α、IFN-γ），且不受 Th2 细胞因子（如 IL-4、IL-10 或 TGF-β）的拮抗。据报道，促炎细胞因子会影响宫颈成熟，导致早产[77]。此外，TNF-α 通过抑制妊娠保护性转化生长因子 β2 引起流产，而后者具有免疫抑制活性[78]。与接受人工流产的女性相比，$CD4^+Treg$ 比例在自然流产患者的蜕膜中显著降低，亦与流产和其他并发症相关[79,80]。相反，在慢性应激中，观察到 Treg 数量增加，这可能是由滋养细胞对炎症过程的反应所介导的[81]。

$CD8^+$ T 细胞群在产前应激反应中出现的频率更高[74]。据报道，细胞毒性 $CD8^+$ T 淋巴细胞增加，伴随耐受性 $CD8^+CD122^+$ Treg 细胞减少，与孕酮水平和胎盘血红素氧合酶 1 表达降低存在因果关系[27]。在小鼠研究中观察到，这些应激诱导的变化可导致宫内生长受限[27]。

由于 B 细胞在胎儿耐受中的作用仍不清楚，它们由于产前应激而引起的改变甚至没有得到很好的研究。然而，在应激女性中 B 细胞水平较低[82]，并且在自然流产中观察到 Breg 细胞减少以及 IL-10 产生受损[47]。

此外，淋巴细胞归巢对于妊娠期间诱导耐受也很重要。生理上，抗炎细胞亚群被募集，并能渗透血管内皮[83]。这种细胞从脉管系统通过内皮转移到组织中的主动过程是由黏附分子介导，如细胞间黏附分子-1(ICAM-1)及其配体淋巴细胞功能相关抗原-1(LFA-1)。小鼠模型显示，在经历妊娠丢失的应激女性中，上皮细胞中的 ICAM-1 和抗原递呈细胞（如巨噬细胞和树突状细胞）上的 LFA-1 表达增强[84]。因此，淋巴细胞被吸引而迁移到子宫组织中诱发炎症反应。促炎细胞因子（如 IL-1、TNF-α 和 IFN-γ）在应激时表现出更高的密度，甚至进一步增加，导致抗原递呈细胞的成熟，例如，DC 离开其未成熟状态，促进向 Th1 型极化。此外，ICAM-1/LFA-1 信号通路诱导滋养细胞凋亡，导致流产，而阻断 ICAM-1 的黏附则可防止流产[84]。

另一种黏附分子是血管细胞黏附蛋白(VCAM)1。与 ICAM-1 相同，其在炎症环境中的表达量更高，同样会吸引白细胞。在高应激小鼠模型中，VCAM 阳性血管明显增多[85]。VCAM 与 α4β1-整合素的相互作用使淋巴细胞、单核细胞、嗜酸性粒细胞和 NK 细胞渗透到组织中，有利于炎症细胞的黏附，从而募集到母胎界面[83]。

黏附分子 P-选择素参与血栓形成，在应激诱导的流产中，可检测到其含量增加[84,86]。研究发现，由于 Th1 细胞增多，蜕膜中 P-选择素表达受凝血酶、组胺和血小板活化因子的调控而上调[86,87]。

5 如何评估应激感知

由于定义方式的差异和研究工具的不同，对应激的评估存在一定难度，造成了研究结果的广泛多样性和数量增加[88]。然而，为了研究应激的影响和病理特征，科学家们开始寻找重大事件（如灾难）后的应激人群，并对诊断为焦虑或其他心理健康问题的人进行调查。此外，日常生活中的困难和个人生活的变化可通过问卷调查来衡量。因此，应激感受量表(perceived stress scale, PSS)，尤其是孕期的产前生活事件量表具有重要意义[48,89]。

PSS 由 Cohen 等[90]开发，是一种基于心理压力概念的自我报告测量方法，侧重于日常烦恼。该量表衡量了在过去 1 个月中，情境被评估为具有压力的程度，包括不可预测性和超负荷感。目前，PSS 是常规和标准化评估日常烦恼的最佳工具之一，并且该问卷已在妊娠期得到了验证[61,90]。

另一种常用的问卷是产前窘迫问卷(PDQ)。1999年由Yali和Lobel设计,2008年由Lobel和Canella修订(NUPDQ)[50]。该问卷不仅包括了典型的应激源,还包括妊娠特有的应激源[55]。产前生活事件量表包含了22项有关个人生活改变事件的信息,如搬迁、离婚、失业和发生在女性或其亲密家庭成员身上的暴力犯罪[89]。

如上所述,应激的严重程度与社会支持密切相关,包括社会关系的稳定和参与[91]。为此,还有一份调查问卷,包含22个项目,涉及感知社会支持的多个维度,如情感支持、工具支持和社会融合。此外,它还评估了女性对其社会支持网络的满意度,并考虑了个人生活中值得信赖的人[91]。

6 如何治疗高应激感知

首先,提高妇产科医生对孕妇整个孕期的监护意识尤为重要。除了关于未出生婴儿的迫在眉睫的医疗问题外,他们还需将视野扩大到女性整体,并密切观察患者是否有超出正常范围的应激迹象。

预防产前应激负面后果的最佳选择是从一开始就予以避免。减少应激源,并通过应激训练和社会支持(一种孕产妇福利的有效调节因素)以增强复原力[91]。应激干预和应对策略(如放松训练、冥想和瑜伽)已在研究中被发现可以改善妊娠结局[61,92,93]。

此外,环境富集(environmental enrichment, EE)被认为是通过社会和物理环境对感觉通路的非侵入性刺激。因此,已有研究表明,EE具有调节代谢并发挥抗炎作用,从而防止小鼠早产[94]。此外,在人类研究中亦表明,充足的闲暇时间、体育活动和抗应激治疗可以减少妊娠相关的损伤[95]。相反,回避策略似乎只会增加应激[61]。

心理压力,如焦虑,也可通过心理治疗来干预。在先前经历过反复妊娠丢失的女性中已经显示出积极的效果[96]。

当然,也可选择旨在对抗应激引起的产科并发症的医疗干预措施。在经历反复妊娠丢失的女性中,补充维生素D在免疫状态方面显示出积极的效果,使其成为潜在的治疗候选药物[97]。此外,外源性给予黄体酮对应激小鼠具有抗流产作用[98]。据报道,有流产倾向的雌性小鼠接受HCG治疗后,流产率降低,CD4$^+$ Treg数量增加[99]。

7 母体应激对生殖结局的影响

如上所述,母体内的性激素会由于应激而发生变化,导致免疫细胞的组成改变。根据应激暴露的特定时间点,对妊娠结局及子代的长期健康影响可能是严重的,并且种类繁多。

高皮质醇水平与影响受孕能力的月经周期不规律有关[100],妊娠早期的应激与流产的病因密切相关[101,102]。妊娠后期,活跃的HPA轴使母体内Th1过剩,阻碍生长激素分泌,引起血压升高,影响胎盘灌注,导致低出生体重、肠道微生物组紊乱和胎儿免疫问题[103]。一般而言,糖皮质激素及其受体的失衡会导致宫内生长迟缓[104]。虽然胎儿通常受到保护,不受过量糖皮质激素的影响,但防止过多糖皮质激素的能力超过了应激所带来的浓度。研究表明,胎儿体内糖皮质激素过量会产生神经毒性作用。大脑发育,尤其是海马系统的发育受损,导致焦虑行为频率增加,认知发育迟缓[105,106]。此外,胎儿HPA轴的变化会破坏神经免疫通信、肠道成熟和微生物群的定植,从而影响行为、免疫和大脑发育[106-108]。母体应激对子代免疫发育的影响也可能是通过直接作用于免疫细胞的发生而引起的。据报道,Th1细胞因子水平(如TNF-α的产生)较低。因此,应激母亲的孩子表现出从Th2到Th1免疫的延迟转化,这在出生后的头两年内生理性发生[108,109]。因此,新生儿的免疫力降低,感染的易感性增加。在以后的生活中,这些儿童患过敏和哮喘的风险增加[110]。

尤其是妊娠晚期,慢性应激可能会导致母亲通过IgG抗体向胎儿传递被动免疫的问题[111]。此外,其他不利因素还包括心脏冠状动脉异常、神经管缺陷和孤立性唇裂,以及心理健康障碍[112]。然而,不仅是应激本身,缺乏社会支持也是导致胎儿平均出生体重降低200g的风险因素[91]。

8 总结和建议

- 精细的内分泌和免疫平衡对于支持耐受性微环境和确保胎儿生长发育至关重要。
- 母体对妊娠的这种复杂而精细的免疫适应极易受到破坏,如应激感知。
- 产前应激影响激素平衡,包括糖皮质激素增加和血清孕酮降低。

- 这种激素变化破坏了免疫细胞组成和细胞因子环境,导致炎症。
- 对产前应激的感知取决于应激源的严重程度、持续时间和现有的应对策略。
- 对于应激的评估,可使用各种问卷,包括PSS、产前生活事件量表和PDQ。
- 产前应激对妊娠结局的影响可能是严重的,且多种多样,包括增加产科并发症的风险,如流产、宫内发育迟缓和早产。
- 产前应激也会影响后代的长期健康,这是由于发育障碍会导致认知发育迟缓和免疫力减弱。
- 预防产前应激负面后果的第一道防线是减少潜在的应激源和可靠的社会支持。
- 对于对抗应激性产科并发症的医疗选择,可考虑补充维生素 D、孕酮和 HCG。

参考文献

[1] Rendell V, Bath NM, Brennan TV. Medawar's paradox and immune mechanisms of fetomaternal tolerance. OBM Transpl 2020;4(1). Available from: https://doi.org/10.21926/obm.transplant.2001104.

[2] Arck PC, Hecher K. Fetomaternal immune cross-talk and its consequences for maternal and offspring's health. Nat Med 2013;19(5):548-56. Available from: https://doi.org/10.1038/nm.3160.

[3] Solano ME. Decidual immune cells: guardians of human pregnancies. Best Pract Res Clin Obstet Gynaecol 2019;60:3-16. Available from: https://doi.org/10.1016/j.bpobgyn.2019.05.009.

[4] Kitazawa J, Kimura F, Nakamura A, et al. Endometrial immunity for embryo implantation and pregnancy establishment. Tohoku J Exp Med 2020;250(1):49-60. Available from: https://doi.org/10.1620/tjem.250.49.

[5] Saito S, Nakabayashi Y, Nakashima A, Shima T, Yoshino O. A new era in reproductive medicine: consequences of third-party oocyte donation for maternal and fetal health. Semin Immunopathol 2016;38(6):687-97. Available from: https://doi.org/10.1007/s00281-016-0577-x.

[6] Papuchova H, Meissner TB, Li Q, Strominger JL, Tilburgs T. The dual role of HLA-C in tolerance and immunity at the maternal-fetal interface. Front Immunol 2019;10:2730. Available from: https://doi.org/10.3389/fimmu.2019.02730.

[7] Moffett A, Loke C. Immunology of placentation in eutherian mammals. Nat Rev Immunol 2006;6(8):584-94. Available from: https://doi.org/10.1038/nri1897.

[8] PrabhuDas M, Bonney E, Caron K, et al. Immune mechanisms at the maternal-fetal interface: perspectives and challenges. Nat Immunol 2015;16(4):328-34. Available from: https://doi.org/10.1038/ni.3131.

[9] Mor G, Cardenas I, Abrahams V, Guller S. Inflammation and pregnancy: the role of the immune system at the implantation site. Ann N Y Acad Sci 2011;1221:80-7. Available from: https://doi.org/10.1111/j.1749-6632.2010.05938.x.

[10] Hanna J, Goldman-Wohl D, Hamani Y, et al. Decidual NK cells regulate key developmental processes at the human fetal-maternal interface. Nat Med 2006;12(9):1065-74. Available from: https://doi.org/10.1038/nm1452.

[11] Heikkinen J, Mottonen M, Komi J, Alanen A, Lassila O. Phenotypic characterization of human decidual macrophages. Clin Exp Immunol 2003;131(3):498-505. Available from: https://doi.org/10.1046/j.1365-2249.2003.02092.x.

[12] Bachy V, Williams DJ, Ibrahim MA. Altered dendritic cell function in normal pregnancy. J Reprod Immunol 2008;78(1):11-21. Available from: https://doi.org/10.1016/j.jri.2007.09.004.

[13] Mjosberg J, Berg G, Jenmalm MC, Ernerudh J. FOXP3+ regulatory T cells and T helper 1, T helper 2, and T helper 17 cells in human early pregnancy decidua. Biol Reprod 2010;82(4):698-705. Available from: https://doi.org/10.1095/biolreprod.109.081208.

[14] Polese B, Gridelet V, Araklioti E, Martens H, Perrier d'Hauterive S, Geenen V. The endocrine milieu and CD4 T-lymphocyte polarization during pregnancy. Front Endocrinol (Lausanne) 2014;5:106. Available from: https://doi.org/10.3389/fendo.2014.00106.

[15] Kane N, Kelly R, Saunders PT, Critchley HO. Proliferation of uterine natural killer cells is induced by human chorionic gonadotropin and mediated via the mannose receptor. Endocrinology 2009;150(6):2882-8. Available from: https://doi.org/10.1210/en.2008-1309.

[16] Kosaka K, Fujiwara H, Tatsumi K, et al. Human chorionic gonadotropin (HCG) activates monocytes to produce interleukin-8 via a different pathway from luteinizing hormone/HCG receptor system. J Clin Endocrinol Metab 2002;87(11):5199-208. Available from: https://doi.org/10.1210/jc.2002-020341.

[17] Furcron AE, Romero R, Mial TN, et al. Human chorionic gonadotropin has anti-inflammatory effects at the maternal-fetal interface and prevents endotoxin-induced preterm birth, but causes dystocia and fetal compromise in mice. Biol Reprod 2016;94(6):136. Available from: https://doi.org/10.1095/biolreprod.116.139345.

[18] Wan H, Versnel MA, Leijten LM, et al. Chorionic gonadotropin induces dendritic cells to express a tolerogenic phenotype. J Leukoc Biol 2008;83(4):894-901. Available from: https://doi.org/10.1189/jlb.0407258.

[19] Khil LY, Jun HS, Kwon H, et al. Human chorionic gonadotropin is an immune modulator and can prevent autoimmune diabetes in NOD mice. Diabetologia 2007;50(10):2147-55. Available from: https://doi.org/10.1007/s00125-007-0769-y.

[20] Rolle L, Memarzadeh Tehran M, Morell-Garcia A, et al. Cutting edge: IL-10-producing regulatory B cells in early human pregnancy. Am J Reprod Immunol 2013;70(6):448-53. Available from: https://doi.org/10.1111/aji.12157.

[21] Xiu F, Anipindi VC, Nguyen PV, et al. High physiological

[21] concentrations of progesterone reverse estradiolmediated changes in differentiation and functions of bone marrow derived dendritic cells. PLoS One 2016；11（4）：e0153304. Available from：https：//doi. org/10. 1371/journal. pone. 0153304.

[22] Tsai YC，Tseng JT，Wang CY，Su MT，Huang JY，Kuo PL. Medroxyprogesterone acetate drives M2 macrophage differentiation toward a phenotype of decidual macrophage. Mol Cell Endocrinol 2017；452；74－83. Available from：https：//doi.org/10.1016/j.mce.2017.05.015.

[23] Arruvito L，Giulianelli S，Flores AC，et al. NK cells expressing a progesterone receptor are susceptible to progesterone-induced apoptosis. J Immunol 2008；180（8）：5746-53. Available from：https：//doi.org/10.4049/jimmunol. 180.8.5746.

[24] Piccinni MP，Giudizi MG，Biagiotti R，et al. Progesterone favors the development of human T helper cells producing Th2-type cytokines and promotes both IL－4 production and membrane CD30 expression in established Th1 cell clones. J Immunol 1995；155（1）；128－33.

[25] Mao G，Wang J，Kang Y，et al. Progesterone increases systemic and local uterine proportions of CD4＋CD25＋Treg cells during midterm pregnancy in mice. Endocrinology 2010；151（11）；5477－88. Available from：https：//doi.org/10. 1210/en.2010-0426.

[26] Xu L，Dong B，Wang H，et al. Progesterone suppresses Th17 cell responses, and enhances the development of regulatory T cells, through thymic stromal lymphopoietin-dependent mechanisms in experimental gonococcal genital tract infection. Microbes Infect 2013；15（12）；796－805. Available from：https：//doi.org/10.1016/j. micinf.2013.06.012.

[27] Solano ME，Kowal MK，O'Rourke GE，et al. Progesterone and HMOX－1 promote fetal growth by CD8＋T cell modulation. J Clin Invest 2015；125（4）；1726－38. Available from：https：//doi.org/10.1172/JCI68140.

[28] Villa A，Rizzi N，Vegeto E，Ciana P，Maggi A. Estrogen accelerates the resolution of inflammation in macrophagic cells. Sci Rep 2015；5；15224. Available from：https：//doi. org/10.1038/srep15224.

[29] Priyanka HP，Krishnan HC，Singh RV，Hima L，Thyagarajan S. Estrogen modulates in vitro T cell responses in a concentration- and receptor-dependent manner：effects on intracellular molecular targets and antioxidant enzymes. Mol Immunol 2013；56（4）；328－39. Available from：https：//doi. org/10.1016/j.molimm.2013.05.226.

[30] Prieto GA，Rosenstein Y. Oestradiol potentiates the suppressive function of human CD4 CD25 regulatory T cells by promoting their proliferation. Immunology 2006；118（1）；58－65. Available from：https：//doi.org/10.1111/j.1365-2567.2006.02339.x.

[31] Piemonti L，Monti P，Allavena P，et al. Glucocorticoids affect human dendritic cell differentiation and maturation. J Immunol 1999；162（11）；6473－81.

[32] Russo-Marie F. Macrophages and the glucocorticoids. J Neuroimmunol 1992；40（2－3）；281－6. Available from：https：//doi.org/10.1016/0165-5728(92)90144-a.

[33] Cooper S，Laird SM，Mariee N，Li TC，Metwally M. The effect of prednisolone on endometrial uterine NK cell concentrations and pregnancy outcome in women with reproductive failure. A retrospective cohort study. J Reprod Immunol 2019；131；1－6. Available from：https：//doi.org/10.1016/j.jri.2018.10.001.

[34] Xu B，Makris A，Thornton C，Hennessy A. Glucocorticoids inhibit placental cytokines from cultured normal and preeclamptic placental explants. Placenta 2005；26（8－9）；654－60. Available from：https：//doi.org/10.1016/j.placenta.2004. 09.011.

[35] Elenkov IJ. Glucocorticoids and the Th1/Th2 balance. Ann N Y Acad Sci 2004；1024；138－46. Available from：https：// doi.org/10.1196/annals.1321.010.

[36] Engler JB，Kursawe N，Solano ME，et al. Glucocorticoid receptor in T cells mediates protection from autoimmunity in pregnancy. Proc Natl Acad Sci U S A 2017；114（2）；E181－90. Available from：https：//doi.org/10.1073/pnas.1617115114.

[37] Fu B，Li X，Sun R，et al. Natural killer cells promote immune tolerance by regulating inflammatory TH17 cells at the human maternal-fetal interface. Proc Natl Acad Sci U S A 2013；110（3）；E231－40. Available from：https：//doi.org/ 10.1073/pnas.1206322110.

[38] Vacca P，Mingari MC，Moretta L. Natural killer cells in human pregnancy. J Reprod Immunol 2013；97（1）；14－19. Available from：https：//doi.org/10.1016/j.jri.2012.10.008.

[39] Blois SM，Ilarregui JM，Tometten M，et al. A pivotal role for galectin-1 in fetomaternal tolerance. Nat Med 2007；13（12）；1450－7. Available from：https：//doi.org/10.1038/nm1680.

[40] Zhang J，Dunk C，Croy AB，Lye SJ. To serve and to protect：the role of decidual innate immune cells on human pregnancy. Cell Tissue Res 2016；363（1）；249－65. Available from：https：//doi.org/10.1007/s00441-015-2315-4.

[41] Tang MX，Hu XH，Liu ZZ，Kwak-Kim J，Liao AH. What are the roles of macrophages and monocytes in human pregnancy？ J Reprod Immunol 2015；112；73－80. Available from：https：//doi.org/10.1016/j.jri.2015.08.001.

[42] Miyazaki S，Tsuda H，Sakai M，et al. Predominance of Th2-promoting dendritic cells in early human pregnancy decidua. J Leukoc Biol 2003；74（4）；514－22. Available from：https：// doi.org/10.1189/jlb.1102566.

[43] Saito S，Nakashima A，Shima T，Ito M. Th1/Th2/Th17 and regulatory T-cell paradigm in pregnancy. Am J Reprod Immunol 2010；63（6）；601－10. Available from：https：//doi. org/10.1111/j.1600-0897.2010.00852.x.

[44] Wu HX，Jin LP，Xu B，Liang SS，Li DJ. Decidual stromal cells recruit Th17 cells into decidua to promote proliferation and invasion of human trophoblast cells by secreting IL－17. Cell Mol Immunol 2014；11（3）；253－62. Available from：https：//doi.org/10.1038/cmi.2013.67.

[45] Nakashima A，Ito M，Yoneda S，Shiozaki A，Hidaka T，Saito S. Circulating and decidual Th17 cell levels in healthy pregnancy. Am J Reprod Immunol 2010；63（2）；104－9. Available from：https：//doi.org/10.1111/j.1600-0897.2009. 00771.x.

[46] Nagaeva O，Jonsson L，Mincheva-Nilsson L. Dominant IL－10 and TGF-beta mRNA expression in gammadelta T cells of human early pregnancy decidua suggests immunoregulatory potential. Am J Reprod Immunol 2002；48（1）；9－17. Available from：https：//doi.org/10.1034/j.1600-0897.2002. 01131.x.

[47] Jensen F，Muzzio D，Soldati R，Fest S，Zenclussen AC. Regulatory B10 cells restore pregnancy tolerance in a mouse model. Biol Reprod 2013；89（4）；90. Available from：https：//doi.org/10.1095/biolreprod.113.110791.

[48] Lobel M. Conceptualizations，measurement，and effects of prenatal maternal stress on birth outcomes. J Behav Med 1994；17（3）；225－72. Available from：https：//doi.org/10.

[49] Coussons-Read ME. Effects of prenatal stress on pregnancy and human development: mechanisms and pathways. Obstet Med 2013;6(2):52-7. Available from: https://doi.org/10.1177/1753495X12473751.

[50] Ibrahim SM, Lobel M. Conceptualization, measurement, and effects of pregnancy-specific stress: review of research using the original and revised prenatal distress questionnaire. J Behav Med 2020;43(1):16-33. Available from: https://doi.org/10.1007/s10865-019-00068-7.

[51] Orr ST, James SA, Casper R. Psychosocial stressors and low birth weight: development of a questionnaire. J Dev Behav Pediatr 1992;13(5):343-7.

[52] Glynn LM, Wadhwa PD, Dunkel-Schetter C, Chicz-Demet A, Sandman CA. When stress happens matters: effects of earthquake timing on stress responsivity in pregnancy. Am J Obstet Gynecol 2001;184(4):637-42. Available from: https://doi.org/10.1067/mob.2001.111066.

[53] Engel SM, Berkowitz GS, Wolff MS, Yehuda R. Psychological trauma associated with the World Trade Center attacks and its effect on pregnancy outcome. Paediatr Perinat Epidemiol 2005;19(5):334-41. Available from: https://doi.org/10.1111/j.1365-3016.2005.00676.x.

[54] Chen T, Laplante DP, Elgbeili G, et al. Coping during pregnancy following exposure to a natural disaster: the QF2011 Queensland flood study. J Affect Disord 2020;273:341-9. Available from: https://doi.org/10.1016/j.jad.2020.03.165.

[55] Coussons-Read M. Stress and immunity in pregnancy. The Oxford Handbook of Psychoneuroimmunology. Publisher: Oxford Universitry Press; 2012. p.3-17. Available from: https://doi.org/10.1093/oxfordhb/9780195394399.013.0001.

[56] Glynn LM, Schetter CD, Wadhwa PD, Sandman CA. Pregnancy affects appraisal of negative life events. J Psychosom Res 2004;56(1):47-52. Available from: https://doi.org/10.1016/S0022-3999(03)00133-8.

[57] Bowers SL, Bilbo SD, Dhabhar FS, Nelson RJ. Stressor-specific alterations in corticosterone and immune responses in mice. Brain Behav Immun 2008;22(1):105-13. Available from: https://doi.org/10.1016/j.bbi.2007.07.012.

[58] Frazier T, Hogue CJR, Bonney EA, Yount KM, Pearce BD. Weathering the storm: a review of pre-pregnancy stress and risk of spontaneous abortion. Psychoneuroendocrinology. 2018;92:142-54. Available from: https://doi.org/10.1016/j.psyneuen.2018.03.001.

[59] Woods SM, Melville JL, Guo Y, Fan MY, Gavin A. Psychosocial stress during pregnancy. Am J Obstet Gynecol 2010;202(1):61. Available from: https://doi.org/10.1016/j.ajog.2009.07.041 e1-7.

[60] Bennett HA, Einarson A, Taddio A, Koren G, Einarson TR. Prevalence of depression during pregnancy: systematic review. Obstet Gynecol 2004;103(4):698-709. Available from: https://doi.org/10.1097/01.AOG.0000116689.75396.5f.

[61] Goletzke J, Kocalevent RD, Hansen G, et al. Prenatal stress perception and coping strategies: insights from a longitudinal prospective pregnancy cohort. J Psychosom Res 2017;102:8-14. Available from: https://doi.org/10.1016/j.jpsychores.2017.09.002.

[62] Neugebauer R, Kline J, Stein Z, Shrout P, Warburton D, Susser M. Association of stressful life events with chromosomally normal spontaneous abortion. Am J Epidemiol 1996;143(6):588-96. Available from: https://doi.org/10.1093/oxfordjournals.aje.a008789.

[63] Joseph DN, Whirledge S. Stress and the HPA axis: balancing homeostasis and fertility. Int J Mol Sci 2017;18(10). Available from: https://doi.org/10.3390/ijms18102224.

[64] Joachim R, Zenclussen AC, Polgar B, et al. The progesterone derivative dydrogesterone abrogates murine stress-triggered abortion by inducing a Th2 biased local immune response. Steroids 2003;68(10-13):931-40. Available from: https://doi.org/10.1016/j.steroids.2003.08.010.

[65] Solano ME, Arck PC. Steroids, pregnancy and fetal development. Front Immunol 2019;10:3017. Available from: https://doi.org/10.3389/fimmu.2019.03017.

[66] Gitau R, Cameron A, Fisk NM, Glover V. Fetal exposure to maternal cortisol. Lancet 1998;352(9129):707-8. Available from: https://doi.org/10.1016/S0140-6736(05)60824-0.

[67] Kalantaridou SN, Makrigiannakis A, Zoumakis E, Chrousos GP. Reproductive functions of corticotropin-releasing hormone. Research and potential clinical utility of antalarmins (CRH receptor type 1 antagonists). Am J Reprod Immunol 2004;51(4):269-74. Available from: https://doi.org/10.1111/j.1600-0897.2004.00155.x.

[68] Arck PC, Rucke M, Rose M, et al. Early risk factors for miscarriage: a prospective cohort study in pregnant women. Reprod Biomed Online 2008;17(1):101-13. Available from: https://doi.org/10.1016/s1472-6483(10)60300-8.

[69] Blois SM, Joachim R, Kandil J, et al. Depletion of CD8+ cells abolishes the pregnancy protective effect of progesterone substitution with dydrogesterone in mice by altering the Th1/Th2 cytokine profile. J Immunol 2004;172(10):5893-9. Available from: https://doi.org/10.4049/jimmunol.172.10.5893.

[70] Antonson AM, Evans MV, Galley JD, et al. Unique maternal immune and functional microbial profiles during prenatal stress. Sci Rep 2020;10(1):20288. Available from: https://doi.org/10.1038/s41598-020-77265-x.

[71] Schedlowski M, Jacobs R, Stratmann G, et al. Changes of natural killer cells during acute psychological stress. J Clin Immunol 1993;13(2):119-26. Available from: https://doi.org/10.1007/BF00919268.

[72] Murphy SP, Fast LD, Hanna NN, Sharma S. Uterine NK cells mediate inflammation-induced fetal demise in IL-10-null mice. J Immunol 2005;175(6):4084-90. Available from: https://doi.org/10.4049/jimmunol.175.6.4084.

[73] King K, Smith S, Chapman M, Sacks G. Detailed analysis of peripheral blood natural killer (NK) cells in women with recurrent miscarriage. Hum Reprod 2010;25(1):52-8. Available from: https://doi.org/10.1093/humrep/dep349.

[74] Arck PC, Rose M, Hertwig K, Hagen E, Hildebrandt M, Klapp BF. Stress and immune mediators in miscarriage. Hum Reprod 2001;16(7):1505-11. Available from: https://doi.org/10.1093/humrep/16.7.1505.

[75] Blois SM, Alba Soto CD, Tometten M, Klapp BF, Margni RA, Arck PC. Lineage, maturity, and phenotype of uterine murine dendritic cells throughout gestation indicate a protective role in maintaining pregnancy. Biol Reprod 2004;70(4):1018-23. Available from: https://doi.org/10.1095/biolreprod.103.022640.

[76] Joachim RA, Handjiski B, Blois SM, Hagen E, Paus R, Arck PC. Stress-induced neurogenic inflammation in murine skin skews dendritic cells towards maturation and migration: key

[76] role of intercellular adhesion molecule-1/leukocyte function-associated antigen interactions. Am J Pathol 2008;173(5): 1379-88. Available from: https://doi.org/10.2353/ajpath.2008.080105.

[77] Zhang W, Wang L, Zhao Y, Kang J. Changes in cytokine (IL-8, IL-6 and TNF-alpha) levels in the amniotic fluid and maternal serum in patients with premature rupture of the membranes. Zhonghua Yi Xue Za Zhi (Taipei) 2000;63(4): 311-15.

[78] Arck PC, Merali FS, Manuel J, Chaouat G, Clark DA. Stress-triggered abortion: inhibition of protective suppression and promotion of tumor necrosis factor-alpha (TNF-alpha) release as a mechanism triggering resorptions in mice. Am J Reprod Immunol 1995;33(1):74-80. Available from: https://doi.org/10.1111/j.1600-0897.1995.tb01141.x.

[79] Sasaki Y, Sakai M, Miyazaki S, Higuma S, Shiozaki A, Saito S. Decidual and peripheral blood CD4+ CD25+ regulatory T cells in early pregnancy subjects and spontaneous abortion cases. Mol Hum Reprod 2004;10(5):347-53. Available from: https://doi.org/10.1093/molehr/gah044.

[80] Winger EE, Reed JL. Low circulating CD4(+) CD25(+) Foxp3(+) T regulatory cell levels predict miscarriage risk in newly pregnant women with a history of failure. Am J Reprod Immunol 2011;66(4):320-8. Available from: https://doi.org/10.1111/j.1600-0897.2011.00992.x.

[81] Ronaldson A, Gazali AM, Zalli A, et al. Increased percentages of regulatory T cells are associated with inflammatory and neuroendocrine responses to acute psychological stress and poorer health status in older men and women. Psychopharmacol (Berl) 2016;233(9):1661-8. Available from: https://doi.org/10.1007/s00213-015-3876-3.

[82] Stefanski V, Raabe C, Schulte M. Pregnancy and social stress in female rats: influences on blood leukocytes and corticosterone concentrations. J Neuroimmunol 2005;162(1-2):81-8. Available from: https://doi.org/10.1016/j.jneuroim.2005.01.011.

[83] Kruse A, Martens N, Fernekorn U, Hallmann R, Butcher EC. Alterations in the expression of homing-associated molecules at the maternal/fetal interface during the course of pregnancy. Biol Reprod 2002;66(2):333-45. Available from: https://doi.org/10.1095/biolreprod66.2.333.

[84] Blois S, Tometten M, Kandil J, et al. Intercellular adhesion molecule-1/LFA-1 cross talk is a proximate mediator capable of disrupting immune integration and tolerance mechanism at the feto-maternal interface in murine pregnancies. J Immunol 2005;174(4):1820-9. Available from: https://doi.org/10.4049/jimmunol.174.4.1820.

[85] Prados MB, Solano ME, Friebe A, Blois S, Arck P, Miranda S. Stress increases VCAM-1 expression at the fetomaternal interface in an abortion-prone mouse model. J Reprod Immunol 2011;89(2):207-11. Available from: https://doi.org/10.1016/j.jri.2011.01.021.

[86] Zenclussen AC, Fest S, Sehmsdorf US, Hagen E, Klapp BF, Arck PC. Upregulation of decidual P-selectin expression is associated with an increased number of Th1 cell populations in patients suffering from spontaneous abortions. Cell Immunol 2001;213(2):94-103. Available from: https://doi.org/10.1006/cimm.2001.1877.

[87] Auvinen K, Jalkanen S, Salmi M. Expression and function of endothelial selectins during human development. Immunology 2014;143(3):406-15. Available from: https://doi.org/10.1111/imm.12318.

[88] Nast I, Bolten M, Meinlschmidt G, Hellhammer DH. How to measure prenatal stress? A systematic review of psychometric instruments to assess psychosocial stress during pregnancy. Paediatr Perinat Epidemiol 2013;27(4):313-22. Available from: https://doi.org/10.1111/ppe.12051.

[89] Lobel M, Dunkel-Schetter C, Scrimshaw SC. Prenatal maternal stress and prematurity: a prospective study of socioeconomically disadvantaged women. Health Psychol 1992;11(1):32-40. Available from: https://doi.org/10.1037//0278-6133.11.1.32.

[90] Cohen S, Kamarck T, Mermelstein R. A global measure of perceived stress. J Health Soc Behav 1983;24(4):385-96.

[91] Elsenbruch S, Benson S, Rucke M, et al. Social support during pregnancy: effects on maternal depressive symptoms, smoking and pregnancy outcome. Hum Reprod 2007;22(3): 869-77. Available from: https://doi.org/10.1093/humrep/del432.

[92] Narendran S, Nagarathna R, Narendran V, Gunasheela S, Nagendra HR. Efficacy of yoga on pregnancy outcome. J Altern Complement Med 2005;11(2):237-44. Available from: https://doi.org/10.1089/acm.2005.11.237.

[93] Khianman B, Pattanittum P, Thinkhamrop J, Lumbiganon P. Relaxation therapy for preventing and treating preterm labour. Cochrane Database Syst Rev 2012;8:CD007426. Available from: https://doi.org/10.1002/14651858.CD007426.pub2.

[94] Schander JA, Aisemberg J, Correa F, et al. The enrichment of maternal environment prevents pre-term birth in a mice model. Reproduction 2020;159(4):479-92. Available from: https://doi.org/10.1530/REP-19-0572.

[95] Hegaard HK, Hedegaard M, Damm P, Ottesen B, Petersson K, Henriksen TB. Leisure time physical activity is associated with a reduced risk of preterm delivery. Am J Obstet Gynecol 2008;198(2):180. Available from: https://doi.org/10.1016/j.ajog.2007.08.038 e1-5.

[96] Stray-Pedersen B, Stray-Pedersen S. Etiologic factors and subsequent reproductive performance in 195 couples with a prior history of habitual abortion. Am J Obstet Gynecol 1984;148(2):140-6. Available from: https://doi.org/10.1016/s0002-9378(84)80164-7.

[97] Goncalves DR, Braga A, Braga J, Marinho A. Recurrent pregnancy loss and vitamin D: a review of the literature. Am J Reprod Immunol 2018;80(5):e13022. Available from: https://doi.org/10.1111/aji.13022.

[98] Haas DM, Hathaway TJ, Ramsey PS. Progestogen for preventing miscarriage in women with recurrent miscarriage of unclear etiology. Cochrane Database Syst Rev 2019;2019 (11). Available from: https://doi.org/10.1002/14651858.CD003511.pub5.

[99] Schumacher A, Heinze K, Witte J, et al. Human chorionic gonadotropin as a central regulator of pregnancy immune tolerance. J Immunol 2013;190(6):2650-8. Available from: https://doi.org/10.4049/jimmunol.1202698.

[100] Nepomnaschy PA, Welch K, McConnell D, Strassmann BI, England BG. Stress and female reproductive function: a study of daily variations in cortisol, gonadotrophins, and gonadal steroids in a rural Mayan population. Am J Hum Biol 2004;16(5):523-32. Available from: https://doi.org/10.1002/ajhb.20057.

[101] Qu F, Wu Y, Zhu YH, et al. The association between psychological stress and miscarriage: a systematic review and meta-analysis. Sci Rep 2017;7(1):1731. Available from:

[102] O'Hare T, Creed F. Life events and miscarriage. Br J Psychiatry 1995;167(6):799-805. Available from: https://doi.org/10.1192/bjp.167.6.799.

[103] Knackstedt MK, Hamelmann E, Arck PC. Mothers in stress: consequences for the offspring. Am J Reprod Immunol 2005;54(2):63-9. Available from: https://doi.org/10.1111/j.1600-0897.2005.00288.x.

[104] Hutter S, Hepp P, Hofmann S, et al. Glucocorticoid receptors alpha and beta are modulated sex specifically in human placentas of intrauterine growth restriction (IUGR). Arch Gynecol Obstet 2019;300(2):323-35. Available from: https://doi.org/10.1007/s00404-019-05189-7.

[105] Jia N, Yang K, Sun Q, et al. Prenatal stress causes dendritic atrophy of pyramidal neurons in hippocampal CA3 region by glutamate in offspring rats. Dev Neurobiol 2010;70(2):114-25. Available from: https://doi.org/10.1002/dneu.20766.

[106] Chagas LA, Batista TH, Ribeiro A, et al. Anxiety-like behavior and neuroendocrine changes in offspring resulting from gestational post-traumatic stress disorder. Behav Brain Res 2021;399:113026. Available from: https://doi.org/10.1016/j.bbr.2020.113026.

[107] Bailey MT, Lubach GR, Coe CL. Prenatal stress alters bacterial colonization of the gut in infant monkeys. J Pediatr Gastroenterol Nutr 2004;38(4):414-21. Available from: https://doi.org/10.1097/00005176-200404000-00009.

[108] Coe CL, Kramer M, Kirschbaum C, Netter P, Fuchs E. Prenatal stress diminishes the cytokine response of leukocytes to endotoxin stimulation in juvenile rhesus monkeys. J Clin Endocrinol Metab 2002;87(2):675-81. Available from: https://doi.org/10.1210/jcem.87.2.8233.

[109] Yabuhara A, Macaubas C, Prescott SL, et al. TH2-polarized immunological memory to inhalant allergens in atopics is established during infancy and early childhood. Clin Exp Allergy 1997;27(11):1261-9.

[110] von Hertzen LC. Maternal stress and T-cell differentiation of the developing immune system: possible implications for the development of asthma and atopy. J Allergy Clin Immunol 2002;109(6):923-8. Available from: https://doi.org/10.1067/mai.2002.124776.

[111] Coe CL, Crispen HR. Social stress in pregnant squirrel monkeys (Saimiri boliviensis peruviensis) differentially affects placental transfer of maternal antibody to male and female infants. Health Psychol 2000;19(6):554-9.

[112] Carmichael SL, Shaw GM. Maternal life event stress and congenital anomalies. Epidemiology 2000;11(1):30-5. Available from: https://doi.org/10.1097/00001648-200001000-00008.

第 8 章

抗磷脂综合征与反复妊娠丢失

Antiphospholipid syndrome and recurrent pregnancy losses

Erra Roberta[1], Trespidi Laura[1], Ossola Wally[1] and Meroni Pier Luigi[2]

[1] Department of Obstetrics and Gynaecology, Fondazione Ca Granda, Ospedale Maggiore Policlinico, Milan, Italy
[2] Istituto Auxologico Italiano, IRCCS, Immunorheumatology Research Laboratory, Milan, Italy

1 引言

1.1 定义

抗磷脂综合征（antiphospholipid syndrome，APS）是一种系统性自身免疫性疾病，其特征是反复妊娠发病或与带负电荷磷脂结合蛋白（aPL）反应的抗体持续存在相关的血管血栓形成。根据悉尼-札幌（Sydney-Sapporo）标准（表8.1），当患者满足至少1个临床症状和1个实验室指标时，可诊断为APS[1]。分类标准的修订过程仍在讨论和定期更新中[2]。

临床分类标准包括两种主要表现：静脉和（或）动脉血栓形成以及妊娠丢失，并定义了3种妊娠病变模式。

（1）在妊娠10周前，出现3次或更多次无法解释的连续自然流产，排除了母亲和父亲因素（如解剖、激素或染色体异常）。

（2）在妊娠10周后，出现至少1次无法解释的形态学正常的胎儿死亡。

（3）在妊娠34周前，出现至少1次重度子痫前期、子痫或严重胎盘功能不全引起的形态正常的新生儿早产[1,3,4]。

aPL可通过3个正式的实验室分类指标进行检测：抗心磷脂抗体（aCL）、抗β2-糖蛋白Ⅰ抗体（anti-β2 GPI）和狼疮抗凝物（LA），并要求必须间隔至少12周连续检测2次，以排除短暂的阳性结果（详见本章2.1）。

抗磷脂综合征可表现为孤立性的（原发性APS），或与其他自身免疫性疾病共同存在，最常见的是系统性红斑狼疮（SLE）或SLE样疾病。APS常同时表现出血管和产科事件，但也已发现了单纯的血栓性APS或产科APS[5]。

1.2 患病率

关于抗磷脂综合征在普通人群中的患病率，目前一些研究在报道中的纳入标准不尽相同，使得关

表8.1 修订版抗磷脂综合征的悉尼-札幌标准[1]

临床标准	
血栓形成	任何组织或器官发生1次或多次动脉、静脉或小血管血栓形成
病理妊娠	胎龄<10周，有≥3次无法解释的连续自然流产，除外母亲和父亲因素（如解剖、激素或染色体异常）
	胎龄≥10周，有≥1次胚胎形态学正常的胎儿死胎
	因重度子痫前期（PE）、子痫或严重胎盘功能不全所致≥1次妊娠34周以前形态正常的新生儿早产
实验室标准	
血浆中存在狼疮抗凝物；抗心磷脂抗体（IgG或IgM）；抗β2-糖蛋白Ⅰ抗体（IgG或IgM）	

注：自身抗体仅在中高滴度时才具相关性，且必须至少间隔12周2次或2次以上的检测加以确认。如果aPL阳性检测结果距临床症状出现不到12周或超过5年，则应避免对APS进行分类。

于抗磷脂综合征实际患病率的最终结论值得怀疑。最近的一项大规模基于人群的研究报道指出，APS每年大约在每10万人中发生2例，估计患病率为每10万人50例[6]。同一研究未具体说明单纯的产科APS患病率。APS尤其影响育龄期女性，aPL是不良产科结局（adverse pregnancy outcomes，APO）最常见的原因[3]。在欧洲磷脂项目（188名孕妇）和PROMISSE研究（144名孕妇）中，APO的患病率分别为27%和19%[7,8]。然而，EURAPS根据较宽松的纳入标准报道了5 229例aPL阳性孕妇中APO为65.1%[9]。实际上，EURAPS包含了早期和晚期流产，尽管有关于早期流产是否应被排除在外的争论，因为它们与APS的相关性并不强[4]。另一份文献综述报道了aPL阳性女性的流产率为9%，重度子痫前期为8%，子痫前期为4%，子痫为16.5%，溶血、肝酶升高、低血小板综合征（HELLP）为3%[10]。第16届抗磷脂会议产科APS工作组最近的一份报道指出，在反复流产且无其他原因的患者中，只有不到5%显示出符合国际共识标准的aPL结果[4]。另一方面，不明原因的胎儿死亡和重度子痫前期和（或）胎盘功能不全的早产似乎是产科APS的更具体特征。aPL-IgG/IgM阳性可能将死胎风险增加5倍[4]。

1.3 潜在的免疫病理机制

虽然血栓事件与血管APS的表现密切相关，但在产科APS的发病机制中，凝血的作用显然没有那么重要。虽然在APS患者的胎盘组织中可以检测到血栓病变，但它们并不具有特异性，因为在与aPL无关的情况下也可能存在。在一些没有血栓病变表现的APS患者中发现存在子宫血管重塑和（或）蜕膜高凝状态[11]。越来越多的证据表明，在APS中，与凝血无关的各种致病机制对于导致APO的胎盘形成缺陷至关重要[5,11]。β2-糖蛋白-Ⅰ（β2GPⅠ）在生理上存在于蜕膜内皮、绒毛和绒毛外滋养层上，可作为母体aPL。β2GPⅠ依赖的aPL与绒毛外胚层上的β2GPⅠ反应，影响其增殖和分化，并诱导凋亡。这些抗体还会干扰血管生成和螺旋动脉发育，并在与蜕膜细胞和绒毛外胚层结合时诱发局部炎症反应（图8.1）[11,12]。

抗磷脂抗体可以激活补体，进而可能与凝血系统相互作用，促进纤维蛋白沉积和胎盘血管血栓形成。已报道在来自APS患者的胎盘中发现了沉积的补体成分。此外，缺乏补体的小鼠（或接受了补体抑制分子处理的小鼠）对通过被动注射人类IgG aPL引起的胎儿死亡具有保护作用[13,14]。由被动注射大量人类IgG aPL的妊娠小鼠所示，补体激活有助于引发胎盘的炎症反应[15]。然而，并非所有研究都报道了人类胎盘组织中的炎症特征[11,14]。此外，在另一个aPL介导的胎儿死亡模型中，少量IgG aPL的被动转移仍会导致流产，而不表现出炎症[16]。总之，尽管补体激活在产科APS中的作用得到广泛认可，但其在促进胎盘炎症或有利于凝血方面的确切作用仍是研究焦点。最后，目前尚不清楚这些致病途径是发生在整个妊娠期，还是在不同的时间发生。例如，在妊娠初期发生并随后消退的炎症反应可以解释其在胎盘损伤中的重要性，同时也可以解释足月胎盘缺乏组织学炎症迹象。抗磷脂抗体对滋养细胞的增殖和分化的影响可能解释了早期流产。另一方面，妊娠晚期的产科表现（如子痫前期、宫内生长受限和宫内胎儿死亡）可能与绒毛外胚层无法重塑螺旋动脉有关，最终导致缺氧损伤、胎儿供应营养不足以及胎盘血流速度及压力增高。

2 评估

2.1 诊断

正如引言部分所述，APS的分类需要至少1个临床标准和1个实验室标准的存在（表8.1）。检测抗阴离子磷脂结合蛋白抗体的正式实验室分类指标包括LA、β2GPI依赖的aCL和抗β2GPI测定[1]。如同其他系统性自身免疫性疾病，我们没有特定的"诊断"标准，APS的诊断目前使用分类标准进行。

"狼疮抗凝物"指的是一系列功能测定，用于检测与不同的磷脂结合蛋白反应的异质性免疫球蛋白，这些免疫球蛋白在体外作为抗凝物的获得性抑制剂。有证据表明，抗β2GPI和凝血酶原（PT）的抗体是最重要的抗体，具有最高的诊断特异性。LA是一个有趣的悖论，因为它会导致PL依赖性的凝血时间延长，但与血栓形成和妊娠发病率的增加有关。LA的检测基于一个三步骤的实验室流程，包括筛查、混合和确认。目前使用两种检测系统，即激活部分凝血时间和稀释罗素蝰蛇毒液时间[17,18]。LA检测结果以阳性或阴性表示，因为尚无证据表明LA效应的强度（凝血试验的延长程度）能否为临床风险分层提供更好的信息。如果三步骤中的至少一个测

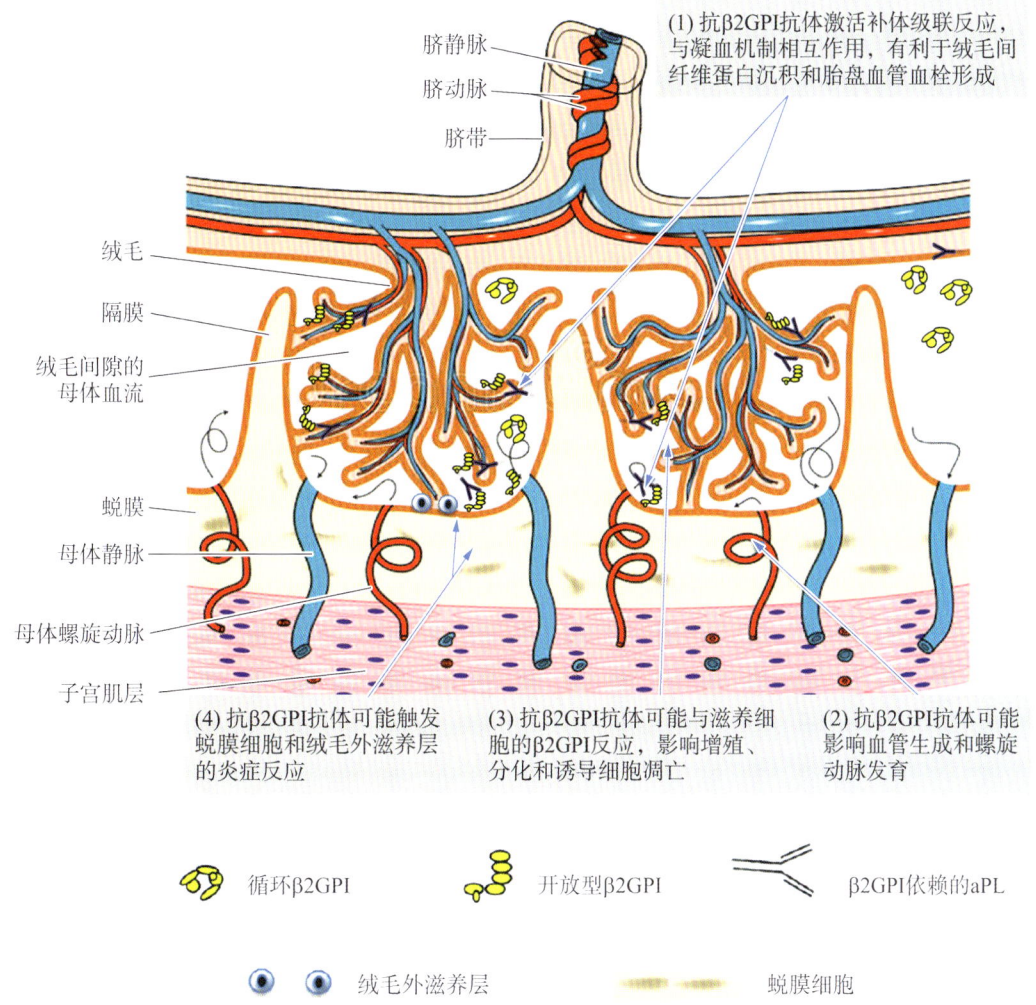

图 8.1 β2GPI 依赖性 aPL 介导胎盘病理的机制。

β2GPI 依赖性 aPL 不与循环的 β2GPI（闭合形式）反应，仅与细胞膜上的开放分子反应。β2GPI 依赖性 aPL 主要通过免疫显性 D1 表位反应。开放型 β2GPI 在生理上存在于蜕膜内皮、绒毛和绒毛外滋养层上，并可与 β2GPI 依赖性 aPL 结合。抗体结合可能导致：①补体激活。②抗血管生成作用。③滋养细胞抑制和凋亡。④蜕膜和绒毛外滋养层炎症反应。

试系统显示标准化比值高于本地截断值，则 LA 被视为阳性。由于存在干扰因素，LA 结果的解释具有挑战性，如伴随抗凝药物和高血浆水平的急性期蛋白，会导致假阳性结果[17,18]。国际血栓与止血学会（the International Society of Thrombosis and Hemostasis，ISTH）近期提供了关于 LA 检测和解释的更新指南[17]。抗 β2GPI 抗体已被证明可以延长 PL 依赖性凝血试验，这在一定程度上是 LA 现象的原因[17-19]。另一方面，抗凝血酶原抗体（aPT），特别是那些与磷脂酰丝氨酸（PS）- PT 复合物（aPS/PT）反应的抗体，能够介导 LA 现象[17-19]。此外，还存在没有任何抗 β2GPI 或 aPS/PT 抗体的"孤立性" LA。在这些病例中，凝血抑制剂（或是抗体）依旧是一个研究问题[17,19,20]。在没有任何 aCL 和抗

β2GPI 的情况下，孤立的 LA 阳性被认为是较低的风险因素[21,22]。

aPL 并不仅仅识别阴离子磷脂本身，还能识别磷脂与磷脂结合蛋白之间的复合物。β2GPI 是 aPL 最相关的辅助因子[19]。β2GPI 依赖的抗体与其抗原结合：①当与 CL 结合时，例如在 aCL 测定中，将 β2GPI 添加到 CL 包被微孔板中。②当微孔板直接包被 β2GPI 时。一旦与 CL 结合，β2GPI 就会表现出构象变化和（或）抗原密度增加，从而有利于抗体结合[19]。将 β2GPI 直接涂覆在 γ-辐照的聚苯乙烯板上，被认为可以再现类似的分子结构，最终为抗体提供正确的抗原结构[19]。因此，β2GPI 依赖性抗体显然是两种固相测定（即 aCL 和抗 β2GPI 检测）阳性结果的原因，这些实验是 APS 的正式实验室分类

标准。由于β2GPI依赖的aPL也与LA现象相关联,这一发现支持了一个观点,即β2GPI依赖的aPL可能造成APS的三个正式实验室分类(和诊断)指标的阳性结果。

与LA不同,aCL和抗β2GPI测定是半定量的固相实验,与正常阈值进行比较,报告分为低度阳性、中度阳性及高度阳性[19]。如本章2.3所讨论的,抗体滴度越高,检测的诊断/预后价值越高。短暂的aPL可以在不同起源的感染性疾病期间检测到,并且通常不与APS的临床表现相关联[19]。同样地,只有在首次检测后至少12周持续aPL阳性才被视为分类和诊断工具(表8.1)。

尽管尚未正式纳入实验室分类标准,但在血管性和产科APS的诊断和风险分层方面,还有其他一些检测方法看起来很有希望。在这些非分类标准中,抗PT抗体,特别是那些可通过PS/PT包被微孔板检测到的抗体,似乎显示出有用的诊断和预后价值[19,23]。然而,它们尚未被正式纳入APS实验室分类标准。抗PS/PT测试可以帮助检测可能导致LA现象的aPL。因此,当存在干扰LA测定的变量时(例如,当患者正在服用抗凝药物或显示循环CRP高水平时),抗PS/PT和抗β2GPI检测可能成为一种替代工具[19]。

β2GPI依赖的aPL针对分子的不同表位,但越来越多的证据表明,在实验模型中,抗体与结构域1(D1)内的构象免疫显性区(跨氨基酸序列的39~43位精氨酸)反应介导致病机制。此外,最近的荟萃分析显示,IgG抗D1 β2GPI的存在比IgG对整个分子具有更高的特异性和预测价值[27]。因此,建议将抗-D1抗体检测作为APS的一项新的实验室标准。然而,一些患者对整个β2GPI分子的抗体检测呈阳性,但在抗-D1检测中呈阴性,这表明抗-D1不能替代针对整个分子的检测。尽管如此,抗-D1抗体在双重/三重aPL阳性的完全型APS患者中更为常见,但通常在其他APS不相关条件下检测不到aPL。因此,寻找抗-D1抗体可用作一种确认性测试[19]。没有可靠的证据表明检测其他aPL(如抗-PS、抗磷脂醇胺)或抗其他凝血蛋白抗体(如抗V型蛋白、抗S/C蛋白)可以提高分类实验的诊断能力[19]。

2.2 何时检测aPL

aPL抗体检测适用于所有有不明原因妊娠相关并发症或动/静脉血栓形成病史的患者。在临床实践中,亦常出于其他原因进行aPL检测,包括:①存在所谓非标准的表现(如网织红细胞增多症、皮肤溃疡、血小板减少等)。②既往诊断为自身免疫性疾病。③既往病理妊娠不符合正式分类标准(例如,少于3次早期流产或不孕)[28]。

2.3 抗磷脂抗体作为一种风险因素

抗磷脂抗体被广泛认为是APS相关临床表现的危险因素,包括产科并发症[12,19]。aPL水平与临床表现的风险相关,中/高滴度比低滴度更具预测性。此外,2个或3个实验室分类指标阳性表示进一步的风险。然而,应该强调的是,即使在低滴度的情况下,两次检测的持续阳性也与显著的流产风险相关。所有患者对治疗(即低剂量阿司匹林和低分子肝素)的反应进一步支持了这一发现的临床意义,而高达20%的中/高aPL滴度患者会复发[19]。虽然IgG型aPL显示出比IgM在血管病变方面更高的预测价值,但对于妊娠并发症的预测价值仍存在争议[9,19,29-31]。

在3个正式的实验室分类指标中,LA被广泛认为是最具预测性的,即使可以找到孤立的LA阳性病例(没有抗β2GPI或抗PS/PT抗体),但与血管和产科APS都没有关联[21,22]。孤立的aCL或抗β2GPI阳性结果的临床意义是存疑的,应该从临床角度进行严格评估。特别是应排除与同时存在的感染相关的短暂阳性结果。检测抗β2GPI结构域1抗体有望作为确认高风险抗体谱的二线方法(详见本章2.1)[27]。产科APS的整体风险谱不仅得到aPL谱(例如滴度、亚型、检测方法)的支持,还包括与aPL无关的变量,如流产的传统风险因素以及存在相关的潜在系统性自身免疫性疾病。此外,既往发生的血栓事件本身就是复发的风险,并进一步受与妊娠相关的血栓倾向风险的影响(图8.2)。

3 临床实践管理

3.1 风险分层

患有APS的孕妇在临床和实验室特征方面表现出不同的产科风险。因此,在孕前咨询期间进行风险分层对于量身定制治疗方案是必要的。如本章2.3所述,"aPL谱"以及临床特征都用于确定APO的最终风险(图8.2)。与这些变量的作用一致,患者必须通过孕前干预进行优化,包括戒烟、减少体重

产科 APS

更高的风险取决于 aPL 谱

aPL 检测类型阳性
三重/双重阳性
LA 阳性
免疫球蛋白亚型(IgG>IgM)
滴度(中/高滴度)

与 aPL 无关的风险因素

既往的产科病史
传统的产科风险因素(年龄、糖尿病、高血压、先天性血栓性疾病、血脂异常、体质指数、吸烟、久坐生活方式等)
潜在的自身免疫性疾病
既往的血栓事件

图 8.2 抗磷脂抗体作为风险因素。

aPL 的类别、亚型、滴度以及 aPL 非相关因素都是产科抗磷脂综合征的风险等级。

指数以及治疗一些已知影响妊娠结局的并发症。

3.1.1 抗体谱

关于抗体谱,2019 年欧洲风湿病联盟(EULAR)关于管理 APS 孕妇的建议将高风险谱定义为持续存在 LA,或双重(任意 LA、aCL 或抗 β2GPI 抗体的组合),或三重(所有三个亚型)aPL 阳性或持续存在高 aPL 滴度[32]。近期已开展了进一步研究以更好地详细阐述 aPL 阳性女性的风险谱。EUREKA 研究表明,除了广泛接受的与中/高 aPL 滴度相关的风险外,低 aPL 滴度也会带来罹患产科并发症的风险。特别是持续的 LA 和低滴度抗 β2GPI IgG 的双重阳性显示出比单独或联合低滴度 aCL 和 IgG 抗

β2GPI 更高的风险[33]。普遍认为,IgG 亚型的 aPL 对于临床表现的预测性比 IgM 更高[29-31]。如本章 2.1 所述,没有抗 β2GPI 或抗 PS/PT 抗体的孤立性 LA 显示出低风险,而 β2GPI 依赖性 aPL 与 D1 的反应则可能支持存在 aPL 相关的 APO 风险[32]。

3.1.2 未满足分类标准的患者

在日常临床环境中存在更为复杂的情况,例如无症状 aPL 阳性女性(所谓的"aPL 携带者")和未满足正式临床或实验室分类标准的女性[28]。事实上,具有风险 aPL 谱但没有任何既往病理妊娠(例如,无症状携带者)或具有病理妊娠但孤立 aPL 阳性和低抗体滴度的患者,常常会被转诊到三级医院进行咨询。由于缺乏特定的临床研究,对这些女性的最佳管理仍然是一个有争议的问题。然而,2019 年 EULAR 和 ACR 关于管理 APS 妊娠管理的建议表明,具有三重阳性的 aPL 携带者或有严重产科病史且 aPL 低风险谱的女性可被视为 APO 高危人群,并最终单独使用低剂量阿司匹林(LDASA)治疗,在特定病例中甚至联合肝素治疗[33,34]。

3.2 治疗

3.2.1 治疗流程

图 8.3 显示了产科 APS 的治疗流程。尽管研究存在异质性,但最近的 Cochrane 系统综述确认,与单独使用阿司匹林相比,普通肝素(UFH)或低分子量肝素(LMWH)与低剂量阿司匹林(LDA)的联合治疗可能会提高持续 aPL 阳性患者的活产率[35]。有证据表明,无论症状类型如何,这种联合治疗可以有效保护 aPL 阳性的孕妇免受妊娠并发症复发的影

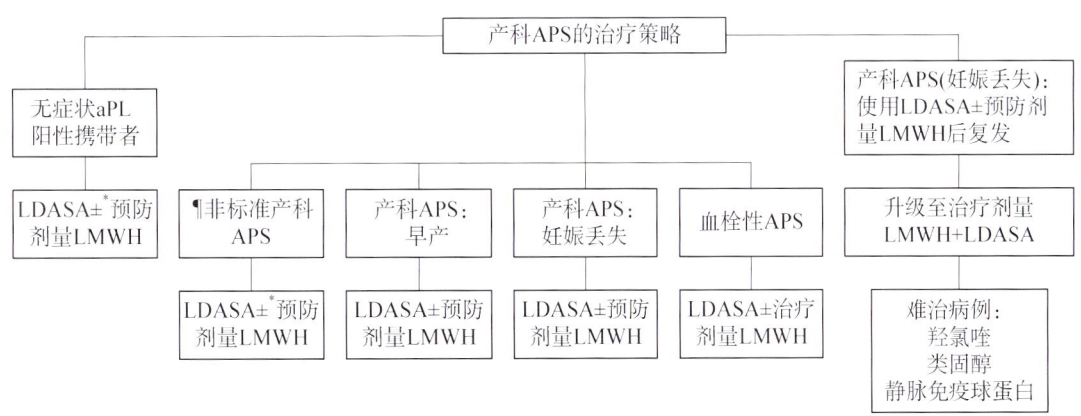

图 8.3 产科 APS 的治疗策略。

* 在低剂量阿司匹林的基础上使用预防性低分子肝素(LMWH)取决于个体的收益/风险。¶非标准 APS:不符合临床和(或)实验室分类标准的妊娠期 APS 女性。aPL,抗磷脂抗体;APS,抗磷脂综合征;LDASA,低剂量阿司匹林;LMWH,低分子肝素;HCQ,羟氯喹;IVIg,静脉免疫球蛋白。

响[3]。理想情况下，LDA 应在妊娠前开始服用，而肝素则在检测到胎儿心跳后立即开始使用。阿司匹林的剂量因各地规范而异，范围从每天 75 mg 到 150 mg，但尚无比较研究以确定最佳剂量[33,34]。对于既往没有血栓事件的 APS 女性建议进行预防性肝素治疗，而对于过去曾有血栓形成的患者，则给予治疗剂量[33,34]。来自 2020 年 Cochrane 综述的数据未发现接受 LDA 和（或）肝素治疗的母亲或孩子（先天畸形、新生儿出血）出现显著的不良事件（出血、肝素诱导的血小板减少症、过敏反应）[35]。

对于未满足分类标准的 APS 孕妇，建议进行个体化治疗。例如，对于无症状 aPL 阳性携带者或未满足产科 APS 分类标准的女性，仅建议使用 LDA；然而，如果风险谱高〔例如，三重阳性和（或）中高 aPL 滴度〕，一些医生也会使用肝素[33,34]。此外，EUREKA 单中心研究显示，对于持续低滴度 aPL 的女性，LDA 加肝素也可改善妊娠结局[36]。非血栓机制在 aPL 相关的胎盘缺陷中发挥了重要作用，这表明肝素和阿司匹林通过干预凝血级联反应之外的机制发挥了保护作用[5]。

3.2.2 难治病例

进行常规治疗后，仍有高达 20%～30% 的 APS 患者的妊娠结局不良[3]。在标准 LDA 和肝素治疗无效的病例中，已报道了其他的治疗方法（图 8.3）。根据证据显示，血栓形成在 APO 中的作用较小，胎盘炎症可能更重要（详见本章 1.3），在妊娠早期添加低剂量强的松对 LDA 和肝素的联合治疗在活产率方面是有益的，并且副作用较少[37]。欧洲多中心研究也支持在难治性产科 APS 患者中添加皮质类固醇具有积极效果[38]。羟氯喹（HCQ）除了具有抗血小板活性和对膜联蛋白-Ⅴ胎盘屏障的保护作用外，在滋养层还具有一些抗炎特性，并能抑制补体活化[39-45]。加上妊娠期良好的安全性，使 HCQ 成为难治病例的一种有吸引力的附加选择。尽管相关随机对照试验仍在进行中，但 EULAR 和 ACR 建议在对 LDA 和肝素无反应的患者中使用 HCQ[33,34]。

在难治病例中，将肝素（特别是低分子肝素）从预防剂量升级为治疗剂量已被建议作为挽救治疗措施，尽管尚未进行专门的临床试验[3]。与免疫球蛋白可能抵消 aPL 致病作用的观点一致，已有报道在特定病例中使用静脉注射免疫球蛋白[46-48]。此外，还有两种额外的治疗方法正在积极研究中：一种是使用肿瘤坏死因子-α（TNF-α）抑制剂来减轻胎盘炎症，另一种是他汀类药物（尤其是普拉伐他汀）对胎盘炎症和血管损伤产生药理效应[3,4,49-51]。

4 监测

妊娠期 APS 患者应被视为高危人群，并每月严格监测一次，必要时则需更为频繁的监测。建议建立一个由产科医生和风湿病学家组成的多学科团队，特别是罹患全身性自身免疫性疾病的患者，应严格评估疾病的活动状态以及相关的免疫抑制治疗情况[33,34]。鉴于补体级联在产科 APS 发病机制中的核心作用，血清补体评估被认为是产科预后的补充预测指标。据报道，一些 APS 孕妇的血清 C3 和 C4 水平较低，尽管它们与不良妊娠结局的关联仍在研究中[14,52]。由于补体水平的生理变异极大，甚至在正常妊娠期间也会升高，因此检测 C3/C4 成分可能不够敏感。与此一致的是，可溶性补体活化产物似乎是一种更为敏感、更有前景的预测生育结局的生物标志物[53,54]。血管生成因子与抗血管生成因子之间的不平衡，如胎盘生长因子（PlGF）和可溶性 fms 样酪氨酸激酶-1（sflt-1），会导致一般人群中的妊娠晚期胎盘相关并发症。到目前为止，关于其在 APS 人群中应用的证据很少，需要进一步研究以支持其潜在的预测作用[55,56]。在 11～13^{+6} 周对所有孕妇常规进行产前胎儿监测，以计算胎龄并行产前诊断；在 19～21 周进行胎儿大排畸检查。对 APS 孕妇则需进行额外的胎儿监测，在妊娠晚期每月行超声检查，评估胎儿生物测量参数、羊水量和多普勒血流速度波形分析（如脐动脉舒张末期无血流）[33,34]。这些方法有助于识别早期或晚期宫内生长受限，并更好地安排分娩时机[57]。

5 分娩和产褥期

分娩的时机和方式应根据母体和胎儿的状况而定。在没有常见的医学或产科指征需要提前终止妊娠的情况下，应在孕 39 周时进行引产或剖宫产，以控制抗凝药物的停用时间，并预防产后血栓风险。目前还没有关于 APS 最佳分娩方式的随机试验。然而，医生应该考虑与阴道分娩相比，剖宫产的血栓栓塞风险更高。在计划剖宫产或引产前 12 小时和 24 小时分别给予预防或治疗剂量的肝素作为最后一剂，以控制血栓形成的风险[58]。APS 患者在给予最后一剂预防性或治疗性肝素后 12 小时和 24 小时可以安全进行阴道分娩或硬膜外麻醉[58]。尽管阿司匹林不会增加脊椎血肿的风险，但麻醉师可能更倾向在进行脊椎穿刺前 3～7 天停用低剂量阿司匹林[3,58]。由于产褥期血栓栓塞风险较高，EULAR 和 ACR 指南都建议在分娩后继续使用阿司匹林和肝素 4～6 周[33,34]。由于阿司匹林和肝素均无哺乳禁忌，如果 APS 患者有意愿，应鼓励母乳喂养[33,34,59]。

6 胎儿和新生儿结局

母体的 IgG 类 aPL 可以穿过胎盘，可在新生儿体内检测到，并持续至分娩后 12 个月[60]。然而，尽管新生儿存在血栓倾向状态，但有关新生儿血栓的报道非常少[60-62]。有人推测，胎盘组织中 β2GPI 的大量存在可能有助于中和致病性的 aPL，最终保护胎儿。此外，阿司匹林可能会穿过胎盘，并发挥其抗血小板的活性。

7 aPL 与不孕症

aPL 在不孕不育中的理论作用可能是由于其对卵母细胞发育、植入前胚胎形态、子宫内膜容受性和适当蜕膜化的负面干扰。除了一些实验模型外，aPL 与不孕症之间的因果关系没有得到很好的支持[63]。例如，最近的一项系统回顾并未发现辅助生殖技术（ART）失败与 aPL 存在之间的关系[64]。与这一发现相一致的是，aPL 检测不应常规纳入不孕女性的诊断中。另一方面，对于 aPL 阳性和 APS 患者，卵巢刺激方案的血栓风险是辅助生殖技术的一个关注点。目前，对于 APS 和 aPL 阳性患者而言，辅助生殖技术被认为是一种普遍安全的方法，并已有指南发布，通过预防性肝素以避免血栓风险[33,34,59]。

8 总结和建议

- aPL 的定义。aPL 是针对 PL 结合蛋白的自身抗体。aPL 与两种主要的自身抗原反应：β2GPI 和 PT。
- 检测方法/实验室分类指标。有三种方法被用作实验室分类指标：LA 是一种定性的功能性 PL 依赖性凝血试验，主要由抗 β2GPI 和（或）抗 PT 抗体介导。aCL 和抗 β2GPI 试验是半定量的固相实验，主要检测 β2GPI 依赖性的 aPL。
- 流行病学。APS 是最常见的可治疗的导致反复妊娠丢失的获得性风险因素之一。
- aPL 的诊断价值。至少一个实验室分类指标持续呈阳性对于 APS 的分类是必需的。目前，相同的标准与临床表现一起被用作诊断工具。尽管在固相实验中，中/高滴度的 aPL 阳性被广泛认为是最具预测性和诊断性的，但低滴度 aPL 也可能与产科并发症有关。
- aPL 作为致病性抗体。实验模型和流行病学研究有充分的证据表明，β2GPI 依赖性 aPL 对 aPL 相关病理妊娠具有致病性。
- aPL 作为风险因素。aPL 检测的双重/三重阳性和固相实验中的中/高滴度 aPL 显示出与产科 APS 相关风险最高。
- 何时进行 aPL 检查？所有存在既往无法解释的病理妊娠以及既往无法解释的动脉或静脉血栓病史，或患有系统性自身免疫疾病并计划妊娠的女性，都应进行 aPL 检查。
- 如何检测 aPL？应检测所有三种正式分类的实验室指标，并在首次检测后 12 周再次进行检测，以排除短暂的阳性结果。
- 产科 APS 的标准疗法。备孕时开始使用低剂量阿司匹林，妊娠确认后使用预防性肝素（通常是低分子肝素）是标准治疗方法。对于因既往血栓事件而使用口服抗凝治疗的孕妇，应使用治疗性肝素。对于标准治疗无效的情况，可升级到治疗性肝素，即使没有既往血栓史，或在标准治疗的基础上添加皮质类固醇、静脉免疫球蛋白和羟氯喹。低剂量阿司匹林和肝素应该在分娩后继续使用 4～6 周。
- APS 孕产妇管理。建议进行严格的多学科临床、实验室和超声监测，包括胎儿生物测量评估和子宫/脐动脉血流测定。

参考文献

[1] Miyakis S, Lockshin MD, Atsumi T, Branch DW, Brey RL, Cervera R, et al. International consensus statement on an update of the classification criteria for definite antiphospholipid syndrome (APS). J Thromb Haemost 2006; 4:295-306.

[2] Barbhaiya M, Zuily S, Ahmadzadeh Y, Amigo MC, Avcin T, Bertolaccini ML. New APS classification criteria collaborators. development of a new international antiphospholipid syndrome classification criteria phase I/II report: generation and reduction of candidate criteria. Arthritis Care Res (Hoboken) 2021; 73(10): 1490-501. Available from: https://doi.org/10.1002/acr.24520.

[3] Beltagy A, Trespidi L, Gerosa M, Ossola MW, Meroni PL, Chighizola CB. Anti-phospholipid antibodies and reproductive failures. Am J Reprod Immunol 2021; 85(4): e13258. Available from: https://doi.org/10.1111/aji.13258.

[4] de Jesús GR, Benson AE, Chighizola B, Sciascia S, Branch DW. 16th International congress on antiphospholipid antibodies task force report on obstetric antiphospholipid syndrome. Lupus 2020; 29(12): 1601-15. Available from: https://doi.org/10.1177/0961203320954520.

[5] Meroni PL, Borghi MO, Grossi C, Chighizola CB, Durigutto P, Tedesco F. Obstetric and vascular antiphospholipid syndrome: same antibodies but different diseases? Nat Rev Rheumatol 2018; 14(7): 433-40. Available from: https://doi.org/10.1038/s41584-018-0032-6.

[6] Duarte-García A, Pham MM, Crowson CS, Amin S, Moder KG, Pruthi RK, et al. The epidemiology of antiphospholipid syndrome: a population-based study. Arthritis Rheumatol 2019; 71(9): 1545-52. Available from: https://doi.org/10.1002/art.40901.

[7] Cervera R, Serrano R, Pons-Estel GJ, Ceberio-Hualde L, Shoenfeld Y, de Ramón E, et al. Morbidity and mortality in the antiphospholipid syndrome during a 10-year period: a multicentre prospective study of 1000 patients. Ann Rheum Dis 2015; 74(6): 1011-18. Available from: https://doi.org/10.1136/annrheumdis-2013-204838.

[8] Yelnik CM, Laskin CA, Porter TF, Branch DW, Buyon JP, Guerra MM, et al. Lupus anticoagulant is the main predictor of adverse pregnancy outcomes in aPL-positive patients: validation of PROMISSE study results. Lupus Sci Med 2016; 3: e000131. Available from: https://doi.org/10.1136/lupus-2015-000131.

[9] Alijotas-Reig J, Esteve-Valverde E, Ferrer-Oliveras R, Sáez-Comet L, Lefkou E, Mekinian A, et al. The European registry on obstetric antiphospholipid syndrome (EUROAPS): a survey of 1000 consecutive cases. Autoimmun Rev 2019; 18(4): 406-14. Available from: https://doi.org/10.1016/j.autrev.2018.12.006.

[10] Andreoli L, Chighizola CB, Banzato A, Pons-Estel GJ, Ramires de Jesus G, Erkan D. Estimated frequency of antiphospholipid antibodies in patients with pregnancy morbidity, stroke, myocardial infarction, and deep vein thrombosis: a critical review of the literature. Arthritis Care Res 2013; 65: 1869e1873.

[11] Viall CA, Chamley LW. Histopathology in the placentae of women with antiphospholipid antibodies: a systematic review of the literature. Autoimmun Rev 2015; 14(5): 446-71. Available from: https://doi.org/10.1016/j.autrev.2015.01.008.

[12] Meroni PL, Borghi MO, Raschi E, Tedesco F. Pathogenesis of antiphospholipid syndrome: understanding the antibodies. Nat Rev Rheumatol 2011; 7(6): 330-9. Available from: https://doi.org/10.1038/nrrheum.2011.52.

[13] Shamonki JM, Salmon JE, Hyjek E, Baergen RN. Excessive complement activation is associated with placental injury in patients with antiphospholipid antibodies. Am J Obst Gynecol 2007; 196(2). Available from: https://doi.org/10.1016/j.ajog.2006 167.e1-5.

[14] Tedesco F, Borghi MO, Gerosa M, Chighizola CB, Macor P, Lonati PA, et al. Pathogenic role of complement in antiphospholipid syndrome and therapeutic implications. Front Immunol 2018; 9: 1388. Available from: https://doi.org/10.3389/fimmu.2018.01388.

[15] Salmon JE, Girardi G. Antiphospholipid antibodies and pregnancy loss: a disorder of inflammation. J Reprod Immunol 2008; 77(1): 51-6. Available from: https://doi.org/10.1016/j.jri.2007.02.007.

[16] Martinez de la Torre Y, Buracchi C, Borroni EM, Dupor J, Bonecchi R, Nebuloni M, et al. Protection against inflammation- and autoantibody-caused fetal loss by the chemokine decoy receptor D6. Proc Natl Acad Sci U S A 2007; 104(7): 2319-24. Available from: https://doi.org/10.1073/pnas.0607514104.

[17] Devreese KMJ, de Groot G, de Laat B, Erkan D, Favaloro EJ, Mackie I, et al. Guidance from the Scientific and Standardization Committee for lupus anticoagulant/antiphospholipid antibodies of the International Society on Thrombosis and Haemostasis: Update of the guidelines for lupus anticoagulant detection and interpretation. J Thromb Haemost 2020; 18(11): 2828-39. Available from: https://doi.org/10.1111/jth.15047.

[18] Chighizola CB, Raschi E, Banzato A, Borghi MO, Pengo V, Meroni PL. The challenges of lupus anticoagulants. Expert Rev Hematol 2016; 9(4): 389-400. Available from: https://doi.org/10.1586/17474086.2016.1140034.

[19] Meroni PL, Borghi MO. Antiphospholipid antibody assays in 2021: looking for a predictive value in addition to a diagnostic one. Front Immunol 2021; 12: 726820. Available from: https://doi.org/10.3389/fimmu.2021.726820.

[20] Oosting JD, Derksen RH, Bobbink IW, Hackeng TM, Bouma BN, de Groot P, et al. Antiphospholipid antibodies directed against a combination of phospholipids with prothrombin, protein C, or protein S: an explanation for their pathogenic mechanism? Blood. 1993; 81(10): 2618-25.

[21] Yin, de Groot PG, Ninivaggi M, Devreese KMJ, de Laat B. Clinical relevance of isolated lupus anticoagulant positivity in patients with thrombotic antiphospholipid syndrome. Thromb Haemost 2021; 121(9): 1220-7. Available from: https://doi.org/10.1055/a-1344-4271.

[22] Pengo V, Testa S, Martinelli I, Ghirarduzzi A, Legnani C, Gresele P, et al. Incidence of a first thromboembolic event in carriers of isolated lupus anticoagulant. Thrombosis Res 2014; 135(1): 46-9. Available from: https://doi.org/10.1016/j.thromres.2014.10.013.

[23] Sciascia S, Sanna G, Murru V, Roccatello D, Khamashta

MA, Bertolaccini ML. Anti-prothrombin (aPT) and anti-phosphatidylserine/prothrombin (aPS/PT) antibodies and the risk of thrombosis in the antiphospholipid syndrome. A systematic review. Thromb Haemost 2014;111(2):354 – 64. Available from: https://doi.org/10.1160/TH13-06-5410509.

[24] de Laat B, de Groot PG. Autoantibodies directed against domain I of 421 beta2-glycoprotein I. Curr Rheumatol Rep 2011;13(1):70 – 6. Available from: https://doi.org/10.1007/s11926-422010-0144-8.

[25] Durigutto P, Grossi C, Borghi MO, Macor P, Pregnolato F, Raschi E, et al. New insight into antiphospholipid syndrome: antibodies to β2glycoprotein I-domain 5 fail to induce thrombi in rats. Haematologica 2019; 104(4): 819 – 26. Available from: https://doi.org/10.3324/haematol.2018.198119.

[26] Agostinis C, Durigutto P, Sblattero D, Borghi MO, Grossi C, Guida F, et al. A non-complement-fixing antibody to β2 glycoprotein I as a novel therapy for antiphospholipid syndrome. Blood 2014;123(22):3478 – 87. Available from: https://doi.org/10.1182/blood-2013-11-537704.

[27] Radin M, Cecchi I, Roccatello D, Meroni PL, Sciascia S. Prevalence and thrombotic risk assessment of anti-β2 glycoprotein i domain i antibodies: a systematic review. Semin Thromb Hemost 2018;44(5):466 – 74. Available from: https://doi.org/10.1055/s-0037-1603936.

[28] Pires da Rosa G, Bettencourt P, Rodríguez-Pintó I, Cervera R, Espinosa G. "Non-criteria" antiphospholipid syndrome: a nomenclature proposal. Autoimmun Rev 2020; 19(12): 102689. Available from: https://doi.org/10.1016/j.autrev.2020.102689.

[29] Chayoua W, Kelchtermans H, Gris JC, Moore GW, Musiał J, Wahl D, et al. The (non-) sense of detecting anti-cardiolipin and anti-b2glycoprotein I IgM antibodies in the antiphospholipid syndrome. J Thromb Haemost 2020;18(1): 169 – 79. Available from: https://doi.org/10.1111/jth.14633.

[30] Bouvier S, Cochery-Nouvellon E, Lavigne-Lissalde G, Mercier E, Marchetti T, Balducchi JP, et al. Comparative incidence of pregnancy outcomes in treated obstetric antiphospholipid syndrome: the NOHAPS observational study. Blood 2014;123(3):404 – 13. Available from: https://doi.org/10.1182/blood-2013-08-522623.

[31] Kelchtermans H, Pelkmans L, de Laat B, Devreese KM. IgG/IgM antiphospholipid antibodies present in the classification criteria for the antiphospholipid syndrome: a critical review of their association with thrombosis. J Thromb Haemost 2016;14(8):1530 – 48. Available from: https://doi.org/10.1111/jth.13379.

[32] Chighizola CB, Pregnolato F, Andreoli L, Bodio C, Cesana L, Comerio C, et al. Beyond thrombosis: anti-β2GPI domain 1 antibodies identify late pregnancy morbidity in anti-phospholipid syndrome. J Autoimmun 2018; 90; 76 – 83. Available from: https://doi.org/10.1016/j.jaut.2018.02.002.

[33] Tektonidou MG, Andreoli L, Limper M, Amoura Z, Cervera R, Costedoat-Chalumeau N, et al. EULAR recommendations for the management of antiphospholipid syndrome in adults. Ann Rheum Dis 2019;78(19):1296 – 304. Available from: https://doi.org/10.1136/annrheumdis-2019-215213.

[34] Sammaritano LR, Bermas BL, Chakravarty EE, Chambers C, Clowse MEB, Lockshin MD, et al. American College of rheumatology guideline for the management of reproductive health in rheumatic and musculoskeletal diseases. Arthritis Rheumatol2020 2020; 72(4): 529 – 56. Available from: https://doi.org/10.1002/art.41191.

[35] Hamulyák EN, Scheres LJ, Marijnen MC, Goddijn M, Middeldorp S. Aspirin or heparin or both for improving pregnancy outcomes in women with persistent antiphospholipid antibodies and recurrent pregnancy loss. Cochrane Database Syst Rev 2020;5(5):CD012852. Available from: https://doi.org/10.1002/14651858. CD012852.

[36] Pregnolato F, Gerosa M, Raimondo MG, Comerio C, Bartoli F, Lonati PA, et al. EUREKA algorithm predicts obstetric risk and response to treatment in women with different subsets of anti-phospholipid antibodies. Rheumatology(Oxf) 2021; 60(3):1114 – 24. Available from: https://doi.org/10.1093/rheumatology/keaa203.

[37] Bramham K, Thomas M, Nelson-Piercy C, Khamashta M, Hunt BJ. First-trimester low-dose prednisolone in refractory antiphospholipid antibody-related pregnancy loss. Blood 2011;117(25):6948 – 51. Available from: https://doi.org/10.1182/blood-2011-02-339234.

[38] Mekinian A, Alijotas-Reig J, Carrat F, Costedoat-Chalumeau N, Ruffatti A, Lazzaroni MG, et al. Refractory obstetrical antiphospholipid syndrome: features, treatment and outcome in a European multicenter retrospective study. Autoimmun Rev 2017;16(7):730 – 4. Available from: https://doi.org/10.1016/j.autrev.2017.05.006.

[39] Edwards MH, Pierangeli S, Liu X, Barker JH, Anderson G, Harris EN. Hydroxychloroquine reverses thrombogenic properties of antiphospholipid antibodies in mice. Circulation 1997;96(12):4380 – 4. Available from: https://doi.org/10.1161/01.cir.96.12.4380.

[40] Rand JH, Wu X-X, Quinn AS, Ashton AW, Chen PP, Hathcock JJ, et al. Hydroxychloroquine protects the annexin A5 anticoagulant shield from disruption by antiphospholipid antibodies: evidence for a novel effect for an old antimalarial drug. Blood 2010; 115(11): 2292 – 9. Available from: https://doi.org/10.1182/blood-2009-04-213520.

[41] Meroni PL. Prevention & treatment of obstetrical complications in APS: is hydroxychloroquine the Holy Grail we are looking for? J Autoimmun 2016;75:1 – 5. Available from: https://doi.org/10.1016/j.jaut.2016.07.003.

[42] Marchetti T, Ruffatti A, Wuillemin C, de Moerloose P, Cohen M. Hydroxychloroquine restores trophoblast fusion affected by antiphospholipid antibodies. J Thromb Haemost 2014;12(6):910 – 20. Available from: https://doi.org/10.1111/jth.12570.

[43] Albert CR, Schlesinger WJ, Viall CA, Mulla MJ, Brosens JJ, Chamley LW, et al. Effect of hydroxychloroquine on antiphospholipid antibody-induced changes in first trimester trophoblast function. Am J Reprod Immunol 2014;71(2):154 – 64. Available from: https://doi.org/10.1111/aji.12184.

[44] Scott RE, Greenwood SL, Hayes DJL, Baker BC, Jones RL, Heazell AEP. Effects of hydroxychloroquine on the human placenta — findings from in vitro experimental data and a systematic review. Reprod Toxicol 2019;87:50 – 9. Available from: https://doi.org/10.1016/j.reprotox.2019.05.056.

[45] Bertolaccini ML, Content G, Lennen R, Sanna G, Blower PJ, Ma MT, et al. Complement inhibition by hydroxychloroquine prevents placental and fetal brain abnormalities in antiphospholipid syndrome. J Autoimmun 2016;75:30 – 8. Available from: https://doi.org/10.1016/j.jaut.2016.04.008.

[46] Hoxha A, Favaro M, Calligaro A, Del Ross T, Ruffatti AT,

Infantolino C, et al. Upgrading therapy strategy improves pregnancy outcome in antiphospholipid syndrome: a cohort management study. Thromb Haemost 2020;120(1):36-43. Available from: https://doi.org/10.1055/s-0039-1697665.

[47] Urban ML, Bettiol A, Serena C, Comito C, Turrini I, et al. Intravenous immunoglobulin for the secondary prevention of stillbirth in obstetric antiphospholipid syndrome: a case series and systematic review of literature. Autoimmun Rev 2020;19(9):102620. Available from: https://doi.org/10.1016/j.autrev.2020.102620.

[48] Ruffatti A, Tonello, Hoxha A, Sciascia S, Cuadrado MJ, Latino JO, et al. Effect of additional treatments combined with conventional therapies in pregnant patients with high-risk antiphospholipid syndrome: a multicentre study. Thromb Haemost 2018;118(4):639-46. Available from: https://doi.org/10.1055/s-0038-1632388.

[49] Lefkou E, Mamopoulos A, Dagklis T, Vosnakis C, Rousso D, Girardi G. Pravastatin improves pregnancy outcomes in obstetric antiphospholipid syndrome refractory to antithrombotic therapy. J Clin Invest 2016;126(8):2933-40. Available from: https://doi.org/10.1172/JCI86957.

[50] Lefkou E, Varoudi K, Pombo J, Jurisic A, Jurisic Z, Contento G, et al. Triple therapy with pravastatin, low molecular weight heparin and low dose aspirin improves placental haemodynamics and pregnancy outcomes in obstetric antiphospholipid syndrome in mice and women through a nitric oxide-dependent mechanism. Biochem Pharmacol 2020;182:114217. Available from: https://doi.org/10.1016/j.bcp.2020.114217.

[51] Vahedian-Azimi A, Karimi L, Reiner Z, Makvandi S, Sahebkar A. Effects of statins on preeclampsia: a systematic review. Pregnancy Hypertension 2021;23:123-30. Available from: https://doi.org/10.1016/j.preghy.2020.11.014.

[52] Nalli C, Lini D, Andreoli L, Crisafulli F, Fredi M, Lazzaroni MG, et al. Low preconception complement levels are associated with adverse pregnancy outcomes in a multicenter study of 260 pregnancies in 197 women with antiphospholipid syndrome or carriers of antiphospholipid antibodies. Biomedicines 2021;9(6):671. Available from: https://doi.org/10.3390/biomedicines9060671.

[53] Kim MY, Guerra MM, Kaplowitz E, Laskin CA, Petri M, Branch DW, et al. Complement activation predicts adverse pregnancy outcome in patients with systemic lupus erythematosus and/or antiphospholipid antibodies. Ann Rheum Dis 2018;77(4):549-55. Available from: https://doi.org/10.1136/annrheumdis-2017-212224.

[54] Scambi C, Ugolini S, Tonello M, Bortolami O, De Franceschi L, Castagna A, et al. Complement activation in the plasma and placentas of women with different subsets of antiphospholipid syndrome. Am J Reprod Immunol 2019;82(6):e13185. Available from: https://doi.org/10.1111/aji.13185.

[55] Kim MY, Buyon JP, Guerra MM, Rana S, Zhang D, Laskin CA, et al. Angiogenic factor imbalance early in pregnancy predicts adverse outcomes in patients with lupus and antiphospholipid antibodies: results of the PROMISSE study. Am J Obstet Gynecol 2016;214(1):108.e101-14. Available from: https://doi.org/10.1016/j.ajog.2015.09.066.

[56] Cochery-Nouvellon É, Mercier É, Bouvier S, Balducchi JP, Quéré I, Perez-Martin A, et al. Obstetric antiphospholipid syndrome: early variations of angiogenic factors are associated with adverse outcomes. Haematologica 2017;102(5):835-42. Available from: https://doi.org/10.3324/haematol.2016.155184.

[57] Alfirevic Z, Stampalija T, Dowswell T. Fetal and umbilical Doppler ultrasound in high-risk pregnancies. Cochrane Database Syst Rev 2017;6(6):Cd007529. Available from: https://doi.org/10.1002/14651858.CD006066.pub3.

[58] Bates SM, Greer JA, Pabinger I, Sofaer SJH. Venous thromboembolism, thrombophilia, antithrombotic therapy, and pregnancy: American College of chest physicians evidence-based clinical practice guidelines (8th edition). Chest 2008;133(6 Suppl.):844Se886S. Available from: https://doi.org/10.1378/chest.08-0761.

[59] Andreoli L, Bertsias GK, Agmon-Levin N, Brown S, Cervera R, Costedoat-Chalumeau N, et al. EULAR recommendations for women's health and the management of family planning, assisted reproduction, pregnancy and menopause in patients with systemic lupus erythematosus and/or antiphospholipid syndrome. Ann Rheum Dis 2017;76(3):476-85. Available from: https://doi.org/10.1136/annrheumdis-2016-209770.

[60] Motta M, Chirico G, Rebaioli CB, Faden D, Lojacono A, Allegri F, et al. Anticardiolipin and anti-beta2 glycoprotein I antibodies in infants born to mothers with antiphospholipid antibody-positive autoimmune disease: a follow-up study. Am J Perinatol 2006;2384:247-51. Available from: https://doi.org/10.1055/s-2006-939533.

[61] Mekinian A, Lachassinne E, Nicaise-Roland P, Carbillon L, Motta M, Vicaut E, et al. European registry of babies born to mothers with antiphospholipid syndrome. Ann Rheum Dis 2013;72(2):217-22. Available from: https://doi.org/10.1136/annrheumdis-2011-201167.

[62] Boffa MC, Lachassinne E. Infant perinatal thrombosis and antiphospholipid antibodies: a review. Lupus 2007;16(8):634-41. Available from: https://doi.org/10.1177/0961203307079039.

[63] Chighizola CB, de Jesus GR, Branch DW. The hidden world of anti-phospholipid antibodies and female infertility: a literature appraisal. Autoimmun Rev 2016;15(6):493-500. Available from: https://doi.org/10.1016/j.autrev.2016.01.018.

[64] Simopoulou M, Sfakianoudis K, Maziotis E, Grigoriadis S, Giannelou P, Rapani A, et al. The impact of auto-antibodies on IVF treatment and outcome: a systematic review. Int J Mol Sci 2019;20(4):892. Available from: https://doi.org/10.3390/ijms20040892.

第 9 章

抗精子抗体与生殖障碍

Antisperm antibodies and reproductive failure

Hiroaki Shibahara, Yuekun Chen, Ayano Yamaya, Yu Wakimoto, Atsushi Fukui and Akiko Hasegawa

Department of Obstetrics and Gynecology, School of Medicine, Hyogo Medical University, Nishinomiya, Hyogo, Japan

1 引言

不孕不育是一种生殖系统疾病，其定义是在 12 个月或更长时间的常规无保护性交后未能实现临床妊娠[1]。不孕不育的发生率为 10%～15%。不孕主要原因有 3 个，包括内分泌、输卵管和男性因素。此外，由于结婚和受孕时间推迟出现卵巢功能下降。

生殖障碍包括不孕不育和反复妊娠丢失（RPL）[2]。妊娠丢失被定义为在胎儿达到生存能力之前的自发死亡。该术语包括从受孕到妊娠 22 周的所有妊娠丢失。指南指出，在发生两次或两次以上妊娠丢失后，可考虑诊断为 RPL[3]。这一定义包括自然受孕和接受辅助生殖技术后的妊娠丢失，但不包括异位妊娠、葡萄胎和种植失败。RPL 的发病率在育龄期女性中高达 2%。RPL 的病因多种多样，然而，约 60% 的 RPL 没有任何风险因素。尽管免疫因素在人类生殖中的相对重要性尚不清楚，但在部分不明原因的不孕不育和 RPL 中可能存在免疫介导的生殖障碍[4]。

作为免疫因素的一个原因，抗精子抗体（antisperm antibodies，ASA）在男性和女性中都会产生。此前，我们已提出了 ASA 免疫不育男性和女性的诊断和治疗[5,6]。据报道，精子表面存在多种对女性而言的外来抗原，因此，可发生同种异体免疫反应。

2 定义

ASA 是针对精子抗原产生的抗体，精子抗原是由 IgG、IgA 和（或）IgM 组成的免疫球蛋白。在女性免疫性不孕中，精子固定抗体与生殖障碍高度相关[7]。不孕女性血清中 ASA 的存在已被证明可以抑制精子在女性生殖道中的迁移，特别是通过精子制动试验（SIT）检测到的精子制动抗体[8,9]。这种抗体还可以对精子-卵子相互作用的各个阶段以及随后的体外胚胎发育产生抑制作用。然而，据报道，ASA 和 RPL 之间的关系仍存在争议[7]。

3 患病率

已有多种检测 ASA 的方法。然而，最重要的考虑因素是不同方法的选择。ASA 在可生育人群中的存在表明，并非所有 ASA 都会导致不孕。因此，建议选择针对女性不孕的临床特异性方法来检测循环 ASA。已明确具有生物活性的 ASA 适合不孕女性进行初步检测，包括精子制动抗体、精子凝集抗体和受精阻断抗体。例如，在第一次去不孕门诊就诊的女性中，血清检测到有精子制动抗体的发病率约为 3%[10]。

4 与生殖相关的潜在免疫病理学

不育女性血清中 ASA 的存在，特别是精子制动抗体，已被证明可以抑制精子在女性生殖道中的迁移。这种抗体还可对精子-卵子相互作用的各个阶段以及随后的体外胚胎发育产生抑制作用。

4.1 抗精子抗体在宫颈黏液水平上抑制精子运输

如果 ASA 对受精过程有任何不利影响，则

ASA应存在于生殖道的分泌液中[11]。ASA可导致处于不同生殖阶段的女性不孕,包括性交后精子在宫颈黏液(CM)中的存活。Koyama等[12]报道称,血清中存在精子制动抗体的患者性交后试验(PCT)结果不良的比例明显高于没有抗体的患者。其他研究也得出了类似的结论[13-15]。这些研究表明了精子制动抗体对于精子穿透宫颈黏液具有抑制作用。

我们通过定量SIT评估了具有精子制动抗体的不孕女性的抗体滴度(50%精子制动单位:SI_{50}单位)是否与PCT结果相关[16,17]。将具有精子固定抗体的患者按SI_{50}滴度分为两组时,所有SI_{50}滴度高(>10)的患者PCT结果异常(10/10),而SI_{50}滴度低(≤10)的患者异常比例为66.7%(14/21)($P<0.05$)。这些结果表明,血清中的SI_{50}滴度可以预测精子制动抗体对不孕女性宫颈黏液精子迁移的抑制作用[18]。为了克服宫颈黏液对精子运输的这种抑制作用,可选择宫腔内人工授精(IUI)治疗具有精子制动抗体的不孕女性[19,20]。然而,其效果有限,这是因为存在其他抑制因素,如精子从宫腔输送到输卵管以及精子与卵子的相互作用。

4.2 抗精子抗体抑制精子从宫腔运输到输卵管

目前尚不清楚抗体是否会损害精子从宫腔到输卵管的运输。腹膜精子回收试验(PSRT)[21]通过腹腔镜检查和IUI后腹膜液中活动精子存在与否以判断精子在输卵管中的迁移是否受到损害[22]。

从Douglas袋中吸出腹膜液并立即离心。用显微镜检查沉积物中是否存在活动精子。存在精子制动抗体的患者有88.9%(24/27)在腹膜液中没有观察到精子,而在没有抗体的患者中该比例为66.0%(140/212),两者存在显著差异($P<0.05$)[22]。将27名具有精子制动抗体的患者根据SI_{50}滴度分为两组,95.7%(22/23)的SI_{50}高滴度(>10)患者和50.0%(2/4)的SI_{50}低滴度(≤10)患者PSRT结果异常($P<0.05$)。这些结果表明,血清中的SI_{50}滴度可以预测具有精子制动抗体的不孕女性对精子从宫腔迁移并通过输卵管的抑制作用。

4.3 抗精子抗体对精子-卵子相互作用的抑制作用

研究表明,精子制动抗体可以在顶体反应[23-25]、透明带识别和穿透[26-32]的水平上对精子-卵子的相互作用产生抑制作用。我们已报道了患者血清和卵泡液间SI_{50}滴度的显著相关性($P<0.0001$)[33]。在该研究中,我们采集了存在血清精子制动抗体的不孕女性在接受体外受精-胚胎移植(IVF-ET)治疗时的血清和卵泡液。因此,在将卵母细胞转移到培养基之前,对收集的卵母细胞进行彻底清洗是重要的,防止培养基受到污染,以获得更好的结果。

例如,我们回顾性研究了不孕女性血清中精子制动抗体对受精率的影响[34]。在引入SIT作为女性不孕的常规检测之前,从9个IVF周期的4名血清中具有精子制动抗体的不孕女性体内采集了85个卵母细胞。随后,在含有患者血清的培养基中用活动精子对卵母细胞进行受精。作为对照,从5个IVF周期的5名血清中具有抗体的不孕女性体内采集了50个卵母细胞,并在加入了人血清白蛋白(HSA)的培养基中用活动精子对卵母细胞进行受精。前一组85个卵母细胞中有41个(48.2%)受精,后一组50个卵母中有43个(86.0%)受精,两组之间存在显著差异($P<0.0001$)。该结果表明,不孕女性血清中的精子制动抗体可能会导致受精率降低[34]。然而,在体外受精前,对采集的卵母细胞进行彻底清洗,并在无患者血清的培养基中培养,卵泡液SI_{50}滴度高(≥10)或低(<10)组的受精率没有差异($P=0.62$)[33]。

4.4 抗精子抗体对早期胚胎发育的损害

由于精子表面抗原已被发现存在于发育中的胚胎,推测ASA可能会损害胚胎发育[35,36]。通过使用免疫荧光染色,Koyama等[36]发现精子特异性抗原被转移到大鼠的受精卵中。它们位于从细胞到囊胚阶段不同发育时期的细胞膜上。在补体存在的情况下,针对大鼠精子的ASA会损害受精卵的体外发育[36]。

Naz[37]研究了64对不孕夫妇的体外受精和胚胎发育过程,发现其中一对夫妇的卵母细胞与精子细胞受精后,受精卵的早期分裂异常。影响受精的异常卵裂不是由于卵母细胞的多精子或孤雌激活,而是由于精子上存在的ASA与人类精子的顶体(强)和尾部(弱)区域反应。设计识别由(14±3)kDa和(18±3)kDa两种糖蛋白组成的双带以及(22±3)kDa蛋白条带的抗体,并在兔体内产生抗双带和抗蛋白的抗体。结果发现,亲和纯化的识别双带而非(22±3)kDa蛋白的人或兔免疫球蛋白对卵母细胞的早期分裂产生显著抑制,但不影响小鼠的原核形成,提示(14±3)kDa 和(18±3)kDa 的精子表面抗原可能为小鼠和人类卵母细胞的分裂提供额外的核外信号。

在人类中,我们发现不孕女性血清中的精子制动抗体会导致体外受精后胚胎质量下降[31]。如上所述,不孕女性血清中的精子制动抗体可能导致受精率降低。在含有患者血清和精子制动抗体的培养基中受精后,根据 Veeck 分类[38],在取卵后的第二天或第三天进行胚胎评级,1 级和 2 级胚胎为质量良好。用含有患者血清培养基孵育的 41 个胚胎中,有 16 个为优胚(39.0%),而加入 HSA 的培养基孵育的 43 个胚胎中有 34 个为优胚(79.1%),两组间有显著性差异($P=0.0003$)。这些发现表明不孕女性血清中的精子制动抗体可能导致体外胚胎质量下降。

出于伦理原因不易获得人类胚胎,研究仅限于探索通过精子制动抗体诱导胚胎破碎的可能机制。因此,我们采集了 8 名具有精子制动抗体的不孕女性和 17 名没有抗体的不孕女性的血清,并使用雄性 ICR 小鼠和雌性 F1 小鼠(BALB/c×C57BL/6J),研究了具有抗人精子抗体的患者血清是否对体外受精和小鼠胚胎发育有抑制作用[39]。在小鼠 IVF 中,将预培养的精子在含有或不含精子制动抗体的培养基中培养,并以含牛血清白蛋白(BSA)的培养基作为对照,比较受精率和囊胚形成率,并测定小鼠 SIT。8 个含精子制动抗体的血清样品中有 5 个(62.5%)、17 个不含抗体的血清样本中有 9 个(52.9%),在小鼠中显示出精子制动活性,两组间无显著性差异。将在人/小鼠中具有精子制动活性的 5 个血清样本和不具有精子制动活性的 5 个血清样本用于后续实验。含 BSA 血清、含精子制动抗体血清和不含抗体血清的受精率分别为 82.5%(746/904)、43.6%(508/1 165)和 64.5%(669/1 037),组间具有显著差异($P<0.001$);囊胚形成率分别为 59.9%(447/746)、31.7%(161/508)和 47.7%(319/669),也具有显著性差异($P<0.01$)。

4.5 抗精子抗体与反复妊娠丢失

ASA 和 RPL 之间的关系仍存争议。一些研究表明,ASA 阳性女性的流产率增加(表 9.1)[40-43],而另一些报道则未发现 ASA 和 RPL 存在相关性(表 9.2)[44-47]。

表 9.1 报道抗精子抗体与反复妊娠丢失正相关的文献

作者	研究对象	患者数	抗精子抗体检测方法	相关性	参考文献
Haas GG 等	RPL(>3)	173	RAA/ELISA/TAT/SIT	是	[40]
Mathur S 等	RPL(>2)与对照组	26(对照组 53)	细胞毒/血细胞凝集	是	[41]
Witkin SS 等	不孕症	109	ELISA	是	[42]
Witkin SS 等	RPL 与对照组	44(对照组 616)	IBT 或 MAR	是	[43]

注:ELISA,酶联免疫吸附试验;IBT,免疫珠试验;MAR,混合抗球蛋白反应试验;RAA,放射性标记的抗球蛋白测定;SIT,精子制动试验;TAT,浅盘凝集试验。

表 9.2 报道抗精子抗体与反复妊娠丢失无相关性的文献

作者	研究对象	患者数	抗精子抗体检测方法	相关性	参考文献
Maier DB 等	RPL(<3)与对照组	34(对照组 24)	IBT	否	[44]
Clarke GN 等	RPL(>3)与对照组	70(对照组 1 133)	IBT	否	[45]
Christiansen OB 等	RPL(<3)	123	SAT/MAR	否	[46]
Al-Hussein K 等	RPL(>3)与对照组	24(对照组 6)	FCA	否	[47]

注:FCA,流式细胞术;IBT,免疫珠试验;MAR,混合抗球蛋白反应试验;SAT,精子凝集试验。

4.6 显示抗精子抗体与反复妊娠丢失呈正相关的研究

Haas 等[40]报道称,ASA 阳性的女性不能妊娠到足月,除非接种了丈夫的白细胞作为她们反复妊娠丢失的以免疫为基础的治疗(与 ASA 无关)。在这篇论文中,研究者使用放射性标记的抗球蛋白测定法(RAA)、改良酶联免疫吸附测定法(ELISA)、浅盘凝集试验(TAT)和 SIT 来检测 173 名有 3 次或 3 次以上反复妊娠丢失史的女性的 ASA(表 9.1)。Mathur 等[41]研究了人白细胞抗原(HLA)A 型和 B 型,并在 26 对有 2 次或 2 次以上早期自然流产的夫妇和 53 对具有正常生育能力的夫妇(对照组)中筛选了精子的细胞毒性和血凝抗体。他们认为,ASA 的存在与早期妊娠丢失有关。组织相容性抗原 B7 和 B35 可能通过与 ASA 和早期自然流产相关而发挥作用。Witkin 等[42]研究了 109 对不孕夫妇的 ASA、受孕和流产之间的关系。通过 ELISA 检测丈夫射精精子表面存在的 ASA,以及丈夫或妻子血清中与丈夫纯化的活动精子反应的抗体。结果发现,女性血清和精液中的 ASA 与妊娠失败和妊娠早期流产有关。此后,他们还报道了 ASA IgG 胞内区的存在与不明原因 RPL 之间的显著相关性($P<0.005$)[43]。ASA 可能是 RPL 女性免疫抑制缺陷的标志物。此外,精子暴露于精子致敏的孕妇可能会激活母体免疫系统,对胚胎上存在的父源抗原做出反应。

4.7 显示抗精子抗体与反复种植失败呈负相关的研究

与上述发现不同的是,一些作者报道了 ASA 和 RPL 之间缺乏相关性(表 9.2)。Maier 等[44]评估了 34 名 RPL 患者是否存在狼疮相关自身抗体、免疫珠试验(IBT)可检测的 ASA,以及补体异常的证据。在这项研究中,没有发现患者的 ASA 呈阳性。他们认为,Haas 等[40]对这项研究的解释很困难,因为使用了很多 ASA 检测方法,两组的阳性率都很高,且没有对照组。此外,大多数阳性结果来自 ELISA 测定。这些方法可检测针对精子内部抗原的抗体,其重要性值得怀疑。他们认为,使用 IBT 无法重复这些结果。Clarke 等[45]报道了 ASA 与 RPL 之间缺乏相关性。他们纳入了 70 名有不明原因 RPL 病史的女性和 1133 名不孕女性作为对照。IBT 用于检测他们血清中的 ASA。反复妊娠丢失患者的循环 ASA 发生率较低(1.4% vs 7.4%)。他们得出的结论是,有 RPL 病史的女性循环 ASA 的发生率明显较低。Christiansen 等[46]研究了 123 名 RPL 女性的人白细胞抗原(HLA)-Ⅱ和抗磷脂抗体(APL)之间的关系。在同一项研究中,还利用这些患者的血清检测了抗核抗体(ANA)、抗透明带抗体和 ASA。19 名(15.4%)患者的抗透明带抗体呈阳性,只有 6 名(4.9%)患者 ASA 呈阳性。其中两个携带 HLA-Dr3 等位基因,这似乎容易形成 ACL 抗体和 ANA。作者认为,由于这些样本数太小,无法进行有意义的统计比较。Al-Hussein 等[47]使用流式细胞术(FCA)检测 24 名 RPL 女性血清中的 ASA,同时检测其丈夫的淋巴细胞和精液样本(组 1)。还从作为对照的 6 对没有流产史的夫妇身上采集了血清、淋巴细胞和精液样本(组 2)。使用敏感的 FCA 分析样本,在组 1 中检测到 IgG 和 IgM 水平升高。然而,与正常妊娠的女性相比,没有发现显著的相关性。作者认为,尽管存在针对三种不同来源的父源抗原的抗体水平升高,但母体 IgG 和 IgM 类抗体在 RPL 中并不起主要作用。

4.8 精子制动抗体阳性的不孕女性的妊娠结局

我们前期在接受 IVF-ET 治疗的不孕女性中研究了精子制动抗体对妊娠结局的影响(图 9.1)[48]。研究比较了 58 名有精子制动抗体不孕女性的 143 个 ET 周期和 363 个输卵管因素不孕女性的 ET 周期。当 hCG 水平升高超过 50 U/L,但未见孕囊,则诊断为生化妊娠。精子制动抗体阳性女性的 143 个周期中有 33 例(23.1%)妊娠,对照组 363 个周期中有 56 例(15.4%)妊娠,两组比较有显著性差异($P<0.05$)。在精子制动抗体阳性的女性中,12 例(36.4%)生化妊娠、5 例(15.2%)流产和 16 例(48.5%)分娩。对照组中有 18 例(32.1%)生化妊娠、10 例(17.9%)临床流产(包括异位妊娠)和 28 例(50.0%)分娩。各组间没有差异。当分析受孕时的 SI_{50} 滴度时,SI_{50} 滴度低于 10 单位的患者生化妊娠率为 22.2%(4/18),SI_{50} 滴度高于 10 单位时为 50.0%(5/10),SI_{50} 滴度高于 100 单位时则为 60.0%(3/5)($P>0.05$)。在 4 个同时有生化妊娠和临床妊娠的患者中,他们生化妊娠周期受孕时的 SI_{50} 滴度高于临床妊娠周期。尽管精子制动抗体阳性患者的妊娠率明显高于输卵管因素不孕的患者,但精子制动抗体滴度较高的患者生化妊娠率也较高。这些结果表明,高滴度的精子制动抗体可能会对人体内胚胎的早期发育造成损害。

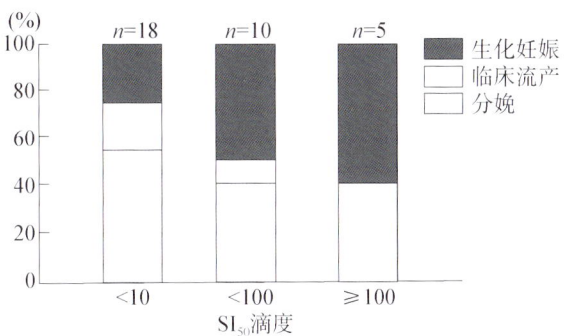

图 9.1 受孕时患者血清中精子制动抗体滴度(SI_{50})与妊娠结局的关系。

根据受孕时血清中的 SI_{50} 滴度,将患者分为三组,比较了 33 个妊娠周期的结局。SI_{50} 滴度低于 10 单位的患者生化妊娠率为 22.2%,SI_{50} 滴度高于 10 单位时为 50.0%,SI_{50} 滴度高于 100 单位时则为 60.0%。

在我们后来的研究中,证明了不孕女性血清中精子制动抗体对受精和胚胎质量的不利影响。尽管患者数量很少,在研究人群中,没有患者在 IVF-ET 成功妊娠后发生流产[34]。

5 评估

5.1 抗精子抗体检测

自 20 世纪 50 年代首次报道血清凝集试验以来,ASA 的检测已经有了很大的发展[49]。Franklin 和 Dukes 发现,在 214 名接受不孕不育调查的女性中,20.1% 的血清可检测到精子凝集活性[50]。在不明原因不孕女性中的阳性率(72.1%)远高于器质性不孕的女性(8.4%)或生育能力正常的女性(5.7%)。值得注意的是,这项研究发现 ASA 的发病率非常高,然而,近期使用 IBT 等方法的报道并不支持这一结果。从历史角度看,该研究值得关注,因为它激发了人们对于女性对精子的免疫反应可能参与了不明原因不孕不育的发展以及抗精子避孕疫苗概念的极大兴趣[51]。

自 20 世纪 70 年代以来,ASA 被认为是不孕的重要原因之一[8,9]。现已经开发了多种检测 ASA 的方法[52-56]。其中,Isojima 等[8,9] 开发了一种补体依赖性 SIT,可检测不孕女性血清中的精子制动抗体。在检测 ASA 的几种方法中,SIT 因其特异性而成为确定不孕最可靠的检测方法。

有研究比较了 SIT、Kibrick 和 Franklin Dukes 精子凝集试验[49,50] 作为在不孕、妊娠和未婚女性中检测血清 ASA 的方法[8,9]。在 17.2% 的不明原因不孕患者的血清中检测到 SIT 阳性反应,而在正常妊娠和未婚女性中没有发现。相比之下,Kibrick 和 Franklin Dukes 试验显示,正常妊娠女性的精子凝集反应阳性率高于不明原因不孕不育的病例,但在未婚女性中的阳性反应率很低。

5.2 计算机辅助精子分析在检测精子制动抗体中的应用

近期,我们团队应用计算机辅助精子分析(CASA)来检测精子制动抗体。如同常规精液检测,SIT 是通过在显微镜下计数活动精子的数量来实现的,可能会由于操作者的主观判断产生不同的结果[57]。我们利用 CASA 开发了一种新的方法,并将检测结果与传统方法进行了比较。基于这两种方法的结果是相同的,78 个测试样本中有 25 个精子制动抗体呈阳性,53 个样本呈阴性。对于 SI 阳性样本,使用这两种方法获得的 SI_{50} 值密切相关。我们认为,使用新的 CASA 方法将有可能客观评估临床 SIT 和 SI_{50} 数据,并增加使用 SIT 作为临床指标的便利性。此外,我们最近开发了一种基于 CASA 的改良 SIT 方法,当无法获得新鲜精子时,可用冷冻保存的精子代替新鲜精子[58]。

6 治疗

6.1 治疗方式

ASA 阳性女性,尤其是精子制动抗体,除了 IVF-ET,传统的方法是难以治疗的。在开展 IVF-ET 之前,基本上有两种治疗 ASA 不孕的策略。一个是减少 ASA 的产生,另一个是增加精子和卵子相遇的概率。对于前者,尝试持续使用避孕套或禁欲以避免精子致敏,或使用免疫抑制治疗,如皮质类固醇抑制抗体产生。然而,由于缺乏疗效和可能的副作用,这些方法已不再使用[59]。对于后者,IUI 和 IVF-ET 已成功用于消除 ASA 对精子通过女性生殖道时所造成的损害[19,48,60]。

如果 ASA 阳性的不孕女性通过 IVF-ET 等方法成功受孕,一旦发生 RPL,则需进一步评估。若没有发现 RPL 的原因,可以考虑在密切观察下通过皮质类固醇治疗以降低 ASA 水平。

6.2 具有精子制动抗体不孕女性的治疗策略

Kobayashi 等[19]根据患者个体 SI_{50} 滴度的波动模式，提出了一种具有精子制动抗体不孕女性的治疗策略。他们根据 SI_{50} 滴度将具有精子制动抗体的患者分为三组。A 组包括具有持续高滴度 SI_{50}（>10 单位）的患者，他们通过常规或反复 IUI 未受孕，但通过 IVF-ET 获得了满意的妊娠率。B 组由具有中等滴度 SI_{50}（10 单位左右）的患者组成，IUI 的成功率较低。C 组是持续低滴度 SI_{50}（<10 单位）的患者，他们通过常规或反复 IUI 受孕，但妊娠率低于 IVF-ET。图 9.2 中展示了基于精子制动抗体的不孕女性治疗策略。该治疗策略强调了评估 SI_{50} 滴度的重要性，以选择治疗具有精子制动抗体不孕女性的方法。

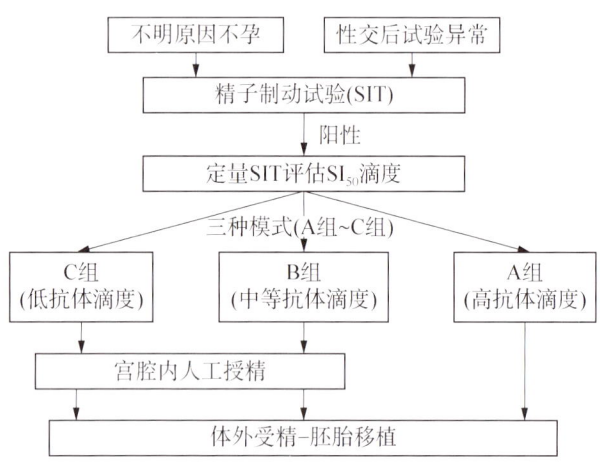

图 9.2 具有精子制动抗体不孕女性的治疗策略。

对具有精子制动抗体的不孕女性，根据个体 SI_{50} 滴度的波动模式，选择不同的治疗方式。A 组：建议持续高滴度 SI_{50}（>10 单位）的患者采用体外受精-胚胎移植（IVF-ET）。B 组：具有中等滴度 SI_{50}（10 单位左右）。C 组：持续低滴度 SI_{50}（<10 单位）的患者建议先通过常规或反复人工授精（IUI）进行治疗。据报道，C 组患者反复 IUI 的妊娠率高于 B 组（25.0% vs 17.6%）。因此，B 组患者如果他们无法通过 IUI 受孕，最好考虑尽早从 IUI 升级为 IVF-ET。

7 生殖结局

众所周知，由于女性生殖道的精子制动抗体抑制了精子在宫颈黏液[12,18]和输卵管[22]内的迁移，导致该类抗体阳性的女性对常规不孕治疗方法（如定时性交或 IUI）反应不佳。为了克服体内这一引起不孕的原因，可通过使用 IVF-ET 技术，给予配子和胚胎适当的培养条件，这已取得令人满意的结果[19,48,60]。建议不孕女性在 IVF 前进行血清 SIT。对具有精子制动抗体的患者，应小心操作配子和胚胎，特别是避免患者血清和卵泡液污染培养基，从而克服由于 ASA 所致女性不孕的免疫因素，在配子和胚胎恰当培养的条件下获得满意效果[19,20,48,60-62]。

8 总结和建议

ASA 与生殖功能障碍之间存在相关性。ASA 具有异质性，包含两种 ASA，与不孕相关的和与不孕无关的。前者可能是生殖障碍的原因。ASA 抑制精子在整个女性生殖道中的迁移，并对精子-卵子相互作用的各个阶段产生抑制。此外，一些 ASA 还显示出对胚胎发育的有害影响。然而，ASA 可能对 RPL 影响不大。在进行 IVF 之前，对不孕女性进行 SIT 的评估是重要的。

- ASA 具有异质性，包含两种 ASA，即与不孕相关的抗体和与不孕无关的抗体。
- 具有生物活性的 ASA，包括精子制动抗体、精子凝集抗体和受精阻断抗体，适合不孕女性进行初步检测。
- 不孕女性血清中 ASA 的存在，特别是精子制动抗体，已被证明可以抑制精子在女性整个生殖道中的迁移。
- ASA 在精子-卵子相互作用的各个阶段发挥抑制作用。一些 ASA 还显示出对胚胎发育的有害影响。
- 为了选择合适的治疗方法，重要的是评估具有精子制动抗体的不孕女性的 SI_{50} 滴度。
- 为了克服 ASA 不孕，通过 IVF-ET 可给予配子和胚胎合适的培养条件以获得满意的结果。
- 关于 RPL 和 ASA，目前的报道存在争议。
- 如果患有 ASA 的不孕女性通过 IVF-ET 等方法成功受孕，一旦出现 RPL，则需进一步评估。
- 在患有 ASA 的不孕女性中，当没有发现引起 RPL 的其他原因时，可以考虑在密切观察下通过皮质类固醇治疗以降低 ASA 水平。

参考文献

[1] Zegers-Hochschild F, Adamson GD, de Mouzon J, et al. International committee for monitoring assisted reproductive technology (ICMART) and the World Health Organization (WHO) revised glossary of ART terminology, 2009. Fertil Steril. 92. 2009. p. 1520-4.

[2] Kokcu A, Yavuz E, Celik H, et al. A panoramic view to relationships between reproductive failure and immunological factors. Arch Gynecol Obstet 2012. Available from: https://doi.org/10.1007/s00404-012-2480-6.

[3] Atik RB, Christiansen OB, Elson J, et al. ESHRE guideline: recurrent pregnancy loss. Hum Reprod Open 2018;1-12.

[4] Choudhury SR, Knapp LA. Human reproductive failure I: immunological factors. Hum Reprod Update 2000;7:113-34.

[5] Shibahara H, Shiraishi Y, Suzuki M. Diagnosis and treatment of immunologically infertile males with antisperm antibodies. Reprod Med Biol 2005;4:133-41.

[6] Shibahara H, Koriyama J, Shiraishi Y, et al. Diagnosis and treatment of immunologically infertile women with sperm-immobilizing antibodies in their sera. J Reprod Immunol 2009;83:139-44.

[7] Shibahara H, Wakimoto Y, Fukui A, et al. Anti-sperm antibodies and reproductive failures. Am J Reprod Immunol 2021;85(4):e13337. Available from: https://doi.org/10.1111/aji.13337.

[8] Isojima S, Li TS, Ashitaka Y. Immunologic analysis of sperm immobilizing factor found in sera of women with unexplained sterility. Am J Obstet Gynecol 1968;101:677-83.

[9] Isojima S, Tsuchiya K, Koyama K, et al. Further studies on sperm-immobilizing antibody found in sera of unexplained cases of sterility in women. Am J Obstet Gynecol 1972;112:199-207.

[10] Shibahara H, Koriyama J. Methods for direct and indirect antisperm antibody testing. Methods Mol Biol 2013;927:51-60.

[11] Isojima S, Koyama K. Techniques for sperm immobilization test. Arch Androl 1989;23:185-99.

[12] Koyama K, Ikuma K, Kubota K, et al. Effects of antisperm antibodies on sperm migration through cervical mucus. Excerpta Med Int Congr Ser 1980;512:705-8.

[13] Cantuaria AA. Sperm immobilizing antibodies in the serum and cervicovaginal secretions of infertile and normal women. Br J Obstet Gynaecol 1977;84:865-8.

[14] Chen C, Jones WR. Application of a sperm micro-immobilization test to cervical mucus in the investigation of immunologic infertility. Fertil Steril 1981;35:542-5.

[15] Jager S, Kremer J, De Wilde-Janssen IW. Are sperm immobilizing antibodies in cervical mucus an explanation for a poor post-coital test? Am J Reprod Immunol 1984;5:56-60.

[16] Isojima S, Koyama K. Quantitative estimation of sperm immobilizing antibody in the sera of women with sterility of unknown etiology: the 50% sperm immobilization unit (SI_{50}). Excerpta Med Int Congr Ser 1974;370:10-15.

[17] Koyama K, Kubota K, Ikuma K, et al. Correlation between quantitative antibody titers of sperm immobilizing antibodies and pregnancy rates by treatments. Fertil Steril 1988;33:201-6.

[18] Shibahara H, Shiraishi Y, Hirano Y, et al. Relationship between level of serum sperm immobilizing antibody and its inhibitory effect on sperm migration through cervical mucus in immunologically infertile women. Am J Reprod Immunol 2007;57:142-6.

[19] Kobayashi S, Bessho T, Shigeta M, et al. Correlation between quantitative antibody titers of sperm immobilizing antibodies and pregnancy rates by treatments. Fertil Steril 1990;54:1107-13.

[20] Hasegawa A, Shigeta M, Shibahara H. Sperm immobilizing antibody and its target antigen. In: Krause WKH, Naz RK, editors. Immune infertility. Switzerland: Springer; 2016. p. 173-84.

[21] Templeton AA, Mortimer D. Laparoscopic sperm recovery in infertile women. Br J Obstet Gynecol 1980;87:1128-31.

[22] Shibahara H, Shigeta M, Toji H, et al. Sperm immobilizing antibodies interfere with sperm migration from the uterine cavity through the Fallopian tubes. Am J Reprod Immunol 1995;34:120-4.

[23] Bandoh R, Yamano S, Kamada M, et al. Effect of sperm-immobilizing antibodies on the acrosome reaction of human spermatozoa. Fertil Steril 1992;57:387-92.

[24] Cheng GY, Shi JL, Wang M, et al. Inhibition of mouse acrosome reaction and sperm-zona pellucida binding by anti-human sperm membrane protein 1 antibody. Asian J Androl 2007;9:23-9.

[25] Zhang J, Ding X, Bian Z, et al. The effect of anti-eppin antibodies on ionophore A23187-induced calcium influx and acrosome reaction of human spermatozoa. Hum Reprod 2010;25:29-36.

[26] Bronson RA, Cooper GW, Rosenfeld DL. Sperm-specific isoantibodies and autoantibodies inhibit the binding of human sperm to the human zona pellucida. Fertil Steril 1982;38:724-9.

[27] Alexander NJ. Antibodies to human spermatozoa impede sperm penetration of cervical mucus or hamster eggs. Fertil Steril 1984;41:433-9.

[28] Kamada M, Daitoh T, Hasebe H, et al. Blocking of human fertilization in vitro by sera with sperm-immobilizing antibodies. Am J Obstet Gynecol 1985;153:328-31.

[29] Mahony MC, Blackmore PF, Bronson RA, et al. Inhibition of human sperm-zona pellucida tight binding in the presence of antisperm antibody positive polyclonal patient sera. J Reprod Immunol 1991;19:287-301.

[30] Tsukui S, Noda Y, Fukuda A, et al. Blocking effect of sperm immobilizing antibodies on sperm penetration of human zonae pellucida. Vitro Fert Embryo Transf 1988;5:123-8.

[31] Shibahara H, Shigeta M, Koyama K, et al. Inhibition of sperm-zona pellucida tight binding by sperm immobilizing antibodies as assessed by the hemizona assay (HZA). Acta Obstet Gynaecol Jpn 1991;43:237-8.

[32] Shibahara H, Burkman LJ, Isojima S, et al. Effects of sperm-immobilizing antibodies on sperm-zona pellucida tight binding. Fertil Steril 1993;60:533-9.

[33] Shibahara H, Hirano Y, Shiraishi Y, et al. Effects of in vivo exposure to eggs with sperm-immobilizing antibodies in follicular fluid on subsequent fertilization and embryo development in vitro. Reprod Med Biol 2006;5:137-43.

[34] Taneichi A, Shibahara H, Hirano Y, et al. Sperm immobilizing antibodies in the sera of infertile women cause low fertilization rates and poor embryo quality in vitro. Am J Reprod Immunol 2002;47:46-51.
[35] Menge AC. Effect of isoimmunization and isoantisera against seminal antigens on fertility processes in female rabbits. Biol Reprod 1971;4:137-44.
[36] Koyama K, Hasegawa A, Isojima S. Effects of antisperm antibody on the rat embryos. Gamete Res 1984;10:143-52.
[37] Naz RK. Effects of antisperm antibodies on early cleavage of fertilized ova. Biol Reprod 1992;46:130-9.
[38] Veeck LL. Atlas of the human oocytes and early conceptus. 1991,2. Baltimore, Williams & Willkins Co.
[39] Taneichi A, Shibahara H, Takahashi K, et al. Effects of sera from infertile women with sperm immobilizing antibodies on fertilization and embryo development in vitro in mice. Am J Reprod Immunol 2003;50:146-51.
[40] Haas GG, Kubota K, Quebbeman JF, et al. Circulating antisperm antibodies in recurrently aborting women. Fertil Steril 1986;45:209-15.
[41] Mathur S, Neff MR, Williamson HO, et al. Sperm antibodies and human leukocyte antigens in couples with early spontaneous abortions. Int J Fertil 1987;32:59-65.
[42] Witkin SS, David SS. Effect of sperm antibodies on pregnancy outcome in a subfertile population. Am J Obstet Gynecol 1988;158:59-62.
[43] Witkin SS, Chaudhry A. Association between recurrent spontaneous abortions and circulating IgG antibodies to sperm tails in women. J Reprod Immunol 1989;15:151-8.
[44] Maier DB, Parke A. Subclinical autoimmunity in recurrent aborters. Fertil Steril 1989;51:280-5.
[45] Clarke GN, Baker HW. Lack of association between sperm antibodies and recurrent spontaneous abortion. Fertil Steril 1993;59:463-4.
[46] Christiansen OB, Ulcova-Gallova Z, Mohapeloa H, et al. Studies on associations between human leukocyte antigen (HLA) class II alleles and antiphospholipid antibodies in Danish and Czech women with recurrent miscarriages. Hum Reprod 1998;13:3326-31.
[47] Al-Hussein K, Al-Mukhalafi Z, Bertilsson P-A, et al. Value of flow cytometric assay for the detection of antisperm antibodies in women with a history of recurrent abortion. Am J Reprod Immunol 2002:31-7.
[48] Shibahara H, Mitsuo M, Ikeda Y, et al. Effects of sperm immobilizing antibodies on pregnancy outcome in infertile women treated with IVF-ET. Am J Reprod Immunol 1996;36:96-100.
[49] Kibrick S, Belding DL, Merrill B. Methods for the detection of antibodies against mammalian spermatozoa. I. A modified macroscopic agglutination test. Fertil Steril 1952;3:419-29.
[50] Franklin RR, Dukes CD. Further studies on sperm-agglutinating antibody and unexplained infertility. JAMA 1964;190:682-3.
[51] Clarke GN. ASA in the female. In Immune infertility. Impact of immune reactions on human fertility, 2nd ed., (Eds) Krause WKH, Naz RK, Springer, 2017:161-172.
[52] Bronson R, Cooper G, Rosenfeld D. Ability of antibody-bound human sperm to penetrate zona-free hamster ova in vitro. Fertil Steril 1981;36:778-83.
[53] Shibahara H, Hirano Y, Takamizawa S, et al. Effects of sperm-immobilizing antibodies bound to the surface of ejaculated human spermatozoa on sperm motility in immunologically infertile men. Fertil Steril 2003;79:641-2.
[54] Jager S, Kremer J, van Slochteren-Draaisma T. A simple method of screening for antisperm antibodies in the human male. Detection of spermatozoal surface IgG with the direct mixed antiglobulin re-action carried out on untreated fresh human semen. Int J Fertil 1978;23:12-21.
[55] Clarke GN, Elliott PJ, Smaila C. Detection of sperm antibodies in semen using the immunobead test: a survey of 813 consecutive patients. Am J Reprod Immunol Microbiol 1985;7:118-23.
[56] Centola GM, Andolina E, Deutsch A. Comparison of the immunobead binding test (IBT) and immunospheres (IS) assay for detecting serum antisperm antibodies. Am J Reprod Immunol 1997;37:300-3.
[57] Wakimoto Y, Fukui A, Kojima T. Application of computer-aided sperm analysis (CASA) for detecting sperm-immobilizing antibody. Am J Reprod Immunol 2018;79(3). Available from: https://doi.org/10.1111/aji.12814.
[58] Wakimoto Y, Fukui A, Kojima T, et al. Sperm immobilization test and quantitative sperm immobilization test using frozen-thawed sperm preparation applied with computer-aided sperm analysis. Reprod Med Biol 2021;20:321-6.
[59] Koyama K. Gamete immunology: infertility and contraception. Reprod Immunol Biol 2009;24:1-17.
[60] Sugimoto Y, Hasegawa A, Yokoyama K, et al. Successful application of in vitro fertilization and embryo replacement in the treatment of infertile women with sperm immobilizing antibody. Acta Obstet Gynaecol Jpn 1987;38:1135-6.
[61] Yovich J, Stranger JD, Kay D, et al. In vitro fertilization of oocytes from women with serum antisperm antibodies. Lancet 1984;1:369-70.
[62] Daitoh T, Kamada M, Yamano S, et al. High implantation rate and consequently high pregnancy rate by in vitro fertilization-embryo transfer in infertile women with antisperm antibody. Fertil Steril 1995;63:87-91.

第 10 章

抗甲状腺抗体与生殖功能
Antithyroid antibodies and reproductive function

Elena Borodina[1,2], Alexander M. Gzgzyan[1,3], Lyailya Kh. Dzhemlikhanova[1,3],
Dariko A. Niauri[1,2,3] and Yehuda Shoenfeld[2,4,5]

[1] Department of Obstetrics, Gynecology and Reproductive Sciences, Saint Petersburg State University, Saint Petersburg, Russia
[2] Laboratory of the Mosaic of Autoimmunity, Saint Petersburg State University, Saint Petersburg, Russia
[3] FSBSI "The Research Institute of Obstetrics, Gynecology and Reproductology named after D.O. Ott," Saint Petersburg, Russia
[4] Ariel University, Ariel, Israel
[5] Zabludowicz Center for Autoimmune Diseases; Sheba Medical Center, Tel-Aviv, Israel

1 引言

现今，甲状腺功能减退对生殖功能的负面影响已是毋庸置疑的事实。甲状腺功能减退可能影响人类妊娠的各个阶段，从排卵功能障碍、早期妊娠丢失，到早产、宫内生长受限[1-3]，甚至影响子代的神经认知功能[4,5]。在发达国家，甲状腺功能减退的最常见原因是自身免疫性甲状腺炎（antoimmune thyroiditis，AIT）[6]，而在甲状腺功能正常的女性中，甲状腺组织自身抗体的直接作用问题仍在讨论之中。

2 自身免疫性甲状腺炎的定义

自身免疫性甲状腺炎（AIT）是一种慢性进行性疾病，在其进展过程中发生对甲状腺腺体的自身免疫反应。这一过程涉及所有淋巴细胞亚群，表现为甲状腺腺体的单核细胞浸润和炎症迹象，导致甲状腺功能逐渐减退并伴有多种并发症。

3 患病率

AIT 在生育年龄的女性中比男性更为常见，是患病率最高的内分泌疾病之一[7]。研究人员现已提出了三种关于未出现明显甲状腺功能减退的 AIT 对生殖功能影响的潜在机制假说。

4 潜在的免疫病理学

4.1 抗甲状腺抗体作为附带现象

一些研究人员认为，抗甲状腺抗体（ATA）（如同其他器官特异性，尤其是非器官特异性抗体一样）是广泛性 T 细胞功能障碍的标志。这一假说提出已有 20 余年，当时科学家们质疑："这些如此不同的抗体是如何导致相同的结果的？"根据这一假说，ATA 和其他自身抗体是在广泛性 T 细胞功能障碍的背景下发生的附带现象[8,9]。已知，Th1/Th2 平衡失调并向 Th1 转化与生殖障碍相关[10-12]，促炎的 Th1 细胞因子（IFN-γ、TNF-α、IL-2）有助于细胞毒性抗体的产生，激活 NK 细胞和效应 T 细胞，导致滋养层破坏[11]。Stewart-Akers 等[13] 报道了 AIT 患者子宫内膜样本中 IFN-γ 明显增加，而抗炎细胞因子如 IL-4 和 IL-10 减少。Kim 等[14] 发现了类似的结果，即患有 AIT 的女性 TNF-α、细胞毒性 NK 细胞计数增加，Th1/Th2 平衡失调并向 Th1 转化，外周血中器官特异性自身抗体更为普遍。其他研究还证明了 AIT 常与抗磷脂抗体[15]、器官特异性自身抗体、其他自身免疫疾病和 NK 细胞毒性增加共同出现[16,17]。此外，AIT 亦与导致不孕的妇科疾病之间存在关联[18,19]。

4.2 抗甲状腺抗体作为甲状腺功能受损的原因

另一种观点解释了 AIT 通过引起甲状腺疾病在不孕和反复妊娠丢失(RPL)中发挥作用。妊娠期间，甲状腺激素的需求平均增加 47%，从妊娠第 5 周开始到 16～20 周达到稳态，直至分娩大致保持在同一水平[19,20]。在 ATA 阳性女性中，有 40% 会出现明显或亚临床甲状腺功能减退[21]，而亚临床甲状腺功能减退的女性大多在刚妊娠时甲状腺功能正常。然而，许多专家认为这些女性的甲状腺功能受损，无法完全满足身体对甲状腺激素的不断增长的需求。

Ashoor 等[22]在分析 TSH、T_4、T_3 和 ATA 水平后认为，甲状腺功能的改变会影响妊娠结局但不会影响 ATA 的存在。在这项研究中，患者激素水平没有超出正常范围。女性的中位 TSH 和游离 T_4 在不良妊娠结局和良好妊娠结局中分别为 1.133 比 1.007 中位数倍数(MoM)和 0.958 比 0.992 MoM。有人认为，与具有良好妊娠结局的女性相比，不良妊娠结局女性的甲状腺功能减退，但仍维持在正常范围。Negro 等[23]的回顾性分析得出了类似的结果，他们分析了甲状腺功能正常的女性在接受辅助生殖技术(ART)时的数据。仅有 ATA 的存在既不影响妊娠率，也不影响流产率。然而，妊娠前的 TSH 水平对妊娠结局有重要影响。在抗甲状腺过氧化物酶抗体(抗-TPO)阳性的女性中，不良妊娠结局的 TSH 水平为 2.8 mU/L，而具有良好妊娠结局的女性 TSH 为 1.6 mU/L；而抗-TPO 阴性的女性 TSH 为 1.1 mU/L。He 等[24]的荟萃分析结果也支持既往的研究发现，即如果女性没有亚临床甲状腺功能减退，ATA 本身并不起作用。此外，Lepoutre 等[25]报道称，对于抗-TPO 阳性的女性，不良妊娠结局只出现在首次产检后没有接受左旋甲状腺素治疗的患者中。一项包含约 8 000 名女性的荟萃分析得出了类似的结论，即左旋甲状腺素治疗降低了抗-TPO 阳性患者的流产和早产风险[26]，其他的研究也获得了类似的结果[27-29]。

4.3 抗甲状腺抗体导致生殖障碍的可能机制

4.3.1 交叉反应抗体理论

目前，已报道了 ATA 可能直接对生殖系统组织产生负面影响的机制。研究表明，在患有 AIT 的女性卵泡液中存在抗-TPO 和抗甲状腺球蛋白抗体(抗-TG)[30,31]。这些抗体在通过血-卵巢屏障后浓度约为血清的一半。与阴性对照组相比，ATA 阳性女性的受精率(63% vs 72%，$P<0.05$)和高质量胚胎的比例(25% vs 48%，$P<0.05$)降低。有趣的是，在 ATA 阳性女性中，只有那些进行体外受精/单精子胞浆内注射(IVF/ICSI)的患者妊娠，而在对照组中，无论 IVF 还是 ICSI 都能妊娠[30]。尽管样本量较小，抗体浓度较低的患者妊娠结局通常更佳。Weghofer 等[32]还研究了 ATA 阳性和阴性女性所得胚胎的质量。该研究包括了卵巢储备功能降低且甲状腺功能正常的高育龄女性。患者根据 TSH 水平分为 TSH<2.5 mU/mL 和 TSH 2.5～4.5 mU/mL 两组。TSH≤2.5 或 TSH>2.5 mU/mL 组中的女性胚胎质量具有可比性。在 TSH≤2.5 mU/mL 组中，抗-TPO 的存在显著影响所获胚胎的质量($P=0.045$)。在 TSH 水平较高且抗-TPO 水平较高的组中，可能由于两个因素叠加，胚胎质量显得更差($P=0.057$)。尽管 Medenica 等[31]的研究没有显示出胚胎质量和数量的变化，但发现 ATA 阳性女性在每个促排周期(30.8% vs 61.5%，$P=0.026$)和胚胎移植周期(34.8% vs 66.7%，$P=0.029$)的妊娠率降低。多元分析显示，ATA 阳性女性实现妊娠的概率低于年龄和体重指数匹配的 ATA 阴性对照组($P=0.004$，$OR=0.036$，95% CI 0.004～0.347)。

这些数据与甲状腺组织和卵巢透明带交叉反应抗体的理论非常一致。这一观察由 Kelkar 等[33]开展，他们研究了自身免疫性卵巢炎患者血清中的抗体交叉反应，并发现抗透明带抗体可以结合到小鼠的甲状腺组织上。据此表明，抗甲状腺抗体可能会结合到透明带上，而透明带的损伤则可能导致早期胚胎发育的异常，包括受精、孵化和种植，以及胚胎的免疫识别受损。这一假设提示 IVF/ICSI 可以预防可能与抗甲状腺抗体相关的并发症。Chen 等[34]评估了 235 名携带抗甲状腺抗体的女性和 214 名携带抗 TPO 的女性进行 IVF/ICSI 的妊娠结局。IVF/ICSI 失败与抗甲状腺抗体的存在没有关联，表明应用 IVF/ICSI 可能弥补了抗甲状腺抗体的负面影响。Tan 等[35]的研究也没有发现抗甲状腺抗体对通过 IVF/ICSI 途径妊娠的负面影响。

此外，Lukaszuk 等[36]评估了甲状腺功能正常的 AIT 对 IVF/ICSI 结果的影响。在接受 ICSI 的女性中，ATA 的存在对受精、种植、妊娠、活产或流产率没有影响。近期由 He 等[37]进行的研究揭示了抗-TPO 对甲状腺功能正常女性的影响。对 1 170 名女性首次进行 IVF/ICSI 的结果分析显示,当 2.5 mU/L≤TSH<4.2 mU/L 时,抗-TPO 阳性患者的受精率显著低于抗-TPO 阴性女性。然而,这一结果可能是由于抗-TPO 和 TSH 水平的协同作用,这是因为该组的受精率显著低于 TSH<2.5 mU/L 组。2.5 mU/L≤TSH<4.2 mU/L 且抗-TPO 阳性的受精率为 73%,而抗-TPO 阴性的受精率为 82%。0.3 mU/L≤TSH<2.5 mU/L 且抗-TPO 阴性的受精率为 83%,而 0.3 mU/L≤TSH<2.5 mU/L 且抗-TPO 阳性的受精率为 84%。

卵巢早衰(通常与卵巢自身免疫损伤有关)患者 ATA 的发生率高于与年龄相关的卵巢储备功能减退的女性(15.3% vs 6%,$P=0.009$)[38]。ATA 的存在被认为是不良生殖结局的危险因素(RR=2.8,95% CI 1.2~6.3)。年龄相关卵巢储备功能减退的女性相对于卵巢早衰患者,妊娠率较高(每周期 16.7% vs 8.7%,$P=0.037$)[38]。有人认为,卵巢早衰患者妊娠率下降可能与生殖器官的自身免疫异常导致子宫内膜受体功能紊乱有关[38]。另一项研究报道指出,甲状腺功能正常的 ATA 阳性患者 IVF/ICSI 妊娠率降低。24 名甲状腺功能正常的 ATA 阳性患者均未妊娠,而 ATA 阴性患者有 23.9% 妊娠。这两组患者在获卵数和胚胎移植数方面没有差异[39]。然而也有其他研究报道,无论采用何种 ART 方式,ATA 或 TSH 水平均不会影响妊娠率、流产率或早产率[40-42]。

4.3.2 动物研究支持交叉反应抗体理论

除了来自透明带可能的交叉反应抗原之外,生殖器官中还存在其他抗-TG 和抗-TPO 的靶标。为了确定抗-TG 在妊娠失败中的作用及其机制,Matalon 等[13]利用甲状腺球蛋白诱导小鼠,使小鼠产生甲状腺抗体。然而,并未在免疫组小鼠中观察到甲状腺功能减退,甲状腺功能与对照组相似。免疫组小鼠的胚胎吸收比例增加($P=0.04$),幼仔平均体重减少[(194±4) mg vs (240±6) mg;$P<0.001$]和胎盘减小[(105±2) mg vs (130±3) mg;$P<0.001$]。抗-TG 与胎盘的结合解释了抗-TG 对妊娠结局的不良影响。为了确定小鼠模型中抗-TG 的靶标,Moravej 等[44]评估了小鼠妊娠早期、中期和晚期卵巢、胎盘和胎膜组织中的甲状腺球蛋白水平。经过组织匀浆,无论是免疫组化还是斑点印迹法,均未检测到组织中的甲状腺球蛋白。此外,通过逆转录-聚合酶链反应(RT-PCR)也未在生殖组织中检测到甲状腺球蛋白基因。这项研究表明,抗-TG 的负面影响可能是由于抗-TG 与生殖器官的其他抗原发生交叉反应,这些抗原具有与甲状腺球蛋白相似的表位结构。根据这项研究,可以假设免疫小鼠胎盘中的抗-TG 与具有相似分子结构的交叉反应抗原结合[43]。

4.3.3 抗甲状腺抗体对胚胎种植的潜在作用

另一个 ATA 的潜在靶点是甲状腺过氧化物酶(TPO),它存在于人类生殖器官中,如子宫内膜和胎盘[45]。在增生期子宫内膜的腺上皮和管腔上皮的细胞质中发现 TPO,其中,子宫内膜上皮管腔表面的表达密度最高。此外,免疫组化也证实了妊娠早期绒毛滋养层中 TPO 的存在[45]。这些研究表明,抗-TPO 可以直接干扰胚胎植入过程,导致早期妊娠丢失。此外,无论 TSH 水平如何,抗-TPO 阳性患者的生化妊娠率为抗-TPO 阴性患者的 5.3 倍($P=0.002$,OR=5.311,95% CI 1.859~15.169)[37],提示抗-TPO 影响胚胎植入过程。

为了研究抗-TPO 的潜在机制,研究人员用重组的小鼠 TPO 免疫小鼠,建立了甲状腺功能正常的 AIT 动物模型[46]。结果发现,产生的抗-TPO 并未导致 T_4 水平的变化;然而,免疫组的 TSH 水平显著高于对照组,但仍保持在参考范围内。该研究还发现甲状腺功能正常的 AIT 小鼠胚胎吸收率增加(14.75% vs 0%;$P<0.05$),幼崽的平均体重减小。由于胚胎种植率没有变化,表明该现象是由胎盘病理造成的。此外,当植入前用抗-TPO 血清冲洗宫腔后,研究组的胚胎种植率与对照组无异。因此推测抗-TPO 是在植入过程结束后发挥作用的[46]。

在小鼠研究中,免疫组化结果显示抗-TPO 可与 3~4 细胞至囊胚阶段的胚胎表面结合[45]。尽管观察到胚胎在 4 细胞阶段发育较慢,但后续的发育阶段,如囊胚形成和孵化,并未与对照组有所不同。可见胚胎能适应这种情况,推测抗-TPO 的有害影响可能不会发生于胚胎植入前。与小鼠胚胎不同,人类植入前的胚胎在囊胚阶段不表达 TPO[45]。这种差异可能与不同的胚胎天数有关:小鼠模型中为 3~4 细胞至桑椹胚阶段的胚胎,人类中则为囊胚期的胚胎。

4.3.4 胎盘是抗甲状腺抗体的潜在靶点

Rahnama 等[45]利用剖宫产所获得的足月妊娠

胎盘，检测抗-TPO 的靶点。免疫组化结果显示，TPO 存在于合体滋养层和侵入性滋养层的表面。此外，通过 RT-PCR 确认了这些组织中存在 TPO 基因。这一发现表明，抗-TPO 可以直接结合到胎盘组织。

抗-TPO 结合到侵入性滋养层表面所存在的 TPO，使侵入性滋养层细胞膜遭到破坏。滋养细胞的侵袭能力降低导致了 AIT 患者的胎盘功能不全。此前，我们在被动免疫的 TPO 小鼠模型中展示了胎盘功能不全[47]。我们认为，小鼠模型所表现的胎盘功能不全可能解释了 AIT 患者的胎盘病理。在小鼠胎盘中，与侵入性滋养层细胞接近的是直接与子宫接触的巨细胞[48]。这些细胞在功能上与人类蜕膜中的多核滋养层巨细胞、合体滋养层细胞相当，代表了侵入性滋养层分化的最后阶段[49]。目前尚不清楚 TPO 是否存在于小鼠胎盘组织中。但是，在接受 TPO 免疫的小鼠组中，滋养层巨细胞及其细胞核的数量减少[47]。这些发现支持了 Rahnama 等的研究，提示胎盘中可能存在 TPO。

抗-TPO 在人类合体滋养层的存在暗示 AIT 可能导致胎盘功能不全，从而减少了胎盘激素的产生，并减少了向胎儿输送营养物质和氧气。这是因为合体滋养层在将营养物质和氧气转运到人类胎盘中起到关键作用，并且是胎盘激素和生长因子的主要来源。

合体滋养层参与向胎儿输送营养和氧气，其位于胎盘屏障的血管间隔层，主要由以下结构组成：胎儿毛细血管的内皮、内皮基底膜、合体滋养层和细胞滋养层，排列在充满母体血液的窦腔中[50]。我们的研究主要观察到，在注射抗 TPO 血清后小鼠胎盘屏障的血管间隔层增厚以及血流异常[47]，而血管间隔层增厚可能是由合体滋养层受损引起的。上述现象表明，抗 TPO 抗体的直接靶标 TPO 可能存在于小鼠合体滋养层上，但这些结果仍需要进一步研究。

5　评估

对甲状腺功能的评估是产前检查的重要组成部分，通常受到国家指南的监管。全球范围内，对甲状腺功能的评估基本相似，许多国家的指南遵循美国甲状腺协会指南[51]，该指南建议对所有寻求妊娠或妊娠初期的女性以及存在甲状腺功能障碍风险因素的患者进行 TSH 水平评估，例如：

（1）已知甲状腺抗体阳性或存在甲状腺肿。
（2）曾经接受头部或颈部辐射或既往甲状腺手术史。
（3）年龄＞30 岁。
（4）1 型糖尿病或其他自身免疫性疾病。
（5）流产、早产或不孕的病史。
（6）多次妊娠的经历。
（7）家族中有自身免疫性甲状腺疾病或甲状腺功能障碍的病史。
（8）病态肥胖。
（9）使用胺碘酮或锂，或最近使用含碘的放射学对比剂。
（10）居住在已知中重度碘缺乏的地区。

此外，对于存在甲状腺功能减退风险的孕妇，特别是抗甲状腺抗体（ATA）阳性的孕妇，应每月监测一次血清 TSH 水平，直至妊娠中期，并在妊娠 30 周左右至少监测一次。

同时，在 TSH＞2.5 mU/L 的情况下应行 ATA 评估。例如，由于俄罗斯几乎整个领土都存在碘缺乏，因此建议所有计划妊娠或妊娠初期的女性进行常规血清 TSH 水平筛查，并由俄罗斯内分泌学协会监督此临床实践[52]。对于 ATA 筛查，TSH＞2.5 mU/L 是进行 ATA 评估的指征。

6　治疗

美国甲状腺协会的指南[51]对于 ATA 阳性的甲状腺功能正常的女性建议如下：对于 TSH 在 2.5 mU/L 以上且低于 4 mU/L 的 ATA 阳性女性，可考虑使用左旋甲状腺素治疗（在大多数情况下，TSH 浓度 4 mU/L 被视为妊娠特定参考范围的上限）。这种方法适用于计划妊娠、妊娠以及正在进行辅助生殖治疗的女性。在所有情况下，使用左旋甲状腺素治疗将孕妇的 TSH 控制在 2.5 mU/L 以下是合理的。此外，对于患有亚临床甲状腺功能减退，尤其是明显甲状腺功能减退的患者，应该接受左旋甲状腺素治疗。不建议对 ATA 阳性的甲状腺功能正常的女性使用糖皮质激素和静脉免疫球蛋白治疗[51]。

7　妊娠结局

目前已有足够信息表明 ATA 是生殖障碍发病机制中的独立危险因素。已发表的研究显示，即使在甲状腺功能正常的情况下，ATA 也可能对生殖功能产生负面影响[53-67]。在一项涉及 90 名 ATA 阳性和 676 名 ATA 阴性患者的研究中，ATA 阳性组的受精率、胚胎种植率和妊娠率显著降低（分别为 64.3% vs 74.6%，$P<0.001$；17.8% vs 27.1%，$P<0.001$；33.3% vs 46.7%，$P=0.002$），而流产率显著增高（26.9% vs 11.8%，$P=0.002$）[53]。然而，在这项研究中，并非所有患者的 TSH 水平都是已知的，应谨慎解释这些数据[53]。

越来越多的研究报道，在甲状腺功能正常的 ATA 阳性女性群体中，流产率和早产率升高[54-59]。此外，该群体女性的围产期死亡风险也增加[60]。相反，Seungdamrong 等[61]的研究通过 logistic 回归分析评估了 1 468 名有流产史的患者。妊娠前抗-TPO 阳性的患者与没有抗-TPO 的患者相比，流产风险增加（43.9% vs 25.3%，OR 2.17，95% CI 1.12~4.22），活产率降低（17.1% vs 25.4%，OR 0.58，95% CI 0.35~0.96）。然而，在这项研究中，两组妊娠的百分比没有显著差异，TSH 水平对妊娠结局没有影响。Meena 等[62]的研究数据证实了 ATA 对妊娠结局的负面影响。与无 ATA 的女性相比，具有 ATA 的亚临床甲状腺功能减退患者的流产率增加（13.33% vs 2.34%，$P<0.001$），出生低体重儿的比例增加（25% vs 5.12%，$P<0.001$），早产率（<34 周）增加（5% vs 1.80%，$P>0.05$）。Poppe 等[63]的研究纳入了接受 IVF 的抗-TPO 阳性（$n=32$）和抗-TPO 阴性（$n=202$）的甲状腺功能正常的患者，抗-TPO 阳性组早期妊娠丢失的风险显著增加（53% vs 23%，OR 3.77，95% CI 1.29~11.05；$P=0.016$），但妊娠率在统计学上与抗-TPO 阴性组没有显著差异。

Dendrinos 等[64]研究表明在 RPL 群体中 ATA 的发生频率明显增加（37% vs 13%，$P<0.05$），Bellver 等[65]发现，ATA 在种植失败的患者中发生频率也有所增加。Dhillon-Smith[66] 和 Chen[67]进行的荟萃分析支持 ATA 对妊娠的负面影响：在甲状腺功能正常的抗 TPO 阳性患者中，流产和早产的比例增加，而服用甲状腺素治疗的患者妊娠结局并没有得到改善[66]。

8 总结和建议

综上所述，尽管已发现 ATA 对生殖功能存在诸多影响，但 ATA 的潜在机制仍不清楚。最有可能的是，人类生殖功能受到了本文所描述的多种机制协同作用的影响。因此，完整且及时的检查至关重要。

- 在备孕阶段（无论是自然妊娠还是辅助生殖），所有女性都应检测血清 TSH 水平，并考虑进行 ATA 筛查。
- 如果血清 TSH 超过 2.5 mU/L，则应进行 ATA 检查。
- 如果女性在妊娠前没有接受评估，则应在第一次孕期检查时检测 TSH。
- 对于 ATA 阳性且 TSH 低于 2.5 mU/L 的女性，建议在妊娠中期之前定期检测 TSH，并在妊娠近 30 周时至少进行一次检测。
- 对于 ATA 阳性且 TSH 高于 2.5 mU/L 的女性，应给予左旋甲状腺素治疗（起始剂量为每天 25~50 μg）。
- 孕妇治疗的目标是将 TSH 降至 2.5 mU/L 以下。

参考文献

[1] Zhang Y, Wang H, Pan X, Teng W, Shan Z. Patients with subclinical hypothyroidism before 20 weeks of pregnancy have a higher risk of miscarriage: a systematic review and meta-analysis. PLoS One 2017;12(4). Available from: https://doi.org/10.1371/journal.pone.0175708.

[2] Maraka S, Ospina NMS, O'Keeffe DT, et al. Subclinical hypothyroidism in pregnancy: a systematic review and meta-analysis. Thyroid 2016;26(4):580-90. Available from: https://doi.org/10.1089/thy.2015.0418.

[3] Shinohara DR, Santos TDS, De Carvalho HC, et al. Pregnancy complications associated with maternal hypothyroidism: a systematic review. Obstet Gynecol Surv 2018;73(4):219-30. Available from: https://doi.org/10.1097/OGX.0000000000000547.

[4] Drover SSM, Villanger GD, Aase H, et al. Maternal thyroid function during pregnancy or neonatal thyroid function and attention deficit hyperactivity disorder: a systematic review. Epidemiology 2019;30(1):130-44. Available from: https://doi.org/10.1097/EDE.0000000000000937.

[5] Liu Y, Chen H, Jing C, Li F. The association between maternal subclinical hypothyroidism and growth, development, and childhood intelligence: a meta-analysis.

JCRPE J Clin Res Pediatr Endocrinol 2018;10(2):153 – 61. Available from: https://doi.org/10.4274/jcrpe.4931.

[6] Petnehazy E, Buchinger W. Hashimoto thyroiditis, therapeutic options and extrathyroidal options-an up-to-date overview. Wiener Medizinische Wochenschrift 2020;170(1 – 2): 26 – 34. Available from: https://doi.org/10.1007/s10354-019-0691-1.

[7] Ralli M, Angeletti D, Fiore M, et al. Hashimoto's thyroiditis: an update on pathogenic mechanisms, diagnostic protocols, therapeutic strategies, and potential malignant transformation. Autoimmun Rev 2020; 19 (10): 102649. Available from: https://doi.org/10.1016/j.autrev.2020.102649.

[8] Gleicher N. Autoimmunity and reproductive failure. Ann N Y Acad Sci 1991;626(1 Frontiers in):537 – 44. Available from: https://doi.org/10.1111/j.1749-6632.1991.tb37945.x.

[9] Gleicher N. Some thoughts on the reproductive autoimmune failure syndrome (RAFS) and Th – 1 vs Th – 2 immune responses. Am J Reprod Immunol 2002; 48 (4): 252 – 4. Available from: https://doi.org/10.1034/j.1600-0897.2002.01111.x.

[10] Kwak-Kim JYH, Chung-Bang HS, Ng SC, et al. Increased T helper 1 cytokine responses by circulating T cells are present in women with recurrent pregnancy losses and in infertile women with multiple implantation failures after IVF. Hum Reprod 2003;18(4):767 – 73. Available from: https://doi.org/10.1093/humrep/deg156.

[11] Raghupathy R, Makhseed M, Azizieh R, Omu A, Gupta M, Farhat R. Cytokine production by maternal lymphocytes during normal human pregnancy and in unexplained recurrent spontaneous abortion. Hum Reprod 2000; 15 (3): 713 – 18. Available from: https://doi.org/10.1093/humrep/15.3.713.

[12] Raghupathy R. Th1-type immunity is incompatible with successful pregnancy. Immunol Today 1997;18(10):478 – 82. Available from: https://doi.org/10.1016/S0167-5699(97)01127-4.

[13] Stewart-Akers AM, Krasnow JS, Brekosky J, DeLoia JA. Endometrial leukocytes are altered numerically and functionally in women with implantation defects. Am J Reprod Immunol 1998; 39 (1): 1 – 11. Available from: https://doi.org/10.1111/j.1600-0897.1998.tb00326.x.

[14] Kim NY, Cho HJ, Kim HY, et al. Thyroid autoimmunity and its association with cellular and humoral immunity in women with reproductive failures. Am J Reprod Immunol 2011;65(1):78 – 87. Available from: https://doi.org/10.1111/j.1600-0897.2010.00911.x.

[15] Promberger R, Walch K, Seemann R, Pils S, Ott J. A retrospective study on the association between thyroid autoantibodies with β2-glycoprotein and cardiolipin antibodies in recurrent miscarriage. 2017;16 <http://ijaai.tums.ac.ir> [accessed 12.03.21].

[16] Kaider AS, Kaider BD, Janowicz PB, Roussev RG. Immunodiagnostic evaluation in women with reproductive failure. Am J Reprod Immunol 1999;42(6):335 – 46. Available from: https://doi.org/10.1111/j.1600-0897.1999.tb00110.x.

[17] Conigliaro P, D'Antonio A, Pinto S, et al. Autoimmune thyroid disorders and rheumatoid arthritis: a bidirectional interplay. Autoimmun Rev 2020; 19 (6): 102529. Available from: https://doi.org/10.1016/j.autrev.2020.102529.

[18] Ho CW, Chen HH, Hsieh MC, et al. Increased risk of polycystic ovary syndrome and it's comorbidities in women with autoimmune thyroid disease. Int J Environ Res Public Health 2020; 17 (7). Available from: https://doi.org/10.3390/ijerph17072422.

[19] Twig G, Shina A, Amital H, Shoenfeld Y. Pathogenesis of infertility and recurrent pregnancy loss in thyroid autoimmunity. J Autoimmun 2012;38(2 – 3). Available from: https://doi.org/10.1016/j.jaut.2011.11.014.

[20] Alexander EK, Marqusee E, Lawrence J, Jarolim P, Fischer GA, Larsen PR. Timing and magnitude of increases in levothyroxine requirements during pregnancy in women with hypothyroidism. N Engl J Med 2004; 351 (3): 241 – 9. Available from: https://doi.org/10.1056/nejmoa040079.

[21] Dhanwal D, Bajaj S, Rajput R, et al. Prevalence of hypothyroidism in pregnancy: an epidemiological study from 11 cities in 9 states of India. Indian J Endocrinol Metab 2016; 20(3): 387 – 90. Available from: https://doi.org/10.4103/2230-8210.179992.

[22] Ashoor G, Maiz N, Rotas M, Jawdat F, Nicolaides KH. Maternal thyroid function at 11 to 13 weeks of gestation and subsequent fetal death. Thyroid 2010; 20 (9): 989 – 93. Available from: https://doi.org/10.1089/thy.2010.0058.

[23] Negro R, Formosa G, Coppola L, et al. Euthyroid women with autoimmune disease undergoing assisted reproduction technologies: the role of autoimmunity and thyroid function. J Endocrinol Invest 2007; 30 (1): 3 – 8. Available from: https://doi.org/10.1007/BF03347388.

[24] He H, Jing S, Gong F, Tan YQ, Lu GX, Lin G. Effect of thyroid autoimmunity per se on assisted reproduction treatment outcomes: a meta-analysis. Taiwan J Obstet Gynecol 2016;55(2):159 – 65. Available from: https://doi.org/10.1016/j.tjog.2015.09.003.

[25] Lepoutre T, Debièvre F, Gruson D, Daumerie C. Reduction of miscarriages through universal screening and treatment of thyroid autoimmune diseases. Gynecol Obstet Invest 2012;74 (4): 265 – 73. Available from: https://doi.org/10.1159/000343759.

[26] Rao M, Zeng Z, Zhou F, et al. Effect of levothyroxine supplementation on pregnancy loss and preterm birth in women with subclinical hypothyroidism and thyroid autoimmunity: a systematic review and meta-analysis. Hum Reprod Update 2019; 25 (3): 344 – 61. Available from: https://doi.org/10.1093/humupd/dmz003.

[27] Velkeniers B, Van Meerhaeghe A, Poppe K, Unuane D, Tournaye H, Haentjens P. Levothyroxine treatment and pregnancy outcome in women with subclinical hypothyroidism undergoing assisted reproduction technologies: systematic review and meta-analysis of RCTs. Hum Reprod Update 2013;19(3):251 – 8. Available from: https://doi.org/10.1093/humupd/dms052.

[28] Thangaratinam S, Tan A, Knox E, Kilby MD, Franklyn J, Coomarasamy A. Association between thyroid auto-antibodies and miscarriage and preterm birth: meta-analysis of evidence. BMJ 2011;342(7806). Available from: https://doi.org/10.1136/bmj.d2616.

[29] Bartáková J, Potluková E, Rogalewicz V, et al. Screening for autoimmune thyroid disorders after spontaneous abortion is cost-saving and it improves the subsequent pregnancy rate. BMC Pregnancy Childbirth 2013; 13. Available from: https://doi.org/10.1186/1471-2393-13-217.

[30] Monteleone P, Parrini D, Faviana P, et al. Female infertility related to thyroid autoimmunity: the ovarian follicle hypothesis. Am J Reprod Immunol 2011;66(2):108 – 14.

Available from: https://doi.org/10.1111/j.1600-0897.2010.00961.x.

[31] Medenica S, Garalejic E, Arsic B, et al. Follicular fluid thyroid autoantibodies, thyrotropin, free thyroxine levels and assisted reproductive technology outcome. PLoS One 2018;13(10). Available from: https://doi.org/10.1371/journal.pone.0206652.

[32] Weghofer A, Himaya E, Kushnir VA, Barad DH, Gleicher N. The impact of thyroid function and thyroid autoimmunity on embryo quality in women with low functional ovarian reserve: a case-control study. Reprod Biol Endocrinol 2015;13(1). Available from: https://doi.org/10.1186/s12958-015-0041-0.

[33] Kelkar RL, Meherji PK, Kadam SS, Gupta SK, Nandedkar TD. Circulating auto-antibodies against the zona pellucida and thyroid microsomal antigen in women with premature ovarian failure. J Reprod Immunol 2005;66(1):53-67. Available from: https://doi.org/10.1016/j.jri.2005.02.003.

[34] Chen X, Mo ML, Huang CY, et al. Association of serum autoantibodies with pregnancy outcome of patients undergoing first IVF/ICSI treatment: a prospective cohort study. J Reprod Immunol 2017;122:14-20. Available from: https://doi.org/10.1016/j.jri.2017.08.002.

[35] Tan S, Dieterle S, Pechlavanis S, Janssen OE, Fuhrer D. Thyroid autoantibodies per se do not impair intracytoplasmic sperm injection outcome in euthyroid healthy women. Eur J Endocrinol 2014;170(4):495-500. Available from: https://doi.org/10.1530/EJE-13-0790.

[36] Łukaszuk K, Kunicki M, Kulwikowska P, et al. The impact of the presence of antithyroid antibodies on pregnancy outcome following intracytoplasmatic sperm injection-ICSI and embryo transfer in women with normal thyreotropine levels. J Endocrinol Invest 2015;38(12):1335-43. Available from: https://doi.org/10.1007/s40618-015-0377-5.

[37] He Q, Zhang Y, Qiu W, Fan J, Zhang C, Kwak-Kim J. Does thyroid autoimmunity affect the reproductive outcome in women with thyroid autoimmunity undergoing assisted reproductive technology? Am J Reprod Immunol 2020;84(6):e13321. Available from: https://doi.org/10.1111/aji.13321 Epub 2020 Sep 9. PMID:33119203.

[38] Beydilli Nacak G, Ozkaya E, Yayla Abide C, Bilgic BE, Devranoglu B, Gokcen Iscan R. The impact of autoimmunity-related early ovarian aging on ICSI cycle outcome. Gynecol Endocrinol 2018;34(11):940-3. Available from: https://doi.org/10.1080/09513590.2018.1469612.

[39] Fumarola A, Grani G, Romanzi D, et al. Thyroid function in infertile patients undergoing assisted reproduction. Am J Reprod Immunol 2013;70(4):336-41. Available from: https://doi.org/10.1111/aji.12113.

[40] Unuane D, Velkeniers B, Bravenboer B, et al. Impact of thyroid autoimmunity in euthyroid women on live birth rate after IUI. Hum Reprod 2017;32(4):915-22. Available from: https://doi.org/10.1093/humrep/dex033.

[41] Unuane D, Velkeniers B, Deridder S, Bravenboer B, Tournaye H, De Brucker M. Impact of thyroid autoimmunity on cumulative delivery rates in in vitro fertilization/intracytoplasmic sperm injection patients. Fertil Steril 2016;106(1):144-50. Available from: https://doi.org/10.1016/j.fertnstert.2016.03.011.

[42] Chai J, Yeung WYT, Lee CYV, Li HWR, Ho PC, Ng HYE. Live birth rates following in vitro fertilization in women with thyroid autoimmunity and/or subclinical hypothyroidism. Clin Endocrinol (Oxf) 2014;80(1):122-7. Available from: https://doi.org/10.1111/cen.12220.

[43] Matalon ST, Blank M, Levy Y, et al. The pathogenic role of anti-thyroglobulin antibody on pregnancy: evidence from an active immunization model in mice. Hum Reprod 2003;18(5):1094-9. Available from: https://doi.org/10.1093/humrep/deg210.

[44] Moravej A, Jeddi-Tehrani M, Salek-Moghaddam AR, et al. Evaluation of thyroglobulin expression in murine reproductive organs during pregnancy. Am J Reprod Immunol 2010;64(2):97-103. Available from: https://doi.org/10.1111/j.1600-0897.2010.00827.x.

[45] Rahnama R, Mahmoudi AR, Kazemnejad S, et al. Thyroid peroxidase in human endometrium and placenta: a potential target for anti-TPO antibodies. Clin Exp Med 2021;21(1):79-88. Available from: https://doi.org/10.1007/s10238-020-00663-y.

[46] Lee YL, Ng HP, Lau KS, et al. Increased fetal abortion rate in autoimmune thyroid disease is related to circulating TPO autoantibodies in an autoimmune thyroiditis animal model. Fertil Steril 2009;91(5 SUPPL):2104-9. Available from: https://doi.org/10.1016/j.fertnstert.2008.07.1704.

[47] Borodina E, Katz I, Antonelli A, et al. The pathogenic role of circulating Hashimoto's thyroiditis-derived TPO-positive IgG on fetal loss in naïve mice. Am J Reprod Immunol 2021;85(1). Available from: https://doi.org/10.1111/aji.13331.

[48] Boltovskaya MN, Artemyeva KA, Nazimova SV, Stepanova II, Starosvetskaya NA, Kalujin OV. Structural and functional comparison of human and mouse placenta as a justification for modeling miscarriage. Clin Exp Morphol 2014;1(9):73-8 Russian.

[49] Ailamazian E, Stepanova O, Selkov S, Sokolov D. Cells of immune system of mother and trophoblast cells: constructive cooperation for the sake of achievement of the joint purpose. Vestnik Rossiǐ skoǐ Akademii Meditsinskikh Nauk 2013;01(1):12-2149 Russian.

[50] Watson ED, Cross JC. Development of structures and transport functions in the mouse placenta. Physiology 2005;20(3):180-93. Available from: https://doi.org/10.1152/physiol.00001.2005.

[51] Alexander EK, Pearce EN, Brent GA, Brown RS, Chen H, Dosiou C, et al. Guidelines of the American thyroid association for the diagnosis and management of thyroid disease during pregnancy and the postpartum. Thyroid 2017;27(3):315-89. Available from: https://doi.org/10.1089/thy.2016.0457.

[52] Russian Association of Endocrinologists. Clinical Recommendations: Hypothyroidism, 2019. 〈https://racorg.ru/system/files/documents/pdf/568_gipotireoz_vzroslye.finalnaya.versiya.pdf〉 Russian.

[53] Zhong YP, Ying Y, Wu HT, et al. Relationship between antithyroid antibody and pregnancy outcome following in vitro fertilization and embryo transfer. Int J Med Sci 2012;9(2):121-5. Available from: https://doi.org/10.7150/ijms.3467.

[54] Rajput R, Yadav T, Seth S, Nanda S. Prevalence of thyroid peroxidase antibody and pregnancy outcome in euthyroid autoimmune positive pregnant women from a tertiary care center in Haryana. Ind J Endocrinol Metab 2017;21(4):577-80. Available from: https://doi.org/10.4103/ijem.IJEM_397_16.

[55] Meena M, Chopra S, Jain V, Aggarwal N. The effect of

[55] antithyroid peroxidase antibodies on pregnancy outcomes in euthyroid women. J Clin Diagnostic Res 2016;10(9):QC04-7. Available from: https://doi.org/10.7860/JCDR/2016/19009.8403.

[56] Han Y, Mao LJ, Ge X, et al. Impact of maternal thyroid autoantibodies positivity on the risk of early term birth: Ma'anshan birth cohort study. Endocrine 2018;60(2):329-38. Available from: https://doi.org/10.1007/s12020-018-1576-6.

[57] Negro R. Thyroid autoimmunity and preterm delivery: brief review and meta-analysis. J Endocrinol Invest 2011;34(2):155-8. Available from: https://doi.org/10.1007/bf03347047.

[58] Negro R, Schwartz A, Gismondi R, Tinelli A, Mangieri T, Stagnaro-Green A. Thyroid antibody positivity in the first trimester of pregnancy is associated with negative pregnancy outcomes. J Clin Endocrinol Metab 2011;96(6). Available from: https://doi.org/10.1210/jc.2011-0026.

[59] Stagnaro-Green A, Roman SH, Cobin RH, Harazy E, Alvarez Marfany M, Davies TF. Detection of at-risk pregnancy by means of highly sensitive assays for thyroid autoantibodies. JAMA J Am Med Assoc 1990;264(11):1422-5. Available from: https://doi.org/10.1001/jama.1990.03450110068029.

[60] Männistö T, Vääräsmäki M, Pouta A, et al. Perinatal outcome of children born to mothers with thyroid dysfunction or antibodies: a prospective population-based cohort study. J Clin Endocrinol Metab 2009;94(3):772-9. Available from: https://doi.org/10.1210/jc.2008-1520.

[61] Seungdamrong A, Steiner AZ, Gracia CR, et al. Preconceptional antithyroid peroxidase antibodies, but not thyroid-stimulating hormone, are associated with decreased live birth rates in infertile women. Fertil Steril 2017;108(5):843-50. Available from: https://doi.org/10.1016/j.fertnstert.2017.08.026.

[62] Meena A, Nagar P. Pregnancy outcome in euthyroid women with antithyroid peroxidase antibodies. J Obstet Gynecol India 2016;66(3):160-5. Available from: https://doi.org/10.1007/s13224-014-0657-6.

[63] Poppe K, Glinoer D, Tournaye H, et al. Assisted reproduction and thyroid autoimmunity: an unfortunate combination? J Clin Endocrinol Metab 2003;88(9):4149-52. Available from: https://doi.org/10.1210/jc.2003-030268.

[64] Dendrinos S, Papasteriades C, Tarassi K, Christodoulakos G, Prasinos G, Creatsas G. Thyroid autoimmunity in patients with recurrent spontaneous miscarriages. Gynecol Endocrinol 2000;14(4):270-4. Available from: https://doi.org/10.3109/09513590009167693.

[65] Bellver J, Soares SR, Álvarez C, et al. The role of thrombophilia and thyroid autoimmunity in unexplained infertility, implantation failure and recurrent spontaneous abortion. Hum Reprod 2008;23(2):278-84. Available from: https://doi.org/10.1093/humrep/dem383.

[66] Dhillon-Smith RK, Coomarasamy A. TPO antibody positivity and adverse pregnancy outcomes. Best Pract Res Clin Endocrinol Metab 2020;34(4). Available from: https://doi.org/10.1016/j.beem.2020.101433.

[67] Chen L, Hu R. Thyroid autoimmunity and miscarriage: a meta-analysis. Clin Endocrinol (Oxf) 2011;74(4):513-19. Available from: https://doi.org/10.1111/j.1365-2265.2010.03974.x.

第 11 章

胎儿和新生儿同种免疫性血小板减少症与反复妊娠丢失

Fetal/neonatal alloimmune-mediated thrombocytopenia and recurrent pregnancy loss

Si won Lee[1], Tiffany Alexis Clinton[2] and Sun Kwon Kim[3]

[1] Department of Obstetrics and Gynecology, Mount Sinai Medical Center, Miami Beach, FL, United States
[2] Department of Obstetrics and Gynecology, Henry Ford Health System, Detroit, MI, United States
[3] Department of Obstetrics and Gynecology, Division of Maternal-Fetal Medicine, Henry Ford Health System, Detroit, MI, United States

1 引言

胎儿和新生儿同种免疫性血小板减少症(fetal and neonatal immune-mediated thrombocytopenia, FNAIT)是一种危及生命的疾病,其特征是母体对胎儿血小板抗原的免疫反应引起的严重血小板减少症,导致胎儿血小板破坏[1]。临床表现多种多样,从无临床症状到胎儿和新生儿严重颅内出血(intracranial hemorrhage, ICH)、反复妊娠丢失、胎儿生长受限(fetal growth restriction, FGR),甚至胎儿和新生儿死亡[1]。母体和胎儿人血小板抗原(human platelet antigens, HPA)不相容性会导致母体针对胎儿血小板形成同种抗体,从而引起胎儿血小板破坏和血小板减少。

2 定义

FNAIT 的定义和分类基于胎儿血小板减少的病史、母体对 HPA 的免疫抗体存在与否,以及既往妊娠中发生的胎儿和新生儿 ICH 病史(表 11.1)[2,3]。

- 未知风险:既往新生儿有血小板减少的病史,病因未知,母体 HPA 抗体检测为阴性。
- 中等风险:既往新生儿有血小板减少的病史,未伴有 ICH,并经血清学确诊为 FNAIT。
- 高风险:既往新生儿有血小板减少和 ICH 的病史,发生在妊娠 28 周后或新生儿期间,并经血清学确诊为 FNAIT。
- 极高风险:既往新生儿有血小板减少和 ICH 的病史,发生在妊娠 28 周前,并经血清学确诊为 FNAIT。

新生儿血小板减少的定义为血小板计数低于 150 000/μL,并可进一步分为轻度(血小板 100 000/μL～150 000/μL)、中度(血小板 50 000/μL～99 000/μL)和重度(血小板 < 50 000/μL)血小板减少[4]。

3 患病率

FNAIT 中严重血小板减少的发生率为每 1000～1200 名活产儿中 1 例[5]。与 FNAIT 相关的 ICH 发生率为每 1000 名活产中 0.02～0.1 例,最早可在妊娠 14～16 周时通过常规超声检查发现。FNAIT 通常在妊娠 28 周前发生,导致致命结果[6-8]。新生儿期 ICH 在 FNAIT 新生儿中占 10%～20%,在 5% 的病例中是导致长期残疾或新生儿死亡的主要原因[9]。一些大型前瞻性研究表明,FNAIT 最常见的触发因素是母体和胎儿 HPA 抗原之间的 HPA-1 组织不相容。在白种女性中,HPA-1b/1b(1a 阴性)的患病率约为 2.5%[3]。

表 11.1　基于病史风险分层的胎儿/新生儿免疫性血小板减少症的定义、监测和管理

风险	定义	监测	医疗管理	分娩
未知	前次妊娠出现胎儿/新生儿血小板减少或原因不明的颅内出血。未检测到 HPA 抗体	妊娠第 8 周开始,每 4 周进行一次抗 HPA 抗体检测和与父亲的血小板交叉配合试验	不建议进行经验性治疗	—
一般	既往胎儿有血小板减少但没有 ICH。血清学确诊为 FNAIT	—	(1) 从妊娠 20 周开始 • IVIG 每周 2 g/kg 或 IVIG 每周 1 g/kg+强的松每天 0.5 mg/kg。 (2) 妊娠 32 周时所有患者调整为 • IVIG 每周 2 g/kg+强的松每天 0.5 mg/kg	在 37～38 周行剖宫产
高	既往胎儿在妊娠 28 周后或新生儿期间发生血小板减少症和 ICH。血清学确诊为 FNAIT	每月监测血红蛋白和红细胞压积。在妊娠 16～20 周进行详细的超声检查。每 4～6 周进行一次超声检查,直至分娩,以检测 ICH	(1) 从妊娠 12 周开始 • IVIG 每周 1 g/kg。 (2) 妊娠 20 周时 • IVIG 每周 1 g/kg+强的松每天 0.5 mg/kg 或增加 IVIG 至每周 2 g/kg。 (3) 孕 28 周时 • IVIG 每周 2 g/kg+强的松每天 0.5 mg/kg	在 37～38 周行剖宫产
极高	既往胎儿出生时伴有血小板减少和发生在妊娠 28 周以前的 ICH,血清学确诊为 FNAIT	—	(1) 在妊娠 12 周开始 • IVIG 每周 2 g/kg。 (2) 在妊娠 20 周 • IVIG 每周 2 g/kg+强的松每天 1 mg/kg,直至分娩	在 36～37 周行剖宫产
修定后的 IVIG 方案	为了更早抑制血小板抗体	每月监测 CBC、抗-HPA 抗体和与父亲的血小板交叉配合试验。在妊娠 16～20 周进行详细的超声检查。每 4 周进行一次超声检查,直至分娩,以检测 ICH	(1) 在妊娠前或妊娠 4～6 周时,开始使用 IVIG 每周 400 mg/kg,同时使用强的松每天 20 mg。 (2) 在妊娠 16 周时,将 IVIG 增加至每周 1 g/kg。 (3) 在妊娠 32 周时,IVIG 增加至每周 2 g/kg,强的松维持在每天 20 mg	—

注:FNAIT,胎儿/新生儿同种免疫性血小板减少症;ICH,颅内出血;GA,胎龄;IVIG,静脉注射免疫球蛋白;HPA,人血小板抗原;CS,剖宫产。

4　与妊娠相关的潜在免疫病理学

4.1　胎儿人血小板抗原引起母体免疫应答

目前,已发现有 37 种抗原与 FNAIT 相关。FNAIT 大多数病例是由 HPA-1 抗原不相容引起的,几乎占到了白种人和非洲血统家族病例中的 85%[1]。这些抗原中约有一半位于整合素 β3 亚单位的结构域上,这些结构域表达于血小板、内皮细胞和滋养层/胎盘细胞[1,10]。整合素是囊胚植入和螺旋动脉重塑的早期参与者,因此在胎盘发育中起着关键作用[1,10]。

怀有 HPA-1a 阳性胎儿的 HPA-1a 阴性(1b/1b)母亲会从胎儿循环中产生针对 HPA-1a 抗原的免疫球蛋白 G 同种抗体。然后这些同种抗体通过 Fc 受体转运经过胎盘并靶向胎儿血小板,导致胎儿血小板被吞噬和破坏[3,10-12]。因此,确定父系杂合性在 FNAIT 的预测中起着重要作用。如果母亲的 HPA-1a(1b/1b)呈阴性,那么 100% 的 HPA-1a 纯合子父亲的胎儿和 50% 的杂合子父亲的胎儿将与母亲的 HPA-1a 抗原不相容。FNAIT 中第二常见的 HPA 是白种人的 HPA-5b 抗原和亚洲人的

HPA-4b 抗原[11]。在一项涉及 569 例 FNAIT 的研究中,75.2%的病例存在抗-HPA-1a 抗体,其次是抗-HPA-5b 抗体(17.8%)、抗-HPA-1a+HPA-5b 抗体(2.3%)、抗-HPA 3a 抗体(1.8%)以及抗低频同种抗原的抗体(HPA-8bW,-11bW,-12bW,-13bW 和-14bW,总计 1.1%)[13]。

4.2 血栓形成和细胞免疫激活

一些使用小鼠 FNAIT 模型的研究表明,与胎儿血小板抗原形成的免疫复合物可以启动血栓形成,导致胎盘病理,从而引起流产、FGR 和死亡[1,9]。这些研究表明,抗-β3 整合素抗体靶向半同种滋养细胞,为自然杀伤细胞(NK 细胞)Fc-δ 受体提供结合位点[9]。在正常妊娠中,子宫 NK 细胞参与螺旋动脉重塑过程,同时保护胎盘免受病原体侵害和随之发生的流产。在 FNAIT 病例中,增加的免疫复合物沉积到母胎界面并激活子宫 NK 细胞,引起母胎交界处的慢性炎症,导致滋养细胞凋亡、螺旋动脉重塑受损和胎盘功能障碍[1,9,14]。相反,NK 细胞介导的胎盘炎症和抗体依赖性细胞介导的侵入性滋养层细胞毒性在 FNAIT、妊娠丢失、FGR、ICH、胎儿宫内死亡或新生儿死亡中发挥着至关重要的作用[1,11]。据报道,活动性 ITP 患者中 CD3⁻CD56⁺ NK 和 CD3⁺CD56⁺ NKT 细胞亚群扩增,与疾病进展或缓解期呈暂时负相关[15,16]。

在 19 名患有 FNAIT 的女性病例中,与对照组相比,TNF-α/IL-10(33.58 ± 7.56 vs 23.93 ± 5.27,$P=0.005$)和分泌 IFN-γ/IL-10 的 Th 细胞比例(18.36 ± 4.51 vs 9.21 ± 4.22,$P=0.000$)显著升高[6]。与正常对照组相比,FNAIT 组中 NK 细胞水平($10.68\%\pm5.01\%$ vs $9.80\%\pm2.01\%$,$P=$ NS)和细胞毒性(23.09 ± 6.21 vs 20.88 ± 3.39,$P=$ NS)更高,但差异并不具有统计学意义[6]。因此,FNAIT 与 Th1/Th2 细胞比值增加以及 NK 细胞数量和细胞毒性增加显著相关,是妊娠丢失和子痫前期的危险因素[6,17]。

5 评估

5.1 诊断标准

围产期出现血小板减少或 ICH,需怀疑 FNAIT。然而,诊断只能基于确凿的实验室证据。

> 临床标准:
> (1) 新生儿出生时或出生后 7 天内血小板减少,低于 100 000/μL。
> (2) 存在胎儿颅内出血[18,19]。
> 实验室诊断标准:
> (1) 母亲和父亲 HPA 抗原的不相容性。
> (2) 母体抗 HPA 抗体对不相容抗原具有特异性[18]。

5.2 临床特征

患有此病的新生儿母亲通常没有症状。患者可能有 FNAIT 的个人史或家族史。轻度血小板减少的新生儿通常不表现任何症状,通常在出生后的检查中被诊断出来。在严重血小板减少的新生儿中,ICH 在产前超声检查中是最常见且最严重的并发症,可以在妊娠 14~16 周时检查发现[6,7]。FNAIT 也可能表现为反复妊娠丢失、FGR 和胎儿死亡[1]。与 Rh 免疫反应不同,FNAIT 在有风险的女性的初次妊娠中检测到的比例超过 50%。随着妊娠次数的增多,FNAIT 的风险和严重程度增加[7,20-22],尤其是 FNAIT 的严重程度取决于母体 HPA-1a 抗体水平[18]。在随后的妊娠中,FNAIT 的复发率接近 100%,并伴有更早的发病时间和更严重的症状[9]。

5.3 检测方法

5.3.1 评估人群

目前鉴于对低发病率和检测费用的考虑,FNAIT 的常规筛查并未在临床实践中进行[2]。然而,由于发病率比既往报道要高,而 PCR 检测的费用已非常合理,可以将筛查检测应用于高风险人群。大多数 FNAIT 病例是在第一次妊娠或分娩时被诊断出来的。在产前检查或新生儿期发现血小板减少时,应评估是否存在细菌和病毒感染、弥散性血管内凝血和其他与血小板减少有关的先天性疾病。在排除这些病因后,应进行诊断检查,包括母亲和父亲的 HPA 分型,以及使用敏感的检测方法进行母亲血小板 HPA 抗体检测。

5.3.2 检测

目前可用的第三代检测方法包括血小板抗原的单克隆抗体固定、改良的抗原捕获酶联免疫吸附检测和特异性血小板抗体的同步分析[23]。除了这些机构内检测之外,还可使用商业化的糖蛋白(GP)特异性检测试剂盒,例如 PakPlus ELISA(Immucor,Dreieich,德国)和基于微珠的 PakLx 免疫检测(Immucor,Dreieich,德国)。可以使用直接和间接的血小板抗体来检测血浆中的游离血小板自身抗体和同种抗体,其中包括完整的血小板或 GP 特异性检测。GP 特异性免疫测定是血小板抗体检测领域最先进的技术。其他可采用的技术包括洗脱、免疫交叉配型和抗 HPA-1a 定量。

抗血小板抗体的筛选和鉴定通常是用血清学/免疫学的血小板交叉配合试验进行。该试验由血小板采集或代表所有相关血小板 GP 的血小板 GP 制剂组成。夫妇间的 HPA 组织相容性可通过基于 DNA 的方法进行 HPA 型别鉴定。当发现 HPA 位点(1、2、3、4、5、6、9 或 15)存在不相容且检测到特异性母体抗 HPA 抗体时,即可诊断 FNAIT[4]。

5.4 筛查和诊断

目前不建议对 FNAIT 进行全面筛查[2]。然而,对风险夫妇进行筛查被认为是合理的。图 11.1 展示了 FNAIT 诊断和处理的流程图。高风险夫妇包括既往妊娠中有 FNAIT 或 ICH 的个人史或家族史。筛查方法包括母亲的血小板计数、母亲和父亲的 HPA 组织相容性筛查,以及母亲的 HPA 抗体检测[24]。

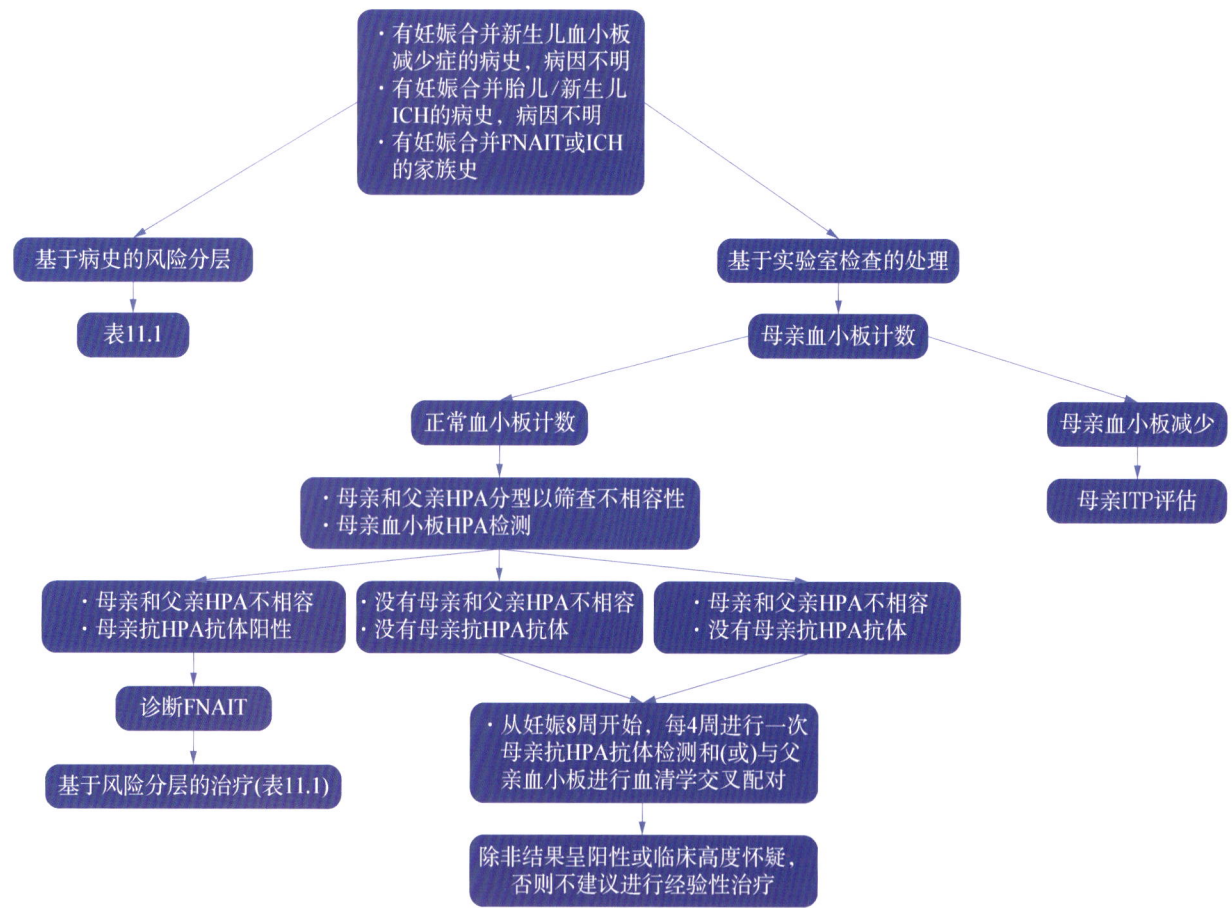

图 11.1 胎儿/新生儿免疫性血小板减少症的诊断和管理推荐策略。

如果夫妇间在 HPA 位点存在不相容,但母亲抗-HPA 抗体呈阴性,则应在妊娠 8 周开始每 4 周重复进行母亲抗-HPA 抗体检测和(或)与父亲的血小板交叉配合试验,以便及早发现致敏反应并进行治疗。以前曾建议在妊娠的 12、24 和 32 周进行筛查;然而,这种方法可能会错过妊娠期间同种免疫的早期检测[4,6]。如果所有结果均为阴性,则可排除 FNAIT[4]。

当怀疑在妊娠期间存在 FNAIT 时,可通过从绒毛膜绒毛取样(CVS)或羊膜穿刺获取胎儿 DNA 以确定胎儿的血小板抗原类型。从理论上讲,无创游离 DNA(cfDNA)检测可能是另一种选择,但目前在美国尚未广泛应用[25,26]。如果血清学检测需要一段时间才能得出结果，则应根据临床疑似表现和胎儿血小板计数启动治疗（表11.1）。

如果存在HPA同种抗体，连续滴度可能有助于确定发生FNAIT的风险，这些患者应被转诊到具有FNAIT管理经验的综合医疗中心。此外，高风险患者应在妊娠8~12周开始，每4周进行一次监测，直至分娩，通过系列抗体检测和超声检查来筛查胎儿ICH[6]。

6 治疗

6.1 药物治疗

FNAIT的管理存在争议，目前尚无专家共识或专业委员会的指南[27]。目前，最可接受的是基于风险分层的方法，涉及静脉注射免疫球蛋白（IVIG），可单独使用，也可与皮质类固醇联合使用。

- 在未知风险的人群中，从妊娠8周开始，每4周进行一次抗HPA抗体检测和与父亲的血小板交叉配合试验。除非检测到HPA抗体或存在高度疑似FNAIT的临床表现，否则不推荐经验性治疗[2,3]。
- 在一般风险人群中，从妊娠20周开始使用IVIG每周2g/kg或IVIG每周1g/kg+强的松每天0.5mg/kg[2,3,28]。数据表明，这两种方案在预防一般风险患者的严重胎儿血小板减少具有相似的作用[24]。无论采用何种方案，建议在妊娠32周时将所有患者的用药调整为IVIG每周2g/kg+强的松每天0.5mg/kg[2,3,28,29]。然而，该方案存在局限性，不能在妊娠20周前预防ICH。
- 在高风险人群中，从妊娠12周开始使用IVIG每周1g/kg，到20周时加入强的松每天0.5mg/kg，或将IVIG增加到每周2g/kg。到28周时，IVIG增加到每周2g/kg，强的松增加到每天0.5mg/kg[2]。
- 在极高风险人群中，从妊娠12周开始使用IVIG每周2g/kg，到20周时加入强的松每天1mg/kg，直至分娩[30]。

对于HPA抗体阳性的患者，可采用修订后的IVIG方案，该方案可在妊娠期间更早抑制血小板抗体并降低IVIG和强的松的副作用。

- 在妊娠前或妊娠4~6周时，使用低剂量IVIG每周400mg/kg+强的松每天20mg[4]。每4周对患者进行一次监测，进行抗HPA抗体检测和与父亲的血小板交叉配合试验，根据检测结果调整强的松剂量。在妊娠16周时，IVIG剂量增加到每周1g/kg，然后在妊娠32周时进一步增加到每周2g/kg，强的松剂量为每天20mg。

这种基于既往妊娠受影响胎儿的风险管理策略的主要目的是避免胎儿采血以减少并发症，同时最大限度降低当前妊娠中ICH的风险[29,30]。然而，应仔细监测与高剂量IVIG和强的松相关的可能副作用，特别是对于高风险和极高风险人群。当治疗后仍发现ICH时，建议采用个体化治疗方法。

6.2 分娩时机和分娩方式

目前对于FNAIT的分娩方式尚无共识。然而，在一般风险、高风险和极高风险的FNAIT患者中，由于胎儿或新生儿ICH的风险增加，更倾向于剖宫产。建议一般和高风险妊娠的分娩时间为妊娠37~38周，而极高风险妊娠的分娩时间为妊娠36~37周[3,31]。允许FNAIT患者经阴道分娩，特别是在妊娠期间接受了IVIG和（或）类固醇治疗的多次妊娠的一般风险女性[32]。需要进一步研究以找到一种更为灵活的分娩策略。在未知胎儿血小板计数的情况下，应避免行阴道分娩手术或涉及胎儿的侵入性操作（如胎儿头皮电极）。此外，应在分娩后立即送检脐带血小板计数。

6.3 围产期和产后管理

大多数有发生FNAIT风险的患者在产前接受了长期类固醇治疗，而妊娠期间长期服用皮质类固醇的影响尚不清楚。理论上，类固醇可能抑制下丘脑垂体肾上腺（HPA）轴，导致分娩或剖宫产时对内源性的应激反应不足[33]。对于中等手术应激的情况（例如下肢血管重建手术、全关节置换手术），在手术前，完成上午计划的类固醇治疗后，静脉注射氢化可的松50mg的应激剂量，然后在接下来的24小时内每8小时注射25mg氢化可的松。在完成应激方案后，继续正常的类固醇剂量。然而，目前没有关于在分娩或剖宫产中是否需要应激剂量类固醇的随机对照研究。由于胎盘分娩后内源性类固醇水平迅速下降，因此建议对类固醇进行控制性减量，并个体化使用应激剂量的氢化可的松[33]。在目前的临床实践中，对于那些接受 3 周以上每天超过 20 mg 强的松治疗的患者，通常会给予应激剂量的类固醇治疗，因为这些患者的 HPA 轴被抑制的可能性很高。然而，最近的研究提出，对于 HPA 轴完好的患者，不需要应激剂量的类固醇[34]。因此，需要进行前瞻性随机研究来阐明这一发现。

对于长期接受强的松治疗的孕妇，是否需要额外使用皮质类固醇以促进胎肺成熟，目前尚不清楚。然而，对于妊娠 23^{+0} 周至 33^{+6} 周且在未来 7 天内有早产风险的患者，建议添加倍他米松或地塞米松以降低新生儿发病率和死亡率[35]。

6.4 潜在的副作用：风险与监测

长期使用全身皮质类固醇可导致母体的不良反应，包括骨质疏松、糖耐量受损、妊娠期糖尿病、免疫抑制和 HPA 轴抑制[18]。因此，建议在治疗 1 个月后进行糖尿病筛查。此前多项荟萃分析显示，使用类固醇也增加了早产、胎膜早破和 FGR 的风险[33]。

母体接受 IVIG 治疗可能的副作用包括注射部位的局部反应、发热、皮疹、免疫改变、无菌性脑膜炎、感染，以及 A、B 或 AB 型血女性的贫血[36]。因此，建议接受 IVIG 的女性补充铁剂，并每月进行血红蛋白和红细胞比容的筛查[36]。

7 生殖结局

7.1 产后管理与评估

除了逐渐减少类固醇以防止 HPA 抑制之外，没有证据表明产后应对产妇立即进行干预。尽管如此，仍应就未来妊娠时筛查和检测的重要性对夫妇进行咨询。

7.2 再次妊娠选择

为避免筛查阳性的夫妇怀上受 FNAIT 影响的胎儿，可考虑使用辅助生殖技术。在无法耐受或有 IVIG 和类固醇治疗禁忌证的高风险和极高风险患者中，使用 HPA 相容的供精可能是最佳选择。如果胎儿的父亲是 HPA 基因的杂合子，也应考虑体外受精，行胚胎植入前遗传学诊断，并选择未受影响的胚胎。

7.3 孕前咨询

有疑似 FNAIT 病史或曾妊娠过病因不明的胎儿/新生儿 ICH 的夫妇，应在后续妊娠时接受孕前咨询。对这些夫妇的评估应首先进行母亲血小板计数，以排除母亲血小板减少症。如果母亲血小板计数正常，应进行母亲抗 HPA 抗体以及母亲和父亲血小板抗原基因分型，以预测未来罹患 FNAIT 的风险。如果检测到 HPA 不相容，且母体血清中存在针对外源父系血小板抗原的特异性 HPA 同种抗体，则可诊断为 FNAIT[3,18,24]。如果患者有家族史而无个人受累的妊娠史，则建议采用相同的检测策略，无须进行 HPA 抗体检测[18]。

7.4 后续妊娠的产前护理

在后续妊娠中，FNAIT 的发展更为严重，且孕周也更早。因此，一旦确认妊娠，高风险患者应立即转诊至具有 FNAIT 管理经验的高危妊娠中心。如果父系情况不明，应在妊娠 10～13 周时行 CVS，或在 16～20 周时行羊膜穿刺术，进行胎儿 HPA 基因分型，以确定胎儿是否具有与母体 HPA 基因型不相容的血小板抗原[8]。如果已知父系情况且检测到 HPA 不相容，下一步则是检测父亲的 HPA 基因型，以评估胎儿是否有 100%（纯合）或 50%（杂合）遗传特定血小板抗原的机会。如果确定胎儿存在风险，应根据风险分层向患者提供孕期治疗建议（表 11.1）。

8 总结和建议

FNAIT 是由于母亲与胎儿 HPA 不相容导致母体产生对胎儿血小板的免疫反应，从而引起胎儿血小板减少和（或）ICH。

- FNAIT 与胎儿/新生儿 ICH、流产、FGR 以及胎儿/新生儿死亡有关。
- 与红细胞免疫反应不同，FNAIT 可在第一次妊娠时发生，且在后续妊娠中的复发率接近 100%，患儿发病更早，症状更为严重。
- 对有风险的夫妇进行筛查，包括母亲和父亲的 HPA 基因型鉴定，以及母体抗血小板抗体评估。目前，由于缺乏经济效益，不建议对所有孕妇进行常规筛查。
- 基于风险分层，建议使用 IVIG 和（或）强的松进行治疗，并建议每 4 周进行重复实验室检查和连续超声随访。

参考文献

[1] Yougbaré I, Tai W-S, Zdravic D, et al. Activated NK cells cause placental dysfunction and miscarriages in fetal alloimmune thrombocytopenia. Nat Commun 2017; 8(1): 1-13.

[2] Pacheco LD, Berkowitz RL, Moise Jr KJ, Bussel JB, McFarland JG, Saade GR. Fetal and neonatal alloimmune thrombocytopenia: a management algorithm based on risk stratification. Obstet Gynecol 2011; 118(5): 1157-63.

[3] Peterson JA, McFarland JG, Curtis BR, Aster RH. Neonatal alloimmune thrombocytopenia: pathogenesis, diagnosis and management. Br J Haematol 2013; 161(1): 3-14.

[4] Fernandes CJ, Mahoney Jr DH. Neonatal immune-mediated thrombocytopenia.

[5] Williamson LM, Hackett G, Rennie J, et al. The natural history of fetomaternal alloimmunization to the platelet-specific antigen HPA-1a (P1A1, Zwa) as determined by antenatal screening. Blood J Am Soc Hematol 1998; 92(7): 2280-7.

[6] Skariah A, Sung N, Salazar Garcia MD, et al. Low-dose prednisone and immunoglobulin G treatment for woman at risk for neonatal alloimmune thrombocytopenia and T helper 1 immunity. Am J Reprod Immunol 2017; 77(6): e12649.

[7] Tiller H, Kamphuis MM, Flodmark O, et al. Fetal intracranial haemorrhages caused by fetal and neonatal alloimmune thrombocytopenia: an observational cohort study of 43 cases from an international multicentre registry. BMJ Open 2013; 3(3).

[8] Lieberman L, Greinacher A, Murphy MF, et al. Fetal and neonatal alloimmune thrombocytopenia: recommendations for evidence-based practice, an international approach. Br J Haematol 2019; 185(3): 549-62.

[9] Yougbaré I, Zdravic D, Ni H. Fetal and neonatal alloimmune thrombocytopenia: Novel mechanisms of miscarriage learned from placental pathology in animal models. J Pediatrics Pediatric Med 2018; 2(1).

[10] Curtis BR, Bussel JB, Manco-Johnson MJ, Aster RH, McFarland JG. Fetal and neonatal alloimmune thrombocytopenia in pregnancies involving in vitro fertilization: a report of four cases. Am J Obstet Gynecol 2005; 192(2): 543-7.

[11] Davoren A, Curtis BR, Aster RH, McFarland JG. Human platelet antigen-specific alloantibodies implicated in 1162 cases of neonatal alloimmune thrombocytopenia. Transfusion 2004; 44(8): 1220-5.

[12] Yougbare I, Wei-She T, Zdravic D, et al. Natural killer cells contribute to pathophysiology of placenta leading to miscarriage in fetal and neonatal alloimmune thrombocytopenia. In: American Society of Hematology, Washington, DC; 2015.

[13] Kroll H, Yates J, Santoso S. Immunization against a low-frequency human platelet alloantigen in fetal alloimmune thrombocytopenia is not a single event: characterization by the combined use of reference DNA and novel allele-specific cell lines expressing recombinant antigens. Transfusion 2005; 45(3): 353-8.

[14] Dubruc E, Lebreton F, Giannoli C, et al. Placental histological lesions in fetal and neonatal alloimmune thrombocytopenia: a retrospective cohort study of 21 cases. Placenta 2016; 48: 104-9.

[15] Talaat R, Elmaghraby A, Barakat S, El-Shahat M. Alterations in immune cell subsets and their cytokine secretion profile in childhood idiopathic thrombocytopenic purpura (ITP). Clin Exp Immunol 2014; 176(2): 291-300.

[16] Xu R, Zheng Z, Ma Y, et al. Elevated NKT cell levels in adults with severe chronic immune thrombocytopenia. Exp Ther Med 2014; 7(1): 149-54.

[17] Garcia MS, Mobley Y, Henson J, et al. Early pregnancy immune biomarkers in peripheral blood may predict preeclampsia. J Reprod Immunol 2018; 125: 25-31.

[18] Paidas MJ, Wilkins-Haug L, Barss V. Fetal and neonatal alloimmune thrombocytopenia: parental evaluation and pregnancy management. In: UpToDate Inc. Waltham, MA; 2020.

[19] Petermann R, Bakchoul T, Curtis BR, et al. Investigations for fetal and neonatal alloimmune thrombocytopenia: communication from the SSC of the ISTH. J Thrombosis Haemost 2018; 16(12): 2526-9.

[20] Kamphuis MM, Paridaans NP, Porcelijn L, Lopriore E, Oepkes D. Incidence and consequences of neonatal alloimmune thrombocytopenia: a systematic review. Pediatrics 2014; 133(4): 715-21.

[21] Delbos F, Bertrand G, Croisille L, Ansart-Pirenne H, Bierling P, Kaplan C. Fetal and neonatal alloimmune thrombocytopenia: predictive factors of intracranial hemorrhage. Transfusion 2016; 56(1): 59-66.

[22] Bussel JB, Sola-Visner M. Current approaches to the evaluation and management of the fetus and neonate with immune thrombocytopenia. Paper presented at Seminars in Perinatology; 2009.

[23] Kiefel V. Platelet antibodies in immune thrombocytopenia and related conditions. J Laboratory Med 2020; 44(5): 273-84.

[24] Lipitz S, Ryan G, Murphy M, et al. Neonatal alloimmune thrombocytopenia due to anti-P1A1 (anti-hpa-1a): Importance of paternal and fetal platelet typing for assessment of fetal risk. Prenat Diagnosis 1992; 12(11): 955-8.

[25] Nogués N. Recent advances in non-invasive fetal HPA-1a typing. Transfus Apheresis Sci 2020; 59(1): 102708.

[26] Ohto H, Kato K, Tohyama Y, et al. Prenatal determination of human platelet antigen type 4 by DNA amplification of amniotic fluid cells. Transfus Sci 1997; 18(1): 85-9.

[27] Winkelhorst D, Oepkes D, Lopriore E. Fetal and neonatal alloimmune thrombocytopenia: evidence based antenatal and postnatal management strategies. Expert Rev Hematol 2017; 10(8): 729-37.

[28] Lakkaraja M, Berkowitz RL, Vinograd CA, et al. Omission of fetal sampling in treatment of subsequent pregnancies in fetal-neonatal alloimmune thrombocytopenia. Am J Obstet Gynecol 2016; 215(4): 471 e471-471. e479.

[29] Berkowitz RL, Lesser ML, McFarland JG, et al. Antepartum treatment without early cordocentesis for standard-risk alloimmune thrombocytopenia: a randomized controlled trial. Obstet Gynecol 2007; 110(2 Part 1): 249-55.

[30] Bussel JB, Berkowitz RL, Hung C, et al. Intracranial hemorrhage in alloimmune thrombocytopenia: stratified management to prevent recurrence in the subsequent affected fetus. Am J Obstet Gynecol 2010; 203(2): 135 e131-

135. e114.

[31] Van den Akker E, Oepkes D, Lopriore E, Brand A, Kanhai H. Noninvasive antenatal management of fetal and neonatal alloimmune thrombocytopenia: safe and effective. BJOG: An Int J Obstet Gynaecol 2007;114(4):469-73.

[32] Ronzoni S, Keunen J, Shah PS, et al. Management and neonatal outcomes of pregnancies with fetal/neonatal alloimmune thrombocytopenia: a single-center retrospective cohort study. Fetal Diagnosis Ther 2019;45(2):85-93.

[33] AlSaad D, Lindow S, Lee BH, Tarannum A, Abdulrouf PV. Maternal, fetal, and neonatal outcomes associated with long-term use of corticosteroids during pregnancy. Obstet Gynaecol 2019;21(2):117-25.

[34] Sylvester-Armstrong KR, Duff P, Genç MR. Are peripartum stress-dose steroids necessary? Obstet Gynecol 2020;135(3):522-5.

[35] Lee M-J, Guinn D, Martin R. Antenatal corticosteroid therapy for reduction of neonatal respiratory morbidity and mortality from preterm delivery. UpToDate Waltham, MA, UpToDate; 2018.

[36] Berger M. Adverse effects of IgG therapy. J Allergy Clin Immunol: Pract 2013;1(6):558-66.

第 12 章

感染性和非感染性子宫内膜炎与反复妊娠丢失

Infections and noninfections endometritis and recurrent pregnancy loss

Fuminori Kimura[1], Aina Morimune[2], Akiko Nakamura[2], Jun Kitazawa[2], Tetsuro Hanada[2] and Takashi Murakami[2]

[1] Department of Obstetrics and Gynecology, Nara Medical University, Kashihara, Nara, Japan
[2] Department of Obstetrics and Gynecology, Shiga University of Medical Science, Otsu, Shiga, Japan

1 引言

子宫内膜炎对于妊娠的建立和维持所造成的不良影响已备受关注。这种炎症并非指严重或迅速发展的疾病,如急性感染,而是指持续且微弱的炎症。微生物引起的子宫内膜感染是引起子宫内膜持续且微弱炎症的典型原因。然而,还应考虑其他影响子宫内膜免疫的疾病。新近研究表明,无论为何原因,持续性炎症对反复妊娠丢失(RPL)有着非常重要的影响。在本章中,我们将讨论感染性和非感染性子宫内膜炎与 RPL 相关的机制。

2 定义

炎症对身体存在有害和有益的效应,这取决于其严重程度和持续时间。对受损组织的有益效应源于机械刺激、化学毒素、微生物入侵和过敏反应[1,2]。炎症可分为急性和慢性阶段。急性炎症是对病原体或物理/化学损伤引起的变化的反应,可消除损伤原因并恢复受影响组织的稳态[1,2]。相反,慢性炎症表示一种持续的炎症反应,可能涉及逐渐发生的变化,导致长期的功能障碍和渐进性破坏。尽管慢性炎症通常较弱,有或没有细微的症状,但渐进性破坏可以部分修复[3]。因此,慢性炎症的特点是在炎症过程中组织同时发生破坏和修复[3,4]。它可能是急性炎症的后继过程,也可能存在长时间的低度反应。慢性感染、自身免疫疾病以及良性妇科疾病,如子宫内膜异位症和子宫腺肌症,常与慢性子宫内膜炎(CE)和炎症反应相关[3,4]。

当炎症发生在子宫内膜时,称为子宫内膜炎,但术语"子宫内膜炎"通常被接受为有感染性病因。因此,描述影响子宫内妊娠建立和维持的轻微炎症状况的表达可能需要更改。在这个意义上,"子宫内膜的炎症受损状态"可能是比"子宫内膜炎"更合适的术语,因为前者直接表明了"子宫内膜的炎症",而不考虑原因[5]。

尽管可能需要进一步讨论这些术语,但在本章中,子宫内膜中的炎症均称为子宫内膜炎。由微生物引起的子宫内膜炎称为感染性子宫内膜炎,而由其他原因引起的则称为非感染性子宫内膜炎。我们将讨论这两种情况对 RPL 的影响。

2.1 感染性子宫内膜炎

2.1.1 感染性子宫内膜炎的病因

在育龄期女性中,子宫内膜在月经期脱落,然后在下一周期中再生。因此,子宫内膜是否持续存在炎症是有争议的。在跨月经周期存在的子宫内膜持续炎症状态称为 CE。只有通过组织学检查才能明确诊断 CE,其特征是在子宫内膜的间质中存在浆细胞[6,7]。除浆细胞外,可能还存在基质细胞高度增殖、上皮和间质成熟不同步以及明显的蜕膜前反应[6,7]。如果考虑到浆细胞的作用(即分泌大量抗体),CE 可能描述的是免疫细胞在宫腔中监测异常病原体的一种状态,以防止其发展成为严重的炎症[8]。因此,CE 可能是急性子宫内膜炎后的陈旧性炎症状态。然而,急性子宫内膜炎和CE之间的关系尚待确定。已经发现CE对胚胎种植存在不良影响。微生物现被认为是CE的主要原因,这是由于大多数情况可通过抗生素治愈。患有CE的不孕女性在接受抗生素治疗时,往往其胚胎种植率有所提高[7,9]。因此,在本章中,CE被描述为感染性子宫内膜炎的同义词。

长期以来一直认为正常女性的宫腔是无菌的。然而,随着二代测序(NGS)技术的发展,可以检测到少量菌种,揭示了女性上生殖器官,包括卵巢、输卵管和子宫,并非无菌,而是存在特定的菌落[10,11]。

以乳酸杆菌等为代表的阴道细菌约占女性体内所有细菌的9%,这表明阴道中存在大量菌落[12,13]。相反,根据Chen等[14]的研究,上生殖器官只有阴道细菌数量的1/10 000。这些细菌被认为可以调节子宫内膜细胞和局部免疫系统的功能,并与病原微生物竞争,产生保护分子以防止子宫感染[15,16]。这表明子宫内存在共生关系。

CE可能是由于宫腔内致病微生物的存在和对它们的轻微免疫反应而破坏防御机制的一种疾病[7]。在CE中,通过微生物培养物、聚合酶链式反应和NGS常检测到链球菌、大肠埃希菌、粪肠球菌、阴道加德纳菌、肺炎克雷伯菌、铜绿假单胞菌、变形杆菌属、葡萄球菌和支原体等。目前认为这些细菌是CE的主要致病病原体[10,17]。

存在于阴道中的微粒可通过子宫蠕动在几分钟内经宫颈转移至宫腔[18]。因此,阴道微生物也可能通过宫颈侵入宫腔。已报道某些菌种,如梭杆菌,能够在小鼠和牛的子宫中寄生[19]。在小鼠中,这种微生物的寄生可通过血液循环发生。此外,口腔或肠道微生物可能通过破坏组织的防御屏障(如牙龈炎和肠炎等局部感染)而进入血管,形成子宫内的菌落。此外,新近研究证实腹腔中存在微生物[14]。来自胃肠道的腹腔微生物可能通过输卵管到达宫腔。因此,需要进一步的探索以阐明导致CE寄生微生物的起源和途径。子宫内膜菌群形成背后的因素也需要在未来进行研究。

2.1.2 慢性子宫内膜炎的患病率和临床特征

CE在RPL女性中的患病率为9.3%～67.6%[20,21]。这些研究之间的巨大差异似乎是由于采用的诊断标准和患者背景的不同。流行病学研究表明,在RPL患者中,CE的诊断率较高。已开展了调查CE危险因素的研究。细菌性阴道病、子宫内膜息肉和子宫内膜异位症是已报告的与CE相关的妇科疾病[22]。非感染性子宫内膜炎与子宫内膜息肉和子宫内膜异位症有关,详见后文。

2.1.3 慢性子宫内膜炎的诊断

CE的诊断是基于对子宫内膜组织切片的病理学评估。尽管在CE中可发现基质细胞的过度增殖、基质和上皮细胞成熟状态的差异,以及明显的蜕膜变化(水肿),但在临床实践中,诊断是通过识别免疫活性细胞的独特分布,尤其是子宫内膜间质中存在的浆细胞[6,23]。

在正常的子宫内膜间质中,除了月经期和月经前期外,一般不存在浆细胞;在HE染色中,浆细胞表现为轴突状的特征形态。然而,在子宫内膜中存在单核细胞浸润、间质分离和浆细胞样基质细胞,由于它们在形态上相似,以致经验丰富的病理学家也很难检测到子宫内膜中的浆细胞。因此,常使用浆细胞的特异性标志物CD138(多配体蛋白聚糖1)通过免疫组化来对其进行鉴定。由于CD138存在于细胞膜上,因此浆细胞的外周常被染色[5,7,21,24],但它们经常在组织中成簇出现(图12.1A和图12.1B)。

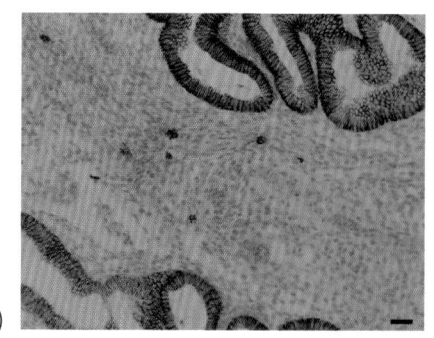 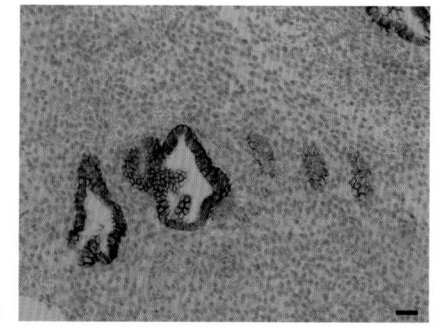

图12.1 伴或不伴慢性子宫内膜炎(CE)的子宫内膜的抗CD138免疫组织化学染色。
(A) CE子宫内膜。CD138⁺浆细胞见于子宫内膜间质。上皮细胞也可见CD138染色。(B)非CE子宫内膜。CD138仅在上皮细胞中染色。标尺=100μm。

应用国际慢性子宫内膜炎标准化工作组制定的"德尔菲法",建立了宫腔镜下 CE 的诊断标准。他们提出了以下标准[25]。

(1) 草莓状外观:大面积充血的子宫内膜,中央有白色点状区域(图 12.2A)。

(2) 局灶性充血:小面积充血的子宫内膜(图 12.2B)。

(3) 出血点:局部红色区域,边界清晰而不规则,可能与毛细血管相连(图 12.2C)。

(4) 微小息肉:小于 1 mm 的宫腔赘生物,具有明显的结缔组织血管轴,分布在局灶区域(图 12.2D)或弥漫整个子宫内膜表面(图 12.2E)。

(5) 卵泡期子宫内膜增厚且苍白:间质水肿的证据(在分泌期是正常的)(图 12.2F)。

诊断需具备至少 1 种上述特征。

目前,这些标准被认为是宫腔镜检测 CE 最可靠的诊断标准,但仍需进一步验证。

2.1.4 慢性子宫内膜炎的病理生理学

孕激素不仅在子宫中具有免疫抑制作用[26],而且还能抑制动物模型中由大肠埃希菌和脂多糖引起的炎症[27]。

因此,当考虑 CE 对胚胎种植和早期妊娠维持的影响时,尚不清楚产后子宫中的炎症是否持续。对 CE 或非 CE 患者流产标本的病理学分析表明,在再次流产的 CE 患者中,超过一半的病例存在具有多个浆细胞的慢性蜕膜炎(CD)[28]。CD 和 CE 一样,是发生在蜕膜内的一种持续性炎症。这一结果表明,即使在妊娠后,炎症也可能持续存在,并导致一些 CE 患者流产。

CE 在生化和形态学上都存在炎症。已清楚显示,经血中的促炎细胞因子,如白细胞介素-6、白细胞介素-1β 和肿瘤坏死因子 α,在 CE 患者中高于非 CE 患者[29]。增加的炎症物质已被证明会影响细胞的增殖、凋亡和功能。由于这种炎症的影响,免疫细胞的分布和组成也发生了变化。正常子宫内膜中 B 细胞的数量较少。然而,在 CE 中,大量 B 细胞浸润功能层的基质和腺上皮,并进入腺管腔[24]。尽管这种 B 细胞浸润可能与间质区域中的浆细胞出现有关,但这些细胞是如何影响妊娠维持的仍不清楚。T 细胞分散在间质和上皮区域。大多数子宫内膜 T 细胞是 $CD8^+$ 细胞、$CD4^+$ 辅助 T 细胞(Th 细胞),它们是建立和维持妊娠重要的亚群。流式细胞分选的结果表明,CE 患者的 Th1 比例增加,而 Th2 的比例减少[30]。免疫组化显示,$CD8^+$ 细胞和 $Foxp3^+$ 调节性 T 细胞的数量显著升高[31]。

自然杀伤(NK)细胞也被认为在妊娠的建立和维持中起着重要作用。NK 细胞的主要表型为 $CD56^{bright}CD16^-$ NK 细胞,具有较低的细胞毒性,在

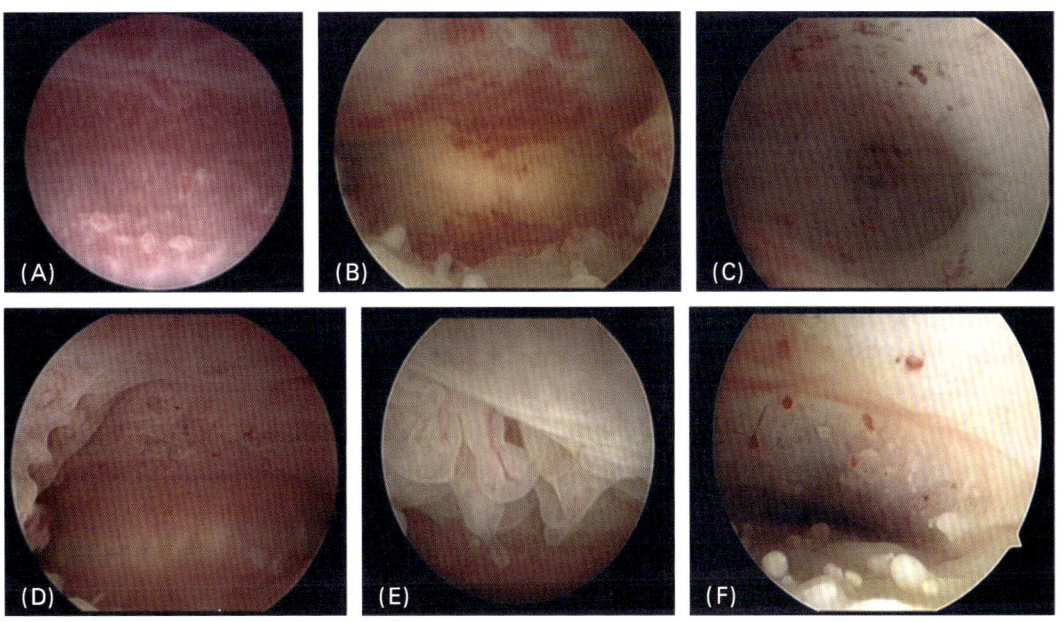

图 12.2 宫腔镜检查慢性子宫内膜炎的诊断标准。

(A)草莓状外观。(B)局灶性充血。(C)出血点。(D)局灶微小息肉。(E)弥漫微小息肉。(F)子宫内膜水肿。来源:Taken from Cicinelli E., Vitagliano A., Kumar A., et al. Unified diagnostic criteria for chronic endometritis at fluid hysteroscopy: proposal and reliability evaluation through an international randomized-controlled observer study. Fertil Steril 2019;112(1):162 – 173.e162。

分泌晚期,可占正常子宫内膜间质区域细胞的30%~40%。最近的研究发现,CD56^{bright}CD16$^-$或CD56$^+$CD16$^-$ NK 细胞亚群在 CE 患者的子宫内膜中随 T 细胞的增加而减少[32]。

为了成功维持妊娠,需要调节影响子宫内膜增殖和分化的性激素。在 CE 中,孕酮对子宫内膜的影响可能是异常的。Ki-67(细胞增殖的标志物)、BCL2 和 BAX(细胞凋亡调节因子)的表达在胚胎种植期子宫内膜中上调[33]。CE 通过雌激素和孕激素受体(PGR)的异常表达改变了蜕膜化[34]。这些结果表明,CE 扰乱了蜕膜化过程,从而影响了妊娠的建立和维持。

2.1.5 慢性子宫内膜炎对妊娠维持的影响和慢性子宫内膜炎治疗的有效性

已在 RPL 患者中研究了 CE 对随后妊娠结局的影响。一项病例对照观察性研究显示,未经治疗的 CE 患者(32.3%,11/34)的流产率高于因其他原因导致 RPL 的无 CE 患者(12.9%,4/31)[35],提示 CE 可能导致 RPL。

McQueen 等[36]报道了对早期 RPL 的 CE 患者的治疗效果。35 名 CE 患者中有 26 名接受了 2 周的氧氟沙星(800 mg)和甲硝唑(1 000 mg)治疗,其余 9 名患者接受了其他抗生素治疗,包括多西环素单药、多西环素和甲硝唑联合治疗,或环丙沙星和甲硝唑联合治疗。31 名患者进行了再次活检以确定治疗效果,其中 7 名被诊断为持续性 CE。这 7 名持续性 CE 患者经第二疗程的抗生素治疗治愈(2/7),或无须额外的抗生素治疗而自然消退(5/7)。因此,单一或两个疗程抗生素治疗后的治愈率分别为 94%(29/31)和 100%(31/31)。当 RPL 患者被诊断为 CE 时,抗生素已被证明可以治愈大多数病例。通过这种方式,在 RPL 患者中,抗生素治疗 CE 的疗效很好[36]。

已报道了抗生素治疗 CE 对随后妊娠的影响。在三组患者中,即无 CE 患者(60%,12/20)、接受治疗的 CE 患者(15%,2/13)和未经治疗的 CE 患者(56%,5/9),流产率存在显著差异($P=0.032$)。与未经治疗的 CE 患者相比,接受治疗的 CE 患者的流产率较高[37]。然而,由于研究参与者数量较少,因此无法得出抗生素对 CE 治愈率和对 RPL 患者随后妊娠维持的确切疗效。在不孕患者中,CE 对胚胎种植和妊娠维持的影响已得到了充分评估。因此,应进一步研究 CE 对流产率的影响。

在未被诊断为种植失败、RPL、子宫腺肌症、子宫黏膜下肌瘤或子宫异常的 IVF-ET 患者中,回顾性分析了 CE 和非 CE 患者的流产率。该研究发现,CE 组(40.0%,14/35)和非 CE 组(12.8%,5/39)的每次妊娠流产率存在显著差异($P<0.03$)[38]。另一项研究报道称,由于采用了不同的诊断标准,CE 和非 CE 患者的流产率没有显著差异[39]。然而,将这些结果汇总后发现,CE 组和非 CE 组的流产率仍存在显著差异(表 12.1)。

表 12.1 慢性子宫内膜炎与非慢性子宫内膜炎患者的流产率

研究对象	CE-流产/总数	非 CE-流产/总数	P	参考文献
接受 IVF 治疗的不孕症患者	14/35	5/39	$P<0.03$	[37]
接受 IVF 治疗的不孕症患者	1/17	53/431	NS	[38]
总计	15/52	58/470	$P<0.003$	

注:CE,慢性子宫内膜炎;IVF,体外受精;NS,无显著差异。

在接受 IVF-ET 治疗的不孕患者中,抗生素对 CE 治愈率的影响已得到很好的研究。一项系统回顾和荟萃分析发现,治愈 CE 的患者显示出较高的持续妊娠率/活产率(OR 6.81)、临床妊娠率(OR 4.02)和种植率(OR 3.24)[9]。在几项涉及生育治疗的研究中,比较了接受 IVF-ET 治疗的治愈和持续 CE 患者的流产率(表 12.2)[40-43]。在这些研究

表 12.2 持续性子宫内膜炎和已治愈慢性子宫内膜炎患者的流产率

研究对象	持续性 CE-流产/总数	治愈 CE-流产/总数	P	参考文献
接受 IVF 治疗的不孕症患者	3/11	15/135	NS	[39]
RIF	2/5	2/30	NS	[40]
RIF	0/0	8/53	—	[41]
RIF	1/3	3/9	NS	[42]
总计	6/19	28/227	$P<0.05$	

注:CE,慢性子宫内膜炎;IVF,体外受精;NS,无显著差异;RIF,反复种植失败。

中,由于抗生素治疗 CE 的治愈率很高,持续 CE 组的患者数量较少,且持续 CE 患者很少妊娠。这些原因可能解释了在先前研究中流产率没有显著差异的原因。当将这些数据汇总时发现,与表 12.2 所示的情况一样,持续 CE 病例的流产率增加。

总之,接受 IVF-ET 的患者如果在未经治疗或持续 CE 的情况下妊娠,流产率可能会增加。抗生素治疗 CE 的治愈率很高,治愈 CE 可以降低流产率并提高种植率。

2.2 非感染性(免疫性)子宫内膜炎

多种情况和疾病都可能导致非感染性子宫内膜炎,包括 Asherman 综合征、子宫内膜息肉、子宫腺肌症和子宫内膜异位症。

2.2.1 Asherman 综合征

Asherman 综合征是指在宫腔或宫颈整个或部分子宫内膜基底层和(或)肌层间形成纤维化和粘连的形态学改变[44,45]。尽管对 Asherman 综合征的具体发病机制知之甚少,但这些变化通常发生在宫腔感染或操作之后,如刮宫术、宫腔手术和处理胎盘残留的产科操作。在这种情况下,急性炎症被认为破坏了子宫内膜的功能性层,引起持续的慢性炎症,随后导致粘连和纤维化,从而改变了子宫内膜的功能。

Asherman 综合征在 RPL 病例中的检出率为 1.3%～9.6%[44,45]。尽管 Asherman 综合征在 RPL 中的患病率较高,但这可能是由于该患者群体接受宫颈扩张和刮宫术的风险增加所致[44,45]。此外,Asherman 综合征的存在可能会影响产科并发症,这是由于缺乏足够的子宫内膜来支持胎儿和胎盘的发育,以及纤维化的子宫内膜血管形成缺陷导致的血供不足,从而引起妊娠丢失[46]。对于 RPL 与 Asherman 综合征之间的关系,目前尚不清楚哪一个是原因,哪一个是结果。既往一项研究报道称,40%(66/165)和 23%(38/165)的后续妊娠分别导致自然流产和早产。然而,根据对未经治疗的 Asherman 综合征患者的分析[47],目前没有足够的证据表明 Asherman 综合征会导致 RPL,并且由于难以进行随机对照试验,这两种情况之间的关联仍存争议[45]。对于合并 Asherman 综合征的 RPL,目前也没有明确的治疗策略。此外,关于手术切除宫腔粘连对妊娠结局的益处,由于手术本身可能促进宫腔内更多粘连的形成,目前也缺乏足够的证据。因此,在首次进行宫腔操作时,动作小心轻柔对于预防 Asherman 综合征的形成非常重要[45]。

2.2.2 子宫内膜息肉

子宫内膜息肉是子宫内膜腺体和间质的局部过度增生,形成从子宫内膜表面突出或带蒂的病变[48]。子宫内膜息肉被认为是由炎症引起的,其自身产生促炎介质,是慢性炎症的原因之一[45]。与 RPL 有关的子宫内膜息肉的患病率为 6.0%～8.5%[49,50]。由于子宫内膜息肉形成了物理障碍,并改变了子宫内膜释放的物质,如胰岛素样生长因子-1 和免疫抑制性糖蛋白,从而对妊娠的维持以及生育能力产生不利影响[51]。尽管在理论上,子宫内膜息肉可能会影响妊娠的维持,但由于缺乏评估息肉切除对流产率影响的研究,目前没有直接证据表明其与 RPL 的关联[52]。因此,目前不足以推荐通过宫腔镜切除息肉以减少 RPL 风险[45,53,54]。然而,值得注意的是,子宫内膜息肉常与慢性子宫内膜炎相关,这种关系应在进一步的研究中加以探讨。

2.2.3 子宫内膜异位症

子宫内膜异位症被定义为子宫外存在子宫内膜或类似子宫内膜的组织[55]。尽管该疾病的根本原因和自然史尚不清楚,但在位子宫内膜存在过度炎症和免疫反应改变,并与临床症状的病因和病理生理相关,包括疼痛、不孕和不良妊娠结局[56]。研究表明,子宫内膜异位症患者的在位子宫内膜产生高水平的 Cox-2、前列腺素和促炎细胞因子,如 IL-6、IL-8 和 IL-17,表明在位子宫内膜存在慢性炎症。因此,子宫内膜异位症的子宫内膜被认为受到慢性炎症的影响[57]。

子宫内膜异位症的最终诊断是通过腹腔镜进行腹腔内检查完成。由于并非所有 RPL 患者都接受腹腔镜检查,因此 RPL 患者中子宫内膜异位症的患病率尚不清楚。因此,目前还无法评估子宫内膜异位症是否会导致 RPL。在我们的日常临床实践中,尚未在 RPL 患者中诊断出子宫内膜异位症的存在。虽然子宫内膜异位症在全球被公认为不孕的原因,但即使根据美国生殖医学学会(ASRM)实践委员会和欧洲人类生殖与胚胎学会(ESHRE)指南[53,54],它也未被认定为导致 RPL 的原因。然而,在腹腔镜诊断的子宫内膜异位症患者中,子宫内膜异位组和非子宫内膜异位组在盆腔环境以及卵子和在位子宫内膜特征的差异已得到充分报道[57-61]。此外,还研究了子宫内膜异位症对临床妊娠结局的影响[62,63]。最近,子宫内膜异位症作为一种影响妊娠结局的不利因素以及导致 RPL 的因素而受到关注。

子宫内膜异位症对流产的影响被认为是由多种机制产生的。首先,子宫内膜异位症引起的炎症可能会影响配子/胚胎周围的环境,并在它们从盆腔转移到宫腔时改变胚胎的质量。这可能会增加胚胎非整倍体的风险。IVF-ET 可以从这些炎症的环境中挽救配子/胚胎。然而,根据最近胚胎植入前染色体分析的结果显示,存在或没有子宫内膜异位症的患者间的非整倍体率没有统计学上的显著差异[64]。其次,子宫内膜的炎症可能会改变子宫内膜的功能。这可能会损害胚胎植入所需的子宫内膜上皮功能和蜕膜化。对子宫内膜异位症患者子宫内膜组织所进行的分子生物学分析显示,上皮和间质中与胚胎植入相关的物质发生了表达改变。子宫内膜异位症中发生的这些变化被认为与炎症引起的雌二醇优势和孕酮抵抗有关[65]。

芳香化酶是一种将雄激素转化为雌激素的酶,存在于子宫内膜异位组织中。此外,在子宫内膜异位症中 17βHSD1 的表达减少,该酶能将雌二醇转化为较弱的雌酮。这使得雌激素在子宫内膜异位症中占优势地位,形成一个促进子宫内膜异位组织增殖和炎症的环境[56,65]。雌二醇通过与其受体结合发挥作用:雌激素受体(ESR)1 和 ESR2。子宫内膜异位组织中 ESR2 的表达增加,ESR1 的表达减少,而雌激素受体的改变会引起炎症[66]。通过雌激素的从头合成促进环氧化酶-2(COX2)和由 COX2 活性产生的前列腺素,这些炎症物质则可能影响子宫内膜的功能[67]。FOXA2 基因在子宫内膜上皮中的表达影响白血病抑制因子(LIF)的表达,并受炎症的影响[68];在子宫内膜异位症患者中也存在这种情况[69]。相反,有报道称在子宫内膜异位症女性的种植窗口期,在位子宫内膜中 ESR2 的表达不变,而 ESR1 的表达增加[66]。ESR 表达在子宫内膜异位症的发病和发展中的作用有待进一步研究。

众所周知,孕酮在子宫内膜异位组织及其在位子宫内膜中的作用减弱。这种现象称为孕酮抵抗。由于减少了对雌激素活性的拮抗作用,孕酮反应性降低会损害蜕膜化并促进细胞增殖。孕酮作用的减弱可能是由于 PGR 表达的改变。在子宫内膜异位组织和这些患者的在位子宫内膜中 PGR 水平降低[70]。因此,PGR 刺激的介质表达减少,包括 Wnt 家族成员 4(WNT4)[71,72]。此外,包括 Notch 同源物 1(NOTCH1)和 FKBP52 在内的孕酮活性增强因子在子宫内膜异位症及其在位子宫内膜中的表达减少。因此,这些基因表达的减少被认为是获得孕酮抵抗的潜在机制[73,74]。

正如前文所提到的,子宫内膜异位症患者的子宫内膜由于基因表达受损,对胚胎的接受能力降低。此外,孕酮抵抗会引起蜕膜化延迟,导致种植窗的开启延迟。近年来的研究表明,种植窗改变的女性有种植失败的风险,而在正常种植窗之外发生胚胎植入的女性流产风险增加[75]。鉴于这一理论背景,子宫内膜异位症患者的流产风险增加。

最近的一项荟萃分析显示,与没有子宫内膜异位症的女性相比,患有子宫内膜异位症的女性流产风险显著增加。例如,一项涵盖 29 个研究的分析包含了 697 984 名女性,结果显示与没有子宫内膜异位症的女性相比,患有子宫内膜异位症的女性流产风险增加(OR:1.81;95% CI,1.44~2.28;I^2=96%)[76]。另一项涵盖 24 个研究的分析包含了 1 924 114 名女性,与健康对照组相比,患有子宫内膜异位症的女性流产风险显著增加(OR 1.75;95% CI,1.29~2.37)[77]。

然而,这些结果是基于自然受孕和 IVF-ET 治疗患者的临床数据。在仅通过 IVF-ET 受孕的患者中比较子宫内膜异位症组和非子宫内膜异位症组时,流产率没有显著差异[78]。在 IVF-ET 中,胚胎在体外发育,且移植前不会接触炎症环境。这与胚胎移植前足量的孕酮支持相结合,可能会克服孕酮抵抗。这些因素可能有助于降低子宫内膜异位症患者的流产率。

2.2.4 子宫腺肌症

子宫腺肌症的定义是在子宫肌层内存在类似于子宫内膜或类似于子宫内膜的腺体和间质。尽管通过对手术切除标本的病理学分析可以明确诊断腺肌症,但有生育意愿的患者通常会接受诊断性成像,如超声和磁共振成像,并接受针对其生育障碍和妊娠并发症的治疗。子宫腺肌症组织和在位子宫内膜的过度炎症和免疫系统的改变可能会对子宫产生影响。

在伴有腺肌症的正常子宫内膜单核细胞中,IFN-γ、TNF-α 和 IL-1β 的产生显著增加[79]。此外,在腺肌症患者的正常子宫内膜中,IL-6、IL-8 和 MCP-1 的分泌量较对照组的子宫内膜更高[80]。因此,子宫内膜炎症的存在可能会改变子宫内膜的功能。腺肌症导致了正常子宫内膜对孕酮正常反应的改变,这也在子宫内膜异位症患者中观察到。在腺肌症患者的正常子宫内膜中,负责内膜容受性、胚胎种植以及蜕膜化的 HOXA10 表达减少[81]。在从腺肌症患者获得的子宫内膜基质细胞的培养上清液中,IGFBP-1 和 PRL 的分泌也减少[80]。这意味着腺肌症患者的正常子宫内膜存在孕酮抵抗。

流产的另一个原因可能是腺肌症对子宫的生理影响,它引起了子宫内膜和子宫肌层中的异常蠕动[82]。腺肌症可引起胚胎植入期间子宫内发生的高频蠕动[83]。芳香化酶存在于子宫腺肌症和子宫内膜异位组织中,由其在子宫肌层产生的异常高水平雌激素被认为会导致子宫的异常蠕动[82]。子宫腺肌症通过这种机制对妊娠的建立和维持产生不利影响。

据报道,子宫腺肌症在 RPL 女性中的患病率为 13.6%[84]。对于存在或没有子宫腺肌症女性的妊娠率和流产率研究主要在接受 IVF 治疗的患者中进行。荟萃分析显示,子宫腺肌症增加了流产率。患有子宫腺肌症的女性流产率(31.9%)高于没有子宫腺肌症的女性(14.1%),相对风险为 2.12(95% CI 1.20~3.75)[85]。这一发现得到了另一项研究的证实,该结果显示患有腺肌症的女性流产风险增加(OR 3.49,95% CI 1.41~8.65)[78]。此外,虽然这些研究难以确定妊娠中期的流产率,但新近的一项回顾性分析显示,患有子宫腺肌症的孕妇在妊娠中期的流产率也高于没有子宫腺肌症的孕妇(12.2% vs 1.2%,OR 11.2,95% CI 2.2~71.2)[86]。

目前已开展子宫腺肌症的保留生育能力手术,但其对流产的预防效果尚未明确。此外,在 IVF 患者中,预处理或长期使用 GnRH 激动剂可以降低子宫腺肌病患者的流产率。在胚胎种植前抑制炎症也可能有助于预防流产[87]。

3 总结与建议

- 在面对 RPL 患者时,需要评估 CE 的存在。
- 对于患有 CE 的 RPL 患者,尽管已有文献报道了在妊娠前进行抗生素治疗有积极效果,但未来仍需进一步验证。
- 子宫内膜异位症和子宫腺肌症可能由于异位和正常子宫内膜中的炎症、雌激素增加及孕酮抵抗相关基因的表达改变而导致流产。
- 当子宫内膜异位症患者通过 IVF-ET 妊娠时,流产率并未增加,这可能是由于生殖细胞脱离于高度炎症环境以及孕酮的强化补充。
- 通过药物长期抑制炎症,如 GnRH 激动剂或抗炎药物,可能有助于预防子宫腺肌症患者的流产。

参考文献

[1] Chen L,Deng H,Cui H,et al. Inflammatory responses and inflammation-associated diseases in organs. Oncotarget 2018;9(6):7204-18.

[2] Pahwa R,Goyal A,Bansal P,Jialal I. Chronic inflammation. StatPearls. FL:Treasure Island;2021.

[3] Kunnumakkara AB,Sailo BL,Banik K,et al. Chronic diseases,inflammation,and spices:how are they linked? J Transl Med 2018;16(1):14.

[4] Katsuyama T,Tsokos GC,Moulton VR. Aberrant T cell signaling and subsets in systemic lupus erythematosus. Front Immunol 2018;9:1088.

[5] Puente E,Alonso L,Lagana AS,Ghezzi F,Casarin J,Carugno J. Chronic endometritis:old problem,novel insights and future challenges. Int J Fertil Steril 2020;13(4):250-6.

[6] Greenwood SM,Moran JJ. Chronic endometritis:morphologic and clinical observations. Obstet Gynecol 1981;58(2):176-84.

[7] Kimura F,Takebayashi A,Ishida M,et al. Review:chronic endometritis and its effect on reproduction. J Obstet Gynaecol Res 2019;45(5):951-60.

[8] Inoue T,Moran I,Shinnakasu R,Phan TG,Kurosaki T. Generation of memory B cells and their reactivation. Immunol Rev 2018;283(1):138-49.

[9] Vitagliano A,Saccardi C,Noventa M,et al. Effects of chronic endometritis therapy on in vitro fertilization outcome in women with repeated implantation failure:a systematic review and meta-analysis. Fertil Steril 2018;110(1):103-12 e101.

[10] Moreno I,Codoner FM,Vilella F,et al. Evidence that the endometrial microbiota has an effect on implantation success or failure. Am J Obstet Gynecol 2016;215(6):684-703.

[11] Kyono K,Hashimoto T,Nagai Y,Sakuraba Y. Analysis of endometrial microbiota by 16S ribosomal RNA gene sequencing among infertile patients:a single-center pilot study. Reprod Med Biol 2018;17(3):297-306.

[12] Gonzalez A,Vazquez-Baeza Y,Knight R. SnapShot:the human microbiome. Cell. 2014;158(3):690 690 e691.

[13] Human Microbiome Project C. Structure,function and diversity of the healthy human microbiome. Nature 2012;486(7402):207-14.

[14] Chen C,Song X,Wei W,et al. The microbiota continuum along the female reproductive tract and its relation to uterine-

related diseases. Nat Commun 2017;8(1):875.
[15] Benner M, Ferwerda G, Joosten I, van der Molen RG. How uterine microbiota might be responsible for a receptive, fertile endometrium. Hum Reprod Update 2018;24(4):393–415.
[16] Crha I, Ventruba P, Zakova J, et al. Uterine microbiome and endometrial receptivity. Ceska Gynekol 2019;84(1):49–54.
[17] Cicinelli E, De Ziegler D, Nicoletti R, et al. Chronic endometritis: correlation among hysteroscopic, histologic, and bacteriologic findings in a prospective trial with 2190 consecutive office hysteroscopies. Fertil Steril 2008;89(3):677–84.
[18] Quayle AJ. The innate and early immune response to pathogen challenge in the female genital tract and the pivotal role of epithelial cells. J Reprod Immunol 2002;57(1–2):61–79.
[19] Santos TM, Bicalho RC. Diversity and succession of bacterial communities in the uterine fluid of postpartum metritic, endometritic and healthy dairy cows. PLoS One 2012;7(12):e53048.
[20] Cicinelli E, Matteo M, Tinelli R, et al. Chronic endometritis due to common bacteria is prevalent in women with recurrent miscarriage as confirmed by improved pregnancy outcome after antibiotic treatment. Reprod Sci 2014;21(5):640–7.
[21] Kitaya K. Prevalence of chronic endometritis in recurrent miscarriages. Fertil Steril 2011;95(3):1156–8.
[22] Takebayashi A, Kimura F, Kishi Y, et al. The association between endometriosis and chronic endometritis. PLoS One 2014;9(2):e88354.
[23] Cicinelli E, Matteo M, Trojano G, et al. Chronic endometritis in patients with unexplained infertility: prevalence and effects of antibiotic treatment on spontaneous conception. Am J Reprod Immunol 2018;79(1).
[24] Kitaya K, Yasuo T. Aberrant expression of selectin E, CXCL1, and CXCL13 in chronic endometritis. Mod Pathol 2010;23(8):1136–46.
[25] Cicinelli E, Vitagliano A, Kumar A, et al. Unified diagnostic criteria for chronic endometritis at fluid hysteroscopy: proposal and reliability evaluation through an international randomized-controlled observer study. Fertil Steril 2019;112(1):162–73 e162.
[26] van der Burg B, van der Saag PT. Nuclear factor-kappa-B/steroid hormone receptor interactions as a functional basis of anti-inflammatory action of steroids in reproductive organs. Mol Hum Reprod 1996;2(6):433–8.
[27] Cui L, Wang H, Lin J, et al. Progesterone inhibits inflammatory response in E. coli-or LPS-Stimulated bovine endometrial epithelial cells by NF-kappaB and MAPK pathways. Dev Comp Immunol 2020;105:103568.
[28] Kaku S, Kubo T, Kimura F, et al. Relationship of chronic endometritis with chronic deciduitis in cases of miscarriage. BMC Women's Health 2020;20(1):114.
[29] Tortorella C, Piazzolla G, Matteo M, et al. Interleukin-6, interleukin-1beta, and tumor necrosis factor alpha in menstrual effluents as biomarkers of chronic endometritis. Fertil Steril 2014;101(1):242–7.
[30] Kitazawa J, Kimura F, Nakamura A, et al. Alteration in endometrial helper T-cell subgroups in chronic endometritis. Am J Reprod Immunol 2021;85(3):e13372.
[31] Li Y, Yu S, Huang C, et al. Evaluation of peripheral and uterine immune status of chronic endometritis in patients with recurrent reproductive failure. Fertil Steril 2020;113(1):187–96 e181.
[32] Matteo M, Cicinelli E, Greco P, et al. Abnormal pattern of lymphocyte subpopulations in the endometrium of infertile women with chronic endometritis. Am J Reprod Immunol 2009;61(5):322–9.
[33] Di Pietro C, Cicinelli E, Guglielmino MR, et al. Altered transcriptional regulation of cytokines, growth factors, and apoptotic proteins in the endometrium of infertile women with chronic endometritis. Am J Reprod Immunol 2013;69(5):509–17.
[34] Wu D, Kimura F, Zheng L, et al. Chronic endometritis modifies decidualization in human endometrial stromal cells. Reprod Biol Endocrinol 2017;15(1):16.
[35] McQueen DB, Perfetto CO, Hazard FK, Lathi RB. Pregnancy outcomes in women with chronic endometritis and recurrent pregnancy loss. Fertil Steril 2015;104(4):927–31.
[36] McQueen DB, Bernardi LA, Stephenson MD. Chronic endometritis in women with recurrent early pregnancy loss and/or fetal demise. Fertil Steril 2014;101(4):1026–30.
[37] Gay C, Hamdaoui N, Pauly V, et al. Impact of antibiotic treatment for chronic endometritis on unexplained recurrent pregnancy loss. J Gynecol Obstet Hum Reprod 2021;50(5):102034.
[38] Morimune A, Kimura F, Nakamura A, et al. The effects of chronic endometritis on the pregnancy outcomes. Am J Reprod Immunol 2021;85(3):e13357.
[39] Li Y, Xu S, Yu S, et al. Diagnosis of chronic endometritis: how many CD138(+) cells/HPF in endometrial stroma affect pregnancy outcome of infertile women? Am J Reprod Immunol 2021;85(5):e13369.
[40] Cicinelli E, Matteo M, Tinelli R, et al. Prevalence of chronic endometritis in repeated unexplained implantation failure and the IVF success rate after antibiotic therapy. Hum Reprod 2015;30(2):323–30.
[41] Kitaya K, Matsubayashi H, Takaya Y, et al. Live birth rate following oral antibiotic treatment for chronic endometritis in infertile women with repeated implantation failure. Am J Reprod Immunol 2017;78(5).
[42] Tersoglio AE, Salatino DR, Reinchisi G, Gonzalez A, Tersoglio S, Marlia C. Repeated implantation failure in oocyte donation. What to do to improve the endometrial receptivity? JBRA Assist Reprod 2015;19(2):44–52.
[43] Xiong Y, Chen Q, Chen C, et al. Impact of oral antibiotic treatment for chronic endometritis on pregnancy outcomes in the following frozen-thawed embryo transfer cycles of infertile women: a cohort study of 640 embryo transfer cycles. Fertil Steril 2021;116(2):413–21.
[44] Hooker AB, Lemmers M, Thurkow AL, et al. Systematic review and meta-analysis of intrauterine adhesions after miscarriage: prevalence, risk factors and long-term reproductive outcome. Hum Reprod Update 2014;20(2):262–78.
[45] Carbonnel M, Pirtea P, de Ziegler D, Ayoubi JM. Uterine factors in recurrent pregnancy losses. Fertil Steril 2021;115(3):538–45.
[46] Yu D, Wong YM, Cheong Y, Xia E, Li TC. Asherman syndrome-one century later. Fertil Steril 2008;89(4):759–79.
[47] Schenker JG, Margalioth EJ. Intrauterine adhesions: an updated appraisal. Fertil Steril 1982;37(5):593–610.
[48] Kim KR, Peng R, Ro JY, Robboy SJ. A diagnostically useful histopathologic feature of endometrial polyp: the long axis of endometrial glands arranged parallel to surface epithelium.

Am J Surg Pathol 2004;28(8):1057-62.

[49] Elsokkary M, Elshourbagy M, Labib K, et al. Assessment of hysteroscopic role in management of women with recurrent pregnancy loss. J Matern Fetal Neonatal Med 2018;31(11):1494-504.

[50] Seckin B, Sarikaya E, Oruc AS, Celen S, Cicek N. Office hysteroscopic findings in patients with two, three, and four or more, consecutive miscarriages. Eur J Contracept Reprod Health Care 2012;17(5):393-8.

[51] Elbehery MM, Nouh AA, Mohamed ML, Alanwar AA, Abd-Allah SH, Shalaby SM. Insulin-like growth factor binding protein-1 and glycodelin levels in uterine flushing before and after hysteroscopic polypectomy. Clin Lab 2011;57(11-12):953-7.

[52] Lieng M, Istre O, Qvigstad E. Treatment of endometrial polyps: a systematic review. Acta Obstet Gynecol Scand 2010;89(8):992-1002.

[53] Practice Committee of the American Society for Reproductive M. Evaluation and treatment of recurrent pregnancy loss: a committee opinion. Fertil Steril 2012;98(5):1103-11.

[54] EGGo RPL, Bender Atik R, Christiansen OB, et al. ESHRE guideline: recurrent pregnancy loss. Hum Reprod Open 2018;2018(2):hoy004.

[55] Saunders PTK, Horne AW. Endometriosis: etiology, pathobiology, and therapeutic prospects. Cell 2021;184(11):2807-24.

[56] Pirtea P, Cicinelli E, De Nola R, de Ziegler D, Ayoubi JM. Endometrial causes of recurrent pregnancy losses: endometriosis, adenomyosis, and chronic endometritis. Fertil Steril 2021;115(3):546-60.

[57] Lessey BA, Kim JJ. Endometrial receptivity in the eutopic endometrium of women with endometriosis: it is affected, and let me show you why. Fertil Steril 2017;108(1):19-27.

[58] Vallve-Juanico J, Houshdaran S, Giudice LC. The endometrial immune environment of women with endometriosis. Hum Reprod Update 2019;25(5):564-91.

[59] Sanchez AM, Vanni VS, Bartiromo L, et al. Is the oocyte quality affected by endometriosis? A review of the literature. J Ovarian Res 2017;10(1):43.

[60] Patel BG, Rudnicki M, Yu J, Shu Y, Taylor RN. Progesterone resistance in endometriosis: origins, consequences and interventions. Acta Obstet Gynecol Scand 2017;96(6):623-32.

[61] Zondervan KT, Becker CM, Missmer SA. Endometriosis. N Engl J Med 2020;382(13):1244-56.

[62] Borisova AV, Konnon SRD, Tosto V, Gerli S, Radzinsky VE. Obstetrical complications and outcome in patients with endometriosis. J Matern Fetal Neonatal Med 2020;1-15.

[63] Lalani S, Choudhry AJ, Firth B, et al. Endometriosis and adverse maternal, fetal and neonatal outcomes, a systematic review and meta-analysis. Hum Reprod 2018;33(10):1854-65.

[64] Juneau C, Kraus E, Werner M, et al. Patients with endometriosis have aneuploidy rates equivalent to their age-matched peers in the in vitro fertilization population. Fertil Steril 2017;108(2):284-8.

[65] Marquardt RM, Kim TH, Shin JH, Jeong JW. Progesterone and estrogen signaling in the endometrium: what goes wrong in endometriosis? Int J Mol Sci 2019;20(15).

[66] Osinski M, Wirstlein P, Wender-Ozegowska E, Mikolajczyk M, Jagodzinski PP, Szczepanska M. HSD3B2, HSD17B1, HSD17B2, ESR1, ESR2 and AR expression in infertile women with endometriosis. Ginekol Pol 2018;89(3):125-34.

[67] Tamura M, Deb S, Sebastian S, Okamura K, Bulun SE. Estrogen up-regulates cyclooxygenase-2 via estrogen receptor in human uterine microvascular endothelial cells. Fertil Steril 2004;81(5):1351-6.

[68] Kelleher AM, Peng W, Pru JK, Pru CA, DeMayo FJ, Spencer TE. Forkhead box a2 (FOXA2) is essential for uterine function and fertility. Proc Natl Acad Sci USA 2017;114(6):E1018-26.

[69] Lin A, Yin J, Cheng C, Yang Z, Yang H. Decreased expression of FOXA2 promotes eutopic endometrial cell proliferation and migration in patients with endometriosis. Reprod Biomed Online 2018;36(2):181-7.

[70] Igarashi TM, Bruner-Tran KL, Yeaman GR, et al. Reduced expression of progesterone receptor-B in the endometrium of women with endometriosis and in cocultures of endometrial cells exposed to 2,3,7,8-tetrachloro-dibenzo-p-dioxin. Fertil Steril 2005;84(1):67-74.

[71] Burney RO, Talbi S, Hamilton AE, et al. Gene expression analysis of endometrium reveals progesterone resistance and candidate susceptibility genes in women with endometriosis. Endocrinology 2007;148(8):3814-26.

[72] Liang Y, Li Y, Liu K, Chen P, Wang D. Expression and significance of WNT4 in ectopic and eutopic endometrium of human endometriosis. Reprod Sci 2016;23(3):379-85.

[73] Yang H, Zhou Y, Edelshain B, Schatz F, Lockwood CJ, Taylor HS. FKBP4 is regulated by HOXA10 during decidualization and in endometriosis. Reproduction 2012;143(4):531-8.

[74] Brown DM, Lee HC, Liu S, et al. Notch-1 signaling activation and progesterone receptor expression in ectopic lesions of women with endometriosis. J Endocr Soc 2018;2(7):765-78.

[75] Wilcox AJ, Baird DD, Weinberg CR. Time of implantation of the conceptus and loss of pregnancy. N Engl J Med 1999;340(23):1796-9.

[76] Huang Y, Zhao X, Chen Y, Wang J, Zheng W, Cao L. Miscarriage on Endometriosis and adenomyosis in women by assisted reproductive technology or with spontaneous conception: a systematic review and meta-analysis. Biomed Res Int 2020;2020:4381346.

[77] Zullo F, Spagnolo E, Saccone G, et al. Endometriosis and obstetrics complications: a systematic review and meta-analysis. Fertil Steril 2017;108(4):667-72 e665.

[78] Horton J, Sterrenburg M, Lane S, Maheshwari A, Li TC, Cheong Y. Reproductive, obstetric, and perinatal outcomes of women with adenomyosis and endometriosis: a systematic review and meta-analysis. Hum Reprod Update 2019;25(5):592-632.

[79] Sotnikova N, Antsiferova I, Malyshkina A. Cytokine network of eutopic and ectopic endometrium in women with adenomyosis. Am J Reprod Immunol 2002;47(4):251-5.

[80] Peng Y, Jin Z, Liu H, Xu C. Impaired decidualization of human endometrial stromal cells from women with adenomyosisdagger. Biol Reprod 2021;104(5):1034-44.

[81] Fischer CP, Kayisili U, Taylor HS. HOXA10 expression is decreased in endometrium of women with adenomyosis. Fertil Steril 2011;95(3):1133-6.

[82] Munro MG. Uterine polyps, adenomyosis, leiomyomas, and endometrial receptivity. Fertil Steril 2019;111(4):629-40.

[83] Zhu L, Che HS, Xiao L, Li YP. Uterine peristalsis before embryo transfer affects the chance of clinical pregnancy in

fresh and frozen-thawed embryo transfer cycles. Hum Reprod 2014;29(6):1238-43.

[84] Atabekoglu CS, Sukur YE, Kalafat E, et al. The association between adenomyosis and recurrent miscarriage. Eur J Obstet Gynecol Reprod Biol 2020;250:107-11.

[85] Vercellini P, Consonni D, Dridi D, Bracco B, Frattaruolo MP, Somigliana E. Uterine adenomyosis and in vitro fertilization outcome: a systematic review and meta-analysis. Hum Reprod 2014;29(5):964-77.

[86] Hashimoto A, Iriyama T, Sayama S, et al. Adenomyosis and adverse perinatal outcomes: increased risk of second trimester miscarriage, preeclampsia, and placental malposition. J Matern Fetal Neonatal Med 2018;31(3):364-9.

[87] Stanekova V, Woodman RJ, Tremellen K. The rate of euploid miscarriage is increased in the setting of adenomyosis. Hum Reprod Open 2018;2018(3):hoy011.

第 13 章

反复妊娠丢失的血栓病理学

Thrombophilic pathologies in recurrent pregnancy losses

Ae Ra Han[1] and Sung Ki Lee[2]

[1]Cha University, Fertility Center, Daegu, Republic of Korea
[2]Department of Obstetrics and Gynecology, Konyang University College of Medicine, Daejeon, Republic of Korea

1 引言

尽管对于反复妊娠丢失（RPL）尚无统一的定义，但在生殖医学领域最有影响力的学术机构美国生殖医学会和欧洲人类生殖与胚胎学会（ESHRE）将 RPL 定义为两次或更多次的妊娠丢失[1,2]。约有 15% 的临床妊娠会偶发流产，2% 的女性经历 2 次连续的流产，≤1% 的女性会经历 3 次或更多次的连续流产[3]。

胎盘形成是在低氧环境下进行的，伴随活跃的血管重塑和适当的凝血。妊娠早期，在胚胎植入和胎盘形成时，子宫内氧饱和度相对较低，而蜕膜中的血管会发生改变，为胎盘提供充足的血液供应做好准备。妊娠期间胎盘的血液供应异常减少，就会导致胎盘形成异常，引起流产、子痫前期（PE）、早产、胎儿宫内生长受限（IUGR）和死胎等多种产科并发症[4]。尽管异常胎盘形成的潜在病理机制尚不清楚，但血管生成标志物的异常表达和高凝状态已被认为是可能的病因[5-8]。

易栓症是一种遗传性或获得性异常形成血栓的倾向，它会增加静脉血栓栓塞症（VTE）和血栓栓塞性疾病的风险[9,10]。抗磷脂综合征（APS）是一种典型的获得性易栓症，以静脉或动脉血栓形成和（或）胎盘介导的妊娠并发症的风险增加为特征[11]。遗传性易栓症是一种遗传突变影响凝血系统蛋白数量或功能的疾病[12]。在本章中，我们将探讨除 RPL 相关的 APS 外其他遗传性和获得性易栓症的病理生理学和管理。

2 易栓症

2.1 遗传性易栓症

最常见的遗传性易栓症包括因子 V Leiden G1691A 突变（FVL）和凝血酶原 G20210A 多态性（PT），以及蛋白 C、蛋白 S 和抗凝血酶（AT）的缺乏。其他遗传性易栓症也被发现与产科并发症（包括 RPL）相关，如因子 V H1299R（R2）多态性，因子 V 的一种错义突变（Y1702C），因子 Ⅷ V34L 多态性，β-纤维蛋白原-455G>A 多态性，以及 HPA1 a/b（L33P）多态性，由四氢叶酸还原酶（MTHFR）C677T 和 A1298C 多态性引起的高同型半胱氨酸血症（Hcy），以及 PAI-1 4G/5G 多态性[5,13-17]。

可按上述病因对 VTE 进行风险划分：①高风险型——AT 缺乏、FVL 纯合、PT 纯合，以及 FVL 和 PT 杂合。②低风险型——FVL 杂合、PT 杂合以及蛋白质 C 和 S 缺乏。尽管有几项研究描述了遗传性易栓症对各种产科并发症发展的影响[18,19]，但关于每种遗传性易栓症对 RPL 或其他产科并发症的风险尚无共识（表 13.1）。

2.2 获得性易栓症

抗磷脂综合征（APS）是最常见的获得性易栓症，将在另一章进行讨论。由叶酸和维生素 B_{12} 缺乏、肥胖和糖尿病引起的叶酸代谢缺陷，是一种可逆转的易栓症，并且是脑静脉血栓形成、先天性畸形和流产的常见危险因素[29]。

表 13.1　遗传性易栓症与反复妊娠丢失的相关性[3,18,20-28]

易栓症	RPL[a]	晚期产科并发症[b]	在一般人群或对照组中的多态性患病率
FVL G1691A	是	是	希腊人和中东裔为13%~15% 欧洲白种人为5%~9%，亚洲人群缺失
PT G20210A	是	是	白种人为2%~4%。亚洲和非洲人群缺失
MTHFR C677T，A1298C	是/否	是(PE)	欧洲人分别为10%~16%和4%~6% 韩国女性分别为20.6%和3.8% 日本女性C677T为19.7%
抗凝血酶	是	否	欧洲白种人为0.02%~1.15% 日本人为0.15%
蛋白C	否	否	欧洲人为0.2%~0.3% 日本人为0.13%
蛋白S	是	是(孕晚期妊娠丢失)	欧洲白种人为0.03%~0.13% 日本男性为1.12%，女性为1.60%

注：[a]反复妊娠丢失。
[b]孕中期和晚期的妊娠丢失，先兆子痫(PE)，胎盘早剥。
来源：Inherited thrombophilia and anticoagulation therapy from women with reproductive failure. J Reprod Immunol 2021；85(4)：e13378。

2.3　遗传性易栓症的患病率

遗传性易栓症的患病率因种族和地理区域而异[30]。与亚洲人相比，白种人FVL和PT多态性的发病率较高，但MTHFR多态性和蛋白S缺乏的发病率较低(表13.1)[3,20-24]。在一项关于特定种族参考范围的研究中，黑种人主体的蛋白C和S水平明显低于白种人[31]。另一项研究显示了亚洲人和中东人之间每种遗传性易栓症患病率的差异[30]。其他因素，如性别、年龄和激素水平，也会影响血浆中天然抗凝物的水平。在一项关于AT、蛋白C和蛋白S正常参考范围的研究中，生育年龄女性的蛋白S水平较同龄男性低[32]。血浆蛋白C水平随年龄增加而升高，但AT和蛋白S则不升高。这些发现得到了Sakata等[20]的证实。激素也可能调节这些标志物。绝经期AT和蛋白S的浓度增加[32-34]。口服避孕药(OC)使用者与非OC使用者相比，AT和蛋白S水平较低，但蛋白C水平较高[32]。由于每种产科疾病的血栓形成倾向标志物的适当范围尚未明确，对遗传性易栓症的诊断应谨慎进行。

3　妊娠期生理性高凝状态

胎盘在妊娠期间允许胚胎进行气体交换并提供营养，同时在妊娠期间控制免疫平衡和凝血系统。早期胎盘形成时，蜕膜基质细胞产生凝血酶，并在毛细血管破裂、随后的血管外滋养层侵入及螺旋动脉重塑过程中形成止血包膜，以防止出血[35]。

在妊娠早期和中期，凝血因子Ⅰ(纤维蛋白原)、Ⅱ(凝血酶，PT)、Ⅶ、Ⅸ和Ⅻ增加，游离蛋白S减少[36]。激活蛋白C的抗性也降低[37]，但蛋白C活性和AT水平变化不大或保持恒定[38]。这种高凝状态持续到产后12周[39]。子宫胎盘循环的低压和低速易引起血栓并发症[35]。妊娠期间的高凝状态有助于减少分娩失血[40-42]；然而，如果生理性高凝状态异常加强，可能导致血栓栓塞和(或)各种胎盘介导的妊娠并发症(如RPL、PE、IUGR、胎盘早剥和死胎)的发生。事实上，流产和死胎的胎盘病理常常表现出血栓改变，如绒毛周围纤维蛋白沉积、蜕膜床的纤维蛋白样坏死，以及绒毛间隙和胎儿血管血栓[43]。妊娠早期蜕膜和绒毛膜循环不足，滋养细胞侵入能力受损，胎盘血管血栓形成过多，妊娠中期和晚期继发性子宫胎盘功能不全，导致中晚期产科并发症的发生[44-47]。为了平衡胎盘循环的高凝状态，血液的抗凝和纤溶活性需在受孕前得到良好维持，并在妊娠期间适当激活。

由于孕妇处于生理性高凝状态，无论是遗传性还是获得性易栓症都可能迅速诱发病理性凝血。此外，自身免疫性疾病中免疫复合物或补体引起的血管内皮损伤，以及活化的免疫效应细胞产生的促炎细胞因子和趋化因子会对血栓形成产生直接刺激。

事实上，研究表明，易栓症或血流动力学参数与RPL多个免疫标志物存在显著相关性[48,49]。众所周知的抗凝药物，如阿司匹林和肝素，具有多种免疫调节功能[50,51]。总之，炎症和凝血相互关联，其中任何一个的异常激活都能导致各种妊娠并发症。

4 遗传性易栓症与反复妊娠丢失

显然，遗传性易栓症在女性和男性中都是VTE的危险因素[9,52]，但每种遗传性易栓症在RPL女性中的作用尚未得到很好阐明。最近的一项荟萃分析描述了RPL女性中各种血栓性疾病的患病率[53]。在研究RPL各种病因的研究中，包括了7项探讨遗传性易栓症（$n=1713$）的研究。FVL的患病率在0%~17.0%，PT基因多态性在RPL女性中为0%~13.6%。蛋白S和蛋白C缺乏在RPL女性中分别为0%~18.2%和1.1%~13.6%。因此，遗传性易栓症在RPL中的患病率根据研究和患者群体的不同而有显著差异。

关于遗传性易栓症在RPL女性和生育能力正常的对照组中的患病率，结果并不一致。Carp等[52]进行的一项病例对照研究中，108名有3次以上流产史的女性和82名健康对照者之间，FVL、PT和MTHFR C677T突变的发生率没有差异。然而，Coulam等[17]观察到，在10个易栓症基因中有超过3个突变的女性中，RPL女性的比例高于生育能力正常的对照组（分别为68% vs 21%，$P=0.02$）。根据对韩国不明原因RPL女性进行的易栓症基因多态性的报道，MTHFR C677T和A1298C、PAI-1 4G/5G、血管紧张素转化酶I/D、p53密码子72和泌乳素受体基因C/T突变的基因型在不明原因RPL女性和生育能力正常的对照组之间没有差异[16,22,54,55]。另一方面，2006年发表的一项系统综述显示，FVL、PT和MTHFR基因突变以及蛋白S缺乏的优势比（OR）在早期妊娠丢失中为1.40~3.55，在反复早期妊娠丢失中为1.91~2.70，在中期妊娠丢失中为4.12~8.60，在晚期妊娠丢失中为1.31~20.09[18]。

5 评估

5.1 谁需要进行检查

不建议在非选择人群中进行常规遗传性易栓症筛查，关于应该对谁进行检查或最佳的筛查方案尚无充分的证据[56]。最新的ESHRE关于RPL的指南反对遗传性易栓症的常规筛查，除非是在研究背景下或在具有其他血栓形成倾向危险因素的女性中[2]。美国妇产科医师学会建议仅对有VTE病史或有高危血栓形成倾向的一级亲属计划妊娠的受试者进行遗传性易栓症筛查[42]。然而，在不明原因RPL的女性中，已有遗传性易栓症和免疫异常的报道。因此，遗传性易栓症检测可能对患有不明病因RPL的女性有所帮助。

5.2 应该进行哪些检测

常见的遗传性易栓症检测包括FVL和PT G20210A多态性、蛋白C和S的功能测试以及AT缺乏检测。此外，还常检测血清同型半胱氨酸水平、MTHFR C667T和PAI-1 4G/5G多态性以及凝血因子Ⅷ水平。遗传性蛋白C和S缺乏以及AT缺乏可能源于基因突变，但突变位点存在差异。因此，使用功能测试来确定这些异常。蛋白S缺乏是最具挑战性的遗传性易栓症，其结果受检测方法和个体状况的影响较大，因此难以确定。筛查蛋白S缺乏最可靠的方法是使用免疫测定法检测游离蛋白S水平[57]。对于蛋白C缺乏，使用酰胺裂解的酶分析法是首选，因为其性能优于凝血分析法[58]。对于AT缺乏，首选色谱法[59]。

5.3 可以应用哪些标准

关于遗传性易栓症在RPL中作用的争议，可能源于影响特定人群中每种易栓症标志物临界值的各种因素。根据我们未发表的数据，每种易栓症标志物的已知参考范围与育龄期女性的均值±2标准差（SD）存在显著差异。具体而言，RPL女性的ATⅢ和蛋白S活性水平比既定的参考范围具有更广的离散度。此外，基于已知参考范围的RPL女性中易栓症的患病率与生育能力正常对照组有显著差异（均值±2 SD）。目前每种易栓症标志物的参考范围最初是为了评估VTE风险而制定的，且来源于95%的18~65岁健康男性和女性[60]。这表明现有的易栓症标志物参考范围可能不适合应用于RPL评估。因此，有必要验证目前参考范围内的这些易栓症标志物是否足以评估RPL女性。我们需要根据临床和实验室标准的要求，为健康育龄期女性建立新的参考范围。

6 遗传性易栓症的治疗

患有遗传性易栓症但尚未发生血栓栓塞(如抗磷脂综合征)的 RPL 女性通常会接受低剂量阿司匹林和预防剂量的低分子肝素(LMWH)治疗。

6.1 抗凝药物

阿司匹林,即乙酰水杨酸,属于非甾体抗炎药,主要用作抗凝血剂[61]。阿司匹林通过与 COX-1 上的长疏水通道结合并抑制花生四烯酸转化为前列腺素(PG)H2——PGD2、PGE2、PGF2a、PGI2 和血栓素 A2(TXA2)的前体[62],从而发挥抗血栓作用。PG 和 TXA2 的产生减少会抑制血小板的激活和聚集。阿司匹林也参与纤维蛋白网络的形成和纤溶过程[61]。阿司匹林这种广谱抗血栓作用,若不慎使用,可能会导致严重的内出血。

肝素是一种糖胺多聚糖,在结构上类似于硫酸肝素,后者是一种内源性大分子,与血液凝固相关的各种蛋白质配体结合。这种相似性赋予了肝素和 LMWH 多种特征。肝素的抗凝作用主要是通过与 AT 结合而产生的。这种肝素-AT 复合物主要灭活因子Ⅹa 和Ⅱa,同时,还能灭活Ⅸa、Ⅺa 和Ⅻa[63]。肝素的高亲和力五糖单元有助于激活 AT,加速其与凝血酶(FⅡa)和活化的因子Ⅹ(因子Ⅹa)的相互作用,从而使因子Ⅹa 失活。除了Ⅹa 因子抑制之外,AT 介导的 FⅡa 失活的催化作用是通过形成肝素-抗凝血酶-凝血酶三元复合物来进行的。LMWH 是分子量从 1 000 Da 到 10 000 Da 不等的聚合混合物,平均分子量在 4 000~5 000 Da,约是普通肝素(UFH)大小的 1/3[64]。LMWH 主要抑制因子Ⅹa,但抑制凝血酶的能力较小。因此,它表现出比 UFH 更低的出血倾向[65]。LMWH 在皮下注射时几乎具有 100% 的生物利用度,且具有剂量非依赖的清除机制,这使其在抗凝方面具有可预测性[66]。由于 LMWH 平均半衰期较 UFH 长,其比 UFH 减少了注射的频率和与注射相关的疼痛[10]。LMWH 的常用剂量见表 13.2。

6.2 反复妊娠丢失女性的遗传性易栓症处理

由于没有一致且有力的证据表明 RPL 女性存在遗传性易栓症,因此几乎所有主要学会的临床指南都建议无论是否存在遗传性易栓症或 RPL,仅对

表 13.2 用于抗凝治疗的低分子肝素剂量

低分子肝素制剂	常用的 LMWH 剂量
预防性 LMWH	依诺肝素,40 mg,皮下注射,每日 1 次; 达肝素,5 000 U,皮下注射,每日 1 次
中等剂量 LMWH	依诺肝素,40 mg,皮下注射,每日 2 次; 达肝素,5 000 U,皮下注射,每日 2 次
治疗性 LMWH	依诺肝素,1 mg/kg,皮下注射,每日 2 次; 达肝素,200 U/kg,每日 1 次

注:LMWH,低分子肝素;SC,皮下注射。在极端体重的情况下可能需要调整剂量。

有家族史(一级亲属)或有 VTE 病史的女性进行 LMWH 预防。Brenner 等[67]首次发表了支持对有流产史和遗传性易栓症女性进行抗凝治疗的研究结果。在这项前瞻性队列研究中,50 名患有遗传性易栓症的不明原因 RPL 女性接受了抗凝治疗,其中具有单一血栓倾向者使用 40 mg/d 的依诺肝素,而合并血栓形成缺陷的患者则使用 80 mg/d 的依诺肝素。依诺肝素组的活产率(LBR)显著高于未治疗组(75% vs 20%)。此后进行了多项研究,均表明 LMWH 联合或不联合阿司匹林可改善患有 RPL 和遗传性易栓症女性的妊娠结局[68-70]。然而,这些研究都有局限性,如样本量小和研究设计(其中多项研究未进行随机分组)。2010 年,第一项关于阿司匹林联合那屈肝素、单独使用阿司匹林和安慰剂治疗的开放标签随机试验(ALIFE1)在携带遗传性凝血异常(FVL、PT、PC、PS 和 AT)的不明原因 RPL 女性中首次报道[71]。所有研究组的流产率均无差异。在这项研究中,使用阿司匹林和那屈肝素治疗的 123 名女性中,仅有 13 人患有遗传性易栓症;120 名使用阿司匹林的女性中有 17 人;121 名接受安慰剂的女性中有 17 人。因此,这项研究的样本量不足以评估遗传性易栓症的亚组效应[71]。这与 HABENOX Ⅰ 试验[72]类似,该试验由于招募量不足而提前结束。

关于抗凝治疗对患有遗传性易栓症的 RPL 女性的影响,多项观察性研究和随机对照试验(RCT)之间存在差异,可能是由于缺乏揭示上述 RPL 适当的易栓症标志物。此外,即使具有相同的遗传性易栓症,在免疫异常激活的情况下,例如慢性炎症或自身免疫性疾病,血栓形成和胎盘血流减少的风险也可能不同。事实上,即使接受抗凝和免疫调节治疗,

患有易栓症且细胞免疫异常的不明原因RPL女性的LBR也不同于那些没有异常细胞免疫的女性[73]。因此，对于患有遗传性易栓症的女性，应考虑评估可能影响凝血的其他因素，例如免疫异常。

另一个障碍是既往研究的异质性。之前的RCT使用了不同的研究方案。选定的遗传性易栓症标志物、受试者的纳入和排除标准、肝素治疗的开始和持续时间，以及肝素的类型和剂量存在不一致。此外，迄今为止，所有关于遗传性易栓症的RPL女性的随机对照试验仅在西方国家进行[71,72]。由于不同种族之间遗传性易栓症的发生率存在差异，非西方国家的研究可能会呈现不同的结果。为了总结遗传性易栓症在RPL中的作用，需要进一步研究来找到合适的遗传性易栓症及其参考范围。根据结果，可以在适当的亚组中进行抗凝治疗。

7 生殖结局

对于患有遗传性易栓症的RPL女性生殖结局的研究仍然不足。我们先前的报道显示，在抗凝治疗后，患有遗传性易栓症的RPL女性的活产率提高，产科并发症的发生率降低[73,74]。在这些回顾性队列研究中，患有免疫病因和（或）凝血异常的RPL女性根据其潜在病因接受治疗，而对照组则是未经治疗，或在未经免疫学和凝血标志物评估的情况下进行经验性治疗的RPL女性。尽管这不是一项随机对照试验，但最近一项在患有易栓症的不明原因RPL女性中进行的多中心队列研究（OTTILTA）显示，在没有抗凝治疗的情况下，流产风险显著增加（OR，2.9；95% CI，1.4～6.1），而使用低分子肝素（单独使用或与阿司匹林联合使用）的活产率提高（OR，10.6；95% CI，5.0～22.3）[75]。此外，该研究还表明在没有凝血异常的RPL女性中，活产率与LMWH预防性治疗（单独使用或与阿司匹林联合使用）无关。结合我们先前的研究[73,74]，支持在患有遗传性易栓症的RPL女性中采用"基于病因的治疗"。

8 总结和建议

与针对患有APS的RPL女性的治疗方案不同，对于患有遗传性易栓症的RPL女性，尚无足够的抗凝治疗数据[76]。然而，最近基于病因的抗凝治疗研究表明，抗凝治疗对患有遗传性易栓症的RPL女性的妊娠结局具有明显益处。需要进一步研究以找到合适的遗传性易栓症标志物及其参考范围，以及抗凝治疗对患有易栓症的RPL女性（而非所有RPL女性）的临床疗效。

- 当防止产时和围产期过多失血的生理性高凝状态异常加剧时，可能会出现母体血栓栓塞和各种胎盘介导的产科并发症，包括RPL。
- 为育龄期健康女性建立参考范围可能有助于对患有遗传性易栓症的RPL女性进行研究。
- 目前的临床指南建议对VTE家族史（一级亲属）或个人史的孕妇进行预防性抗凝治疗，无论是否有易栓症。
- 尽管由于证据不足，临床指南不建议对患有遗传性易栓症的RPL女性进行抗凝治疗，但最近的研究表明，预防性LMWH抗凝治疗在患有遗传性易栓症的RPL女性具有良好效果。
- LMWH和阿司匹林，作为VTE预防药物，在妊娠前和妊娠期间使用相对安全。

参考文献

[1] Practice Committee of the American Society for Reproductive M. Evaluation and treatment of recurrent pregnancy loss: a committee opinion. Fertil Steril 2012;98(5):1103-11.

[2] ESHRE Guideline Group on RPL, et al. ESHRE guideline: recurrent pregnancy loss. Hum Reprod Open 2018;2018(2):hoy004.

[3] Pritchard AM, Hendrix PW, Paidas MJ. Hereditary thrombophilia and recurrent pregnancy loss. Clin Obstet Gynecol 2016;59(3):487-97.

[4] Adu-Gyamfi EA, Ding YB, Wang YX. Regulation of placentation by the transforming growth factor beta superfamily. Biol Reprod 2020;102(1):18-26.

[5] Bogdanova N, et al. A common haplotype of the annexin A5 (ANXA5) gene promoter is associated with recurrent pregnancy loss. Hum Mol Genet 2007;16(5):573-8.

[6] Tiscia G, et al. Haplotype M2 in the annexin A5 (ANXA5) gene and the occurrence of obstetric complications. Thromb Haemost 2009;102(2):309-13.

[7] Alfaidy N, et al. The emerging role of the prokineticins and homeobox genes in the vascularization of the placenta:

[7] physiological and pathological aspects. Front Physiol 2020;11:591850.
[8] Sugimura M, et al. Intraplacental coagulation in intrauterine growth restriction: cause or result? Semin Thromb Hemost 2001;27(2):107-13.
[9] Khan S, Dickerman JD. Hereditary thrombophilia. Thromb J 2006;4:15.
[10] Arachchillage DRJ, Makris M. Inherited thrombophilia and pregnancy complications: should we test? Semin Thromb Hemost 2019;45(1):50-60.
[11] Alijotas-Reig J, et al. Inherited thrombophilia in women with poor aPL-related obstetric history: prevalence and outcomes. Survey of 208 cases from the European registry on obstetric antiphospholipid syndrome cohort. Am J Reprod Immunol 2016;76(2):164-71.
[12] Stevens SM, et al. Guidance for the evaluation and treatment of hereditary and acquired thrombophilia. J Thromb Thrombolysis 2016;41(1):154-64.
[13] Zhao L, et al. Association between the SERPINE1 (PAI-1) 4G/5G insertion/deletion promoter polymorphism (rs1799889) and pre-eclampsia: a systematic review and meta-analysis. Mol Hum Reprod 2013;19(3):136-43.
[14] Wu X, et al. Folate metabolism gene polymorphisms MTHFR C677T and A1298C and risk for preeclampsia: a meta-analysis. J Assist Reprod Genet 2015;32(5):797-805.
[15] Park CW, et al. The role of methylenetetrahydrofolate reductase C677T polymorphism on the peripheral blood natural killer cell proportion in women with unexplained recurrent miscarriages. Clin Exp Reprod Med 2011;38(3):168-73.
[16] Kim JJ, et al. The PAI-1 4G/5G and ACE I/D polymorphisms and risk of recurrent pregnancy loss: a case-control study. Am J Reprod Immunol 2014;72(6):571-6.
[17] Coulam CB, et al. Multiple thrombophilic gene mutations rather than specific gene mutations are risk factors for recurrent miscarriage. Am J Reprod Immunol 2006;55(5):360-8.
[18] Robertson L, et al. Thrombophilia in pregnancy: a systematic review. Br J Haematol 2006;132(2):171-96.
[19] Rey E, et al. Thrombophilic disorders and fetal loss: a meta-analysis. Lancet 2003;361(9361):901-8.
[20] Sakata T, et al. Prevalence of protein S deficiency in the Japanese general population: the Suita Study. J Thromb Haemost 2004;2(6):1012-3.
[21] Ivanov P, et al. Inherited thrombophilia and IVF failure: the impact of coagulation disorders on implantation process. Am J Reprod Immunol 2012;68(3):189-98.
[22] Hwang KR, et al. Methylenetetrahydrofolate reductase polymorphisms and risk of recurrent pregnancy loss: a case-control study. J Korean Med Sci 2017;32(12):2029-34.
[23] Makino A, et al. No association of C677T methylenetetra-hydrofolate reductase and an endothelial nitric oxide synthase polymorphism with recurrent pregnancy loss. Am J Reprod Immunol 2004;52(1):60-6.
[24] Tait RC, et al. Prevalence of protein C deficiency in the healthy population. Thromb Haemost 1995;73(1):87-93.
[25] Bennett SA, Bagot CN, Arya R. Pregnancy loss and thrombophilia: the elusive link. Br J Haematol 2012;157(5):529-42.
[26] Di Nisio M, et al. Thrombophilia and outcomes of assisted reproduction technologies: a systematic review and meta-analysis. Blood 2011;118(10):2670-8.
[27] Wu X, et al. Association between the MTHFR C677T polymorphism and recurrent pregnancy loss: a meta-analysis. Genet Test Mol Biomarkers 2012;16(7):806-11.
[28] Hansda J, Roychowdhury J. Study of thrombophilia in recurrent pregnancy loss. J Obstet Gynaecol India 2012;62(5):536-40.
[29] Gogineni S, et al. Deep cerebral venous thrombosis-a clinicoradiological study. J Neurosci Rural Pract 2021;12(3):560-5.
[30] Dugalic S, et al. Perinatal complications related to inherited thrombophilia: review of evidence in different regions of the world. J Matern Fetal Neonatal Med 2021;34(15):2567-76.
[31] Jerrard-Dunne P, et al. Ethnic differences in markers of thrombophilia: implications for the investigation of ischemic stroke in multiethnic populations: the South London ethnicity and stroke study. Stroke 2003;34(8):1821-6.
[32] Franchi F, et al. Normal reference ranges of antithrombin, protein C and protein S: effect of sex, age and hormonal status. Thromb Res 2013;132(2):e152-7.
[33] Rodeghiero F, Tosetto A. The VITA project: population-based distributions of protein C, antithrombin III, heparin-cofactor II and plasminogen-relationship with physiological variables and establishment of reference ranges. Thromb Haemost 1996;76(2):226-33.
[34] Gari M, et al. The influence of low protein S plasma levels in young women, on the definition of normal range. Thromb Res 1994;73(2):149-52.
[35] Lanir N, Aharon A, Brenner B. Haemostatic mechanisms in human placenta. Best Pract Res Clin Haematol 2003;16(2):183-95.
[36] Brenner B. Haemostatic changes in pregnancy. Thromb Res 2004;114(5-6):409-14.
[37] Bremme KA. Haemostatic changes in pregnancy. Best Pract Res Clin Haematol 2003;16(2):153-68.
[38] Leaf RK, Connors JM. The role of anticoagulants in the prevention of pregnancy complications. Clin Appl Thromb Hemost 2017;23(2):116-23.
[39] Kamel H, et al. Risk of a thrombotic event after the 6-week postpartum period. N Engl J Med 2014;370(14):1307-15.
[40] Bennett SA, et al. Women with unexplained recurrent pregnancy loss do not have evidence of an underlying prothrombotic state: experience with calibrated automated thrombography and rotational thromboelastometry. Thromb Res 2014;133(5):892-9.
[41] Papadakis E, et al. Low molecular weight heparins use in pregnancy: a practice survey from Greece and a review of the literature. Thromb J 2019;17:23.
[42] American College of, O. and B.-O. Gynecologists' Committee on Practice. ACOG practice bulletin no. 197: inherited thrombophilias in pregnancy. Obstet Gynecol 2018;132(1):e18-34.
[43] Salafia C, et al. Placental and decidual histology in spontaneous abortion: detailed description and correlations with chromosome number. Obstet Gynecol 1993;82(2):295-303.
[44] Arias F, et al. Thrombophilia: a mechanism of disease in women with adverse pregnancy outcome and thrombotic lesions in the placenta. J Matern Fetal Med 1998;7(6):277-86.
[45] Mousa HA, Alfirevic Z. Do placental lesions reflect thrombophilia state in women with adverse pregnancy outcome? Hum Reprod 2000;15(8):1830-3.

[46] Rand JH, et al. Antiphospholipid immunoglobulin G antibodies reduce annexin-V levels on syncytiotrophoblast apical membranes and in culture media of placental villi. Am J Obstet Gynecol 1997;177(4):918-23.

[47] Kuperman A, Di Micco P, Brenner B, et al. Fertility, infertility and thrombophilia. Women's Health (Lond) 2011;7(5):545-53.

[48] Ota K, et al. Effects of MTHFR C677T polymorphism on vitamin D, homocysteine and natural killer cell cytotoxicity in women with recurrent pregnancy losses. Hum Reprod 2020;35(6):1276-87.

[49] Koo HS, et al. Resistance of uterine radial artery blood flow was correlated with peripheral blood NK cell fraction and improved with low molecular weight heparin therapy in women with unexplained recurrent pregnancy loss. Am J Reprod Immunol 2015;73(2):175-84.

[50] Köller M, et al. Influence of low molecular weight heparin (certoparin) and unfractionated heparin on the release of cytokines from human leukocytes. Inflammation 2001;25(5):331-7.

[51] Kharbanda RK, et al. Prevention of inflammation-induced endothelial dysfunction: a novel vasculoprotective action of aspirin. Circulation 2002;105(22):2600-4.

[52] Carp H, et al. Prevalence of genetic markers for thrombophilia in recurrent pregnancy loss. Hum Reprod 2002;17(6):1633-7.

[53] van Dijk MM, et al. Recurrent pregnancy loss: diagnostic workup after two or three pregnancy losses? A systematic review of the literature and meta-analysis. Hum Reprod Update 2020;26(3):356-67.

[54] Yoon SH, et al. No association of p53 codon 72 polymorphism with idiopathic recurrent pregnancy loss in Korean population. Eur J Obstet Gynecol Reprod Biol 2015;192:6-9.

[55] Kim JJ, et al. Prolactin receptor gene polymorphism and the risk of recurrent pregnancy loss: a case-control study. J Obstet Gynaecol 2018;38(2):261-4.

[56] Haemostasis, B. C. f. S. i. H. Thrombosis Task Force, Investigation and management of heritable thrombophilia. Br J Haematol 2001;114(3):512-28.

[57] Smock KJ, et al. Protein S testing in patients with protein S deficiency, factor V Leiden, and rivaroxaban by North American Specialized Coagulation Laboratories. Thromb Haemost 2016;116(1):50-7.

[58] Sala N, Owen WG, Collen D. A functional assay of protein C in human plasma. Blood 1984;63(3):671-5.

[59] Van Cott EM, et al. Recommendations for clinical laboratory testing for antithrombin deficiency: communication from the SSC of the ISTH. J Thromb Haemost 2020;18(1):17-22.

[60] CLSI. Defining, establishing, and verifying reference intervals in the clinical laboratory: approved guideline. CLSI document EP28-A3c. 3rd ed. Wayne, PA: Clinical and Laboratory Standards Institute; 2008.

[61] Undas A, Brummel-Ziedins KE, Mann KG. Antithrombotic properties of aspirin and resistance to aspirin: beyond strictly antiplatelet actions. Blood 2007;109(6):2285-92.

[62] Picot D, Loll PJ, Garavito RM. The X-ray crystal structure of the membrane protein prostaglandin H2 synthase-1. Nature 1994;367(6460):243-9.

[63] Hirsh J, et al. Guide to anticoagulant therapy: Heparin: a statement for healthcare professionals from the American Heart Association. Circulation 2001;103(24):2994-3018.

[64] Nelson SM, Greer IA. The potential role of heparin in assisted conception. Hum Reprod Update 2008;14(6):623-45.

[65] Kim JH, Lim KM, Gwak HS. New anticoagulants for the prevention and treatment of venous thromboembolism. Biomol Ther (Seoul) 2017;25(5):461-70.

[66] Weitz JI. Low-molecular-weight heparins. N Engl J Med 1997;337(10):688-98.

[67] Brenner B, et al. Gestational outcome in thrombophilic women with recurrent pregnancy loss treated by enoxaparin. Thromb Haemost 2000;83(5):693-7.

[68] Carp H, Dolitzky M, Inbal A. Thromboprophylaxis improves the live birth rate in women with consecutive recurrent miscarriages and hereditary thrombophilia. J Thromb Haemost 2003;1(3):433-8.

[69] Brenner B, et al. Efficacy and safety of two doses of enoxaparin in women with thrombophilia and recurrent pregnancy loss: the LIVE-ENOX study. J Thromb Haemost 2005;3(2):227-9.

[70] Folkeringa N, et al. Reduction of high fetal loss rate by anticoagulant treatment during pregnancy in antithrombin, protein C or protein S deficient women. Br J Haematol 2007;136(4):656-61.

[71] Kaandorp SP, et al. Aspirin plus heparin or aspirin alone in women with recurrent miscarriage. N Engl J Med 2010;362(17):1586-96.

[72] Visser J, et al. Thromboprophylaxis for recurrent miscarriage in women with or without thrombophilia. HABENOX: a randomised multicentre trial. Thromb Haemost 2011;105(2):295-301.

[73] Lee SK, et al. Intravenous immunoglobulin G improves pregnancy outcome in women with recurrent pregnancy losses with cellular immune abnormalities. Am J Reprod Immunol 2016;75(1):59-68.

[74] Han AR, et al. Obstetrical outcome of anti-inflammatory and anticoagulation therapy in women with recurrent pregnancy loss or unexplained infertility. Am J Reprod Immunol 2012;68(5):418-27.

[75] Grandone E, et al. Findings from a multicentre, observational study on reproductive outcomes in women with unexplained recurrent pregnancy loss: the OTTILIA registry. Hum Reprod 2021;36(8):2083-90.

[76] Royal College of Obstetricians and Gynaecologists. The Investigation and Treatment of Couples with Recurrent Firsttrimester and Second-trimester Miscarriage (Green-top Guideline No. 17). [cited 2020]. Available from: 〈https://www.rcog.org.uk/globalassets/documents/guidelines/gtg_17.pdf〉;2011.

第 14 章

风湿病与生殖结局

Rheumatic diseases and reproductive outcomes

Brooke Mills and Bonnie L. Bermas

Division of Rheumatic Diseases, University of Texas Southwestern Medical Center, Dallas, TX, United States

1 引言

风湿病主要影响育龄期女性。鉴于风湿病是自身免疫性疾病，而免疫系统在妊娠期间会发生变化，因此风湿病对生育的影响是不可避免的，反之亦然。在本章中，我们将讨论较为常见的风湿病，包括类风湿关节炎(RA)、系统性红斑狼疮(SLE)、系统性硬化症和抗磷脂综合征，以及它们对生育结局的影响。我们还将讨论抗Ro(SSA)和抗La(SSB)抗体在新生儿狼疮(NL)中的作用。

妊娠是免疫耐受的自然试验。母体必须对胎儿表达的父系抗原具有耐受性。这种耐受性是通过胎盘将胎儿与母体分离、胎儿细胞逃避母体免疫系统的识别以及妊娠引起的母体免疫系统的变化而产生的。诺贝尔奖获得者Peter Medawar首次提出，胎儿作为半同种异体移植物，可诱导母体免疫耐受，从而避免妊娠失败[1]。人白细胞抗原(HLA)不匹配是诱导免疫耐受的一个重要因素。事实上，母体与胎儿之间的HLA差异越大，妊娠成功的可能性就越大[2]。在过去的几十年里，生殖免疫学研究纳入了从我们对免疫系统的理解中所获得的知识。例如，在20世纪90年代，科学家描述了两种不同类型的T辅助细胞：辅助性T细胞1(TH1)和辅助性T细胞2(TH2)。他们假设细胞介导的免疫反应由TH1细胞调节，体液免疫反应由TH2细胞调节[3]。Wegmann和Mosman将这一理论应用于对生殖的理解，并提出妊娠是一种TH2现象，其中TH2型细胞因子调节对胎儿的保护，而TH1型细胞因子则会引起妊娠丢失[4]。最新的数据表明，该理论过于简单，TH1、TH2、辅助性T细胞17(TH17)和调节性T细胞(Treg)都参与其中[5]。此外，妊娠成功不太可能是TH2类型转变的结果，而是促炎性细胞因子可溶性拮抗剂的作用[6]。有关细胞因子在妊娠成功中所起作用的研究取得进展的同时，细胞因子还被发现在自身免疫性疾病活动的调节中起关键作用[7]。这些研究结果已经推动了生物药物的开发，从而改变了风湿病的治疗管理方式[8]。有关免疫系统在妊娠成功和风湿病活动中的信息不断涌现，揭示了关于妊娠如何影响风湿病活动以及风湿病如何影响妊娠结局的重要见解。几十年来的临床观察也为这些见解提供了佐证。

2 类风湿关节炎

2.1 定义和患病率

RA是一种典型的慢性炎症性疾病，产生促炎细胞因子，导致引起全身和局部关节炎症。全身性炎症可引起不适和疲劳等症状，还可导致血管炎和炎症性肺病。局部炎症会引起关节滑膜肥厚，导致关节肿胀，进而破坏关节[9]。炎症细胞因子如IL-6和IL-1被认为驱动这一过程[10]。RA在女性中更为常见，患病率约为1%[11]。

2.2 类风湿关节炎影响生殖结局的潜在免疫机制

在胎儿生长阶段，促炎细胞因子IL-6和IL-1的相对下调可改善RA[12]。这与文献报道一致。Hench首次观察到多达70%的RA患者在妊娠期间疾病活动度有所改善[13]。一项系统回顾和荟萃分析发现，60%患有 RA 的孕妇疾病活动度有所改善，46.7%的孕妇在产后病情复发[14]。与疾病改善相关的因素包括不存在类风湿因子或抗瓜氨酸蛋白抗体[15]。研究发现，母体和胎儿间的 HLA 差异与妊娠期疾病活动度减弱有关[16]。此外，还有数据表明，与 RA 发病风险相关的 HLA-DRB1 等位基因可通过母胎交换产生的微嵌合体获得[17]。

2.3 评估

如果出现一个或多个关节肿胀超过 6 周，且无法用其他疾病过程解释，则需评估 RA。应进行类风湿因子和抗环瓜氨酸肽（抗 ccp）抗体的检测，因为在大多数 RA 患者中，这两项检测中的 1 项或 2 项呈阳性，尽管不存在这些自身抗体也不能排除 RA 的诊断。还应检查炎症标志物、红细胞沉降率（ESR）和 C 反应蛋白。如果患者至少有一个关节出现滑膜炎，并且在 4 个项目的评分中达到 6 分，包括受累关节的数量、血清阳性[存在 RF 和（或）抗 ccp]、炎症标志物升高以及症状持续时间至少 6 周，则认为患有 RA（2010 年 ACR/EULAR 标准）[18]。

2.4 治疗

妊娠期 RA 的治疗重点是控制疾病，因为活动性疾病会增加不良妊娠结局的风险。许多（但不是全部）常用于治疗 RA 的药物可以继续使用[19]。这些药物包括羟氯喹、柳氮磺胺吡啶和 TNF-α 抑制剂；后者通常在妊娠晚期停用。非甾体抗炎药（NSAID）可使用至妊娠 20 周，此时发育中的胎儿有发生肾脏问题的风险，可能导致羊水过少[20]。30 周后，非甾体抗炎药会增加动脉导管过早闭合的风险。低剂量阿司匹林没有这些限制，可以在整个妊娠期使用。关于 NSAID 是否会干扰胚胎植入导致早期妊娠丢失，存在相互矛盾的数据[21,22]。其他生物制剂如阿巴西普、托珠单抗和利妥昔单抗可在受孕期间继续使用[19]。目前的数据不足以判定小分子药物（如 JAK 激酶抑制剂）是否适用于妊娠期。甲氨蝶呤和来氟米特不能用于妊娠期，前者具有致畸性，后者的安全性尚不清楚。在受孕前 1～3 个月应停用甲氨蝶呤。来氟米特应在受孕前 2 年停用，或是利用消胆胺将其从母体内清除，直至无法检测到。疾病发作时，应尽量使用非氟化的糖皮质激素，并尽可能低剂量使用，因为这些药物可导致妊娠期高血压、糖尿病，以及小于胎龄儿和未足月胎膜早破[19]。

2.5 生殖结局

据报道，与分娩后诊断 RA 的患者相比，在分娩前诊断出 RA 的家庭较少[23]。其原因是多因素的，包括由于疾病活动而延迟尝试受孕，担心照顾孩子的能力，以及需要更长的时间来实现妊娠[24]。关于 RA 患者不孕风险的数据存在矛盾。虽然报道有 42%的 RA 患者不孕，但原因尚不清楚。研究表明，通过抗苗勒管激素测定，她们的卵巢储备功能正常[25,26]。罹患 RA 的女性发生其他不良妊娠结局的风险更高，包括子痫前期、早产、小于胎龄儿和更高的剖宫产率[27,28]。子痫前期发病率的增加，特别是在疾病活动度高的女性中，尤为有趣，这是因为肿瘤坏死因子-α 和 IL-6 水平在 RA 疾病活动期和子痫前期中均有所升高[29]。

3 系统性红斑狼疮

3.1 定义和患病率

SLE 是一种多器官系统性疾病，主要影响育龄期女性。全球约有千分之一的人受累，非洲血统、亚洲种族和西班牙裔女性的患病率较高。SLE 可表现为轻度，患者出现轻度皮疹、关节疼痛和良性细胞减少；也可能具有与高发病率和死亡率相关的重度表现，如肾脏、肺、神经和心血管系统的广泛器官受累[30]。

3.2 系统性红斑狼疮影响生殖结局的潜在免疫机制

妊娠期间从促炎状态转变为抗炎抗体介导的状态可能会增加抗体介导疾病（如 SLE）的疾病活动度。此外，妊娠期间的激素变化也可能诱发 SLE[31]。事实上，一些患有狼疮的女性在妊娠期间会出现疾病发作[32]。此外，患有狼疮的女性更易发生子痫前期。其潜在机制尚不清楚，但可能与胎盘中的补体沉积以及局部胎盘炎症有关[33]。区分 SLE 发作和子痫前期可能具有挑战性，并且最终的诊断通常仍不清楚。

3.3 评估

育龄期女性出现多器官症状，包括皮疹、血细胞减少、关节炎、浆膜炎、肾脏疾病和神经系统疾病，应评估系统性红斑狼疮。应进行抗核抗体（ANA）检测，1∶80 或更高滴度视为阳性。ANA 检测呈阳性本身并不能诊断 SLE，因为 ANA 可能存在于超过 10% 的人群中。当个体 ANA 阳性并累积满足包括 7 个临床领域（包括全身状况、血液系统、神经精神症状、皮肤黏膜、浆膜腔、肌肉骨骼、肾脏）和 3 个免疫学领域（包括抗磷脂抗体、补体成分和 SLE 特异性抗体）在内的加权标准 ≥10 分时（译者注：欧洲抗风湿病联盟/美国风湿病学会的 SLE 诊断标准），即可被诊断为 SLE。临床和免疫学领域的组合是必要的[34]。

3.4 孕期治疗

SLE 患者妊娠管理的首要原则是疾病控制。患者在尝试妊娠的前几个月应处于病情缓解状态或疾病活动度较低，因为妊娠时的活动性疾病预示着不良妊娠结局。此外，曾患有系统性红斑狼疮肾病的患者在妊娠期间更易发作[35]。所有 SLE 患者在妊娠期间都应该服用羟氯喹，该药已被证明可降低子痫前期的风险，并改善妊娠结局[36]。对于妊娠期的复燃，可使用非氟化的糖皮质激素；然而，临床医生应尽可能开具最低剂量的处方，因为糖皮质激素会导致妊娠期高血压和妊娠期糖尿病，以及小于胎龄儿和胎膜早破。免疫抑制剂，如硫唑嘌呤、环孢菌素和他克莫司，可用于治疗复燃，或在尝试妊娠前作为过渡药物。霉酚酸酯和环磷酰胺具有致畸性，不适用于妊娠期[37]。

3.5 生殖结局

SLE 女性的原发性生育能力似乎没有受损。既往接受过环磷酰胺治疗的患者可能因药物诱导的卵巢早衰而导致不孕。继发性不孕是由于抗磷脂抗体的存在（见下文）。这些抗体在 SLE 患者中很常见。SLE 患者发生子痫前期的风险更高，胎儿死亡率也更高。小于胎龄儿和胎膜早破常见于 SLE 患者；然而，从疾病活动中剖析出药物使用的影响是具有挑战性的。

4 系统性硬化症

4.1 定义和患病率

系统性硬化症（SSc）是一种罕见的异质性自身免疫性疾病，其特征是皮肤和内脏的血管病变和进行性纤维化[38]。SSc 的年发病率为每百万成年人 10~20 例。SSc 的患病率因性别、地理区域和种族而异。在女性中的流行率是男性的 4 倍多。SSc 可发生在任何年龄，发病高峰年龄为 35~65 岁[39]。

4.2 系统性硬化症影响生殖结局的潜在免疫机制

患有 SSc 的女性在全身性疾病发病前流产率增加。据推测，这部分是由于母胎微嵌合体[40]。微嵌合体被定义为来自一个个体的细胞存在于基因不同的另一个体中。微嵌合体最常见的来源是妊娠期间的母胎细胞交换，包括妊娠失败和终止妊娠。在分娩后的健康女性中发现了胎儿来源的可存活的免疫干细胞，并发现 SSc 患者比健康对照者有更多的循环胎儿细胞[41]。一些综述将 SSc 的发展归因于对这些持续存在的胎儿细胞缺乏免疫耐受，类似于移植物抗宿主病[42]。这在一定程度上解释了 SSc 患病率增加的原因，特别是在女性和生育后。但是，未生育的女性也可能患有 SSc。因此，可能存在遗传和环境因素，在未来 SSc 的发展中起到一定作用。

4.3 评估

对于有手指皮肤增厚表现的患者，应由风湿病或皮肤科医生评估其是否患有系统性硬化症。该疾病的诊断是临床性的，并且需要存在雷诺现象的相关特征、特征性的指甲褶皱改变、钙质沉积、毛细血管扩张和胃灼热等症状来支持。应进行基本的肾功能和肺功能检查。抗着丝点抗体和抗 scl‑70 抗体分别提示局限性系统性硬化症和弥漫性系统性硬化症，但即便没有这些抗体的存在，只要有临床特征，也可做出诊断；反之，如果没有临床特征，仅这些抗体的存在并不能确诊该疾病[43]。

4.4 治疗方式

目前尚无关于 SSc 和妊娠的正式治疗指南。常用于治疗 SSc 皮肤硬化的药物，如甲氨蝶呤和霉酚酸酯，在妊娠期是禁用的。SSc 通常与 APS 和干燥综合征重叠；因此，应对 SSc 患者进行抗磷脂抗体和 SSA 抗体的检测。如果这些检测呈阳性，患者应分别开始服用羟氯喹和（或）低剂量阿司匹林[19]。

4.5 生殖结局

关于 SSc 与妊娠的数据很少，因为这是一种罕见疾病，其发病高峰期处于生育年龄末段。2020 年的一项荟萃分析发现,系统性硬化症患者的流产率明显高于健康对照组[44]。然而,过去的小型综述并未发现 SSc 患者的妊娠丢失率增加。研究还表明,患者在发病前妊娠丢失的风险增加[45]。系统性硬化症患者易患肺动脉高压(pulmonary artery hypertension,PAH),需要在妊娠前对此进行监测。虽然 PAH 是妊娠的相对禁忌证,但最近的数据表明,患有 PAH 的女性妊娠结局比此前认为的要好[46]。然而,病情稳定的患者可以顺利妊娠,并有良好的母婴结局。从关于妊娠和 SSc 有限的文献中发现,这些患者的流产(为健康对照组的 1.6 倍)、宫内生长受限和早产的风险增加[44]。

5 抗磷脂综合征

5.1 定义和患病率

抗磷脂综合征(APS)是一种自身免疫性疾病,其特征是在抗磷脂抗体(APL)持续阳性存在的情况下出现血栓形成和(或)妊娠并发症。APL 包括狼疮抗凝物、抗 β2-糖蛋白 1 抗体和抗心磷脂抗体。产科 APS 是指在相隔 12 周两次检查发现 APL 阳性,并伴有以下情况之一:3 次或 3 次以上在妊娠 10 周前发生反复妊娠丢失;1 次或多次在妊娠 10 周后发生妊娠丢失,且产前超声检查胎儿解剖结构正常;妊娠 34 周前由重度子痫前期、子痫或与胎盘功能不全导致的 1 次或多次早产,新生儿形态正常[47]。APS 可作为一种孤立性疾病发生,也可作为其他系统性疾病的表现,其中最常见的是 SLE。据报道,APS 的患病率为每 10 万人中 2~50 人[48]。约 35%的 APS 病例伴有 SLE[49]。在反复妊娠丢失患者中,APL 阳性的发病率是正常妊娠者的 3 倍[50]。

5.2 与生殖相关的潜在免疫病理学

APS 发生反复妊娠丢失的机制尚不完全清楚,可能是多因素的。APL 阳性患者的胎盘组织病理学显示存在胎盘梗死、螺旋动脉重塑受损、蜕膜炎症、合体结节增多、血管合体膜减少和补体沉积,但胎盘很少出现血管内凝血的证据[51]。炎症在 APS 反复妊娠丢失中比血栓形成起到更大的作用。抗磷脂抗体直接靶向滋养层和蜕膜细胞,导致补体激活和滋养细胞凋亡[52]。滋养细胞无法充分重塑螺旋动脉,这可能导致子痫前期、宫内生长受限和死胎[53]。由于上述因素,反复妊娠丢失被认为与胎盘形成缺陷有关。胎盘功能不全的表现包括胎儿监护异常、多普勒波形异常、羊水过少和出生体重低于第 10 百分位。

在 APS 中可见过量的中性粒细胞胞外诱捕网(NET),并在 APS 发病机制中发挥作用[50,54]。NET 的存在导致促炎状态,随后内皮功能障碍,以及胎盘绒毛间间隙出现 NET。NET 与蜕膜坏死、母体血管炎、母胎界面出血和血栓性血管病变有关[55]。

5.3 评估

对于有不明原因或诱发性血栓事件史、反复的早期妊娠丢失、妊娠中期流产或死胎史的女性,应进行 APL 评估。检查狼疮抗凝血、抗 β2-糖蛋白 1 抗体和抗心磷脂抗体。如果其中任何一项呈阳性,应在 12 周后复查以确诊。

5.4 妊娠期抗磷脂综合征的治疗

在考虑妊娠期间是否需要预防性抗凝或抗血小板治疗时,需要考虑三种情况:APL 阳性但无产科 APS 或血栓病史的患者、产科 APS 但无血栓病史的患者,以及有 APS 和血栓病史的患者[56]。这三组患者的初级血栓预防和治疗有所不同,概述如下。

5.4.1 无症状抗磷脂抗体阳性

APL 阳性的无症状患者通常无须预防性抗凝治疗以预防血栓形成。2007 年的一项随机、双盲安慰剂对照试验显示,接受低剂量阿司匹林治疗的无症状 APL 阳性患者与接受安慰剂治疗的患者之间的血栓形成率没有差异[57]。然而,APL 的存在是子痫前期的一个独立危险因素。有重要证据表明,低剂量阿司匹林有益于预防子痫前期[58]。因此,美国风湿病学会有条件建议该类患者服用低剂量阿司匹林以预防子痫前期[56]。

观察性研究表明,羟氯喹可能对 SLE 及合并 APL 患者的血栓形成具有保护作用[59,60]。然而,目前尚不清楚在没有相关 SLE 诊断的情况下,羟氯喹是否能有效预防 APL 阳性患者的血栓形成。由于患者招募率低,羟氯喹价格上涨和短缺,为研究这一假设而进行的唯一随机对照试验提前终止[54,61]。目前,不建议使用羟氯喹作为该患者群体血栓形成的一级预防[56]。

5.4.2 产科抗磷脂综合征

对于符合产科 APS 标准的患者,美国风湿病学会强烈建议联合使用低剂量阿司匹林和预防性低分子量肝素（LMWH）直至产后 6~12 周[56]。与单独使用低剂量阿司匹林相比，该组合已被证明可以提高反复妊娠丢失患者的活产数[62]。

除标准疗法外，静脉注射免疫球蛋白（IVIG）、羟氯喹、普伐他汀和强的松也已用于治疗难治性 APS[63]。强的松可提高产科 APS 患者的活产率。然而，其与早产和子痫前期发生率增加有关，因此不推荐用于产科 APS 的治疗[64]。没有足够的数据支持在难治性产科 APS 中使用 IVIG 和普伐他汀，目前不推荐使用这些治疗方法[56,63]。两项回顾性研究（其中一项排除了 SLE 患者）表明，羟氯喹可能有益于提高难治性产科 APS 的活产率，目前推荐用于产科 APS 患者[56,65,66]。

5.4.3 血栓性抗磷脂综合征

对于有 APS 血栓形成史的孕妇，除了低剂量阿司匹林外，建议使用肝素进行治疗性抗凝治疗[56]。除抗凝作用外，肝素还具有抗炎和抗补体特性，使其能够有效治疗妊娠期 APS。由于前述原因，也建议该组患者在妊娠期间接受羟氯喹治疗。

5.4.4 其他注意事项

尽管有关于妊娠期 APS 治疗的一般指南，但许多患者有特殊的情况需要考虑。APL 滴度的数量和水平具有不同的风险。高滴度 APL 三重阳性患者的临床结局比 APL 单阳性或双阳性患者差[63]。对于不完全符合产科 APS 标准的 APL 三重阳性患者，应在个体化基础上决定使用预防性肝素治疗。

对于计划通过辅助生殖技术（ART）妊娠的患者，由于她们会暴露于激素治疗（如雌激素），会增加血栓形成的风险。建议对接受 ART 的 APL 阳性患者进行预防性低分子肝素治疗，无论其是否符合产科 APS 标准[56]。

5.5 生殖结局

APS 妊娠并发症包括反复的早期妊娠丢失、胎儿死亡以及可能导致子痫前期、子痫和宫内生长受限的胎盘功能不全。狼疮抗凝物和 APL 三重阳性的存在与不良妊娠结局有关[67,68]。在一项多中心回顾性队列研究（PREGNANTS）中，尽管使用了预防性肝素和低剂量阿司匹林[68]，但只有 30% 的 APL 三重阳性患者最终活产。适当的药物治疗可改善 APS 患者的生殖结局。然而，APS 仍与显著的妊娠并发症相关。此外，20%~30% 的患者出现治疗失败[69]。需要更多的研究来确定其他治疗方法。

6 新生儿狼疮

6.1 定义和患病率

NL 发生于抗体从母体被动转移到发育中的胎儿。大多数病例涉及抗 Ro/SSA 和抗 La/SSB，NL 也可由抗 RNP 抗体引起[70]。这些抗体出现在各种风湿性疾病中，包括干燥综合征、类风湿关节炎和 SLE。在 0.2%~0.86% 的人群中，它们也可能在没有已知风湿病诊断的情况下存在[71,72]。上述抗体通常出现在没有风湿病诊断的 NL 受累患儿的母亲体内；然而，这些无症状母亲中有一半最终会发展为风湿病[73]。NL 的表现包括皮肤和（或）心脏表现。皮肤 NL 发生在约 10% 的抗 Ro 和（或）抗 La 阳性母亲所生的儿童中。婴儿表现为光敏性皮疹，可伴有肝酶升高和血小板减少症。这些症状可在 6 月龄时消退[74]。心脏 NL 的发生率约为 1:15 000 活产婴儿，并出现在 1%~2% Ro/La 抗体阳性患者的妊娠中[75]。先天性完全性心脏传导阻滞（CCHB）在随后妊娠中的复发率约为 18%[76]。胎儿在妊娠 18 周至 25 周之间会出现Ⅰ度、Ⅱ度或Ⅲ度心脏传导阻滞。在Ⅲ度心脏传导阻滞中，心房和心室之间没有传导。患有这种疾病的婴儿在出生时可能需要起搏器[77]。

6.2 与生殖结局相关的潜在免疫机制

在皮肤 NL 中，暴露于紫外线下会释放新生儿皮肤中的抗原，这些抗原与循环中的抗 Ro/SSA 和抗 La/SSB 抗体发生反应，导致皮疹[74]。在发生 CCHB 时，抗 Ro 和抗 La 抗体穿过胎盘，结合胎儿心脏细胞上表达的 SSA/Ro 和 SSB/La 抗原，释放促炎细胞因子，导致发育中的胎儿心脏组织损伤和房室结纤维化[78]。

6.3 评估

若有可能，患有 SLE、RA 和干燥综合征的女性应在妊娠前检查抗 Ro/SSA 和抗 La/SSB 抗体。对于没有已知风湿病诊断的孕妇，如果胎儿或子代患有 CCHB，应检查这些抗体，如果呈阳性，应进行风湿病评估。抗体阳性的患者需要在 16~26 周进行胎儿超声心动图以评估 CCHB。

6.4 治疗方式

不幸的是，逆转心脏传导阻滞的治疗方法仍令人失望。虽然使用大剂量地塞米松和 IVIG 的病例报道显示了Ⅱ度心脏传导阻滞的逆转,但随机对照研究没有阳性结果[79,80]。最新的数据表明,羟氯喹可以降低这种疾病的发病率,尤其是作为二级预防[81]。

6.5 生殖结局

母体存在抗 Ro 和抗 La 抗体的妊娠中有 10% 会发生新生儿皮肤狼疮,1%～2% 发生 CCHB。当 CCHB 发生时,胎儿死亡的概率为 17%[82]。在有一个罹患 CCHB 孩子的女性中,她们下一个孩子有 18% 的风险会发生 CCHB。

7 结论

风湿病在育龄期女性中很常见。疾病的活动度可受妊娠影响,RA 可能会改善,SLE 可能会恶化。总的来说,原发性生育能力似乎不受风湿病的影响,尽管当存在 APL 时,可看到以反复妊娠丢失为表现的继发性不孕。不良妊娠结局在风湿病患者中更为常见,包括子痫前期、胎膜早破和小于胎龄儿的风险更高。在疾病静止期受孕对于改善妊娠结局至关重要。抗 Ro 和抗 La 阳性的女性有 1%～2% 的概率会怀上患有 CCHB 的胎儿,有 5%～10% 的概率生出患有 NL 的孩子。

8 总结和建议

- RA 在妊娠期间趋于改善。
- SLE 在妊娠期间趋于加重。
- 在系统性硬化症诊断前和诊断后,流产率均增加;然而,关于系统性硬化症与妊娠的文献是有限的。
- 无论潜在诊断如何,风湿性疾病的活动度都与不良妊娠结局相关,包括子痫前期、小于胎龄儿和胎膜早破。
- 所有抗磷脂抗体阳性的患者,无论是否诊断为 APS,都应在整个妊娠期服用阿司匹林。
- 产科 APS 患者与血栓性 APS 患者在妊娠期的 APS 治疗不同。
- APL 三重阳性患者的妊娠结局比只有 1 个或 2 个 APL 阳性的患者差。
- 抗 Ro(SSA)和抗 La(SSB)抗体与 NL 相关。
- NL 可表现以皮疹为主要症状的自限性疾病,少部分也可表现为 CCHB。
- 妊娠前,应使用适用于妊娠的药物对风湿性疾病进行良好控制。

参考文献

[1] Deshmukh H, Way SS. Immunological basis for recurrent fetal loss and pregnancy complications. Annu Rev Pathol Mech Dis 2019;14(1):185–210. Available from: https://doi.org/10.1146/annurev-pathmechdis-012418-012743.

[2] Ober C. Current topic: HLA and reproduction: lessons from studies in the Hutterites. Placenta 1995;16(7):569–77. Available from: https://doi.org/10.1016/0143-4004(95)90026-8.

[3] Mosmann TR, Cherwinski H, Bond MW, Giedlin MA, Coffman RL. Two types of murine helper T cell clone. I. Definition according to profiles of lymphokine activities and secreted proteins. J Immunol 1986;136(7):2348–57. Available from: http://www.ncbi.nlm.nih.gov/pubmed/2419430.

[4] Wegmann TG, Lin H, Guilbert L, Mosmann TR. Bidirectional cytokine interactions in the maternal-fetal relationship: is successful pregnancy a TH2 phenomenon? Immunol Today 1993;14(7):353–6. Available from: https://doi.org/10.1016/0167-5699(93)90235-D.

[5] Saito S, Nakashima A, Shima T, Ito M. Th1/Th2/Th17 and regulatory T-Cell paradigm in pregnancy. Am J Reprod Immunol 2010;63(6):601–10. Available from: https://doi.org/10.1111/j.1600-0897.2010.00852.x.

[6] Ostensen M. Cytokines and pregnancy in rheumatic disease. Ann N Y Acad Sci 2006;1069(1):353–63. Available from: https://doi.org/10.1196/annals.1351.033.

[7] Brennan FM, Feldmann M. Cytokines in autoimmunity. Curr Opin Immunol 1992;4(6):754–9. Available from: https://doi.org/10.1016/0952-7915(92)90057-L.

[8] Maini RN, Brennan FM, Williams R, et al. TNF-alpha in rheumatoid arthritis and prospects of anti-TNF therapy. Clin Exp Rheumatol 1993;11(Suppl 8):S173–5. Available from: http://www.ncbi.nlm.nih.gov/pubmed/8391952.

[9] Lee DM, Weinblatt ME. Rheumatoid arthritis. Lancet 2001;358(9285):903–11. Available from: https://doi.org/10.1016/S0140-6736(01)06075-5.

[10] McInnes IB, Schett G. Cytokines in the pathogenesis of rheumatoid arthritis. Nat Rev Immunol 2007;7(6):429–42. Available from: https://doi.org/10.1038/nri2094.

[11] Alamanos Y, Voulgari PV, Drosos AA. Incidence and prevalence of rheumatoid arthritis, based on the 1987 American College of Rheumatology criteria: a systematic review. Semin Arthritis Rheum 2006;36(3):182–8. Available from: https://doi.org/10.1016/j.semarthrit.2006.08.006.

[12] Förger F, Villiger PM. Immunological adaptations in

[13] Hench PS. The amelorating effect of pregnancy on chronic atrophic (infectious, rheumatoid) arthritis, fibrositis, and intermittent hydrarthrosis. Mayo Clin Proc 1938;13:161-7.

[14] Jethwa H, Lam S, Smith C, Giles I. Does rheumatoid arthritis really improve during pregnancy? A systematic review and metaanalysis. J Rheumatol 2019;46(3):245-50. Available from: https://doi.org/10.3899/jrheum.180226.

[15] de Man YA, Bakker-Jonges LE, Goorbergh CMDd, et al. Women with rheumatoid arthritis negative for anticyclic citrullinated peptide and rheumatoid factor are more likely to improve during pregnancy, whereas in autoantibody-positive women autoantibody levels are not influenced by pregnancy. Ann Rheum Dis 2010;69(2):420-3. Available from: https://doi.org/10.1136/ard.2008.104331.

[16] Nelson JL, Hughes KA, Smith AG, Nisperos BB, Branchaud AM, Hansen JA. Remission of rheumatoid arthritis during pregnancy and maternal-fetal class II alloantigen disparity. Am J Reprod Immunol 1992;28(3-4):226-7. Available from: https://doi.org/10.1111/j.1600-0897.1992.tb00798.x.

[17] Yan Z, Aydelotte T, Gadi VK, Guthrie KA, Nelson JL. Acquisition of the rheumatoid arthritis HLA shared epitope through microchimerism. Arthritis Rheum 2011;63(3):640-4. Available from: https://doi.org/10.1002/art.30160.

[18] Aletaha D, Neogi T, Silman AJ, et al. 2010 rheumatoid arthritis classification criteria: an American College of Rheumatology/European League Against Rheumatism collaborative initiative. Ann Rheum Dis 2010;69(9):1580-8. Available from: https://doi.org/10.1136/ard.2010.138461.

[19] Sammaritano LR, Bermas BL, Chakravarty EE, et al. 2020 American College of Rheumatology guideline for the management of reproductive health in rheumatic and musculoskeletal diseases. Arthritis Rheumatol (Hoboken, NJ) 2020;72(4):529-56. Available from: https://doi.org/10.1002/art.41191.

[20] US FDA Drug Safety Communication. FDA recommends avoiding use of NSAIDs in pregnancy at 20 weeks or later because they can result in low amniotic fluid. ⟨https://www.fda.gov/media/142967/download⟩.

[21] Li D-K, Ferber JR, Odouli R, Quesenberry C. Use of nonsteroidal anti-inflammatory drugs during pregnancy and the risk of miscarriage. Am J Obstet Gynecol 2018;219(3):275.e1-8. Available from: https://doi.org/10.1016/j.ajog.2018.06.002.

[22] Edwards DRV, Aldridge T, Baird DD, Funk MJ, Savitz DA, Hartmann KE. Periconceptional over-the-counter nonsteroidal anti-inflammatory drug exposure and risk for spontaneous abortion. Obstet Gynecol 2012;120(1):113-22. Available from: https://doi.org/10.1097/AOG.0b013e3182595671.

[23] Katz PP. Childbearing decisions and family size among women with rheumatoid arthritis. Arthritis Rheum 2006;55(2):217-23. Available from: https://doi.org/10.1002/art.21859.

[24] Jawaheer D, Zhu JL, Nohr EA, Olsen J. Time to pregnancy among women with rheumatoid arthritis. Arthritis Rheum 2011;63(6):1517-21. Available from: https://doi.org/10.1002/art.30327.

[25] Clowse MEB, Chakravarty E, Costenbader KH, Chambers C, Michaud K. Effects of infertility, pregnancy loss, and patient concerns on family size of women with rheumatoid arthritis and systemic lupus erythematosus. Arthritis Care Res (Hoboken) 2012;64(5):668-74. Available from: https://doi.org/10.1002/acr.21593.

[26] Brouwer J, Laven JSE, Hazes JMW, Schipper I, Dolhain RJEM. Levels of serum anti-Müllerian hormone, a marker for ovarian reserve, in women with rheumatoid arthritis. Arthritis Care Res (Hoboken) 2013;65(9):1534-8. Available from: https://doi.org/10.1002/acr.22013.

[27] Aljary H, Czuzoj-Shulman N, Spence AR, Abenhaim HA. Pregnancy outcomes in women with rheumatoid arthritis: a retrospective population-based cohort study. J Matern Fetal Neonatal Med 2020;33(4):618-24. Available from: https://doi.org/10.1080/14767058.2018.1498835.

[28] Chakravarty EF, Nelson L, Krishnan E. Obstetric hospitalizations in the United States for women with systemic lupus erythematosus and rheumatoid arthritis. Arthritis Rheum 2006;54(3):899-907. Available from: https://doi.org/10.1002/art.21663.

[29] Pinheiro MB, Carvalho MG, Martins-Filho OA, et al. Severe preeclampsia: are hemostatic and inflammatory parameters associated? Clin Chim Acta 2014;427:65-70. Available from: https://doi.org/10.1016/j.cca.2013.09.050.

[30] Kiriakidou M, Ching CL. Systemic lupus erythematosus. Ann Intern Med 2020;172(11):ITC81-96. Available from: https://doi.org/10.7326/AITC202006020.

[31] Oktem O, Yagmur H, Bengisu H, Urman B. Reproductive aspects of systemic lupus erythematosus. J Reprod Immunol 2016;117:57-65. Available from: https://doi.org/10.1016/j.jri.2016.07.001.

[32] Ruiz-Irastorza G, Lima F, Alves J, et al. Increased rate of lupus flare during pregnancy and the puerperium: a prospective study of 78 pregnancies. Br J Rheumatol 1996;35(2):133-8. Available from: http://www.ncbi.nlm.nih.gov/pubmed/8612024.

[33] Abramson SB, Buyon JP. Activation of the complement pathway: comparison of normal pregnancy, preeclampsia, and systemic lupus erythematosus during pregnancy. Am J Reprod Immunol 1992;28(3-4):183-7. Available from: https://doi.org/10.1111/j.1600-0897.1992.tb00787.x.

[34] Aringer M, Costenbader K, Daikh D, et al. 2019 European League against rheumatism/American College of Rheumatology classification criteria for systemic lupus erythematosus. Arthritis Rheumatol (Hoboken, NJ) 2019;71(9):1400-12. Available from: https://doi.org/10.1002/art.40930.

[35] Jara LJ, Medina G, Cruz-Dominguez P, Navarro C, Vera-Lastra O, Saavedra MA. Risk factors of systemic lupus erythematosus flares during pregnancy. Immunol Res 2014;60(2-3):184-92. Available from: https://doi.org/10.1007/s12026-014-8577-1.

[36] Clowse MEB, Magder L, Witter F, Petri M. Hydroxychloroquine in lupus pregnancy. Arthritis Rheum 2006;54(11):3640-7. Available from: https://doi.org/10.1002/art.22159.

[37] Andreoli L, Bertsias GK, Agmon-Levin N, et al. EULAR recommendations for women's health and the management of family planning, assisted reproduction, pregnancy and menopause in patients with systemic lupus erythematosus and/or antiphospholipid syndrome. Ann Rheum Dis 2017;76(3):476-85. Available from: https://doi.org/10.1136/annrheumdis-2016-209770.

[38] van den Hoogen F, Khanna D, Fransen J, et al. 2013 classification criteria for systemic sclerosis: an American

College of Rheumatology/European League against rheumatism collaborative initiative. Ann Rheum Dis 2013;72 (11):1747-55. Available from: https://doi.org/10.1136/annrheumdis-2013-204424.

[39] Mayes MD, Lacey JV, Beebe-Dimmer J, et al. Prevalence, incidence, survival, and disease characteristics of systemic sclerosis in a large US population. Arthritis Rheum 2003;48 (8):2246-55. Available from: https://doi.org/10.1002/art.11073.

[40] Abbot S, Bossingham D, Proudman S, de Costa C, Ho-Huynh A. Risk factors for the development of systemic sclerosis: a systematic review of the literature. Rheumatol Adv Pract 2018;2(2). Available from: https://doi.org/10.1093/rap/rky041.

[41] Di Cristofaro J, Karlmark KR, Kanaan SB, et al. Soluble HLA-G expression inversely correlates with fetal microchimerism levels in peripheral blood from women with scleroderma. Front Immunol 2018; 9. Available from: https://doi.org/10.3389/fimmu.2018.01685.

[42] Nelson JL. Maternal-fetal immunology and autoimmune disease. Is some autoimmune disease auto-alloimmune or allo-autoimmune? Arthritis Rheum 1996;39(2):191-4. Available from: https://doi.org/10.1002/art.1780390203.

[43] Poormoghim H, Lucas M, Fertig N, Medsger TA. Systemic sclerosis sine scleroderma: demographic, clinical, and serologic features and survival in forty-eight patients. Arthritis Rheum 2000;43(2):444-51 10.1002/1529-0131 (200002)43:2(444::AID-ANR27)3.0.CO;2-G.

[44] Blagojevic J, AlOdhaibi KA, Aly AM, et al. Pregnancy in systemic sclerosis: results of a systematic review and metaanalysis. J Rheumatol 2020;47(6):881-7. Available from: https://doi.org/10.3899/jrheum.181460.

[45] Silman AJ, Black C. Increased incidence of spontaneous abortion and infertility in women with scleroderma before disease onset: a controlled study. 1988;441-444.

[46] Ekici H, Imamoglu M, Okmen F, Ogultarhan R, Yeniel AO. Pulmonary hypertension in pregnancy: experience from 45 cases at a tertiary care center. J Matern Fetal Neonatal Med 2020;1-6. Available from: https://doi.org/10.1080/14767058.2020.1770216.

[47] Miyakis S, Lockshin MD, Atsumi T, et al. International consensus statement on an update of the classification criteria for definite antiphospholipid syndrome (APS). J Thromb Haemost 2006;4(2):295-306. Available from: https://doi.org/10.1111/j.1538-7836.2006.01753.x.

[48] Duarte-García A, Pham MM, Crowson CS, et al. The epidemiology of antiphospholipid syndrome: a population-based study. Arthritis Rheumatol (Hoboken, NJ) 2019;71 (9):1545-52. Available from: https://doi.org/10.1002/art.40901.

[49] Cervera R, Serrano R, Pons-Estel GJ, et al. Morbidity and mortality in the antiphospholipid syndrome during a 10-year period: a multicentre prospective study of 1000 patients. Ann Rheum Dis 2015;74(6):1011-18. Available from: https://doi.org/10.1136/annrheumdis-2013-204838.

[50] D'Ippolito S, Ticconi C, Tersigni C, et al. The pathogenic role of autoantibodies in recurrent pregnancy loss. Am J Reprod Immunol 2020;83(1). Available from: https://doi.org/10.1111/aji.13200.

[51] Viall CA, Chamley LW. Histopathology in the placentae of women with antiphospholipid antibodies: a systematic review of the literature. Autoimmun Rev 2015;14(5):446-71. Available from: https://doi.org/10.1016/j.autrev.2015.01.008.

[52] Garcia D, Erkan D. Diagnosis and management of the antiphospholipid syndrome. Longo DL, (ed.) N Engl J Med. 2018;378(21):2010-2021. doi:10.1056/NEJMra1705454

[53] Abrahams VM, Chamley LW, Salmon JE. Emerging treatment models in rheumatology: antiphospholipid syndrome and pregnancy: pathogenesis to translation. Arthritis Rheumatol 2017;69(9):1710-21. Available from: https://doi.org/10.1002/art.40136.

[54] Sammaritano LR. Anti-phospholipid syndrome. Best Pract Res Clin Rheumatol 2020;34(1):101463. Available from: https://doi.org/10.1016/j.berh.2019.101463.

[55] Marder W, Knight JS, Kaplan MJ, et al. Placental histology and neutrophil extracellular traps in lupus and preeclampsia pregnancies. Lupus Sci Med 2016;3(1):e000134. Available from: https://doi.org/10.1136/lupus-2015-000134.

[56] Sammaritano LR, Bermas BL, Chakravarty EE, et al. 2020 American College of Rheumatology guideline for the management of reproductive health in rheumatic and musculoskeletal diseases. Arthritis Care Res (Hoboken) 2020; 72(4):461-88. Available from: https://doi.org/10.1002/acr.24130.

[57] Erkan D, Harrison MJ, Levy R, et al. Aspirin for primary thrombosis prevention in the antiphospholipid syndrome: a randomized, double-blind, placebo-controlled trial in asymptomatic antiphospholipid antibody-positive individuals. Arthritis Rheum 2007;56(7):2382-91. Available from: https://doi.org/10.1002/art.22663.

[58] LeFevre ML. Low-dose aspirin use for the prevention of morbidity and mortality from preeclampsia: U.S. preventive services task force recommendation statement. Ann Intern Med 2014;161(11):819. Available from: https://doi.org/10.7326/M14-1884.

[59] Kaiser R, Cleveland CM, Criswell LA. Risk and protective factors for thrombosis in systemic lupus erythematosus: results from a large, multiethnic cohort. Ann Rheum Dis 2009;68 (2):238-41. Available from: https://doi.org/10.1136/ard.2008.093013.

[60] Jung H, Bobba R, Su J, et al. The protective effect of antimalarial drugs on thrombovascular events in systemic lupus erythematosus. Arthritis Rheum 2010;62(3):863-8. Available from: https://doi.org/10.1002/art.27289.

[61] Erkan D, Unlu O, Sciascia S, et al. Hydroxychloroquine in the primary thrombosis prophylaxis of antiphospholipid antibody positive patients without systemic autoimmune disease. Lupus 2018;27(3):399-406. Available from: https://doi.org/10.1177/0961203317724219.

[62] Mak A, Cheung MW-L, Cheak AA, Ho RC-M. Combination of heparin and aspirin is superior to aspirin alone in enhancing live births in patients with recurrent pregnancy loss and positive antiphospholipid antibodies: a meta-analysis of randomized controlled trials and meta-regression. Rheumatology (Oxf) 2010;49(2):281-8. Available from: https://doi.org/10.1093/rheumatology/kep373.

[63] Arslan E, Fellow V, Medicine M, Branch DW, James R, Endowed JS. Best practice & research clinical obstetrics and gynaecology antiphospholipid syndrome: diagnosis and management in the obstetric patient. Best Pract Res Clin Obstet Gynaecol 2020;64:31-40. Available from: https://doi.org/10.1016/j.bpobgyn.2019.10.001.

[64] Cowchock FS, Reece EA, Balaban D, Branch DW, Plouffe

L. Repeated fetal losses associated with antiphospholipid antibodies: a collaborative randomized trial comparing prednisone with low-dose heparin treatment. Am J Obstet Gynecol 1992;166(5):1318 - 23. Available from: http://www.ncbi.nlm.nih.gov/pubmed/1595785.

[65] Sciascia S, Hunt BJ, Talavera-Garcia E, Lliso G, Khamashta MA, Cuadrado MJ. The impact of hydroxychloroquine treatment on pregnancy outcome in women with antiphospholipid antibodies. Am J Obstet Gynecol 2016;214 (2):273.e1 - 8. Available from: https://doi.org/10.1016/j.ajog.2015.09.078.

[66] Mekinian A, Lazzaroni MG, Kuzenko A, et al. The efficacy of hydroxychloroquine for obstetrical outcome in antiphospholipid syndrome: Data from a European multicenter retrospective study. Autoimmun Rev 2015;14(6):498 - 502. Available from: https://doi.org/10.1016/j.autrev.2015.01.012.

[67] Lockshin MD, Kim M, Laskin CA, et al. Prediction of adverse pregnancy outcome by the presence of lupus anticoagulant, but not anticardiolipin antibody, in patients with antiphospholipid antibodies. Arthritis Rheum 2012;64(7):2311 - 18. Available from: https://doi.org/10.1002/art.34402.

[68] Saccone G, Berghella V, Maruotti GM, et al. Antiphospholipid antibody profile based obstetric outcomes of primary anti-phospholipid syndrome: the PREGNANTS study. Am J Obstet Gynecol 2017;216(5):525.e1 - 525.e12. Available from: https://doi.org/10.1016/j.ajog.2017.01.026.

[69] Schreiber K, Hunt BJ. Managing antiphospholipid syndrome in pregnancy. Thromb Res 2019;181;S41 - 6. Available from: https://doi.org/10.1016/S0049-3848(19)30366-4.

[70] Izmirly PM, Rivera TL, Buyon JP. Neonatal lupus syndromes. Rheum Dis Clin North Am 2007;33(2):267 - 85. Available from: https://doi.org/10.1016/j.rdc.2007.02.005.

[71] Fritzler MJ, Pauls JD, Kinsella TD, Bowen TJ. Antinuclear, anticytoplasmic, and anti-Sjogren's syndrome antigen A (SS-A/Ro) antibodies in female blood donors. Clin Immunol Immunopathol 1985;36(1):120 - 8. Available from: https://doi.org/10.1016/0090-1229(85)90045-5.

[72] Satoh M, Chan EKL, Ho LA, et al. Prevalence and sociodemographic correlates of anti-nuclear antibodies in the United States. Arthritis Rheum 2012; 64(7): 2319 - 27. Available from: https://doi.org/10.1002/art.34380.

[73] Rivera TL, Izmirly PM, Birnbaum BK, et al. Disease progression in mothers of children enrolled in the research registry for neonatal lupus. Ann Rheum Dis 2009;68(6):828 - 35. Available from: https://doi.org/10.1136/ard.2008.088054.

[74] Neiman AR, Lee LA, Weston WL, Buyon JP. Cutaneous manifestations of neonatal lupus without heart block: characteristics of mothers and children enrolled in a national registry. J Pediatr 2000;137(5):674 - 80. Available from: https://doi.org/10.1067/mpd.2000.109108.

[75] Brucato A, Frassi M, Franceschini F, et al. Risk of congenital complete heart block in newborns of mothers with anti-Ro/SSA antibodies detected by counterimmunoelectrophoresis: a prospective study of 100 women. Arthritis Rheum 2001;44(8):1832 - 5. Available from: https://doi.org/10.1002/1529-0131(200108)44:8〈1832::AID-ART320〉3.0.CO;2-C.

[76] Llanos C, Izmirly PM, Katholi M, et al. Recurrence rates of cardiac manifestations associated with neonatal lupus and maternal/fetal risk factors. Arthritis Rheum 2009;60(10):3091 - 7. Available from: https://doi.org/10.1002/art.24768.

[77] Waltuck J, Buyon JP. Autoantibody-associated congenital heart block: outcome in mothers and children. Ann Intern Med 1994;120(7):544 - 51. Available from: https://doi.org/10.7326/0003-4819-120-7-199404010-00003.

[78] Miranda-Carús ME, Askanase AD, Clancy RM, et al. Anti-SSA/Ro and anti-SSB/La autoantibodies bind the surface of apoptotic fetal cardiocytes and promote secretion of TNF-alpha by macrophages. J Immunol 2000;165(9):5345 - 51. Available from: https://doi.org/10.4049/jimmunol.165.9.5345.

[79] Jaeggi ET, Fouron J-C, Silverman ED, Ryan G, Smallhorn J, Hornberger LK. Transplacental fetal treatment improves the outcome of prenatally diagnosed complete atrioventricular block without structural heart disease. Circulation 2004;110(12):1542 - 8. Available from: https://doi.org/10.1161/01.CIR.0000142046.58632.3A.

[80] Eliasson H, Sonesson S-E, Sharland G, et al. Isolated atrioventricular block in the fetus: a retrospective, multi-national, multicenter study of 175 patients. Circulation 2011;124(18):1919 - 26. Available from: https://doi.org/10.1161/CIRCULATIONAHA.111.041970.

[81] Barsalou J, Costedoat-Chalumeau N, Berhanu A, et al. Effect of in utero hydroxychloroquine exposure on the development of cutaneous neonatal lupus erythematosus. Ann Rheum Dis 2018;77(12):1742 - 9. Available from: https://doi.org/10.1136/annrheumdis-2018-213718.

[82] Izmirly PM, Saxena A, Kim MY, et al. Maternal and fetal factors associated with mortality and morbidity in a multi-racial/ethnic registry of anti-SSA/Ro-associated cardiac neonatal lupus. Circulation 2011;124(18):1927 - 35. Available from: https://doi.org/10.1161/CIRCULATIONAHA.111.033894.

第 3 篇

反复种植失败

Repeated implantation failures

第 15 章

生殖免疫学在反复妊娠丢失和反复种植失败中的作用

The role of reproductive immunology in recurrent pregnancy loss and repeated implantation failure

Jenny S. George, Roisin Mortimer and Raymond M. Anchan

Center for Infertility and Reproductive Surgery, Brigham and Women's Hospital, Harvard Medical School, Boston, MA, United States

1 引言

尽管临床上有15%~25%的妊娠发生流产,但只有1%~5%的流产可归因于反复妊娠丢失(RPL)。PRL是一个特殊的疾病,定义为两次或更多次的临床妊娠丢失。绝大多数偶发流产是由于染色体的错误分离,导致三倍体、单倍体和多倍体[1]。尽管通过全面的评估,仍有50%的RPL病因不明。随着植入前遗传学检测(PGT-A)和单基因病检测(PGT-M)的出现,现在有机会筛选并选择没有特定突变的染色体核型正常的胚胎。虽然优先移植了染色体核型正常的胚胎,但某些患者仍会经历反复种植失败(RIF)。RIF被定义为高质量胚胎三次移植失败[2]。管理这些患者在临床上具有挑战性,因为这些妊娠丢失和种植失败的潜在病因尚不明确。近年来,多个生殖免疫学研究组发现免疫调节在成功植入和妊娠结局方面具有核心作用。在本章中,我们将回顾在不明原因RPL和染色体核型正常胚胎移植后仍发生RIF的患者中进行全面生殖免疫学评估的作用。根据当前的文献,我们提出由生殖内分泌学家和生殖免疫学家共同管理RPL和RIF,以帮助患者实现成功的妊娠。

2 定义和术语

妊娠丢失被定义为在孕20周之前自发终止的妊娠[1]。偶发的妊娠丢失很常见,发生在15%~25%的妊娠中[1]。大部分偶发妊娠丢失是由于染色体错误导致的,包括三倍体、单倍体和多倍体。这些染色体错误与母亲年龄增加密切相关。因此,单次临床丢失不一定会在随后的妊娠中增加流产风险,也不意味着是之后流产的复发病因。相反,RPL是一种以3次或更多次临床妊娠丢失为流行病学定义的疾病[1],通过妊娠早期超声或子宫内膜病理见绒毛的存在得以证实。因此,该定义不包括异位妊娠、葡萄胎妊娠和种植失败[3]。此外,需要注意的是,3次或3次以上妊娠丢失的阈值仅适用于流行病学研究,而在早期妊娠2次丢失后就应进行临床评估[3,4]。RPL可以进一步分为原发性和继发性RPL:原发性RPL是指从未有活产史的患者,而继发性RPL指的是在反复妊娠丢失之前至少有1次活产的患者。

相比之下,RIF的定义仍存争议。在一项使用了不同RIF定义的系统回顾中,Polanski等将RIF定义为一种在体外受精(IVF)或卵胞浆内单精子注射(ICSI)周期中反复失败的医源性疾病。他们提出"前3次IVF胚胎移植失败"作为RIF最常见的定义。一小部分临床医生认为必须考虑移植胚胎的数量和质量[5],而其他人则提出了严格的诊断标准,将RIF定义为40岁以下在至少3个新鲜或冷冻周期中移植≥4个优质胚胎仍失败[6]。由于缺乏定义为"优质"胚胎的标准,进一步增加了定义RIF的复杂性。在一项新发表的研究中，Ata 等阐释了女性年龄和预期的胚胎整倍体率对累积种植率的影响，认为 RIF 应该是一个指导进一步管理的功能术语[7]。研究表明，当移植胚胎的整倍体状态未知时，必须移植至少 7 个囊胚，才能获得 95% 的累积概率以种植至少 1 个胚胎。因此，作者提出，RIF 应该是种植失败的一个术语，它不太可能是由胚胎非整倍体引起，而胚胎非整倍数体是种植失败的主要原因。

3 患病率

RPL 的患病率被定义为在特定时间点，人群中经历了 3 次或更多次临床妊娠丢失的患者数量。RPL 的患病率较低，只有不到 5% 的患者经历了 2 次连续的流产，不足 1% 的患者经历了 3 次或更多次的流产[8,9]。在一项回顾性研究中，Rasmark 等[10]利用瑞典国家患者登记提供的数据，展示了 2003 年 18~42 岁女性中 RPL 的平均发病率为每 10 万人 42 例（0.042%）；值得注意的是，到 2012 年，平均发病率上升到每 10 万人 73 例（0.073%）。作者推测，RPL 发病率显著上升可能是由多种因素引起的，包括母亲年龄增长、环境因素和免疫影响。

与 RPL 相比，RIF 的发病率和患病率难以阐明，因为 RIF 仍是一个没有统一明确定义的重要临床疾病。在一项旨在研究 RIF 真实患病率的回顾性队列研究中，Pirtea 等[11]评估了具有正常子宫解剖结构的女性（$n=4\,429$），她们进行了最多 3 次连续的冷冻胚胎移植，均为染色体核型正常的单胚胎移植。作者发现真实的 RIF 发病率很低，如果连续移植了 3 个染色体核型正常的胚胎，不到 5% 的患者无法实现临床妊娠。

4 与生殖相关的免疫病理

女性生殖道由卵巢、输卵管、子宫、宫颈和阴道组成，在妊娠和非妊娠状态下都有独特的免疫调节要求[12]。在非妊娠状态下，生殖道上皮细胞调节黏膜免疫，保护组织免受微生物感染和由此产生的炎症。与生殖道上皮细胞相比，卵巢利用巨噬细胞来协调月经周期：卵巢巨噬细胞促进细微的炎症反应，促使排卵和黄体溶解。此外，巨噬细胞分泌生长因子，促进血管生成和细胞增殖，并吞噬卵泡闭锁后凋亡的颗粒细胞和黄体细胞[13]。显然，巨噬细胞对于卵巢免疫至关重要，因为卵巢巨噬细胞的紊乱和失调已被认为与多囊卵巢综合征[14]、卵巢早衰[13]和子宫内膜异位症[15]有关。

在妊娠期间，适应性和固有免疫系统需经历广泛的调整，以确保胎儿和胎盘组织不会被排斥为"外来"实体。通过与滋养细胞进行交叉信号传递，子宫自然杀伤细胞（uNK）下调其自身细胞毒活性，有效为胎儿和胎盘创造免疫抑制环境。uNK 细胞在早孕期的蜕膜内达到峰值，然后在妊娠过程中逐渐减少，至分娩时仅少量存在[16]。作为胎盘内主要的免疫细胞，uNK 细胞占胎盘炎症细胞的 75%，对于促进滋养层对蜕膜和螺旋动脉的侵袭、血管生成以及抑制巨噬细胞和 T 细胞等具有重要作用[17]。

蜕膜巨噬细胞占蜕膜粒细胞的 15%，可分为 M2 型（与免疫调节和组织重塑有关）或 M1 型（促炎性）[18]。大部分蜕膜巨噬细胞属于 M2 型，旨在通过产生抗炎细胞因子、发挥吞噬作用和分泌血管生成因子来减少炎症[17]。蜕膜巨噬细胞对于正常的生殖功能和妊娠也至关重要，因为它们具有吞噬凋亡滋养细胞的功能[12]。虽然这些凋亡细胞通常出现在发育胎盘中，但凋亡的滋养细胞可能会被识别为外来组织，从而引起强烈的母体免疫反应[19]。蜕膜巨噬细胞通过吞噬凋亡细胞、阻止促炎物质释放以防止这种反应。

5 评估

评估者面临的主要挑战是区分偶发流产与 RPL。在考虑评估对象时，需要注意 3 次或 3 次以上妊娠丢失的阈值仅适用于评估 RPL 的流行病学研究，而在临床上，妊娠早期 2 次流产后就需进行评估[3,4]。对 RPL 的评估可以根据潜在病因进行分类：染色体异常、解剖异常、抗磷脂综合征（APLAS）、激素紊乱、同种免疫异常、环境因素和感染（表 15.1）。然而，全面评估仍未能对高达 50% 的 RPL 患者做出诊断。

5.1 细胞遗传学异常

遗传异常是早期妊娠丢失的最常见原因，在高达 60% 的流产物中检测出零星的核型异常。具体而言，在 RPL 队列中，29%~46% 的流产是由非整倍体引起的[20]，而这个风险随着流产次数的增加而减少[21]。非整倍体的风险随着母亲年龄的增加而

表 15.1 反复妊娠丢失的潜在病因

病因	对 PRL 的影响	评估
细胞遗传	2%～5%	平衡易位 流产组织分子遗传检测(核型、微阵列分析)
抗磷脂综合征	8%～42%	狼疮抗凝物、抗心磷脂 IgG 或 IgM 抗体、抗β2糖蛋白Ⅰ IgG 或 IgM
解剖结构	1.8%～37.6%	碘油造影，子宫输卵管超声造影，磁共振成像，宫腔镜
内分泌和代谢	17%～20%	TSH、泌乳素、HbA1c、卵巢储备功能检测
同种免疫和细胞免疫	20%	外周和子宫 NK 细胞比例、NK 细胞毒性、细胞因子谱、辅助 T 细胞比例、封闭抗体、HLA 分型、抗配偶淋巴细胞抗体
环境	—	病史
感染	0.5%～5%	细菌性阴道炎的分泌物培养、宫颈分泌物培养、PCR 检测子宫内膜微生物基因
血栓形成倾向	40%～50%	凝血因子 Ⅴ Leiden 突变、凝血因子 Ⅱ (凝血酶原)基因突变、高同型半胱氨酸症、活化蛋白 C 抵抗和蛋白 S 缺乏
不明原因	高达 50%	

注：改编自 Practice Committee of the American Society for Reproductive Medicine, Evaluation and treatment of recurrent pregnancy loss: a committee opinion. Fertil Steil. 2012;98(5):1103-11。

增加[1]，这被认为是整个人群和 RPL 患者未来流产的最大单一风险因素[22]。此外，随着流产次数的增加，正常染色体的妊娠丢失风险也增加。因此，在 RPL 病例中应对流产物进行染色体遗传学分析。如果检测到染色体异常，未来的妊娠预后会得到改善[23]。

双亲染色体核型异常的发生频率要低得多，但在评估 RPL 原因时仍需考虑这一因素。可以通过对双亲的核型分析来评估，特别是评估是否存在平衡易位或罗伯逊易位，占 RPL 病例的 2%～5%[24]。

5.2 解剖结构异常

子宫解剖异常的患病率在普通人群中约为 6.7%，在不孕症患者中为 7.3%，而在 RPL 患者中则为 12.6%～16.7%[25,26]。子宫解剖异常与妊娠中期的流产密切相关，尽管其与妊娠早期流产的关联性不如与妊娠中晚期流产的关联性那么明确[1]。可能导致 RPL 的先天苗勒管畸形包括纵隔子宫和双角子宫。对纵隔子宫的矫正与 RPL 患者妊娠结局的改善相关[26]。可用于评估子宫畸形的方法包括三维超声、磁共振、子宫输卵管超声造影(HyCoSy)和碘油造影(HSG)。诊断性和治疗性宫腔镜可在带或不带辅助腹腔镜的情况下进行明确诊断并予以治疗。

5.3 抗磷脂综合征

关于 APLAS 分类标准的国际共识已经发布[27]。据报道，有 8%～42% 的 RPL 患者抗磷脂抗体检测结果呈阳性，一般认为该范围在 5%～20%[28]。尽管有很多抗磷脂抗体，但只有狼疮抗凝物、抗心磷脂抗体(IgM 或 IgG)或抗β2糖蛋白Ⅰ(IgM 或 IgG)具有标准化的临床检测方法和足够的证据，用于 RPL 患者的常规筛查。

5.4 激素紊乱

多种激素与 RPL 相关。对甲状腺激素的评估应从 TSH 水平开始。如果 TSH>2.5，则应进行 T_4 检测[29]。糖尿病控制不佳与妊娠丢失有关，可通过检测糖化血红蛋白(HbA1c)水平来诊断[30]。高泌乳素血症与 RPL 相关。下丘脑-垂体-卵巢轴的改变导致卵泡发育不良和(或)黄体功能不足，也与高泌乳素血症相关。在一项研究中，将患有高泌乳素血症的 RRL 患者在妊娠后随机分配到溴隐亭治疗组和无治疗组，治疗组的活产率显著提高(87% vs 52%)[31]。

5.5 凝血异常

对 31 项凝血因子与妊娠丢失的研究进行荟萃

分析发现，凝血因子Ⅴ Leiden突变、凝血因子Ⅱ（凝血酶原）基因突变、活化蛋白C抵抗和蛋白S缺乏与早期和晚期RPL风险显著增加相关[32]。然而，前瞻性研究未能证实这种风险的增加[33,34]。对于有VTE个人病史或显著家族史的患者，建议进行遗传性凝血异常筛查。

6 治疗

6.1 反复妊娠丢失的治疗

对于反复妊娠丢失的患者，临床管理着重于解决潜在的病因。平衡易位和罗伯逊易位在反复妊娠丢失患者中占2%～5%[35]。如果这些患者或其伴侣的外周核型分析发现有平衡易位，则要进行遗传咨询，这是由于活产的可能性取决于重排的类型以及涉及的具体染色体。胚胎植入前遗传学检测（PGT）是一种需要通过体外受精（IVF）形成胚胎并进行囊胚滋养层活检的遗传学检测方法。PGT也可用于识别受易位影响夫妇的结构重排（PGT-SR）。多年来，PGT-SR已从荧光原位杂交（FISH）、实时定量PCR（qPCR）发展到包括基于阵列的比较基因组杂交（CGH）和二代测序（NGS）等方法。最显著的变化是能够在第5天进行滋养层活检，而不是在第3天对卵裂球细胞进行检测。在一项对575对染色体易位夫妇（169对行SNP-PGD，406对行FISH-PGD）的回顾性研究中，Tan等[36]发现，与接受FISH-PGD的患者相比，接受SNP-PGD的患者妊娠率更高，流产率更低。在一项评估PGT-SR前后平衡易位携带者妊娠结局的研究中，Huang等[37]发现，在PGT-SR之后，之前经历过两次或更多次反复妊娠丢失的平衡易位携带者的流产风险降低，活产率提高。基于文献，我们推荐对由于平衡易位引起的反复妊娠丢失的患者进行IVF和PGT-SR。

纠正子宫畸形对于治疗RPL至关重要。通过子宫输卵管造影、超声造影或三维超声识别先天苗勒管畸形，包括单角子宫、双角子宫和纵隔子宫。对可疑的发现可通过成像的金标准，即盆腔MRI加以确认。既往的研究已经证实了子宫解剖异常在生殖结局中的作用：纵隔子宫与生育力降低、流产率增加和早产率增加相关[38]。子宫纵隔切除的深度阈值仍存在争议：美国生殖医学协会（ASRM）将弓形子宫定义为宫角内膜顶点连线中点至凹陷顶点的深度＜1 cm，而纵隔子宫的深度＞1.5 cm。因此，深度在1.0～1.5 cm范围下缺乏临床指导。在子宫纵隔切除试验（TRUST）中，Rikken等[39]将患者随机分配到宫腔镜切除组或期待管理组；主要研究结果包括活产率、持续妊娠、临床妊娠和流产。共有80名患者被随机分配，其中39名分配到子宫纵隔切除组，活产率为31%（12/39），40名分配到期待管理组，活产率为35%（14/40）。因此得出结论，宫腔镜切除不会改善纵隔子宫患者的生殖结局。然而，需要注意的是，在这80名随机分配的患者中，71名为部分子宫纵隔，深度＜1.5 cm。因此，如果深度＞1.5 cm，则宫腔镜切除子宫纵隔可能会在生殖方面带来显著的益处。

根据已确定的APLAS分类标准，标准治疗包括低剂量阿司匹林和每日两次的普通肝素[40]，这种治疗方案可将APLAS患者的妊娠丢失减少54%。尽管一些医生可能会每天开一次低分子量肝素以代替普通肝素，但类似的疗效尚未确定。在一项新的双盲安慰剂对照试验中，Pasquier等[41]发现，与安慰剂相比，每日40 mg的依诺肝素不能改善无血栓形成患者的不明原因RPL的活产机会。同样，一项比较低剂量阿司匹林与低分子量肝素和阿司匹林联合治疗的随机对照试验（RCT）发现，与单用阿司匹林相比，联合治疗对活产率没有额外的益处[42]。

6.2 反复种植失败的治疗

RIF和RPL在治疗方面存在一些重叠，其中包括利用宫腔镜对宫腔进行评估和纠正子宫病理、激素水平的评估（TSH、HbA1c、泌乳素），以及血栓倾向性筛查。然而，目前RIF的治疗选择仍然有限，许多疗法被认为是试验性的。最近的一项荟萃分析将针对RIF治疗和干预分为四类（表15.2）。

6.3 子宫干预

子宫干预包括旨在通过各种机制调节子宫炎性因子和刺激免疫调节因子的治疗方法。

6.3.1 主动子宫内膜损伤

主动子宫内膜损伤或"内膜搔刮"理论上可通过诱导免疫调节因子来增加妊娠率和活产率。然而，已有的研究存在差异，涉及的因素包括所使用的工具（Pipelle活检、Karman活检、宫腔镜导管）、搔刮的时机（周期的不同阶段，是否在移植的同一周期或先前的周期），以及研究结果都有所不同。从两项观察性研究的结果中汇总显示对种植率和妊娠率存在

表 15.2 反复种植失败的建议治疗方法

类别	方法
子宫干预	主动子宫内膜损伤
	子宫内膜活检，治疗慢性子宫内膜炎
	阿托西班
	含铜宫内节育器
	支架放置
实验室和移植策略及干预措施	序贯移植
	卵胞浆内形态学选择精子注射
	囊胚移植
	输卵管内受精卵移植（ZIFT）
	辅助孵化
	PGT-A
	胚胎时差成像
免疫调节疗法	低分子肝素
	静脉注射免疫球蛋白 G
	宫腔内外周血单核细胞输注
	皮下注射粒细胞集落刺激因子
	宫腔内输注粒细胞集落刺激因子
	宫腔内自体富血小板血浆（PRP）输注
	淋巴细胞免疫治疗（LIT）
	脂肪乳剂
子宫内膜治疗	雌二醇
	孕酮
	阿司匹林
	戊酮可可碱+/−维生素 E
	生长激素
	西地那非
	子宫内膜容受性检测
	宫腔镜
	骨髓干细胞子宫内膜移植
其他	子宫移植
	代孕

注：改编自 Busnelli, Andrea, et al. "Efficacy of therapies and interventions for repeated embryo implantation failure: a systematic review and meta-analysis." Scientific Reports vol. 11, 1 1747. 18 Jan. 2021, doi:10.1038/s41598-021-81439-6。

有益的效果[43,44]，但另外三项 RCT 的荟萃分析并未显示妊娠或活产的机会增加，也没有在流产率方面有任何差异[45-47]。

6.3.2 慢性子宫内膜炎

长期以来，慢性子宫内膜炎一直被认为是反复种植失败的原因，这是由于它会产生炎性子宫内环境。其定义各异，但通常为子宫样本中浆细胞（>5个/高倍视野）的存在增加[48]。最近的一项回顾性研究评估了 RIF 和 RPL 患者的外周血和子宫样本。子宫样本被用于诊断患有慢性子宫内膜炎的患者。这类患者在血液免疫细胞水平方面与其他患者相似，但内膜细胞因子和淋巴细胞水平较高，经过抗生素治疗后显著降低[49]。然而，治疗的临床益处尚未得到确切的证实。一项比较研究发现，被诊断为慢性子宫内膜炎的 RIF 患者在接受抗生素治疗后，种植率较低，但持续临床妊娠率与没有在活检中发现子宫内膜炎或未行子宫内膜活检的患者相似[50]。

6.3.3 阿托西班

阿托西班是一种复合的催产素/加压素 V1A 受体拮抗剂，据推测可用于 RIF 的治疗，这是因为与自然周期相比，促排卵的 IVF 周期中子宫收缩增加，且与明显降低的妊娠成功率相关。有一项前瞻性队列研究调查了阿托西班对 RIF 的影响[51]。这项研究显示，具有 2 次或更多次胚胎移植失败的患者在接受阿托西班治疗后，胚胎植入的机会增加（OR 3.14,95% CI 1.54～6.28），而流产的风险没有降低（OR 1.66,95% CI 0.43～6.35, $P=0.46$）。用于重复结果并进一步评估的 RCT 正在进行。

6.3.4 含铜宫内节育器

一项非随机研究评估了接受宫腔镜检查的 RIF 患者。在手术完成后，可选择放置含铜宫内节育器（Copper IUD），研究假设短期放置铜宫内节育器能够改变子宫内膜的细胞因子分布情况，这在小鼠中已得到证实。在这项研究中，放置宫内节育器的女性具有较高的种植率和临床妊娠率[52]。

6.4 实验室和移植策略及干预措施

6.4.1 囊胚移植、序贯胚胎移植和受精卵输卵管内移植

序贯胚胎移植是指在同一周期的第 2～3 天首先移植卵裂期胚胎，然后在同一周期的第 5 天移植囊胚。一项随机对照试验未显示接受序贯移植与单囊胚移植相比的生化或临床妊娠率有所增加[53]。然而，另一项观察性研究的荟萃分析则显示了序贯胚胎移植的益处，其具有较高的临床妊娠机会（OR

2.64，95% CI 1.56～4.47，$I^2=0$)[5]。囊胚移植在 RIF 患者中也被认为具有更好的妊娠结局。与 D2～D3 阶段胚胎移植相比，一项研究显示该策略的种植率显著增加，但在临床妊娠率或活产率方面没有差异。受精卵输卵管内移植(ZIFT)也被作为 RIF 的一种治疗方法进行了研究[54]，因为理论上天然的输卵管内环境可以使胚胎发育和子宫内膜更好的同步，但尚未证明其能够增加临床妊娠率或活产率，并且在观察性研究中其与囊胚移植相比结局更差[54]。

6.4.2 植入前遗传学检测(PGT-A)

植入前遗传学检测(PGT-A)被提出作为一种减少 RIF 风险的技术，这是因为染色体异常的胚胎成功植入的可能性较小。然而，迄今为止，没有证据支持这一发现，两项随机对照试验和多项观察性研究均未发现接受 PGT-A 的 RIF 患者在临床妊娠率或活产率方面存在差异[55,56]。

6.4.3 辅助孵化

在植入之前，囊胚必须从透明带中"孵化"出来。辅助孵化是指人为削薄或穿破透明带，早期多项研究表明，这种技术可以增加种植率和临床妊娠率[57]。然而在一项已进行的随机试验中未显示接受辅助孵化的患者临床妊娠率增加[58]。

6.4.4 卵胞浆内形态学选择精子注射

卵胞浆内形态学选择精子注射(IMSI)是一种针对伴有男性因素不育及相关 RIF 患者的解决方案。与卵胞浆内单精子注射(ICSI)相比，IMSI 利用高达 6000× 的放大倍数检测潜在异常，如精子细胞核中液泡数量的异常。这种"超微形态检测"在观察性研究中显示，与 ICSI 相比，RIF 患者的临床妊娠和活产率得到了改善，但这些研究的规模较小且为回顾性，仍需进一步的研究[59-61]。

6.5 免疫调节疗法

免疫调节疗法是 RPL 和 RIF 管理中新颖且令人兴奋的临床医学前沿。正在进行的随机对照试验使用了皮质类固醇进行免疫调节，Sung 等[62]综述了该治疗模式。本部分内容将讨论其中的一些疗法。

6.5.1 静脉免疫球蛋白(IVIG)

已有一项研究评估了 IVIG 治疗对于 RIF 患者的影响[63]。IVIG 的作用机制既包括直接抗体效应又包括免疫调节效应。在这项研究中，Ho 等首先检测了 RIF 患者的外周血单个核细胞水平(包括自然杀伤细胞水平)。与卵泡期 NK 细胞水平较高的患者相比，NK 细胞水平较低的患者种植率较低。此外，在 NK 细胞水平较低的患者中，接受 IVIG 治疗后的临床妊娠率和活产率提高。

6.5.2 宫腔内外周血单个核细胞(PMBC)输注

宫腔内输注 PBMC 治疗 RIF 也具有一定潜力。一般来说，该方法是在预定胚胎移植之前的 1～3 天内宫腔输注 PBMC。已进行的多项观察性研究和 3 项随机对照试验都显示 PBMC 治疗提高了种植率和临床妊娠率[63-69]。这些研究的影响程度很大，尽管只有一项研究报道了活产率[64]，并且关于这种疗法的安全性数据仍然很少。

6.5.3 宫腔内自体富血小板血浆(PRP)输注

富血小板血浆也被提出作为 RIF 的治疗方法，于前一周期的黄体期使用。一项新近的研究比较了子宫内膜下层注射 PRP 和宫腔内输注 PRP 与标准冻胚移植在 RIF 患者中的疗效，结果发现接受 PRP 治疗的患者有着更高的持续妊娠率和活产率[70]，但子宫内膜下层注射和宫腔内输注之间没有差异。值得注意的是，PRP 方案还包括了 PRP 输注后连续 3 天皮下注射 G-CSF。

6.5.4 皮下注射或宫腔内输注粒细胞集落刺激因子

粒细胞集落刺激因子(G-CSF)通过影响淋巴细胞、巨噬细胞和 T 辅助细胞在早期妊娠中发挥抑制免疫反应的作用[71]。在 RIF 治疗中，现已对皮下和宫腔内两种给药途径开展了研究，并进行了 6 项随机对照试验。总体而言，对这些随机对照试验的固定效应荟萃分析显示，在接受 G-CSF 治疗的患者中，临床妊娠率增加，尽管只有一项研究考虑了活产率，且未发现差异[72]。在亚组分析中，皮下 G-CSF 给药仍与种植率和临床妊娠率增加相关，效应幅度较大，但宫腔内 G-CSF 给药则没有此效应。

6.5.5 低分子肝素

鉴于易栓症与 RPL 相关，已报道了抗血小板和抗凝治疗作为 RIF 的潜在治疗方法。然而，多项随机对照试验未显示出低分子肝素对临床妊娠率或活产率有益的影响[73-77]。最近的一项荟萃分析包含了 5 项随机对照试验，亦未发现低分子肝素的益处。由于这些随机对照试验的参与者数量较少，仍需要进行多中心试验来进行论证[78]。

6.5.6 宫腔内 hCG 输注

两项观察性研究的荟萃分析显示，宫腔输注

hCG显著增加临床妊娠和活产的机会[79,80]。

6.6 子宫内膜治疗

雌二醇。

孕酮支持。

阿司匹林。

己酮可可碱(pentoxifylline)+/−维生素E。

宫腔镜检查。

骨髓干细胞移植。

肌内注射生长激素。

6.6.1 阴道用西地那非

一项小规模的随机对照试验评估了阴道用西地那非对因子宫内膜厚度不足而导致RIF的影响[81]。西地那非是一种PDE抑制剂,可以增加一氧化氮的功能,从而产生血管扩张作用。这项涉及105名患者的试验显示,在接受西地那非治疗的患者中,种植率和持续妊娠率明显提高。然而,该试验未对慢性子宫内膜炎这一因素进行控制,而这在各组之间有着显著差异。

6.6.2 子宫内膜活检

评估子宫内膜可以通过多种方式进行,包括宫腔镜检查和子宫内膜活检[82]。目前,有三种可用的商业化子宫内膜容受性阵列,用于评估胚胎是否能够植入。研究表明,人类的"种植窗"范围为月经周期的第19～23天(排卵日为周期的第14天)。因此,子宫内膜容受性分析试验旨在确定子宫内膜的精确时间,以优化移植时机,结果喜忧参半[83]。子宫内膜功能检测由两部分组成:对子宫内膜进行组织学评估和对子宫内膜进行时间标定(于月经周期的第15天和第24天活检)[84]。ReceptivaDx采用了不同的方法,检测与子宫内膜异位症相关的炎性标志物(BCL6),这是由于子宫内膜异位症与RIF有关[85]。这些检测的成本高,而迄今支持其应用的数据仍很少。未来,这些检测可能会与上述部分免疫调节的检测相结合,以在复杂情况下清晰描绘子宫内膜。

6.7 综合治疗

多种因素可能叠加导致RIF和RPL,包括细胞因素、体液因素和凝血因素[86],这表明可能需要结合多种治疗方法才能取得成功。一项回顾性队列研究比较了有RPL和RIF病史的患者,在IVF治疗过程中同时接受免疫调节治疗(强的松和IVIG)和抗凝治疗(低分子肝素和阿司匹林)与同期对照组的情况。结果显示,与对照组相比,RIF和(或)RPL的患者,PR和LBR均显著提高[62]。

7 生殖结局

7.1 反复妊娠丢失

已有的研究报道一致表明,未来流产的风险随着既往流产的次数增加而增加:在连续3次流产后,随后1次妊娠的流产风险约为29%,在既往流产次数达到6次或更多时,这一风险增加到约53%[22]。然而,这种关联的原因仍不清楚。为了确定在继发性RPL患者中,连续和非连续早期流产是否对预后产生不同的影响,Egerup等[87]进行了一项回顾性队列分析,研究了在1991—2014年丹麦进行的3项双盲安慰剂对照试验中(包含无明显原因继发性RPL患者)的妊娠结果。在纳入试验的168名患者中,127名患有继发性RPL,并在妊娠期间经历了随后的活产或不明显原因的流产。在继发性RPL患者中,末次妊娠前的晚期和早期流产对下一次妊娠中再次发生流产的风险没有显著影响。晚期流产的发生率比(IRR)为1.31(95% CI 0.62～2.77),早期流产的IRR为0.88(95% CI 0.70～1.11)。因此,作者认为,在继发性RPL患者中分娩消除了既往妊娠丢失对预后的负面影响。

7.2 反复种植失败

尽管新兴的RIF疗法开始显现出希望,但在诊断RIF后实现活产的预后仍不清楚。因此,医生必须就继续进行胚胎移植的效果向患者提供咨询。Koot等[88]进行了一项回顾性队列分析,评估了在接受IVF/ICSI治疗时发生不明原因RIF的女性中,后续通过IVF/ICSI或自然受孕的累积活产率和平均妊娠时间,该研究涵盖了2008年1月至2012年12月间经历RIF的223名年龄不超过39岁的患者。结果表明,5.5年内累积的活产率为49%(95% CI 39%～59%);在可生育的女性中,计算出的中位妊娠时间是经历RIF后9个月,其中18%为自然受孕。

8 总结与建议

- RPL是一种以3次或更多次临床妊娠失败(<24周孕龄)为特征的疾病,通过妊娠早期

超声或在子宫内膜检查中发现绒毛来验证。在经历了 2 次早期妊娠丢失后,就需进行临床评估。
- RIF 的定义仍存争议;如果定义为连续 3 次冷冻的整倍体单胚胎移植后仍未能妊娠,RIF 的发生率<5%。
- 妊娠需要广泛改变适应性和固有免疫反应,包括卵巢巨噬细胞、uNK 细胞、胎盘和蜕膜的巨噬细胞。
- 对 RPL 的评估可根据其潜在病因进行分类:染色体异常、解剖异常、抗磷脂综合征(APLAS)、激素失调、同种免疫异常、环境因素和感染。
- 全面的评估在多达 50% 的 RPL 患者中仍无法得出诊断。
- RPL 的治疗包括对有平衡易位的患者进行 PGT-SR,纠正子宫异常,对 APLAS 患者使用低剂量阿司匹林和每日 2 次的普通肝素。
- RIF 的治疗仍存在争议,尽管宫腔内自体 PRP 输注和皮下/宫腔内应用 G-CSF 能提高临床妊娠率。
- 未来妊娠失败的风险会随着既往流产次数的增加而增加。然而,新近的数据表明,继发性 RPL 患者在成功分娩后会消除既往流产对预后的负面影响。
- 在 RIF 被诊断后,实现活产的预后尚不清楚,因此,关于进行额外胚胎移植的咨询仍然是治疗的主要内容。

参考文献

[1] Practice Committee of the American Society for Reproductive Medicine. Evaluation and treatment of recurrent pregnancy loss: a committee opinion. Fertil Steril 2012 Nov;98(5):1103-11.

[2] Polanski LT, Baumgarten MN, Quenby S, Brosens J, Campbell BK, Raine-Fenning NJ. What exactly do we mean by "recurrent implantation failure"? A systematic review and opinion. Reprod Biomed Online 2014;28(4):409-23.

[3] Practice Committee of the American Society for Reproductive Medicine. Electronic address: asrm@asrm.org. Definitions of infertility and recurrent pregnancy loss: a committee opinion. Fertil Steril 2020 Mar;113(3):533-5.

[4] ESHRE Guideline: Recurrent Pregnancy Loss. Human reproduction [Open]. Oxford Academic [Internet]. [cited 2021 Sep 13]. 〈https://academic.oup.com/hropen/article/2018/2/hoy004/4963604〉.

[5] Busnelli A, Somigliana E, Cirillo F, Baggiani A, Levi-Setti PE. Efficacy of therapies and interventions for repeated embryo implantation failure: a systematic review and meta-analysis. Sci Rep 2021;11(1):1747.

[6] Coughlan C. What to do when good-quality embryos repeatedly fail to implant. Best Pract Res Clin Obstet Gynaecol 2018;53:48-59.

[7] Ata B, Kalafat E, Somigliana E. A new definition of recurrent implantation failure on the basis of anticipated blastocyst aneuploidy rates across female age. Fertil Steril 2021;S0015-0282(21):00558-6.

[8] Stirrat GM. Recurrent miscarriage. Lancet Lond Engl 1990;336(8716):673-5.

[9] Jauniaux E, Farquharson RG, Christiansen OB, Exalto N. Evidence-based guidelines for the investigation and medical treatment of recurrent miscarriage. Hum Reprod Oxf Engl 2006;21(9):2216-22.

[10] Is the incidence of recurrent pregnancy loss increasing? A retrospective register-based study in Sweden, Rasmark Roepke, 2017. Acta Obstetricia et Gynecologica Scandinavica. Wiley Online Library [Internet]. [cited 2021 Sep 13]. 〈https://obgyn.onlinelibrary.wiley.com/doi/full/10.1111/aogs.13210〉.

[11] Pirtea P, De Ziegler D, Tao X, Sun L, Zhan Y, Ayoubi JM, et al. Rate of true recurrent implantation failure is low: results of three successive frozen euploid single embryo transfers. Fertil Steril 2021;115(1):45-53.

[12] Picut CA, Dixon D, de Rijk EPCT. Immunopathology of the female reproductive tract and mammary gland In: Parker GA, editor. Immunopathology in toxicology and drug development, Volume 2. Cham: Springer International Publishing; 2017. p.541-614 [cited 2021 Sep 13] (Molecular and Integrative Toxicology). Available from. Available from: https://doi.org/10.1007/978-3-319-47385-7_11.

[13] Wu R, Van der Hoek KH, Ryan NK, Norman RJ, Robker RL. Macrophage contributions to ovarian function. Hum Reprod Update 2004;10(2):119-33.

[14] Lima PDA, Nivet A-L, Wang Q, Chen Y-A, Leader A, Cheung A, et al. Polycystic ovary syndrome: possible involvement of androgen-induced, chemerin-mediated ovarian recruitment of monocytes/macrophages. Biol Reprod 2018;99(4):838-52.

[15] Li Q, Yuan M, Jiao X, Huang Y, Li J, Li D, et al. M1 Macrophage-derived nanovesicles repolarize M2 macrophages for inhibiting the development of endometriosis. Front Immunol 2021;12:707784.

[16] Gaynor LM, Colucci F. Uterine natural killer cells: functional distinctions and influence on pregnancy in humans and mice. Front Immunol 2017;8:467.

[17] Picut CA, Swanson CL, Parker RF, Scully KL, Parker GA. The metrial gland in the rat and its similarities to granular cell tumors. Toxicol Pathol 2009;37(4):474-80.

[18] Pinhal-Enfield G, Vasan NS, Leibovich SJ. The role of macrophages in the placenta [Internet]. Embryology — updates and highlights on classic topics. IntechOpen; 2012 [cited 2021 Sep 13]. 〈https://www.intechopen.com/

chapters/34561〉.

[19] Cao L, Tang Y, Niu X, Guo Q, Huang L. Mifepristone regulates macrophage-mediated natural killer cells function in decidua. Reprod Biol 2021;21(3):100541.

[20] Stephenson MD, Awartani KA, Robinson WP. Cytogenetic analysis of miscarriages from couples with recurrent miscarriage: a case-control study. Hum Reprod Oxf Engl 2002;17(2):446-51.

[21] Carp H, Toder V, Aviram A, Daniely M, Mashiach S, Barkai G. Karyotype of the abortus in recurrent miscarriage. Fertil Steril 2001;75(4):678-82.

[22] Clifford K, Rai R, Regan L. Future pregnancy outcome in unexplained recurrent first trimester miscarriage. Hum Reprod Oxf Engl 1997;12(2):387-9.

[23] Recurrent Miscarriage, Investigation and Treatment of Couples (Green-top Guideline No. 17) [Internet]. Royal College of Obstetricians and Gynaecologists. [cited 2021 Sep 13]. 〈https://www.rcog.org.uk/en/guidelines-research-services/guidelines/gtg17/〉

[24] Stephenson MD, Sierra S. Reproductive outcomes in recurrent pregnancy loss associated with a parental carrier of a structural chromosome rearrangement. Hum Reprod Oxf Engl 2006;21(4):1076-82.

[25] Saravelos SH, Cocksedge KA, Li T-C. Prevalence and diagnosis of congenital uterine anomalies in women with reproductive failure: a critical appraisal. Hum Reprod Update 2008;14(5):415-29.

[26] Grimbizis GF, Camus M, Tarlatzis BC, Bontis JN, Devroey P. Clinical implications of uterine malformations and hysteroscopic treatment results. Hum Reprod Update 2001;7(2):161-74.

[27] Miyakis S, Lockshin MD, Atsumi T, Branch DW, Brey RL, Cervera R, et al. International consensus statement on an update of the classification criteria for definite antiphospholipid syndrome (APS). J Thromb Haemost JTH 2006;4(2):295-306.

[28] ACOG Practice Bulletin No.118: antiphospholipid syndrome. Obstet Gynecol. 2011 Jan;117(1):192-9.

[29] Abalovich M, Gutierrez S, Alcaraz G, Maccallini G, Garcia A, Levalle O. Overt and subclinical hypothyroidism complicating pregnancy. Thyroid J Am Thyroid Assoc 2002;12(1):63-8.

[30] Jovanovic L, Knopp RH, Kim H, Cefalu WT, Zhu X-D, Lee YJ, et al. Elevated pregnancy losses at high and low extremes of maternal glucose in early normal and diabetic pregnancy: evidence for a protective adaptation in diabetes. Diabetes Care 2005;28(5):1113-17.

[31] Hirahara F, Andoh N, Sawai K, Hirabuki T, Uemura T, Minaguchi H. Hyperprolactinemic recurrent miscarriage and results of randomized bromocriptine treatment trials. Fertil Steril 1998;70(2):246-52.

[32] Rey E, Kahn SR, David M, Shrier I. Thrombophilic disorders and fetal loss: a meta-analysis. Lancet Lond Engl 2003;361(9361):901-8.

[33] Silver RM, Zhao Y, Spong CY, Sibai B, Wendel G, Wenstrom K, et al. Prothrombin gene G20210A mutation and obstetric complications. Obstet Gynecol 2010;115(1):14-20.

[34] Dizon-Townson D, Miller C, Sibai B, Spong CY, Thom E, Wendel G, et al. The relationship of the factor V Leiden mutation and pregnancy outcomes for mother and fetus. Obstet Gynecol 2005;106(3):517-24.

[35] Verdoni A, Hu J, Surti U, Babcock M, Sheehan E, Clemens M, et al. Reproductive outcomes in individuals with chromosomal reciprocal translocations. Genet Med J Am Coll Med Genet 2021; May 10.

[36] Tan Y-Q, Tan K, Zhang S-P, Gong F, Cheng D-H, Xiong B, et al. Single-nucleotide polymorphism microarray-based pre-implantation genetic diagnosis is likely to improve the clinical outcome for translocation carriers. Hum Reprod 2013;28(9):2581-92.

[37] Huang C, Jiang W, Zhu Y, Li H, Lu J, Yan J, et al. Pregnancy outcomes of reciprocal translocation carriers with two or more unfavorable pregnancy histories: before and after pre-implantation genetic testing. J Assist Reprod Genet 2019;36(11):2325-31.

[38] Chan YY, Jayaprakasan K, Tan A, Thornton JG, Coomarasamy A, Raine-Fenning NJ. Reproductive outcomes in women with congenital uterine anomalies: a systematic review. Ultrasound Obstet Gynecol J Int Soc Ultrasound Obstet Gynecol 2011;38(4):371-82.

[39] Rikken JFW, Kowalik CR, Emanuel MH, Bongers MY, Spinder T, Jansen FW, et al. Septum resection vs expectant management in women with a septate uterus: an international multicentre open-label randomized controlled trial. Hum Reprod Oxf Engl 2021;36(5):1260-7.

[40] Empson M, Lassere M, Craig JC, Scott JR. Recurrent pregnancy loss with antiphospholipid antibody: a systematic review of therapeutic trials. Obstet Gynecol 2002;99(1):135-44.

[41] Pasquier E, de Saint Martin L, Bohec C, Chauleur C, Bretelle F, Marhic G, et al. Enoxaparin for prevention of unexplained recurrent miscarriage: a multicenter randomized double-blind placebo-controlled trial. Blood 2015;125(14):2200-5.

[42] Laskin CA, Spitzer KA, Clark CA, Crowther MR, Ginsberg JS, Hawker GA, et al. Low molecular weight heparin and aspirin for recurrent pregnancy loss: results from the randomized, controlled HepASA Trial. J Rheumatol 2009;36(2):279-87.

[43] Matsumoto Y, Kokeguchi S, Shiotani M. Effects of endometrial injury on frozen-thawed blastocyst transfer in hormone replacement cycles. Reprod Med Biol 2017;16(2):196-9.

[44] Raziel A, Schachter M, Strassburger D, Bern O, Ron-El R, Friedler S. Favorable influence of local injury to the endometrium in intracytoplasmic sperm injection patients with high-order implantation failure. Fertil Steril 2007;87(1):198-201.

[45] Gürgan T, Kalem Z, Kalem MN, Ruso H, Benkhalifa M, Makrigiannakis A. Systematic and standardized hysteroscopic endometrial injury for treatment of recurrent implantation failure. Reprod Biomed Online 2019;39(3):477-83.

[46] Olesen MS, Hauge B, Ohrt L, Olesen TN, Roskær J, Bæk V, et al. Therapeutic endometrial scratching and implantation after in vitro fertilization: a multicenter randomized controlled trial. Fertil Steril 2019;112(6):1015-21.

[47] Baum M, Yerushalmi GM, Maman E, Kedem A, Machtinger R, Hourvitz A, et al. Does local injury to the endometrium before IVF cycle really affect treatment outcome? Results of a randomized placebo controlled trial. Gynecol Endocrinol J Int Soc Gynecol Endocrinol 2012;28(12):933-6.

[48] Zargar M, Ghafourian M, Nikbakht R, Mir Hosseini V, Moradi Choghakabodi P. Evaluating chronic endometritis in

women with recurrent implantation failure and recurrent pregnancy loss by hysteroscopy and immunohistochemistry. J Minim Invasive Gynecol 2020;27(1):116-21.

[49] Li Y, Yu S, Huang C, Lian R, Chen C, Liu S, et al. Evaluation of peripheral and uterine immune status of chronic endometritis in patients with recurrent reproductive failure. Fertil Steril 2020;113(1):187-196.e1.

[50] Johnston-MacAnanny EB, Hartnett J, Engmann LL, Nulsen JC, Sanders MM, Benadiva CA. Chronic endometritis is a frequent finding in women with recurrent implantation failure after in vitro fertilization. Fertil Steril 2010;93(2):437-41.

[51] He Y, Wu H, He X, Xing Q, Zhou P, Cao Y, et al. Application of atosiban in frozen-thawed cycle patients with different times of embryo transfers. Gynecol Endocrinol J Int Soc Gynecol Endocrinol 2016;32(10):811-15.

[52] Mao X, Zhang J, Chen Q, Kuang Y, Zhang S. Short-term copper intrauterine device placement improves the implantation and pregnancy rates in women with repeated implantation failure. Fertil Steril 2017;108(1)55-61.e1.

[53] Tehraninejad ES, Raisi E, Ghaleh FB, Rashidi BH, Aziminekoo E, Kalantari V, et al. The sequential embryo transfer compared to blastocyst embryo transfer in in vitro fertilization (IVF) cycle in patients with the three repeated consecutive IVF. A randomized controlled trial. Gynecol Endocrinol J Int Soc Gynecol Endocrinol 2019;35(11):955-9.

[54] Shahrokh Tehraninejad E, Azimi Nekoo E, Ghaffari F, Hafezi M, Karimian L, Arabipoor A. Zygote intrafallopian tube transfer vs intrauterine cleavage or blastocyst stage transfer after intracytoplasmic sperm injection cycles in patients with repeated implantation failure: a prospective follow-up study. J Obstet Gynaecol Res 2015;41(11):1779-84.

[55] Rubio C, Bellver J, Rodrigo L, Bosch E, Mercader A, Vidal C, et al. Pre-implantation genetic screening using fluorescence in situ hybridization in patients with repetitive implantation failure and advanced maternal age: two randomized trials. Fertil Steril 2013;99(5):1400-7.

[56] Blockeel C, Schutyser V, De Vos A, Verpoest W, De Vos M, Staessen C, et al. Prospectively randomized controlled trial of PGS in IVF/ICSI patients with poor implantation. Reprod Biomed Online 2008;17(6):848-54.

[57] Simon A, Laufer N. Assessment and treatment of repeated implantation failure (RIF). J Assist Reprod Genet 2012;29(11):1227-39.

[58] Rufas-Sapir O, Stein A, Orvieto R, Avrech OM, Kotler N, Pinkas H, et al. Is assisted hatching beneficial in patients with recurrent implantation failures? Clin Exp Obstet Gynecol 2004;31(2):110-12.

[59] Tasaka A, Doshida M, Sato Y, Kyoya T, Nakajo Y, Kyono K. Outcome of IMSI (intracytoplasmic morphologically selected sperm injection) in patients with repeated ICSI failures. Fertil Steril 2009;92(3):S76.

[60] Delaroche L, Yazbeck C, Gout C, Kahn V, Oger P, Rougier N. Intracytoplasmic morphologically selected sperm injection (IMSI) after repeated IVF or ICSI failures: a prospective comparative study. Eur J Obstet Gynecol Reprod Biol 2013;167(1):76-80.

[61] Karabulut S, Aksunger O, Korkmaz O, Gozel HE, Keskin I. Intracytoplasmic morphologically selected sperm injection, but for whom? Zygote 2019;27(5):299-304.

[62] Sung N, Khan SA, Yiu ME, Jubiz G, Salazar MD, Skariah A, et al. Reproductive outcomes of women with recurrent pregnancy losses and repeated implantation failures are significantly improved with immunomodulatory treatment. J Reprod Immunol 2021;148:103369.

[63] Ho Y-K, Chen H-H, Huang C-C, Lee C-I, Lin P-Y, Lee M-S, et al. Peripheral CD56+ CD16+ NK cell populations in the early follicular phase are associated with successful clinical outcomes of intravenous immunoglobulin treatment in women with repeated implantation failure. Front Endocrinol 2019;10:937.

[64] Madkour A, Bouamoud N, Louanjli N, Kaarouch I, Copin H, Benkhalifa M, et al. Intrauterine insemination of cultured peripheral blood mononuclear cells prior to embryo transfer improves clinical outcome for patients with repeated implantation failures. Zygote Camb Engl 2016;24(1):58-69.

[65] Nobijari FF, Arefi SS, Moini A, Taheripanah R, Fazeli E, Kharazi H, et al. Endometrium immunomodulation by intrauterine insemination administration of treated peripheral blood mononuclear cell prior frozen/thawed embryos in patients with repeated implantation failure. Zygote Camb Engl 2019;27(4):214-18.

[66] Yu N, Zhang B, Xu M, Wang S, Liu R, Wu J, et al. Intrauterine administration of autologous peripheral blood mononuclear cells (PBMCs) activated by HCG improves the implantation and pregnancy rates in patients with repeated implantation failure: a prospective randomized study. Am J Reprod Immunol N Y N 1989 2016;76(3):212-16.

[67] Okitsu O, Kiyokawa M, Oda T, Miyake K, Sato Y, Fujiwara H. Intrauterine administration of autologous peripheral blood mononuclear cells increases clinical pregnancy rates in frozen/thawed embryo transfer cycles of patients with repeated implantation failure. J Reprod Immunol 2011;92(1-2):82-7.

[68] Li S, Wang J, Cheng Y, Zhou D, Yin T, Xu W, et al. Intrauterine administration of hCG-activated autologous human peripheral blood mononuclear cells (PBMC) promotes live birth rates in frozen/thawed embryo transfer cycles of patients with repeated implantation failure. J Reprod Immunol 2017;119:15-22.

[69] Yoshioka S, Fujiwara H, Nakayama T, Kosaka K, Mori T, Fujii S. Intrauterine administration of autologous peripheral blood mononuclear cells promotes implantation rates in patients with repeated failure of IVF-embryo transfer. Hum Reprod Oxf Engl 2006;21(12):3290-4.

[70] Noushin MA, Ashraf M, Thunga C, Singh S, Singh S, Basheer R, et al. A comparative evaluation of subendometrial and intrauterine platelet-rich plasma treatment for women with recurrent implantation failure. FS Sci 2021;2(3):295-302.

[71] Moldenhauer LM, Keenihan SN, Hayball JD, Robertson SA. GM-CSF is an essential regulator of T cell activation competence in uterine dendritic cells during early pregnancy in mice. J Immunol Baltim Md 1950 2010;185(11):7085-96.

[72] Kalem Z, Namli Kalem M, Bakirarar B, Kent E, Makrigiannakis A, Gurgan T. Intrauterine G-CSF administration in recurrent implantation failure (RIF): an RCT. Sci Rep 2020;10(1):5139.

[73] Urman B, Ata B, Yakin K, Alatas C, Aksoy S, Mercan R, et al. Luteal phase empirical low molecular weight heparin administration in patients with failed ICSI embryo transfer cycles: a randomized open-labeled pilot trial. Hum Reprod Oxf Engl 2009;24(7):1640-7.

[74] Noci I, Milanini MN, Ruggiero M, Papini F, Fuzzi B, Artini PG. Effect of dalteparin sodium administration on IVF outcome in non-thrombophilic young women: a pilot study. Reprod Biomed Online 2011;22(6):615-20.

[75] Lodigiani C, Dentali F, Banfi E, Ferrazzi P, Librè L, Quaglia I, et al. The effect of parnaparin sodium on in vitro fertilization outcome: a prospective randomized controlled trial. Thromb Res 2017;159:116-21.

[76] Berker B, Takin S, Kahraman K, Takin EA, Atabekogglu C, Sönmezer M. The role of low-molecular-weight heparin in recurrent implantation failure: a prospective, quasi-randomized, controlled study. Fertil Steril 2011;95(8):2499-502.

[77] Xiong. Low-molecularweight heparin in women with ... Google Scholar [Internet]. [cited 2021 Sep 13]. 〈https://scholar.google.com/scholar_lookup?hl=en&volume=31&publication_year=2015&pages=614-7&journal=J+Pract+Obstet+Gynecol&author=ZF+Xiong&author=XH+Dang&author=B+Li&author=LY+Wang&title=Low%E2%80%90molecular%E2%80%90weight+heparin+in+women+with+repeated+implantation+failure+%28in+Chinese%29〉.

[78] Yang X-L, Chen F, Yang X-Y, Du G-H, Xu Y. Efficacy of low-molecular-weight heparin on the outcomes of in vitro fertilization/intracytoplasmic sperm injection pregnancy in non-thrombophilic women: a *meta*-analysis. Acta Obstet Gynecol Scand 2018;97(9):1061-72.

[79] Huang P, Wei L, Li X, Qin A. Effects of intrauterine perfusion of human chorionic gonadotropin in women with different implantation failure numbers. Am J Reprod Immunol N Y N 1989 2018;79(2).

[80] Liu X, Ma D, Wang W, Qu Q, Zhang N, Wang X, et al. Intrauterine administration of human chorionic gonadotropin improves the live birth rates of patients with repeated implantation failure in frozen-thawed blastocyst transfer cycles by increasing the percentage of peripheral regulatory T cells. Arch Gynecol Obstet 2019;299(4):1165-72.

[81] Sher G, Fisch JD. Effect of vaginal sildenafil on the outcome of in vitro fertilization (IVF) after multiple IVF failures attributed to poor endometrial development. Fertil Steril 2002;78(5):1073-6.

[82] Kliman HJ, Frankfurter D. Clinical approach to recurrent implantation failure: evidence-based evaluation of the endometrium. Fertil Steril 2019;111(4):618-28.

[83] Tan J, Kan A, Hitkari J, Taylor B, Tallon N, Warraich G, et al. The role of the endometrial receptivity array (ERA) in patients who have failed euploid embryo transfers. J Assist Reprod Genet 2018;35(4):683-92.

[84] Young SL. Evaluation of endometrial function: a Heraclean or Sisyphean task? Fertil Steril 2017;108(4):604-5.

[85] Almquist LD, Likes CE, Stone B, Brown K, Savaris R, Forstein DA, et al. Endometrial BCL6 testing for the prediction of IVF outcomes: a cohort study. Fertil Steril 2017;108(6):1063-9.

[86] Kwak-Kim J, Skariah A, Wu L, Salazar D, Sung N, Ota K. Humoral and cellular autoimmunity in women with recurrent pregnancy losses and repeated implantation failures: a possible role of vitamin D. Autoimmun Rev 2016;15(10):943-7.

[87] Egerup P, Kolte AM, Larsen EC, Krog M, Nielsen HS, Christiansen OB. Recurrent pregnancy loss: what is the impact of consecutive vs non-consecutive losses? Hum Reprod Oxf Engl 2016;31(11):2428-34.

[88] Koot YEM, Hviid Saxtorph M, Goddijn M, de Bever S, Eijkemans MJC, Wely MV, et al. What is the prognosis for a live birth after unexplained recurrent implantation failure following IVF/ICSI? Hum Reprod Oxf Engl 2019;34(10):2044-52.

第 16 章

生殖障碍中的胚胎：免疫学视角

The embryo in reproductive failure: immunological view

Tia Brodeur and Navid Esfandiari

Division of Reproductive Endocrinology and Infertility, Department of Obstetrics and Gynecology and Reproductive Sciences, Larner College of Medicine at the University of Vermont, Burlington, VT, United States

1 引言

体外受精（IVF）是 20 世纪最重要的医学进展之一。美国每年出生的婴儿中，约有 2% 是通过辅助生殖技术（ART）受孕的[1]。女性伴侣或卵子捐赠者的年龄是 IVF 成功的最重要指标；然而，自从辅助生殖技术诞生 40 年以来，IVF 的成功率逐渐提高，这在很大程度上要归功于胚胎实验室技术的进步。IVF 可能是严重男性因素不孕症的首选治疗方法，包括那些需要提取睾丸精子或附睾抽吸术的患者。此外，IVF 还可为不孕夫妇提供额外的诊断信息，如卵母细胞受精后的受精不良或失败，卵母细胞形态异常以及胚胎发育不良等。

在获取卵母细胞后，可以进行传统的人工授精或卵胞质内单精子注射（ICSI）使卵母细胞受精。受精技术的选择取决于诊断、精子的来源和质量、卵母细胞的数量和质量，以及既往周期的受精结果（如果有）。受精评估通常在卵母细胞受精或 ICSI 后的 16~18 小时内进行。从此时开始，形态学评估被用来对发育胚胎的质量进行分级（图 16.1）。在实践中，优质胚胎通常在卵裂阶段（受精后第 3 天）或囊

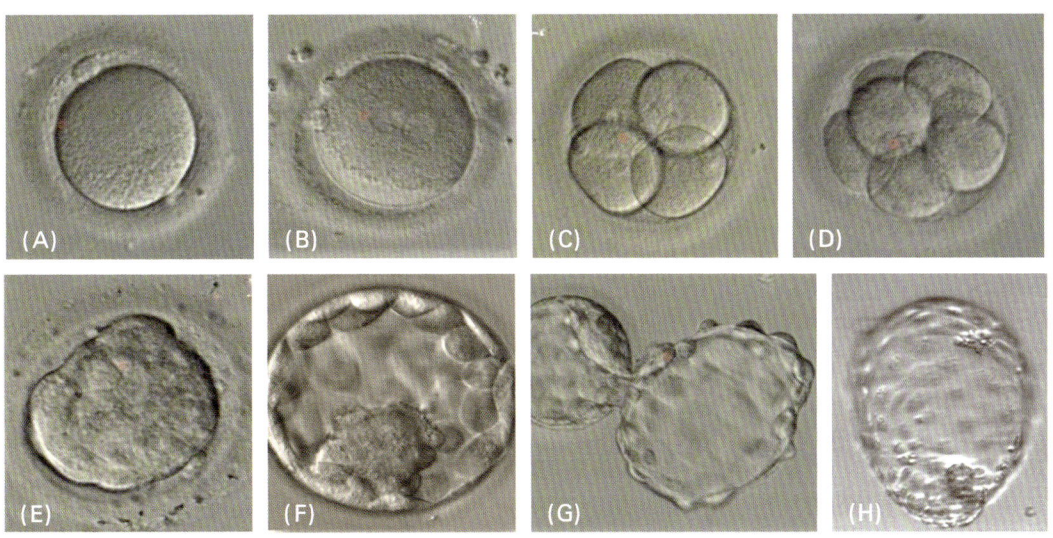

图 16.1 人卵母细胞和胚胎。

(A)中期Ⅱ卵母细胞（MⅡ）。(B)受精卵母细胞。含 2 个原核。(C)4 细胞期胚胎。(D)8 细胞期胚胎。(E)桑椹胚。(F)囊胚。(G)孵化囊胚。(H)完全孵化的囊胚。

胚阶段(受精后第 5 或 6 天)移植到子宫中。有人提出,将培养延长到囊胚阶段有助于选择具有更高生殖潜力的胚胎,并且囊胚可能与子宫内膜具有更好的同步性,从而获得更高的种植率。然而,临床妊娠率和活产率的荟萃分析显示,囊胚移植的改善幅度较小[2]。

卵裂期胚胎和囊胚均有分级系统,这些分级系统有助于选择活产率更高的胚胎[3]。卵裂期胚胎根据卵裂球数量、对称性和碎片程度进行分级,而 Gardner 系统则是一种常用的囊胚分级系统。囊胚分级基于三部分评分,包括:①描述囊胚扩张程度的 1~6 数值评分。②内细胞团的定性和定量评估。③滋养层(TE)的定性评估。这些综合评分与胚胎种植潜力相关[4,5]。

生物化学和代谢组学方法也被提出作为选择高质量胚胎的方法;然而,这些方法目前仍处于实验阶段,可能会带来相当大的成本和人力投入。时差显微镜(TLM)技术可以通过测量胚胎发育的动力学来评估胚胎的生殖潜力[6]。胚胎植入前非整倍体基因检测(PGT-A)也可用于选择染色体正常的胚胎。对于尽管移植了优质或整倍体胚胎但仍出现反复种植失败(RIF)的患者,研究评估胚胎生殖潜力的替代方法可能有助于为未来的治疗提供信息。

2 影响局部免疫环境的胚胎源性信号

2.1 人绒毛膜促性腺激素

人绒毛膜促性腺激素(hCG)是胚胎产生的主要妊娠血清蛋白标志物。由囊胚产生的 hCG 最早可于受精后 7 天在母体血清中检测到[7]。除了为黄体提供维持孕酮分泌所需的关键支持外,hCG 还诱导细胞滋养层细胞的增殖和侵袭。它通过控制基质金属蛋白酶、血管内皮生长因子(VEGF)和巨噬细胞集落刺激因子(M-CSF)来调节子宫内膜的微结构。此外,hCG 还影响固有和适应性免疫细胞的活动,包括巨噬细胞、自然杀伤(NK)细胞和 T 细胞[7,8]。尽管 NK 细胞不表达 hCG 受体,但 hCG 通过甘露糖受体介导这些细胞的增殖[9]。

2.2 早孕因子

早孕因子(EPF)由早期胚胎在受精后数小时内分泌[10],具有免疫抑制特性[11,12]。有研究表明,EPF 可能具有促进胚胎发育和植入的作用[13]。EPF 的发现源于近期受精女性血清能够增强玫瑰花环抑制试验的能力。玫瑰花环抑制试验是一种体外试验,使用抗血清对外周血淋巴细胞进行抑制,在外周血单个核细胞与绵羊红细胞混合时,抑制了玫瑰花环的形成[14]。EPF 抑制淋巴细胞增殖和(或)激活的机制尚未确立。然而,这些研究表明,植入前胚胎分泌 EPF,从而影响局部免疫细胞的表型,并可能限制 T 细胞的扩增,这可能导致过度的免疫应答。

2.3 血小板活化因子

血小板活化因子(PAF)属于磷脂家族,能够介导血小板释放组胺。PAF 由胚胎和子宫内膜共同产生,具有广泛的生物学功能。在人类体外受精中,PAF 早在受精时就开始产生[15]。PAF 被认为是胚胎活力的预测因子,因为培养基中的 PAF 水平与临床妊娠率相关[16,17]。PAF 拮抗剂能抑制小鼠胚胎种植,这部分研究支持了 PAF 在胚胎植入中的作用。PAF 还能增强前列腺素 E2(PGE2)的合成和 PGF2α 的释放,这为 PAF 在胚胎植入中的作用提供了一个潜在机制[16-18]。PAF 也可能在生殖道的其他区域发挥作用,有趣的是,它似乎对精子的运动具有促进作用[16]。

3 胚胎与子宫内膜的相互作用

3.1 炎症细胞因子

炎症细胞因子,如 IL-1β 和前列腺素(PG),在早期妊娠子宫内膜中的表达水平较非妊娠子宫内膜高[19]。白细胞的精细平衡以及子宫内膜和局部白细胞分泌的低水平促炎症细胞因子可能有助于胚胎种植。事实上,较高水平的 IL-1β 和 TNF-α 与 IVF 患者的临床妊娠率相关[20]。IL-1β 由囊胚和子宫内膜产生,可在体外刺激子宫内膜细胞产生 PG[21]。

3.2 前列腺素

PG 是急性炎症的介质,同时在转录水平上增强免疫细胞的响应[22]。环氧合酶-1(COX-1)和 COX-2 是介导 PG 从花生四烯酸产生的酶。大多数组织能产生 PG,可以在基础条件下表达或对损伤刺激做出反应[23]。PG 是胚胎种植所必需的,PGE2 是蜕膜反应的介质。子宫内膜基质中的 PGE2 受体能以孕激素依赖的方式诱导[24]。COX-1 的产生会在孕激素和 17β-雌二醇的刺激下减少,因此在植入前其水平会下降。COX-2 的表达受限于小鼠的种植部位[25],提示胚胎种植微环境中的 PG 可能受到严格的控制,以防止免疫反应过度激活。

3.3 白血病抑制因子

白血病抑制因子(LIF)是 IL-6 家族细胞因子的一员,具有高度多效性[26]。LIF 由子宫内膜腺体和基质表达,似乎在胚胎植入中具有跨物种保守的作用。小鼠的相互胚胎移植研究表明,母体 LIF 对胚胎植入至关重要。胚胎表达 LIF 受体,在胚胎培养基中加入外源性 LIF 可以改善人类的囊胚形成[27]。在体外小鼠胚胎中敲减 LIF 会降低囊胚形成率和囊胚直径[28]。然而,LIF 受体缺陷的胚胎可以发育到囊胚阶段[29]。蜕膜 NK 细胞和 T 细胞已被证明表达 LIF 信使 RNA[30]。这表明在植入过程中 LIF 可能介导了子宫内膜-白细胞的相互作用以及胚胎-子宫内膜的相互作用。

4 反复种植失败

胚胎植入是一个复杂的过程,需要胚胎和子宫内膜的共同指导,免疫因素在这一过程中具有相互允许和限制的作用。蜕膜化的特征是白细胞显著增加,蜕膜组织中约有 40% 的细胞是白细胞,主要是 NK 细胞[31]。在人类中,蜕膜化是由升高的孕激素触发的,并不需要胚胎来源的信号[32]。在植入过程中,囊胚的滋养细胞附着于子宫内膜的上皮层,然后增殖并侵入子宫内膜基质。滋养细胞侵袭受损也会导致胎儿生长受限和子痫前期等产科疾病[7]。

4.1 定义

反复种植失败的定义各不相同,可能会随着辅助生殖技术的发展而不断演变。RIF 定义的变化导致了这一领域研究的异质性。然而,我们建议,3 次优质胚胎移植(无论是单胚胎移植还是多胚胎移植)出现种植失败是 RIF 的一种可接受的定义。

4.2 患病率

反复种植失败的患病率很难确定,尽管可能相对罕见,但它可能对患者造成毁灭性的打击,并困扰 IVF 团队。Pirtea 等[33]最近的一项研究表明,92.6% 的患者在最多 3 次整倍体单胚胎移植后能够获得妊娠,第 1 次、第 2 次和第 3 次整倍体单胚胎移植后的活产率分别为 64.8%、54.4% 和 54.1%,这表明当整倍体胚胎移植时,真正的 RIF 并不常见。

4.3 评估

那些经历了多次优质胚胎移植失败的患者应被视为评估 RIF 的潜在人群。不幸的是,一些接受多次胚胎移植失败的患者可能是由于胚胎发育不良、非整倍体或子宫内膜不理想而未能受孕。这些患者可能不属于 RIF 的诊断范围,因为胚胎质量差可能最终解释了种植失败的原因,也可能是其不孕的基础。

4.3.1 胚胎植入前遗传学检测

非整倍体是一种偏离正常染色体的现象。由于许多接受 IVF 的女性生育年龄较大,更容易发生卵母细胞非整倍体,因此种植失败的很大一部分与胚胎的遗传能力相关。

胚胎植入前遗传学检测(PGT)是一种用于筛查高危患者卵母细胞和胚胎非整倍体(PGT-A)的检测技术。PGT 允许选择正常胚胎,以避免种植失败和妊娠丢失。有两种基本的方法可获取用于遗传分析的材料:来自卵母细胞和体外发育的胚胎。对于卵母细胞,需要从成熟的 MII 卵中抽取第一极体,或从正常受精的卵母细胞中抽取第二极体,或者两者都抽取。极体活检可以间接评估相关卵母细胞的染色体组成,因此,该方法仅检测了后续发育胚胎的母体成分(图 16.2)[34]。对于胚胎,涉及从卵裂期胚

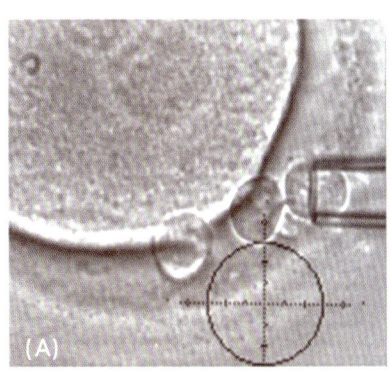
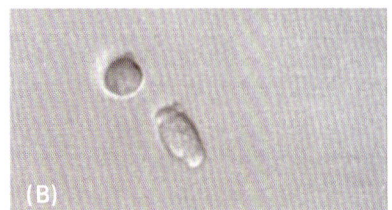

图 16.2 极体活检。
(A)从受精卵母细胞中移除极体。(B)极体(×400 倍)。

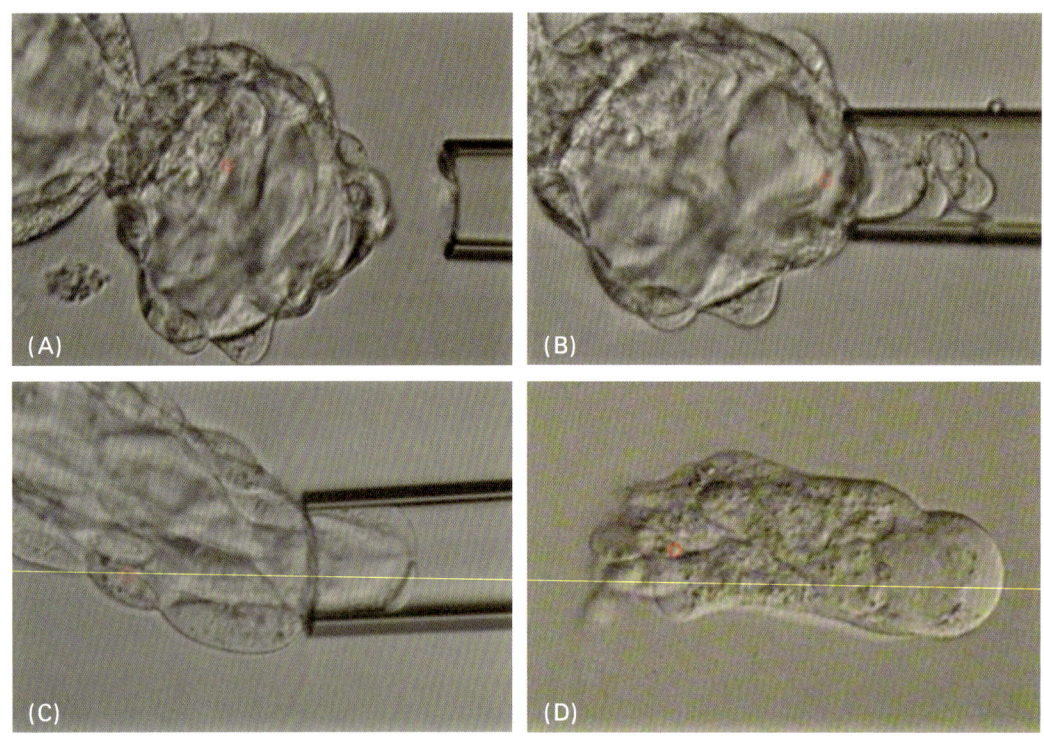

图 16.3 滋养层(TE)活检过程。
(A)第 5 天扩张的囊胚,滋养细胞通过 2 天前使用激光在透明带上打出的开口膨出。(B)用固定管将囊胚固定,将少量滋养细胞吸入活检管。(C)使用激光脉冲从囊胚中活检 3~5 个滋养细胞。(D)活检后的滋养细胞。

胎(受精后第 3 天)中取出 1 个或 2 个卵裂球,或从囊胚期胚胎(受精后第 5 天或第 6 天)中取出几个滋养细胞(图 16.3)。卵裂期胚胎具有较高的嵌合率,如果胚胎是嵌合的,则对 1 个或 2 个卵裂球进行活检行遗传学检测可能会产生错误的结果[35]。然而,对几个滋养细胞进行活检能提供更多用于检测的 DNA,可减少由于嵌合现象而导致误诊的机会。

PGT-A 可能在 RIF 或 RPL 患者中有一定益处,但这尚未得到明确的结论[36]。值得注意的是,胚胎形态与染色体状态之间没有直接关联,因为非整倍体胚胎可能具有良好的胚胎形态,而整倍体胚胎的质量可能并不理想。Sato 等[37]的研究比较了接受 PGT-A 或接受未经检测胚胎移植的 RIF 患者的妊娠率。共有 92 名 RIF 患者参与了研究,其中 42 名患者接受了 PGT-A。在 PGT-A 组中,24 名患者行胚胎移植,而在对照组的 50 名患者中,有 42 名接受了未经检测的胚胎移植。PGT-A 组每名患者的活产率为 35.7%,而对照组为 26%,两者之间没有统计学差异。然而,PGT-A 组的每次胚胎移植的活产率为 62.5%,对照组则为 31.7%($P = 0.016$)。这项研究包括了 42 岁的高育龄女性,这些患者更易因非整倍体而导致移植失败,而 PGT-A 是否为年轻患者的最佳策略尚不清楚。

平衡易位或倒位等遗传异常也可能导致 RPL。Raziel 等[38]的一项研究表明,在 65 名重度 RIF 患者(6~16 个周期未实现临床妊娠,平均 7.8 个周期)中,15.4% 存在染色体异常,包括易位、嵌合、倒位和缺失。有趣的是,染色体异常患者的胚胎形态没有差异。然而,这种小样本量和相当重度 RIF 的适用性可能并不广泛。

4.3.2 精子 DNA 损伤和非整倍体

DNA 损伤对精子质量的影响是一个正在积极研究的领域,尽管目前在 RIF 中关于精子 DNA 损伤的信息还很少。有趣的是,一项纳入 637 对夫妇的研究,包括了 387 个人工授精(IUI)周期、388 个 IVF 周期和 223 个 ICSI 周期,结果显示,精子 DNA 断裂水平较高的患者生化妊娠率更高。在这项研究中,纳入标准是未洗涤精液中的精子浓度为 1×10^6/mL,女性伴侣年龄小于 40 岁,BMI 小于 30 kg/m^2,基线 FSH 低于 12 U/L[39]。一项有关男性因素不孕症的病例研究中,使用射精精子进行 ICSI 后出现 RIF 的 4 对夫妇,当使用睾丸精子时,所有 4 对夫妇均成功妊娠,作者提出精子可能在睾丸后发生了 DNA 损伤[40]。精子 DNA 完整性检测目前在临床上尚未广泛使用,而在资源消耗方面的效益可能不如预期的改善显著[41]。美国生殖医学会的实践委员会不建议常规检测精子 DNA 损伤,并指出在不孕夫妇的评估和治疗中常规使用精子DNA 完整性检测的证据不足[42]。如果存在精索静脉曲张或感染,经治疗可能会改善不育男性的精子DNA 完整性,而有关补充抗氧化剂和改变生活方式的数据仍不清楚[43]。与卵母细胞非整倍体相比,精子非整倍体并不常见,但在不育男性中更为常见。此外,研究表明,精子非整倍体与胚胎非整倍体相关。然而,非整倍体精子存在于其他正常精液样本中[44]。

4.3.3 胚胎-子宫内膜不同步

与自然周期相比,接受促性腺激素卵巢刺激的患者种植窗口期提前 1~2 天[45]。卵巢刺激方案的选择[46,47],或 GnRH 激动剂与 hCG 扳机的选择可能会影响子宫内膜的容受性[16]。子宫内膜容受性分析(ERA)通过检测月经周期不同时间点表达的基因转录本,在某些临床情况下用于评估胚胎-子宫内膜的不同步性。这项检测旨在识别子宫内膜容受性的"偏移",意味着调整胚胎移植时间可能会改善子宫内膜接收胚胎的同步性。当 RIF 患者与 IVF 对照组患者进行比较时,ERA 异常的发生率分别为 25% 和 14%(四项研究分别涉及 50、62、80 和 85 名 RIF 患者)[48]。对 50 名经历约 5 次冷冻囊胚移植失败的 RIF 患者进行的一项回顾性研究显示,其中 24% 的患者"不容受(提前容受或延后容受)";而对检测中被判定为"提前容受"的患者,通过个体化的胚胎移植时间,第一次移植后的临床妊娠率达到 50%,而容受组为 35.3%[49]。Tan 等[50]的一项研究回顾了 88 名进行 ERA 检查的患者。其中 38 名患者曾经历整倍体胚胎移植失败,排除了非整倍体对种植失败的影响。在这项研究中,ERA 显示种植窗口期偏移的患者比例为 22.5%。虽然个体化的胚胎移植时间与增加的活产率之间存在相关性,但无统计学意义。

4.3.4 子宫内膜异位症(B 细胞 CLL/淋巴瘤 6 检测)

B 细胞 CLL/淋巴瘤 6(BCL6)是在生发中心 B 细胞和滤泡辅助性 T 细胞中表达的主要转录调节因子[51]。BCL6 已被提出作为不明原因不孕症患者子宫内膜容受性的标志物,也是子宫内膜异位症的生物标志物[52],表明部分不明原因不孕症患者可能患有亚临床子宫内膜异位症。子宫内膜异位症患者的在位子宫内膜可能通过多种途径受到炎症环境的影响,包括孕酮抵抗,因为孕酮可以减少子宫内膜的炎症[53]。这可能是子宫内膜容受性和子宫内膜异位症之间相关性的潜在解释。BCL6 低表达女性的临床妊娠率高于 BCL6 高表达女性(64.7% vs 17.3%),活产率也更高(58.8% vs 11.5%)[54]。

4.3.5 慢性子宫内膜炎和子宫内膜微生物失调

慢性子宫内膜炎很可能是由子宫内膜微生物失调引起的。在免疫组化检查子宫内膜活检标本时,其典型的病理特征是存在浆细胞[55,56]。在 RIF 和 RPL 患者中,慢性子宫内膜炎的发生率较高(分别为 14% 和 27%)[57]。Cicinelli 等[58]的一项研究试图确定慢性子宫内膜炎治疗是否会改善妊娠结局。在这项研究中,106 例 RIF 患者中 70 例诊断为慢性子宫内膜炎,所有患者均给予抗生素治疗;然而,24.6% 的患者在再次评估时仍有慢性子宫内膜炎。慢性子宫内膜炎治愈的患者活产率为 60.8%,而难治性慢性子宫内膜炎患者的活产率为 13.3%。将难治性慢性子宫内膜炎作为对照组很有意思;然而,该组患者在基线时可能有更严重的病理,这可能会给研究带来偏倚。

5 提高胚胎种植率的方法

5.1 胚胎选择

虽然包括原核期、卵裂期和囊胚期在内的胚胎形态学提供了关于单个胚胎生殖潜力的有用信息,但仍有超过一半的胚胎移植不会导致妊娠。评估胚胎种植潜力的辅助方法是一个活跃的研究领域。

5.2 胚胎形态动力学

时差显微镜已被用于研究胚胎发育,而胚胎发育的形态动力学也已被提出作为预测单个胚胎生殖潜力的方法;然而,这种方法是否能够改善种植率和活产率尚未得到证实。与 PGT 相比,时差显微镜具有非侵入性的优势。然而,目前的技术水平可能无法接近 PGT-A 在胚胎染色体倍性方面的敏感性[34,59]。

5.3 代谢组学和胚胎培养液中的代谢物浓度

废胚培养液的代谢组学分析已被提出作为评估胚胎生殖潜力的非侵入性手段。Seli 等[60]的一项研究使用了废胚培养液,并记录这些胚胎在第 3 天单胚胎移植后是否临床妊娠。然后，他们将培养液用近红外光谱进行分析，产生一个生存力指数，该指数可以独立于形态学预测第 2 天和第 3 天胚胎的生存力。谷氨酸、丙氨酸和亮氨酸水平也被用作评价胚胎质量的标志物[34]。血清水平的代谢组学研究也已开展，包括 RoyChoudhury 等[61]进行的一项有趣的研究，将患有 RIF 的女性与每次胚胎移植都成功植入的女性进行了比较。结果发现，反复植入成功女性的缬氨酸、己二酸、L-赖氨酸、肌酸、鸟氨酸、甘油、D-葡萄糖和尿素的水平都显著低于 RIF 患者。该研究还证明，RIF 患者的血清内皮型一氧化氮合酶（eNOS）水平较低。eNOS 在黄体期的子宫内膜中存在，而 NOS 抑制剂可能会影响子宫内膜的容受性和胚胎种植[62]。

5.4　胚胎培养条件

开发胚胎共培养系统是为了在体外为早期胚胎提供生长因子和细胞因子的来源，以模拟体内环境，促进胚胎的持续发育[63]。一项荟萃分析回顾了 17 项关于胚胎与多种细胞类型共培养的研究，显示了在植入和临床妊娠方面的有利结果[64]。在过去 30 年，虽然有不少研究已完成，尚无关于共培养胚胎后代长期健康影响的报道。然而，要确定两者之间的关系非常困难。在共培养体系中释放的细胞因子和生长因子可能并不完全知晓，而添加细胞因子和生长因子确实具有优于共培养的优势。一项随机对照试验比较了常规培养与添加了 GM-CSF、肝素结合性表皮生长因子（HB-EGF）和 LIF 等细胞因子的培养情况，结果显示在囊胚的发育和质量方面略有改善，种植率增加，活产率增加（45% vs 33%），而早产和活产儿体重没有改变[65]。虽然这些结果令人鼓舞，但对后代的长期健康影响很难评估。

5.5　序贯胚胎移植

序贯胚胎移植用于 RIF 患者的应用已有文献报道。相关研究通常采用先卵裂期胚胎后囊胚的顺序进行序贯移植，但这种方法被认为不太可能改善子宫内膜-胚胎不同步的问题[66,67]。Esfandiari 等[68]采用了一种不同的方法，他们描述了一例曾经历 5 次失败 IVF 周期的患者，进行了自然周期冷冻胚胎移植（FET）（黄体期补充孕酮）。该患者进行了两次双胚胎移植，共使用了 4 个裂解期第 3 天的胚胎，每次移植 2 枚胚胎，分别在 LH 峰后的第 5 天和第 7 天进行，最终单胎活产。值得注意的是，该患者的月经周期为 21 天；然而，她在之前的激素替代 FET 周期中均未取得成功[68]。采用这种方式进行序贯移植可能会克服子宫内膜-胚胎不同步问题，因为移植的胚胎处于相同的发育阶段，植入到两个具有不同准备程度的子宫内膜中。

5.6　辅助孵化

辅助孵化包括一系列机械、化学或激光方法，用于剥脱或变薄透明带。方法、患者群体和诊断的异质性可能会混淆辅助孵化和活产之间的关联。然而，一项大型荟萃分析得出的结论是，目前没有足够的证据支持常规进行辅助孵化[69]。关于辅助孵化在 RIF 中益处的数据存在不一致[70,71]。一项 RCT 试验的荟萃分析显示，在接受新鲜胚胎移植并进行辅助孵化的 RIF 患者中，临床妊娠率增加（$RR=1.73, CI=1.37 \sim 2.17$），而在进行辅助孵化的非选择性患者组中没有益处[72]。这表明一部分患者可能存在与透明带有关的植入障碍。

5.7　改善精子非整倍体的疗法

关于改善精子非整倍体的疗法的研究有限。在一项针对 31 名具有高频精子非整倍体的不育男性患者的小型研究中，22 名患者接受了重组 FSH 治疗（150 U，每周 3 次）。重组 FSH 治疗降低了总体精子的非整倍体率（$P<0.001$）；然而，未报道妊娠率[73]。Young 等[74]进行的一项针对 97 名健康志愿者的研究旨在确定营养与精子非整倍体之间的关联。参与者填写了膳食问卷，然后根据该问卷估算出平均每日营养摄入量。研究结果显示，每日叶酸摄入量每增加 100 mg，精子非整倍体率就降低 $3.6\% (95\% CI: -6.3\% \sim -0.8\%)$。值得注意的是，这不是一个不育群体，且未评估妊娠率。第三项研究包括了接受 ICSI 治疗的严重少弱精症患者夫妇。该研究中纳入的 33 对夫妇既往至少有过一次 ICSI 周期不成功的经历。治疗为期 3 个月，每天 2 次服用左旋肉碱 1 g，每天 2 次服用乙酰左旋肉碱 500 mg，再加上每 4 天服用 1 粒 30 mg 辛诺昔康（cinnoxicam）片。治疗前后评估多项指标，包括精子浓度、活力和形态、非整倍体精子的百分比、受精卵母细胞数量、移植胚胎数量以及妊娠率和活产率。33 名患者中有 22 名的精子非整倍体减少（基线为 15%，干预后为 2%，$P<0.01$）和正常精子形态增加

（基线为3%，干预后为7.5%，$P<0.01$）。在精子参数得到改善的22名患者中，临床妊娠率为50%，而在同样接受干预但精子参数无明显改善的11名患者中，临床妊娠率为9.1%（$P<0.01$），活产率分别为45.4%和9.1%（$P<0.01$）[75]。这些初步研究表明了改善精子非整倍体的潜在治疗方法。

6 免疫调节

6.1 粒细胞集落刺激因子

在过去的几十年里，人们提出了针对不同免疫靶点的治疗策略，以改善胚胎种植和妊娠结局。粒细胞集落刺激因子（G-CSF）是一种主要负责干细胞分化和迁移的细胞因子，由造血细胞和一小部分非造血细胞产生。G-CSF 在胚胎植入过程中具有免疫调节功能，例如抑制白细胞活性。最近的一项荟萃分析表明，局部和全身应用 G-CSF 均能提高临床妊娠率[76]。然而，一项针对 RIF 患者（定义为年龄小于40岁，在至少3个新鲜或冷冻周期移植4个高质量胚胎后未能妊娠）的随机临床试验并没有显示临床妊娠率、活产率或子宫内膜厚度存在显著差异[77]。

6.2 富血小板血浆

富血小板血浆（PRP）已在多项研究中作为 RIF 患者的治疗手段。PRP 含有多种生长因子，包括血小板衍生生长因子、胰岛素样生长因子和 VEGF[78]。一项针对30名行 FET 的 RIF 患者的小型研究并未发现胚胎移植前48小时接受 PRP 治疗的患者与未接受治疗的患者之间存在差异[79]。Nazari 等[80]进行了一项单臂 PRP 研究，报道了20名 RIF 患者中有18例妊娠，其中16例为持续妊娠，1例为葡萄胎，1例为流产。该研究由于缺乏对照组和缺乏妊娠结局数据，局限性较大。

6.3 粒细胞集落刺激因子和富血小板血浆

一项针对 RIF 患者（定义为至少2次胚胎移植，移植至少5枚形态学良好的胚胎）和首次 IVF/ICSI 对照组（未接受辅助药物）的初步研究使用 PRP 和 G-CSF 的联合方案（"PRIMER"）以改善子宫内膜容受性。每组有33名患者。两组的持续妊娠率和活产率均为27.3%。作者认为他们的结果表明，使用 PRIMER 的 RIF 患者与对照组的活产率相当；

然而，PRIMER 组的流产率为25%，而对照组为9%。尽管由于样本量小，差异没有统计学意义[81]，但仍对 PRIMER 在重度 RIF 患者亚组中的疗效提出了质疑。

6.4 脂肪乳剂

脂肪乳剂（intralipid）是一种最早且目前仍在用于肠外营养的大豆油乳剂，作为免疫调节剂的疗效报道存在差异[82]。脂肪乳剂已被用于治疗 RIF 和 RPL，其原理是降低 NK 细胞的细胞毒性[83]。NK 细胞是固有淋巴细胞，负责杀伤肿瘤细胞和病毒感染细胞，并产生细胞因子以募集和影响其他淋巴细胞[84,85]。NK 细胞与 RIF 和 RPL 均有关[83]。一项回顾性单中心研究显示，使用脂肪乳剂的活产成本增加了681美元，但活产率却没有获益[86]。相比之下，一项针对具有至少1次种植失败史的 IVF/ICSI 患者的单盲随机临床试验显示，脂肪乳剂组的活产率为28.8%，对照组为10%[87]。由于至少有1次种植失败的标准，该研究人群可能并不能代表真正的 RIF 患者群体。在一中位数为9.5次（3~19次）胚胎移植失败的 RIF 患者研究中，9名接受脂肪乳剂治疗的患者实现了临床妊娠（56%）。在这项研究中，活产率是根据实现临床妊娠后活产的患者比例计算，而不是与所有接受胚胎移植的患者进行比较。脂肪乳剂组的活产率为55%（9名妊娠患者中有5名活产），而对照组的活产率为33%（6名患者中有2名），但差异没有统计学意义。这篇报道中使用包括他们自己的数据在内的三项研究（共107名 RPL 患者和47名对照组）进行文献回顾，支持使用脂肪乳剂治疗[88]。

6.5 人白细胞抗原

人白细胞抗原（HLA）是一种具有免疫调节功能的细胞表面蛋白。人类合体滋养层细胞上的 HLA 表达受到严格调控，以避免对半同种基因的胚胎产生免疫反应。HLA-G 在滋养细胞表面表达，并据推测在调节巨噬细胞、NK 细胞和胚胎间的相互作用中发挥作用，因为这些细胞均表达 HLA-G 受体[25]。因此提出，可溶性 HLA-G 的检测可作为生殖潜力的标志。Sher 等和 Kotze 等在独立研究中发现，培养液中含有可溶性 HLA-G 的胚胎具有更高的种植率和临床妊娠率[89]以及持续妊娠率[90]。

6.6 宫腔内人绒毛膜促性腺激素治疗

由于 hCG 在胚胎植入过程中起着关键作用,已对接受胚胎移植前宫腔内 hCG 治疗的患者进行了多项研究。无论是初步研究还是荟萃分析,结果均不一致。有人提出,宫腔内 hCG 可能改善 IVF 周期中可能发生的子宫内膜不同步的问题。在一项由 Strug 等[91]进行的研究中,卵母细胞捐赠者在宫腔内输注 hCG 2 天后进行了子宫内膜活检。与对照组相比,她们的 α-平滑肌肌动蛋白水平更高,对 Notch1 和 C3 的影响可能更温和。在该研究中纳入了年轻的卵母细胞捐赠者,可能由于强烈的反应和由此产生的更高雌激素水平,子宫内膜的效应可能更为显著。Mansour 等和 Santibañez 等[92,93]的前瞻性研究表明,在宫腔内 hCG 治疗后移植卵裂期胚胎可以改善临床妊娠率和活产率。Zarei 等[94]进行的一项随机对照试验也显示,在胚胎移植前应用宫腔内 hCG 治疗可以提高临床妊娠率和活产率。然而,囊胚移植的研究并未显示 hCG 对临床妊娠率有这种有益影响[95,96]。Volovsky 等[97]的研究表明,宫腔内 hCG 治疗对非 RIF 患者的临床妊娠率和活产率有负面影响,对 RIF 患者没有影响。考虑到这些相互矛盾的结果,还需要进一步研究以确定哪些患者群体(如果有的话)可以从 hCG 治疗中获益。

6.7 子宫内膜损伤("搔刮")

多项研究评估了 IUI 和 IVF 患者的妊娠率,均显示子宫内膜损伤或"搔刮"(通常使用子宫内膜活检刮匙进行)有益处[98-100]。近期一项针对接受新鲜胚胎移植或冷冻胚胎移植的 IVF 患者的系统评价和荟萃分析并没有发现接受子宫内膜搔刮的患者的临床妊娠率或活产率存在显著差异[101]。另一项针对接受新鲜胚胎移植或冷冻胚胎移植患者的大型随机对照试验表明,子宫内膜搔刮与活产率无关[102]。这种方法可能对特定易于子宫内膜微结构紊乱的患者亚群有效;然而,识别这些患者可能困难重重。基于现有证据,目前不推荐将子宫内膜搔刮作为 RIF 的常规治疗方法。

7 总结与建议

- 胚胎与子宫内膜之间的相互作用可能受到免疫因素和内在因素的双重影响。
- 胚胎非整倍体可能是 RIF 的原因之一,可以考虑对胚胎或患者及配偶进行遗传检测。
- 免疫调节剂的使用仍在积极探索中,鉴于免疫系统在胚胎植入过程中发挥重要作用,有必要进行严谨的研究。

参考文献

[1] ART Success Rates. CDC; 2021. 〈https://www.cdc.gov/art/artdata/index.html〉[accessed 2.20.2021].

[2] Glujovsky D, Farquhar C, Quinteiro Retamar AM, Alvarez Sedo CR, Blake D. Cleavage stage vs blastocyst stage embryo transfer in assisted reproductive technology. Cochrane Database Syst Rev 2016;(6) CD002118.

[3] Balaban B, Urman B, Sertac A, Alatas C, Aksoy S, Mercan R. Blastocyst quality affects the success of blastocyst-stage embryo transfer. Fertil Steril 2000;74(2):282-7.

[4] Gardner DK, Lane M, Stevens J, Schlenker T, Schoolcraft WB. Blastocyst score affects implantation and pregnancy outcome: towards a single blastocyst transfer. Fertil Steril 2000;73(6):1155-8.

[5] Elder K, Cohen J. Human preimplantation embryo selection. Boca Raton, Fla: CRC Press; 2008.

[6] Armstrong S, Bhide P, Jordan V, Pacey A, Marjoribanks J, Farquhar C. Time-lapse systems for embryo incubation and assessment in assisted reproduction. Cochrane Database Syst Rev 2019;5 CD011320.

[7] Schumacher A, Zenclussen AC. Human chorionic gonadotropin-mediated immune responses that facilitate embryo implantation and placentation. Front Immunol 2019;10:2896.

[8] Gridelet V, Perrier d'Hauterive S, Polese B, Foidart JM, Nisolle M, Geenen V. Human chorionic gonadotrophin: new pleiotropic functions for an "old" hormone during pregnancy. Front Immunol 2020;11:343.

[9] Kane N, Kelly R, Saunders PT, Critchley HO. Proliferation of uterine natural killer cells is induced by human chorionic gonadotropin and mediated via the mannose receptor. Endocrinology 2009;150(6):2882-8.

[10] Fan XG, Zheng ZQ. A study of early pregnancy factor activity in preimplantation. Am J Reprod Immunol 1997;37(5):359-64.

[11] Bose R, Cheng H, Sabbadini E, McCoshen J, MaHadevan MM, Fleetham J. Purified human early pregnancy factor from preimplantation embryo possesses immunosuppressive properties. Am J Obstet Gynecol 1989;160(4):954-60.

[12] Morton H. Early pregnancy factor: an extracellular chaperonin 10 homologue. Immunol Cell Biol 1998;76(6):483-96.

[13] Athanasas-Platsis S, Corcoran CM, Kaye PL, Cavanagh AC, Morton H. Early pregnancy factor is required at two important stages of embryonic development in the mouse. Am J Reprod Immunol 2000;43(4):223-33.

[14] Bach JF, Dormont J, Dardenne M, Balner H. In vitro rosette

[14] inhibition by antihuman antilymphocyte serum. Correlation with skin graft prolongation in subhuman primates. Transplantation 1969;8(3):265-80.

[15] Nakatsuka M, Yoshida N, Kudo T. Platelet activating factor in culture media as an indicator of human embryonic development after in-vitro fertilization. Hum Reprod 1992;7(10):1435-9.

[16] Harper MJ. Platelet-activating factor: a paracrine factor in preimplantation stages of reproduction? Biol Reprod 1989;40(5):907-13.

[17] Harper MJ, Kudolo GB, Alecozay AA, Jones MA. Platelet-activating factor (PAF) and blastocyst-endometrial interactions. Prog Clin Biol Res 1989;294:305-15.

[18] Tiemann U. The role of platelet-activating factor in the mammalian female reproductive tract. Reprod Domest Anim 2008;43(6):647-55.

[19] Calleja-Agius J, Jauniaux E, Pizzey AR, Muttukrishna S. Investigation of systemic inflammatory response in first trimester pregnancy failure. Hum Reprod 2012;27(2):349-57.

[20] Boomsma CM, Kavelaars A, Eijkemans MJ, et al. Endometrial secretion analysis identifies a cytokine profile predictive of pregnancy in IVF. Hum Reprod 2009;24(6):1427-35.

[21] Huang JC, Liu DY, Yadollahi S, Wu KK, Dawood MY. Interleukin-1 beta induces cyclooxygenase-2 gene expression in cultured endometrial stromal cells. J Clin Endocrinol Metab 1998;83(2):538-41.

[22] Tilley SL, Coffman TM, Koller BH. Mixed messages: modulation of inflammation and immune responses by prostaglandins and thromboxanes. J Clin Invest 2001;108(1):15-23.

[23] Ricciotti E, FitzGerald GA. Prostaglandins and inflammation. Arterioscler Thromb Vasc Biol 2011;31(5):986-1000.

[24] Psychoyos A, Nikas G, Gravanis A. The role of prostaglandins in blastocyst implantation. Hum Reprod 1995;10(Suppl 2):30-42.

[25] Norwitz ER, Schust DJ, Fisher SJ. Implantation and the survival of early pregnancy. N Engl J Med 2001;345(19):1400-8.

[26] Nicola NA, Babon JJ. Leukemia inhibitory factor (LIF). Cytokine Growth Factor Rev 2015;26(5):533-44.

[27] Dunglison GF, Barlow DH, Sargent IL. Leukaemia inhibitory factor significantly enhances the blastocyst formation rates of human embryos cultured in serum-free medium. Hum Reprod 1996;11(1):191-6.

[28] Cheng TC, Huang CC, Chen CI, et al. Leukemia inhibitory factor antisense oligonucleotide inhibits the development of murine embryos at preimplantation stages. Biol Reprod 2004;70(5):1270-6.

[29] Paria BC, Song H, Dey SK. Implantation: molecular basis of embryo-uterine dialogue. Int J Dev Biol 2001;45(3):597-605.

[30] Jokhi PP, King A, Sharkey AM, Smith SK, Loke YW. Screening for cytokine messenger ribonucleic acids in purified human decidual lymphocyte populations by the reverse-transcriptase polymerase chain reaction. J Immunol 1994;153(10):4427-35.

[31] Ander SE, Diamond MS, Coyne CB. Immune responses at the maternal-fetal interface. Sci Immunol 2019;4(31):1-22.

[32] Taylor HS, Pal L, Seli E, Fritz MA. Speroff's clinical gynecologic endocrinology and infertility. 9th ed. Philadelphia: Wolters Kluwer; 2020.

[33] Pirtea P, De Ziegler D, Tao X, et al. Rate of true recurrent implantation failure is low: results of three successive frozen euploid single embryo transfers. Fertil Steril 2021;115(1):45-53.

[34] Nagy ZP, Varghese, Alex C., Agarwal, A. In vitro fertilization. A Textb Curr Emerg Meth Dev. 2019.

[35] Esfandiari N, Bunnell ME, Casper RF. Human embryo mosaicism: did we drop the ball on chromosomal testing? J Assist Reprod Genet 2016;33(11):1439-44.

[36] Coughlan C. What to do when good-quality embryos repeatedly fail to implant. Best Pract Res Clin Obstet Gynaecol 2018;53:48-59.

[37] Sato T, Sugiura-Ogasawara M, Ozawa F, et al. Preimplantation genetic testing for aneuploidy: a comparison of live birth rates in patients with recurrent pregnancy loss due to embryonic aneuploidy or recurrent implantation failure. Hum Reprod 2019;34(12):2340-8.

[38] Raziel A, Friedler S, Schachter M, Kasterstein E, Strassburger D, Ron-El R. Increased frequency of female partner chromosomal abnormalities in patients with high-order implantation failure after in vitro fertilization. Fertil Steril 2002;78(3):515-19.

[39] Bungum M, Humaidan P, Axmon A, et al. Sperm DNA integrity assessment in prediction of assisted reproduction technology outcome. Hum Reprod 2007;22(1):174-9.

[40] Weissman A, Horowitz E, Ravhon A, Nahum H, Golan A, Levran D. Pregnancies and live births following ICSI with testicular spermatozoa after repeated implantation failure using ejaculated spermatozoa. Reprod Biomed Online 2008;17(5):605-9.

[41] Collins JA, Barnhart KT, Schlegel PN. Do sperm DNA integrity tests predict pregnancy with in vitro fertilization? Fertil Steril 2008;89(4):823-31.

[42] Schlegel PN, Sigman M, Collura B, et al. Diagnosis and treatment of infertility in men: AUA/ASRM guideline part I. Fertil Steril 2021;115(1):54-61.

[43] Esteves SC, Santi D, Simoni M. An update on clinical and surgical interventions to reduce sperm DNA fragmentation in infertile men. Andrology 2020;8(1):53-81.

[44] Garcia-Mengual E, Trivino JC, Saez-Cuevas A, Bataller J, Ruiz-Jorro M, Vendrell X. Male infertility: establishing sperm aneuploidy thresholds in the laboratory. J Assist Reprod Genet 2019;36(3):371-81.

[45] Nikas G, Develioglu OH, Toner JP, Jones Jr. HW. Endometrial pinopodes indicate a shift in the window of receptivity in IVF cycles. Hum Reprod 1999;14(3):787-92.

[46] Rackow BW, Kliman HJ, Taylor HS. GnRH antagonists may affect endometrial receptivity. Fertil Steril 2008;89(5):1234-9.

[47] Bashiri A, Halper KI, Orvieto R. Recurrent implantation failure-update overview on etiology, diagnosis, treatment and future directions. Reprod Biol Endocrinol 2018;16(1):121.

[48] Lessey BA, Young SL. What exactly is endometrial receptivity? Fertil Steril 2019;111(4):611-17.

[49] Hashimoto T, Koizumi M, Doshida M, et al. Efficacy of the endometrial receptivity array for repeated implantation failure in Japan: a retrospective, two-centers study. Reprod Med Biol 2017;16(3):290-6.

[50] Tan J, Kan A, Hitkari J, et al. The role of the endometrial receptivity array (ERA) in patients who have failed euploid

embryo transfers. J Assist Reprod Genet 2018;35(4):683-92.
[51] Ise W, Fujii K, Shiroguchi K, et al. T follicular helper cell-germinal center b cell interaction strength regulates entry into plasma cell or recycling germinal center cell fate. Immunity 2018;48(4):702-715 e704.
[52] Evans-Hoeker E, Lessey BA, Jeong JW, et al. Endometrial BCL6 overexpression in eutopic endometrium of women with endometriosis. Reprod Sci 2016;23(9):1234-41.
[53] Lessey BA, Kim JJ. Endometrial receptivity in the eutopic endometrium of women with endometriosis: it is affected, and let me show you why. Fertil Steril 2017;108(1):19-27.
[54] Almquist LD, Likes CE, Stone B, et al. Endometrial BCL6 testing for the prediction of in vitro fertilization outcomes: a cohort study. Fertil Steril 2017;108(6):1063-9.
[55] Liu Y, Ko EY, Wong KK, et al. Endometrial microbiota in infertile women with and without chronic endometritis as diagnosed using a quantitative and reference range-based method. Fertil Steril 2019;112(4):707-717 e701.
[56] Liu L, Yang H, Guo Y, Yang G, Chen Y. The impact of chronic endometritis on endometrial fibrosis and reproductive prognosis in patients with moderate and severe intrauterine adhesions: a prospective cohort study. Fertil Steril 2019;111(5):1002-1010 e1002.
[57] Bouet PE, El Hachem H, Monceau E, Gariepy G, Kadoch IJ, Sylvestre C. Chronic endometritis in women with recurrent pregnancy loss and recurrent implantation failure: prevalence and role of office hysteroscopy and immunohistochemistry in diagnosis. Fertil Steril 2016;105(1):106-10.
[58] Cicinelli E, Matteo M, Tinelli R, et al. Prevalence of chronic endometritis in repeated unexplained implantation failure and the IVF success rate after antibiotic therapy. Hum Reprod 2015;30(2):323-30.
[59] Zaninovic N, Irani M, Meseguer M. Assessment of embryo morphology and developmental dynamics by time-lapse microscopy: is there a relation to implantation and ploidy? Fertil Steril 2017;108(5):722-9.
[60] Seli E, Vergouw CG, Morita H, et al. Noninvasive metabolomic profiling as an adjunct to morphology for noninvasive embryo assessment in women undergoing single embryo transfer. Fertil Steril 2010;94(2):535-42.
[61] RoyChoudhury S, Singh A, Gupta NJ, et al. Repeated implantation failure vs repeated implantation success: discrimination at a metabolomic level. Hum Reprod 2016;31(6):1265-74.
[62] Chwalisz K, Garfield RE. Role of nitric oxide in implantation and menstruation. Hum Reprod 2000;15(Suppl 3):96-111.
[63] Vajta G, Rienzi L, Cobo A, Yovich J. Embryo culture: can we perform better than nature? Reprod Biomed Online 2010;20(4):453-69.
[64] Kattal N, Cohen J, Barmat LI. Role of coculture in human in vitro fertilization: a meta-analysis. Fertil Steril 2008;90(4):1069-76.
[65] Fawzy M, Emad M, Elsuity MA, et al. Cytokines hold promise for human embryo culture in vitro: results of a randomized clinical trial. Fertil Steril 2019;112(5):849-857 e841.
[66] Ashkenazi J, Yoeli R, Orvieto R, Shalev J, Ben-Rafael Z, Bar-Hava I. Double (consecutive) transfer of early embryos and blastocysts: aims and results. Fertil Steril 2000;74(5):936-40.
[67] Loutradis D, Drakakis P, Dallianidis K, et al. A double embryo transfer on days 2 and 4 or 5 improves pregnancy outcome in patients with good embryos but repeated failures in IVF or ICSI. Clin Exp Obstet Gynecol 2004;31(1):63-6.
[68] Esfandiari N, Coogan-Prewer J, Gotlieb L, Claessens EA, Casper RF. Successful pregnancy following double-frozen embryo transfer in a patient with repeated implantation failure. Fertil Steril 2008;90(4) 1199 e1113-1195.
[69] Carney SK, Das S, Blake D, Farquhar C, Seif MM, Nelson L. Assisted hatching on assisted conception in vitro fertilisation (IVF) and intracytoplasmic sperm injection (ICSI). Cochrane Database Syst Rev 2012;12 CD001894.
[70] Stein A, Rufas O, Amit S, et al. Assisted hatching by partial zona dissection of human pre-embryos in patients with recurrent implantation failure after in vitro fertilization. Fertil Steril 1995;63(4):838-41.
[71] Valojerdi MR, Eftekhari-Yazdi P, Karimian L, Ashtiani SK. Effect of laser zona pellucida opening on clinical outcome of assisted reproduction technology in patients with advanced female age, recurrent implantation failure, or frozen-thawed embryos. Fertil Steril 2008;90(1):84-91.
[72] Martins WP, Rocha IA, Ferriani RA, Nastri CO. Assisted hatching of human embryos: a systematic review and meta-analysis of randomized controlled trials. Hum Reprod Update 2011;17(4):438-53.
[73] Piomboni P, Serafini F, Gambera L, et al. Sperm aneuploidies after human recombinant follicle stimulating hormone therapy in infertile males. Reprod Biomed Online 2009;18(5):622-9.
[74] Young SS, Eskenazi B, Marchetti FM, Block G, Wyrobek AJ. The association of folate, zinc and antioxidant intake with sperm aneuploidy in healthy non-smoking men. Hum Reprod 2008;23(5):1014-22.
[75] Cavallini G, Magli MC, Crippa A, Ferraretti AP, Gianaroli L. Reduction in sperm aneuploidy levels in severe oligoasthenoteratospermic patients after medical therapy: a preliminary report. Asian J Androl 2012;14(4):591-8.
[76] Zhang L, Xu WH, Fu XH, et al. Therapeutic role of granulocyte colony-stimulating factor (G-CSF) for infertile women under in vitro fertilization and embryo transfer (IVF-ET) treatment: a meta-analysis. Arch Gynecol Obstet 2018;298(5):861-71.
[77] Kalem Z, Namli Kalem M, Bakirarar B, Kent E, Makrigiannakis A, Gurgan T. Intrauterine G-CSF administration in recurrent implantation failure (RIF): an Rct. Sci Rep 2020;10(1):5139.
[78] Dawood AS, Salem HA. Current clinical applications of platelet-rich plasma in various gynecological disorders: an appraisal of theory and practice. Clin Exp Reprod Med 2018;45(2):67-74.
[79] Aghajanzadeh F, Esmaeilzadeh S, Basirat Z, Mahouti T, Heidari FN, Golsorkhtabaramiri M. Using autologous intrauterine platelet-rich plasma to improve the reproductive outcomes of women with recurrent implantation failure. JBRA Assist Reprod 2020;24(1):30-3.
[80] Nazari L, Salehpour S, Hoseini S, Zadehmodarres S, Ajori L. Effects of autologous platelet-rich plasma on implantation and pregnancy in repeated implantation failure: a pilot study. Int J Reprod Biomed 2016;14(10):625-8.
[81] Dieamant F, Vagnini LD, Petersen CG, et al. New therapeutic protocol for improvement of endometrial receptivity (PRIMER) for patients with recurrent

implantation failure (RIF) — a pilot study. JBRA Assist Reprod 2019;23(3):250-4.
[82] Wanten GJ, Calder PC. Immune modulation by parenteral lipid emulsions. Am J Clin Nutr 2007;85(5):1171-84.
[83] Roussev RG, Acacio B, Ng SC, Coulam CB. Duration of intralipid's suppressive effect on NK cell's functional activity. Am J Reprod Immunol 2008;60(3):258-63.
[84] Poznanski SM, Ashkar AA. What defines NK cell functional fate: phenotype or metabolism? Front Immunol 2019;10:1414.
[85] Cooper MA, Fehniger TA, Caligiuri MA. The biology of human natural killer-cell subsets. Trends Immunol 2001;22(11):633-40.
[86] Martini AE, Jasulaitis S, Fogg LF, Uhler ML, Hirshfeld-Cytron JE. Evaluating the utility of intralipid infusion to improve live birth rates in patients with recurrent pregnancy loss or recurrent implantation failure. J Hum Reprod Sci 2018;11(3):261-8.
[87] Singh N, Davis AA, Kumar S, Kriplani A. The effect of administration of intravenous intralipid on pregnancy outcomes in women with implantation failure after IVF/ICSI with non-donor oocytes: a randomised controlled trial. Eur J Obstet Gynecol Reprod Biol 2019;240:45-51.
[88] Placais L, Kolanska K, Kraiem YB, et al. Intralipid therapy for unexplained recurrent miscarriage and implantation failure: case-series and literature review. Eur J Obstet Gynecol Reprod Biol 2020;252:100-4.
[89] Sher G, Keskintepe L, Fisch JD, et al. Soluble human leukocyte antigen G expression in phase I culture media at 46 hours after fertilization predicts pregnancy and implantation from day 3 embryo transfer. Fertil Steril 2005;83(5):1410-13.
[90] Kotze D, Kruger TF. HLA-G as a marker for embryo selection in assisted reproductive technology. Fertil Steril 2013;100(6):e44.
[91] Strug MR, Su R, Young JE, et al. Intrauterine human chorionic gonadotropin infusion in oocyte donors promotes endometrial synchrony and induction of early decidual markers for stromal survival: a randomized clinical trial. Hum Reprod 2016;31(7):1552-61.
[92] Santibanez A, Garcia J, Pashkova O, et al. Effect of intrauterine injection of human chorionic gonadotropin before embryo transfer on clinical pregnancy rates from in vitro fertilisation cycles: a prospective study. Reprod Biol Endocrinol 2014;12:9.
[93] Mansour R, Tawab N, Kamal O, et al. Intrauterine injection of human chorionic gonadotropin before embryo transfer significantly improves the implantation and pregnancy rates in vitro fertilization/intracytoplasmic sperm injection: a prospective randomized study. Fertil Steril 2011;96(6) 1370-1374 e1371.
[94] Zarei A, Parsanezhad ME, Younesi M, et al. Intrauterine administration of recombinant human chorionic gonadotropin before embryo transfer on outcome of in vitro fertilization/intracytoplasmic sperm injection: a randomized clinical trial. Iran J Reprod Med 2014;12(1):1-6.
[95] Wirleitner B, Schuff M, Vanderzwalmen P, et al. Intrauterine administration of human chorionic gonadotropin does not improve pregnancy and life birth rates independently of blastocyst quality: a randomised prospective study. Reprod Biol Endocrinol 2015;13:70.
[96] Hong KH, Forman EJ, Werner MD, et al. Endometrial infusion of human chorionic gonadotropin at the time of blastocyst embryo transfer does not impact clinical outcomes: a randomized, double-blind, placebo-controlled trial. Fertil Steril 2014;102(6) 1591-1595 e1592.
[97] Volovsky M, Healey M, MacLachlan V, Vollenhoven BJ. Should intrauterine human chorionic gonadotropin infusions ever be used prior to embryo transfer? J Assist Reprod Genet 2018;35(2):273-8.
[98] Nastri CO, Lensen SF, Gibreel A, et al. Endometrial injury in women undergoing assisted reproductive techniques. Cochrane Database Syst Rev 2015;(3) CD009517.
[99] Goel T, Mahey R, Bhatla N, Kalaivani M, Pant S, Kriplani A. Pregnancy after endometrial scratching in infertile couples undergoing ovulation induction and intrauterine insemination cycles-a randomized controlled trial. J Assist Reprod Genet 2017;34(8):1051-8.
[100] Barash A, Dekel N, Fieldust S, Segal I, Schechtman E, Granot I. Local injury to the endometrium doubles the incidence of successful pregnancies in patients undergoing in vitro fertilization. Fertil Steril 2003;79(6):1317-22.
[101] Vitagliano A, Andrisani A, Alviggi C, et al. Endometrial scratching for infertile women undergoing a first embryo transfer: a systematic review and meta-analysis of published and unpublished data from randomized controlled trials. Fertil Steril 2019;111(4) 734-746 e732.
[102] Lensen S, Venetis C, Ng EHY, et al. Should we stop offering endometrial scratching prior to in vitro fertilization? Fertil Steril 2019;111(6):1094-101.

第 17 章

自然杀伤细胞病理学与反复种植失败
Natural killer cell pathology and repeated implantation failures

Atsushi Fukui[1,2], Ayano Yamaya[1], Shinichiro Saeki[1], Ryu Takeyama[1], Toru Kato[1], Yu Wakimoto[1] and Hiroaki Shibahara[1]

[1] Department of Obstetrics and Gynecology, School of Medicine, Hyogo Medical University, Nishinomiya, Hyogo, Japan
[2] Fukushima Medical Center for Child and Woman, Fukushima Medical University, Fukushima, Japan

1 引言

1.1 反复种植失败

反复种植失败（RIF）通常被定义为在多次高质量胚胎移植后仍发生种植失败。然而，关于失败的胚胎移植周期数、移植的胚胎数、移植的胚胎发育阶段（卵裂期与囊胚期）、移植的胚胎形态质量以及是否包括进行胚胎植入前遗传学诊断（如胚胎植入前的非整倍体检测、PGT-A）等方面，尚无统一的定义。

已有多项研究将这些变量纳入 RIF 的诊断中。例如，Polanski 等[1]将 RIF 定义为连续 2 个新鲜或冷冻胚胎移植周期，累计移植 4 个及以上卵裂期优质胚胎或 2 个及以上优质囊胚后仍未植入。Coughlan 等[2]将 RIF 定义为年龄不超过 40 岁的女性在至少 3 个新鲜或冷冻胚胎移植周期中，移植至少 4 个优质胚胎后仍未能实现临床妊娠。最近，加拿大的 RIF 指南[3]和 ESHRE 特别小组[4]将 RIF 定义为在进行 2～3 次及更多次胚胎移植后，或移植 3～4 个及更多个优质胚胎后种植失败。

RIF 与反复妊娠丢失（RPL）有一些共同的病因。因此，一般将 RIF 与 RPL 进行相似的评估。然而，最近的研究表明，RPL 和 RIF 在某些程度上具有相似但不同的病理条件。因此，在未经恰当评估的情况下，建议不要将 RPL 的筛查或治疗方式应用于 RIF 患者。

1.2 反复种植失败的患病率

由于迄今为止对 RIF 的定义尚无全球统一的共识，因此很难估计 RIF 的真实患病率。然而，据报道在全球范围内进行 IVF-ET 的患者中，RIF 的患病率为 10%。Busnelli 等[5]使用基于 3 次高质量胚胎移植失败的 RIF 定义显示，估计 RIF 的患病率为 15%。

在移植 PGT-A 筛选过的优质整倍体胚胎时，消除了胚胎的遗传病因，即所谓的"卵母细胞或胚胎质量差"，可将 RIF 的潜在原因限制在子宫或母体上。据报道，一项针对 PGT-A 后使用整倍体胚胎进行 3 次移植的大规模研究显示[6]，第一次移植的累计妊娠率和活产率分别为 69.9% 和 64.8%，第二次移植分别为 87.9% 和 83.9%，第三次移植分别为 95.2% 和 92.6%。因此，根据这项研究，排除因胚胎非整倍导致种植失败的病例，真正的 RIF 患病率可能低于 5%。

2 自然杀伤细胞与妊娠

自然杀伤（NK）细胞在人类妊娠中发挥着重要作用，而对 NK 细胞的系统调节有助于成功妊娠。大部分外周血 NK（pNK）细胞是常规 NK 细胞，而组织驻留 NK 细胞存在于子宫中，称为子宫 NK（uNK）、子宫内膜 NK（eNK）或蜕膜 NK（dNK）细胞。NK 细胞占外周血淋巴细胞（PBL）的 5%～10%，妊娠早期蜕膜免疫细胞中 70%～90% 通过表达 NK 特异性表面标志物（即 CD56）来区别于其他细胞类型。人类 NK 细胞亚群包括 CD56^{bright} 和 CD56^{dim} NK 细胞。CD56^{dim} 细胞的主要功能是对靶细胞（如肿瘤细胞或外来病原体）进行细胞毒性作用，而 CD56^{bright} 细胞则主要分泌细胞因子，如肿瘤坏死因子（TNF）- α 和干扰素 - γ（IFN - γ）。CD56^{bright} 细胞主要存在于子宫内膜和蜕膜，而 CD56^{dim} 细胞主要存在于外周血。

NK 细胞属于固有免疫细胞，可利用其激活性和抑制性受体攻击靶细胞，而无须记忆。表达主要组织相容性复合体（MHC）分子的细胞可以逃避 NK 细胞的攻击，因为 MHC 与 NK 细胞上的抑制性受体结合可抑制 NK 细胞的细胞毒性作用。在人类中，绒毛外滋养层细胞表达经典 MHC Ⅰ 类抗原，即人白细胞抗原（HLA）- C，以及非经典 Ⅰ 类抗原，包括 HLA - G，HLA - F 和 HLA - E。因此，这些细胞可以逃避 NK 细胞的细胞毒性。然而，合体滋养层细胞不表达 MHC 分子，使其易受 NK 细胞的细胞毒性攻击。已报道 MHC Ⅰ 类相关蛋白 A 和 B（MIC - A 和 MIC - B）以及可溶性 HLA - G 参与控制 pNK 细胞的细胞毒性。因此，NK 细胞（无论是 uNK 细胞，还是 pNK 细胞）或其他 NK 细胞控制机制的紊乱都可能会导致生殖障碍和产科并发症，如 RPL、种植失败或子痫前期[7]。

蜕膜中细胞毒性 NK 细胞的增加可能不利于胚胎种植和早期妊娠中的胎儿存活。已在各种生殖障碍性疾病中报道了 NK 细胞数量和比例的异常、NK 细胞表面受体的表达异常以及细胞因子分泌失调[8-14]。因此，适当调节免疫细胞，尤其是 NK 细胞及其功能，对于实现成功妊娠至关重要[15]。

3 与生殖相关的潜在免疫病理学

评估 NK 细胞功能最广泛的方法是使用 pNK 细胞的 NK 细胞毒性检测。利用 K562 细胞系作为靶细胞，通过 ^{51}Cr 释放试验或流式细胞术进行测定。评估 NK 细胞功能的另一种方法是使用多种 NK 细胞表面标志物（CD16、CD56 等）分析 NK 细胞亚群，并检测 pNK 细胞和 uNK 细胞分泌的细胞因子、趋化因子和其他因子。

NK 细胞在建立和维持妊娠的子宫中含量丰富。uNK 细胞的主要群体是 CD56^{bright} NK 细胞。与 pNK（CD56^{dim}）不同，CD56^{bright} uNK 细胞不具备细胞毒性，并通过分泌细胞因子、生长促进蛋白和血管生成因子参与胎盘形成和血管重塑。据报道，uNK 细胞的细胞毒性增加和异常细胞因子分泌会导致妊娠失败，如 RIF[9,10]。因此，在 RIF 患者中，免疫治疗调节 NK 细胞可能对成功的生殖结局至关重要。

3.1 外周血自然杀伤细胞的细胞毒性和比例

研究显示，如果妊娠前在 ^{51}Cr 释放试验中 pNK 细胞的细胞毒性超过 46%，流式细胞术测得的 pNK 细胞（CD56$^+$ 细胞）比例超过 16.4%，RPL 患者的妊娠可能以生化妊娠或流产告终[16]。此外，胚胎移植时 pNK 细胞的细胞毒性或 pNK 细胞的异常比例可以预测接受 IVF 的女性随后的妊娠结局[17]。胚胎植入失败患者的 CD56$^+$ 和 CD56$^+$/CD16$^+$ NK 细胞百分比显著高于胚胎植入成功者[17]。此外，^{51}Cr 释放试验显示，胚胎植入成功者在胚胎移植时的 NK 细胞毒性低于既往 IVF 周期失败或植入失败的患者[17]。

另一方面，Moffett 等[18]报道称，pNK 细胞的检测不能告诉我们在子宫中发生了什么。相反，Park 等[19]发现，外周血 pNK 细胞反映了 RPL 患者子宫内 dNK 细胞的变化。NKp46 是一种天然的细胞毒性受体，其表达与 pNK 和 uNK 细胞的细胞因子分泌有关。外周血 CD56$^+$/NKp46$^+$ 细胞百分比与黄体中期子宫内膜 CD56^{bright}/NKp46$^+$ 细胞百分比显著相关[20,21]。这表明，pNK 和 uNK 细胞之间存在特异性 NK 细胞标志物的表达。因此，对 pNK 细胞功能的评估可能反映了 uNK 细胞的功能，基于 pNK 细胞评估选择的治疗策略可能有助于改善生育障碍女性的妊娠结局。

3.2 子宫和蜕膜自然杀伤细胞的细胞毒性和比例

子宫内 NK 细胞或 dNK 细胞的比例可通过流式细胞术来测定。使用子宫内膜取样器在黄体中期（即种植窗口期）收集子宫内膜组织。将 uNK 或 dNK 细胞机械分散，用单克隆抗体染色，并通过流式细胞术进行分析[17]。在 RIF 或 RPL 患者的子宫内膜或蜕膜中，具有高度细胞毒性的 CD16$^+$/CD56^{dim} 细胞增加[17,22]。Tuckerman 等[23]利用免疫组化发现，RIF 患者的子宫内膜中 CD56$^+$ 细胞比例[中位数（范围）CD56$^+$ 细胞密度 = 14.5%（1.5% ~ 71.4%）]显著高于对照组[5%（2.1% ~

19.2%)]。

该研究得出的结论是,RIF患者子宫内膜中CD56$^+$ NK细胞的增加直接参与了胚胎植入失败的过程。据报道,患有特发性RIF的女性黄体中期CD56$^+$ uNK细胞的比例高于对照组或已知病因的RIF组(如染色体异常、甲状腺疾病、易栓症)[24],且uNK细胞与CD56$^+$ pNK细胞呈正相关(r=0.707,$P<0.001$)[24]。基于这些发现,建议对患有特发性RIF的女性进行NK细胞分析。由于NK细胞和RIF之间的关联在子宫内膜中更为明显,因此在黄体中期也应考虑进行子宫内膜活检以评估uNK细胞。

另一方面,uNK细胞通过分泌细胞因子、趋化因子和血管生成因子,对于蜕膜化以及螺旋动脉的形成和重塑至关重要[25,26]。Kofod等[27]报道,植入前子宫内膜的uNK细胞丰度似乎对于正常生育和成功妊娠很重要。因此,除了简单的uNK细胞计数外,uNK细胞的功能分析对于评估NK细胞相关的病理学也很关键。

3.3 自然杀伤细胞的激活和抑制受体

NK细胞表达多种激活性和抑制性受体。这些受体间的平衡决定了NK细胞的功能,即NK细胞的细胞毒作用。在激活性受体方面,已有研究在正常和包括RPL及RIF的异常妊娠中检测了杀伤细胞免疫球蛋白样受体(KIR:KIR2DS1、KIR2DS2、KIR2DL4等)、C型凝集素受体(CD94/NKG2C和CD94/NKG2D)、天然细胞毒性受体(NCRs:NKp46、NKp44和NKp30)以及CD16的表达水平。同时,研究还评估了NK细胞上的抑制性受体表达,如KIR [KIR2DL1(CD158a)、KIR2DL2/3(CD158b)等]和c-型凝集素受体(CD94/NKG2A)[28-36]。此外,NKp46作为NK细胞激活性受体之一,是参与细胞毒性和细胞因子分泌的主要触发受体[8,10-12,37,38]。NKp46$^+$ NK细胞可分为NKp46^{bright}和NKp46^{dim} NK细胞。特别是NKp46^{bright}/CD56^{bright} NK细胞相较于NKp46^{dim} NK细胞能分泌更高水平的IFN-γ[37]。根据不孕症的原因,未能受孕者外周血中NKp46^{bright} NK细胞比例明显低于自然受孕或IVF-ET受孕成功者,而NKp46^{dim} NK细胞比例明显较高。NKp46^{bright} NK细胞与分泌转化生长因子-β(TGF-β)的NK细胞呈正相关,NKp46^{dim} NK细胞与分泌Ⅰ型细胞因子(干扰素-γ和肿瘤坏死因子-α)的NK细胞呈正相关,提示未能受孕者的TGF-β水平较低,Ⅰ型细胞因子水平较高[11]。这些发现表明,NKp46可能是预测生殖结局(如RIF和RPL)的一个潜在有用的标志物。

3.4 自然杀伤细胞分泌的细胞因子

NK细胞能分泌多种细胞因子,但主要为Ⅰ型细胞因子,如IFN-γ和TNF-α。然而,NK细胞亦能分泌其他细胞因子,如IL-4、IL-10、TGF-β、GM-CSF、M-CSF、LIF等。妊娠与辅助T细胞1(Th1)免疫反应的减少以及Th2反应的偏倚有关[39]。类似于Th1/Th2概念,已经提出NK1/NK2模型来描述NK细胞,在细胞因子分泌谱中显示出类似的极性[9,40-42]。NK1细胞因子对维持妊娠至关重要[43-46],在促进血管生成和动脉重塑中发挥作用,而螺旋动脉未能完全重塑则会导致RPL和子痫前期[47]。我们报道了在生殖障碍(如RPL和RIF)女性中,分泌TNF-α和IFN-γ的NK细胞数量显著增多。因此,NK细胞分泌炎性细胞因子(尤其是TNF-α和IFN-γ)的失调控可能与生殖障碍的免疫病理学密切相关[9]。

4 患者评估

最近报道了一种基于子宫内膜免疫细胞的评分来预测胚胎移植的妊娠结局[48,49]。利用免疫组化技术检测子宫内膜免疫细胞标志物的表达,包括CD56$^+$ NK细胞、CD68$^+$泛巨噬细胞、CD163$^+$ M2型巨噬细胞、Foxp3$^+$调节性T细胞、CD1a$^+$未成熟树突状细胞、CD83$^+$成熟树突状细胞、CD8$^+$细胞毒性T细胞,以及CD57$^+$成熟NK和T细胞。子宫内膜样本是在月经周期的黄体中期,控制性卵巢刺激周期之前采集的。在首个IVF-ET周期中,妊娠患者和胚胎种植失败患者间的CD56$^+$ NK细胞和调节性T细胞的表达没有差异。然而,用泛巨噬细胞和M2型巨噬细胞开发了一个用于制定胚胎移植策略的诺模图[48]。

通过二代测序技术的靶向RNA测序分析RPL和不明原因不孕症患者与对照组女性间的黄体中期子宫内膜活检样品。对在蜕膜化过程中子宫内膜转化所必需的NK细胞相关基因(*FOXO1*、*GZMB*、*IL15*、*SCNN1A*、*SGK1*和*SLC2A1*)的表达进行测定和评分。将这6个基因的综合评分指定为蜕膜化评分,其中最大得分为"6",最小得分为"0"。得分小于4表示蜕膜化过程异常[49]。

可通过以下策略来评估NK细胞病理:用$_{51}$Cr释放试验或流式细胞术评估pNK细胞的细胞毒性,用多种NK细胞标志物进行pNK和uNK细胞比例分析。这些检测都是相当标准化和直接的,且结果一致,有助于确定治疗适应证。此外,NK细胞和uNK细胞上的NKp46表达,以及NK1/NK2比值,类似于Th1/Th2比值,都是有待进一步研究和临床验证的潜在生物标志物。

5 治疗

5.1 抗凝治疗(阿司匹林和肝素)

尽管目前尚不清楚易栓症或抗磷脂综合征是否为RIF的原因,但有报道称,植入前应用阿司匹林和肝素能有效预防RIF[50]。此外,RPL患者的子宫动脉阻力指数(URa-RI)较高,且其水平随pNK细胞数量的增加而增加[51],而低分子量肝素治疗能有效降低RPL患者的URa-RI,并改善其妊娠结局[51]。另有研究报道,RPL和URa-RI较高的患者在备孕期使用低分子量肝素[根据患者体重,依诺肝素,20～40 mg(lovenox)=2 000～4 000 U(Clexane)/天]、低剂量阿司匹林(81 mg/d)和强的松(10 mg/d)治疗[53],也有积极的妊娠结局[52]。因此,阿司匹林-肝素疗法可能对RIF有效。

药品说明书指出,阿司匹林不应在妊娠28周后使用,因为它可能导致孕期延长、动脉导管早期闭锁、抑制子宫收缩、增加分娩时的出血。然而,81 mg/d剂量的阿司匹林用于某些特定的妊娠相关疾病,在妊娠任何阶段都可作为FDA建议(避免在妊娠20周或之后使用NSAID)的例外情况。与此同时,肝素亦可使用至分娩开始前。

5.2 类固醇

强的松已被证明可降低NK细胞的细胞毒性并抑制TNF-α的分泌,用于具有高Th1/Th2比值和高NK细胞毒性的RIF患者。然而,一份Cochrane综述报告称,没有明确证据表明糖皮质激素可显著改善IVF-ET的临床结局[54]。美国生殖医学会的指南指出,从控制性卵巢刺激到围胚胎移植期使用糖皮质激素可提高活产率[55]。强的松从母体转移到胎儿的能力较低,尚无关于其致畸性的报道。因此,在≤10 mg/d时可安全使用,但≥20 mg/d应谨慎,因为会增加妊娠期糖尿病、高血压和感染的风险[56]。

5.3 免疫球蛋白

免疫球蛋白被称为免疫调节剂,并已被用于RIF,因为它们通过免疫调节作用(如使NK细胞的细胞毒性和Th1/Th2比值正常化),在建立和维持妊娠方面发挥着有益的作用。韩国生殖免疫学会关于静脉注射免疫球蛋白G(IVIG)治疗生殖障碍(如RIF和RPL)的指南指出,应进行免疫学检测,如NK细胞水平和细胞毒性,以及Th1/Th2,以决定免疫球蛋白的给药和治疗方案,以及对RIF患者的随访间隔和持续时间[57]。

对于IgA缺乏症患者,应谨慎使用免疫球蛋白G,因为它可能导致抗IgA抗体阳性患者发生过敏反应。因此,在使用前应检测血清IgA水平。由于免疫球蛋白的半衰期为18～25天,从胚胎移植前开始,应每3～4周按400 mg/kg给药一次,直至妊娠至少10周。根据患者的情况确定IVIG治疗的终点以及是否需要进一步的实验室检查。RPL或RIF等生殖障碍患者注射IVIG后NK细胞的细胞毒性变化如图17.1所示。NK细胞的细胞毒性通常随着妊娠过程而降低。在具有高NK细胞毒性的生殖障碍患者中,NK细胞的细胞毒性在IVIG治疗后下降,但在IVIG半衰期后再次升高,表明需要重复给予IVIG。对RIF患者IVIG治疗的有效性已进行了综述[58]。在这篇综述中,IVIG治疗对于改善RIF患者的妊娠率和活产率是有效的。因此,对于根据NK、NKT和T细胞等相关免疫紊乱选择的RIF患者,IVIG可能是一种有益的治疗策略。此外,通过免疫调节治疗,包括强的松、IVIG以及低分子量肝素和低剂量阿司匹林的抗凝治疗,可显著改善具有细胞免疫异常和血栓形成倾向的RPL和RIF患者的IVF-ET成功率[15]。与历史对照组相比,接受免疫调节治疗的所有患者的IVF周期妊娠率和每个胚胎移植周期的活产率均显著增加[15]。最近,Saab等[59]回顾了RIF患者IVIG治疗的4个荟萃分析,并得出结论,IVIG对于提高RIF患者的临床妊娠率和活产率是有价值的。然而,美国生殖医学会的指南指出,尚无足够的证据建议接受IVF-ET治疗的患者使用免疫球蛋白,需要进一步研究来阐明免疫球蛋白适用的病例[55]。

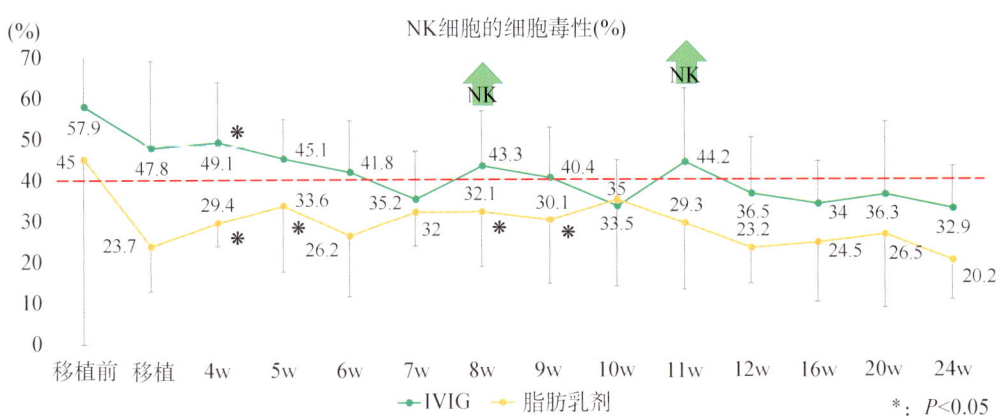

图 17.1 接受静脉注射免疫球蛋白 G(IVIG)和脂肪乳剂治疗的反复种植失败(RIF)患者的自然杀伤(NK)细胞的细胞毒性。

IVIG 抑制外周血 NK 细胞的细胞毒性(绿线)。IVIG 的半衰期为 3 周,IVIG 治疗 4 周后 NK 细胞的细胞毒性再次升高,故应定期予以 IVIG 治疗。妊娠期间输注脂肪乳剂也可抑制外周血 NK 细胞的细胞毒性(黄线),并且重复使用脂肪乳剂可维持 NK 细胞的细胞毒性。

5.4 脂肪乳剂输注疗法

由大豆油和蛋黄卵磷脂组成的脂肪乳剂(intralipid)输注疗法,对 NK 细胞的细胞毒性和炎症细胞因子具有免疫抑制作用,已用于术前和术后营养支持以及 RIF[60,61]。关于脂肪乳剂输注疗法的荟萃分析[62]和综述[63]表明,脂肪乳剂输注疗法可提高 RIF 的临床妊娠率和活产率。同时,也有相互矛盾的报道[64]。美国生殖医学会指南指出,没有足够的证据支持接受 IVF-ET 的患者使用脂肪乳剂输注疗法。需要进一步研究来阐明脂肪乳剂的使用适应证[55]。脂肪乳剂输注疗法适用于 NK 细胞异常等免疫异常的患者。接受脂肪乳剂输注疗法的生殖障碍患者的 NK 细胞毒性如图 17.1 所示。

未稀释的脂肪乳剂(10%～20%)在市场上是可购得的。将 2～4 mL 的 20% 脂肪乳剂溶液与 250 mL 无菌静脉注射生理盐水混合,以每小时 250 mL 的速度输注给患者[65]。应小心进行稀释以避免配方发生变化。此外,未稀释的脂肪乳剂(20%, 250 mL)也可用于治疗[66-68]。胚胎移植前每 2～3 周输注一次脂肪乳剂,直至妊娠 10 周或更长时间[66-68]。

5.5 羟氯喹

羟氯喹是一种抗疟药物,临床已使用多年,也可用于治疗自身免疫性疾病,包括系统性红斑狼疮、皮肤红斑狼疮和类风湿关节炎。羟氯喹因其对不孕症和 RIF 的影响而受到关注。一项针对具有高 Th1/Th2 的 RIF 患者的研究显示[69],在羟氯喹治疗后,血液和子宫内膜中的 Th1/Th2[69] 以及 Th17/调节性 T 细胞比值[70]降低。妊娠期间使用羟氯喹不存在致畸性问题。而氯喹与羟氯喹具有相似的化学结构和药理作用,具有遗传毒性和生殖毒性。因此,氯喹在妊娠期间使用存在致畸和胎儿毒性风险增加的问题。

5.6 肿瘤坏死因子抑制剂

肿瘤坏死因子(TNF)抑制剂被用于治疗类风湿关节炎、白塞病、川崎病、克罗恩病和溃疡性结肠炎,并且越来越多的患者在接受 TNF 抑制剂治疗时怀孕。与未接受治疗的风湿性疾病患者相比,虽然在接受英夫利昔单抗(infliximab)和阿达木单抗(adalimumab)治疗的患者中观察到流产率增加,但早产、低出生体重或胎儿畸形的发生率没有差异[71]。此外,在一项关于妊娠期意外使用 TNF 抑制剂的研究中,胎儿畸形的发生率也未发现差异[72,73]。在具有高 Th1/Th2 的 RIF 患者中,接受 TNF 抑制剂治疗与 Th1/Th2 降低相关,并显著提高了胚胎种植率、临床妊娠率和活产率[74]。Fu 等[75]报道,相比使用安慰剂的对照组,接受依那西普(etanercept)治疗的 RPL 患者的 NK 细胞毒性和 TNF-α 水平降低。基于这些研究,TNF 抑制剂治疗可能对具有高 Th1/Th2 或 NK 细胞毒性的 RIF 患者有益,进一步研究 TNF 抑制剂治疗在 RIF 患者中的应用是必要的。

5.7 维生素 D

维生素 D 缺乏(25-羟基维生素 D＜30 ng/mL)可导致 NK 细胞异常,如细胞毒性 NK 细胞的数量增加和细胞毒性提高。在维生素 D(1 000～2 000 U/d)治疗后,NK 细胞的细胞毒性抑制,NK 细胞激活性受体的表达降低以及 NK 细胞 I 型细胞因子的分泌减少[76,77]。此外,活性维生素 D(1,25-二羟基维生素 D)也被报道可降低 NK 细胞的细胞毒性和 NK 细胞分泌的 I 型细胞因子[77]。至少可以说,维生素 D 对妊娠和胎儿至关重要,因为它能控制异常的促炎免疫反应。目前,维生素 D 可以作为补充剂轻松获得,当维生素 D 水平较低时,可以进行补充。

6 总结与建议

- RIF 目前还没有普遍接受的定义。
- RIF 一般定义为 2～3 次胚胎移植失败或移植 3～4 个优质胚胎后失败。
- 真正的 RIF 比例可能低于 5%。
- NK 细胞在人类妊娠中起着重要作用,对 NK 细胞的调节对于生殖成功至关重要。
- NK 细胞的一般功能可通过 NK 细胞的细胞毒性和细胞因子的分泌来衡量。
- 使用子宫内膜组织和外周血来评估和诊断免疫性 RIF 患者的 NK 细胞水平(比例)和细胞毒性是很好的选择。
- 对于 NK 细胞毒性较高或细胞因子分泌异常的 RIF 患者,有多种免疫调节治疗可供选择。
- 对于多普勒超声检测到子宫螺旋动脉血流指数异常的 RIF 患者,阿司匹林和肝素治疗是一个好的选择。
- 对于 NK 细胞异常的 RIF 患者,IVIG 和(或)类固醇是其主要治疗方法。
- 脂肪乳剂、羟氯喹、TNF 抑制剂和维生素 D 已经在具有 NK 细胞异常的 RIF 患者中得到应用(图 17.2)。

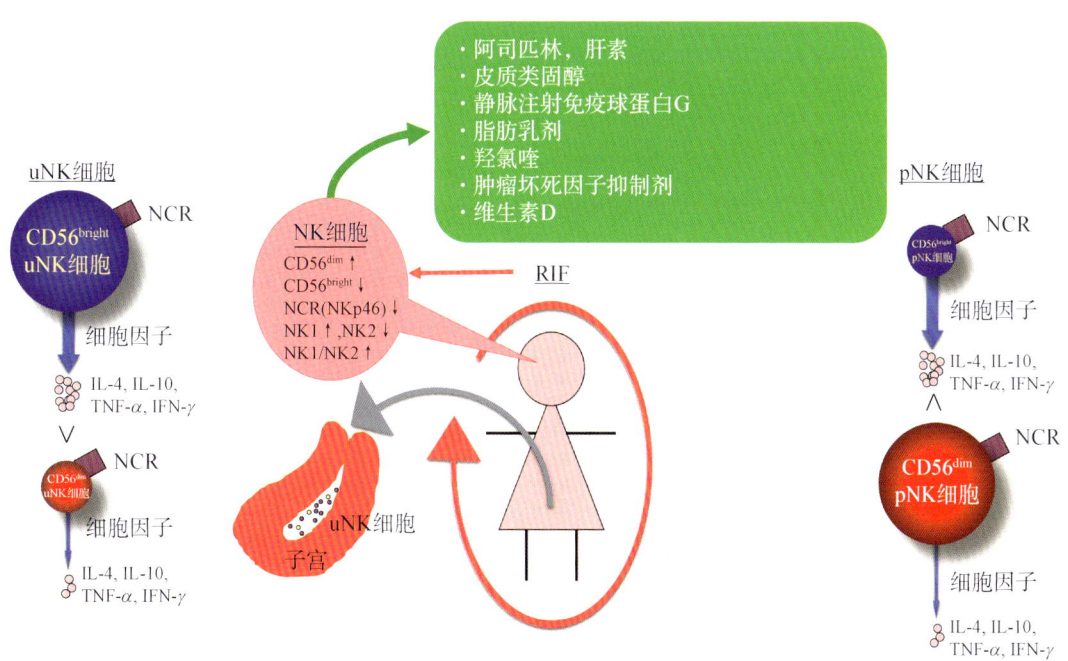

图 17.2 反复种植失败患者的自然杀伤(NK)细胞异常及其治疗。

有两种类型的 NK 细胞,CD56^{bright} NK 细胞和 CD56^{dim} NK 细胞。CD56^{bright} NK 细胞的主要功能是分泌细胞因子,而 CD56^{dim} NK 细胞的主要功能是细胞毒性。在患有 RIF 的女性中,细胞毒性 CD56^{dim} NK 细胞增加,而分泌细胞因子的 CD56^{bright} NK 细胞减少。NK 细胞表面 NKp46 的表达降低。分泌 I 型细胞因子的 NK 细胞(NK1)增加,而分泌 II 型细胞因子的 NK 细胞(NK2)减少。因此,RIF 患者的 NK1/NK2 升高。肝素、阿司匹林、皮质类固醇、静脉注射免疫球蛋白 G、脂肪乳剂、羟氯喹、肿瘤坏死因子抑制剂和维生素 D 等免疫治疗可能有助于使 RIF 患者的 NK 细胞异常正常化。

参考文献

[1] Polanski LT, Baumgarten MN, Quenby S, Brosens J, Campbell BK, Raine-Fenning NJ. What exactly do we mean by 'recurrent implantation failure'? A systematic review and opinion. Reprod Biomed Online 2014;28:409-23.

[2] Coughlan C, Ledger W, Wang Q, Liu F, Demirol A, Gurgan T, et al. Recurrent implantation failure: definition and management. Reprod Biomed Online 2014;28:14-38.

[3] Shaulov T, Sierra S, Sylvestre C. Recurrent implantation failure in IVF: a Canadian fertility and andrology society clinical practice guideline. Reprod Biomed Online 2020;41:819-33.

[4] Cimadomo D, Craciunas L, Vermeulen N, Vomstein K, Toth B. Definition, diagnostic and therapeutic options in recurrent implantation failure: an international survey of clinicians and embryologists. Hum Reprod 2021;36:305-17.

[5] Busnelli A, Reschini M, Cardellicchio L, Vegetti W, Somigliana E, Vercellini P. How common is real repeated implantation failure? An indirect estimate of the prevalence. Reprod Biomed Online 2020;40:91-7.

[6] Pirtea P, De Ziegler D, Tao X, Sun L, Zhan Y, Ayoubi JM, et al. Rate of true recurrent implantation failure is low: results of three successive frozen euploid single embryo transfers. Fertil Steril 2021;115:45-53.

[7] Fukui A, Yokota M, Funamizu A, Nakamua R, Fukuhara R, Yamada K, et al. Changes of NK cells in preeclampsia. Am J Reprod Immunol 2012;67:278-86.

[8] Fukui A, Ntrivalas E, Gilman-Sachs A, Kwak-Kim J, Lee SK, Levine R, et al. Expression of natural cytotoxicity receptors and a2V-ATPase on peripheral blood NK cell subsets in women with recurrent spontaneous abortions and implantation failures. Am J Reprod Immunol 2006;56:312-20.

[9] Fukui A, Kwak-Kim J, Ntrivalas E, Gilman-Sachs A, Lee SK, Beaman K. Intracellular cytokine expression of peripheral blood natural killer cell subsets in women with recurrent spontaneous abortions and implantation failures. Fertil Steril 2008;89:157-65.

[10] Fukui A, Funamizu A, Fukuhara R, Shibahara H. Expression of natural cytotoxicity receptors and cytokine production on endometrial natural killer cells in women with recurrent pregnancy loss or implantation failure, and the expression of natural cytotoxicity receptors on peripheral blood natural killer cells in pregnant women with a history of recurrent pregnancy loss. J Obstet Gynaecol Res 2017;43:1678-86.

[11] Mai C, Fukui A, Takeyama R, Yamamoto M, Saeki S, Yamaya A, et al. NK cells that differ in expression of NKp46 might play different roles in endometrium. J Reprod Immunol 2021;147:103367.

[12] Takeyama R, Fukui A, Mai C, Yamamoto M, Saeki S, Yamaya A, et al. Co-expression of NKp46 with activating or inhibitory receptors on, and cytokine production by, uterine endometrial NK cells in recurrent pregnancy loss. J Reprod Immunol 2021;145:103324.

[13] Lachapelle MH, Miron P, Hemmings R, Roy DC. Endometrial T, B, and NK cells in patients with recurrent spontaneous abortion. Altered profile and pregnancy outcome. J Immunol 1996;156:4027-34.

[14] Gilman-Sachs A, DuChateau BK, Aslakson CJ, Wohlgemuth GP, Kwak JY, Beer AE, et al. Natural killer (NK) cell subsets and NK cell cytotoxicity in women with histories of recurrent spontaneous abortions. Am J Reprod Immunol 1999;41:99-105.

[15] Sung N, Khan SA, Yiu ME, Jubiz G, Salazar MD, Skariah A, et al. Reproductive outcomes of women with recurrent pregnancy losses and repeated implantation failures are significantly improved with immunomodulatory treatment. J Reprod Immunol 2021;148:103369.

[16] Yamada H, Morikawa M, Kato EH, Shimada S, Kobashi G, Minakami H. Pre-conceptional natural killer cell activity and percentage as predictors of biochemical pregnancy and spontaneous abortion with normal chromosome karyotype. Am J Reprod Immunol 2003;50:351-4.

[17] Fukui A, Fujii S, Yamaguchi E, Kimura H, Sato S, Saito Y. Natural killer cell subpopulations and cytotoxicity for infertile patients undergoing in vitro fertilization. Am J Reprod Immunol 1999;41:413-22.

[18] Moffett A, Regan L, Braude P. Natural killer cells, miscarriage, and infertility. BMJ 2004;329:1283-5.

[19] Park DW, Lee HJ, Park CW, Hong SR, Kwak-Kim J, Yang KM. Peripheral blood NK cells reflect changes in decidual NK cells in women with recurrent miscarriages. Am J Reprod Immunol 2010;63:173-80.

[20] Fukui A. Uterine and circulating natural killer cells and their roles in women with recurrent pregnancy losses, implantation failures or preeclampsia. J Reprod Immunol 2010;86:14.

[21] Fukui A. NK cells and its role in reproduction. Am J Reprod Immunol 2010;64:1.

[22] Fukui A. Role of NK cells in women with recurrent pregnancy loss and implantation failure. Acta obstet gynaec Jpn 2011;63:2167-84.

[23] Tuckerman E, Mariee N, Prakash A, Li TC, Laird S. Uterine natural killer cells in peri-implantation endome-trium from women with repeated implantation failure after IVF. J Reprod Immunol 2010;87:60-6.

[24] Santillan I, Lozano I, Illan J, Verdu V, Coca S, Bajo-Arenas JM, et al. Where and when should natural killer cells be tested in women with repeated implantation failure? J Reprod Immunol 2015;108:142-8.

[25] Russell P, Anderson L, Lieberman D, Tremellen K, Yilmaz H, Cheerala B, et al. The distribution of immune cells and macrophages in the endometrium of women with recurrent reproductive failure I: techniques. J Reprod Immunol 2011;91:90-102.

[26] Kofod L, Lindhard A, Hviid TVF. Implications of uterine NK cells and regulatory T cells in the endometrium of infertile women. Hum Immunol 2018;79:693-701.

[27] Kofod L, Lindhard A, Bzorek M, Eriksen JO, Larsen LG, Hviid TVF. Endometrial immune markers are potential predictors of normal fertility and pregnancy after in vitro fertilization. Am J Reprod Immunol 2017;78.

[28] Yamada H, Shimada S, Morikawa M, Iwabuchi K, Kishi R, Onoe K, et al. Divergence of natural killer cell receptor and related molecule in the decidua from sporadic miscarriage with normal chromosome karyotype. Mol Hum Reprod 2005;11:451-7.

[29] Verma S, King A, Loke YW. Expression of killer cell

inhibitory receptors on human uterine natural killer cells. Eur J Immunol 1997;27;979-83.

[30] Fukui A, Fujii S, Kasai G, Kimura H, Yamaguchi E, Mizunuma H. Correlation with endometrial NK cell, KIRs and NKT cells. IFFS 2001 Sel Commun 2001;65-71.

[31] Acar N, Ustunel I, Demir R. Uterine natural killer (uNK) cells and their missions during pregnancy: a review. Acta Histochem 2011;113:82-91.

[32] Varla-Leftherioti M, Spyropoulou-Vlachou M, Niokou D, Keramitsoglou T, Darlamitsou A, Tsekoura C, et al. Natural killer (NK) cell receptors' repertoire in couples with recurrent spontaneous abortions. Am J Reprod Immunol 2003; 49: 183-91.

[33] Ntrivalas EI, Bowser CR, Kwak-Kim J, Beaman KD, Gilman-Sachs A. Expression of killer immunoglobulin-like receptors on peripheral blood NK cell subsets of women with recurrent spontaneous abortions or implantation failures. Am J Reprod Immunol 2005;53;215-21.

[34] Hong Y, Wang X, Lu P, Song Y, Lin Q. Killer immunoglobulin-like receptor repertoire on uterine natural killer cell subsets in women with recurrent spontaneous abortions. Eur J Obstet Gynecol Reprod Biol 2008; 140: 218-23.

[35] Yan WH, Lin A, Chen BG, Zhou MY, Dai MZ, Chen XJ, et al. Possible roles of KIR2DL4 expression on uNK cells in human pregnancy. Am J Reprod Immunol 2007;57:233-42.

[36] Wang XL, Wang Q, Sun CJ, Zhang WY. Genetic polymorphisms of killer cell immunoglobulin-like receptor 3DL2 in preeclampsia. J Perinat Med 2011;39;273-8.

[37] Yokota M, Fukui A, Funamizu A, Nakamura R, Kamoi M, Fuchinoue K, et al. Role of NKp46 expression in cytokine production by CD56-positive NK cells in the peripheral blood and the uterine endometrium. Am J Reprod Immunol 2013; 69:202-11.

[38] Fukui A, Kamoi M, Funamizu A, Fuchinoue K, Chiba H, Yokota M, et al. NK cell abnormality and its treatment in women with reproductive failures such as recurrent pregnancy loss, implantation failures, pre-eclampsia, and pelvic endometriosis. Reprod Med Biol 2015;14;151-7.

[39] Kwak-Kim JY, Gilman-Sachs A, Kim CE. T helper 1 and 2 immune responses in relationship to pregnancy, nonpregnancy, recurrent spontaneous abortions and infertility of repeated implantation failures. Chem Immunol Allergy 2005; 88; 64-79.

[40] Carter LL, Dutton RW. Relative perforin-and Fas-mediated lysis in T1 and T2 CD8 effector populations. J Immunol 1995; 155:1028-31.

[41] Peritt D, Robertson S, Gri G, Showe L, Aste-Amezaga M, Trinchieri G. Differentiation of human NK cells into NK1 and NK2 subsets. J Immunol 1998;161;5821-4.

[42] Higuma-Myojo S, Sasaki Y, Miyazaki S, Sakai M, Siozaki A, Miwa N, et al. Cytokine profile of natural killer cells in early human pregnancy. Am J Reprod Immunol 2005;54;21-9.

[43] Bulmer JN, Lash GE. Human uterine natural killer cells: a reappraisal. Mol Immunol 2005;42;511-21.

[44] Ashkar AA, Di Santo JP, Croy BA. Interferon gamma contributes to initiation of uterine vascular modification, decidual integrity, and uterine natural killer cell maturation during normal murine pregnancy. J Exp Med 2000;192;259-70.

[45] Terranova PF, Hunter VJ, Roby KF, Hunt JS. Tumor necrosis factor-alpha in the female reproductive tract. Proc Soc Exp Biol Med 1995;209;325-42.

[46] Toder V, Fein A, Carp H, Torchinsky A. TNF-alpha in pregnancy loss and embryo maldevelopment: a mediator of detrimental stimuli or a protector of the fetoplacental unit? J Assist Reprod Genet 2003;20;73-81.

[47] Brosens IA, Robertson WB, Dixon HG. The role of the spiral arteries in the pathogenesis of preeclampsia. Obstet Gynecol Annu 1972;1;177-91.

[48] Diao L, Cai S, Huang C, Li L, Yu S, Wang L, et al. New endometrial immune cell-based score (EI-score) for the prediction of implantation success for patients undergoing IVF/ICSI. Placenta 2020;99;180-8.

[49] Dambaeva S, Bilal M, Schneiderman S, Germain A, Fernandez E, Kwak-Kim J, et al. Decidualization score identifies an endometrial dysregulation in samples from women with recurrent pregnancy losses and unexplained infertility. F S Rep 2021;2;95-103.

[50] Bohlmann MK. Effects and effectiveness of heparin in assisted reproduction. J Reprod Immunol 2011;90;82-90.

[51] Koo HS, Kwak-Kim J, Yi HJ, Ahn HK, Park CW, Cha SH, et al. Resistance of uterine radial artery blood flow was correlated with peripheral blood NK cell fraction and improved with low molecular weight heparin therapy in women with unexplained recurrent pregnancy loss. Am J Reprod Immunol 2015;73;175-84.

[52] Bao SH, Chigirin N, Hoch V, Ahmed H, Frempong ST, Zhang M, et al. Uterine radial artery resistance index predicts reproductive outcome in women with recurrent pregnancy losses and thrombophilia. BioMed Res Int 2019; 2019;8787010.

[53] Han AR, Ahn H, Vu P, Park JC, Gilman-Sachs A, Beaman K, et al. Obstetrical outcome of anti-inflammatory and anticoagulation therapy in women with recurrent pregnancy loss or unexplained infertility. Am J Reprod Immunol 2012; 68;418-27.

[54] Boomsma CM, Keay SD, Macklon NS. Peri-implantation glucocorticoid administration for assisted reproductive technology cycles. Cochrane database Syst Rev 2012;CD005996.

[55] Practice Committee of the American Society for Reproductive Medicine. Electronic address Aao, Practice Committee of the American Society for Reproductive M: the role of immunotherapy in vitro fertilization: a guideline. Fertil Steril 2018;110;387-400.

[56] Mekinian A, Cohen J, Alijotas-Reig J, Carbillon L, Nicaise-Roland P, Kayem G, et al. Unexplained recurrent miscarriage and recurrent implantation failure: is there a place for immunomodulation? Am J Reprod Immunol 2016; 76;8-28.

[57] Sung N, Han AR, Park CW, Park DW, Park JC, Kim NY, et al. Ivig Task Force KSfRI: Intravenous immuno-globulin G in women with reproductive failure: the Korean Society for reproductive immunology practice guidelines. Clin Exp Reprod Med 2017;44;1-7.

[58] Abdolmohammadi-Vahid S, Pashazadeh F, Pourmoghaddam Z, Aghebati-Maleki L, Abdollahi-Fard S, Yousefi M. The effectiveness of IVIG therapy in pregnancy and live birth rate of women with recurrent implantation failure (RIF): a systematic review and meta-analysis. J Reprod Immunol 2019;134-135;28-33.

[59] Saab W, Seshadri S, Huang C, Alsubki L, Sung N, Kwak-Kim J. A systemic review of intravenous immuno-globulin G treatment in women with recurrent implantation failures and

recurrent pregnancy losses. Am J Reprod Immunol 2021;85:e13395.

[60] Achilli C, Duran-Retamal M, Saab W, Serhal P, Seshadri S. The role of immunotherapy in vitro fertilization and recurrent pregnancy loss: a systematic review and meta-analysis. Fertil Steril 2018;110:1089-100.

[61] Fukui A, Funamizu A, Yokota M, Yamada K, Nakamua R, Fukuhara R, et al. Uterine and circulating natural killer cells and their roles in women with recurrent pregnancy loss, implantation failure and preeclampsia. J Reprod Immunol 2011;90:105-10.

[62] Zhou P, Wu H, Lin X, Wang S, Zhang S. The effect of intralipid on pregnancy outcomes in women with previous implantation failure in vitro fertilization/intracytoplasmic sperm injection cycles: a systematic review and meta-analysis. Eur J Obstet Gynecol Reprod Biol 2020;252:187-92.

[63] Coulam CB. Intralipid treatment for women with reproductive failures. Am J Reprod Immunol 2020;e13290.

[64] Canella P, Barini R, Carvalho PO, Razolli DS. Lipid emulsion therapy in women with recurrent pregnancy loss and repeated implantation failure: the role of abnormal natural killer cell activity. J Cell Mol Med 2021.

[65] Roussev RG, Acacio B, Ng SC, Coulam CB. Duration of intralipid's suppressive effect on NK cell's functional activity. Am J Reprod Immunol 2008;60:258-63.

[66] Meng L, Lin J, Chen L, Wang Z, Liu M, Liu Y, et al. Effectiveness and potential mechanisms of intralipid in treating unexplained recurrent spontaneous abortion. Arch Gynecol Obstet 2016;294:29-39.

[67] W E-K, M ES. Intralipid for repeated implantation failure (RIF): a randomized controlled trial. Fertil Steril 2015;104:e26.

[68] I G, MF G, A S, V A. Intralipid infusion does not improve live birth rates in women with unexplained recurrent implantation failure and may increase the risk of congenital malformations, a double-blinded randomised controlled trial. BJOG-Int J Obstet Gynaecol 2018;125.

[69] Ghasemnejad-Berenji H, Ghaffari Novin M, Hajshafiha M, Nazarian H, Hashemi SM, Ilkhanizadeh B, et al. Immunomodulatory effects of hydroxychloroquine on Th1/Th2 balance in women with repeated implantation failure. Biomed Pharmacother 2018;107:1277-85.

[70] Sadeghpour S, Ghasemnejad Berenji M, Nazarian H, Ghasemnejad T, Nematollahi MH, Abroon S, et al. Effects of treatment with hydroxychloroquine on the modulation of Th17/Treg ratio and pregnancy out-comes in women with recurrent implantation failure: clinical trial. Immunopharmacol Immunotoxicol 2020;42:632-42.

[71] Komoto S, Motoya S, Nishiwaki Y, Matsui T, Kunisaki R, Matsuoka K, et al. Japanese study group for pregnant women with IBD: pregnancy outcome in women with inflammatory bowel disease treated with anti-tumor necrosis factor and/or thiopurine therapy: a multicenter study from Japan. Intest Res 2016;14:139-45.

[72] Roux CH, Brocq O, Breuil V, Albert C, Euller-Ziegler L. Pregnancy in rheumatology patients exposed to anti-tumour necrosis factor (TNF)-alpha therapy. Rheumatology (Oxf) 2007;46:695-8.

[73] Hyrich KL, Symmons DP, Watson KD, Silman AJ. British Society fRBR: Pregnancy outcome in women who were exposed to anti-tumor necrosis factor agents: results from a national population register. Arthritis Rheum 2006;54:2701-2.

[74] Winger EE, Reed JL, Ashoush S, Ahuja S, El-Toukhy T, Taranissi M. Treatment with adalimumab (Humira) and intravenous immunoglobulin improves pregnancy rates in women undergoing IVF. Am J Reprod Immunol 2009;61:113-20.

[75] Fu J, Li L, Qi L, Zhao L. A randomized controlled trial of etanercept in the treatment of refractory recurrent spontaneous abortion with innate immune disorders. Taiwan J Obstet Gynecol 2019;58:621-5.

[76] Ota K, Dambaeva S, Han AR, Beaman K, Gilman-Sachs A, Kwak-Kim J. Vitamin D deficiency may be a risk factor for recurrent pregnancy losses by increasing cellular immunity and autoimmunity. Hum Reprod 2014;29:208-19.

[77] Ota K, Dambaeva S, Kim MW, Han AR, Fukui A, Gilman-Sachs A, et al. 1,25-dihydroxy-vitamin D3 regulates NK-cell cytotoxicity, cytokine secretion and degranulation in women with recurrent pregnancy losses. Eur J Immunol 2015.

第 18 章

辅助性 T 细胞病理学与反复种植失败
Helper T cell pathology and repeated implantation failures

Koji Nakagawa[1], Keiji Kuroda[2] and Rikikazu Sugiyama[3]

[1] Director, Center for Reproductive Medicine and Implantation Research, Sugiyama Clinic Shinjuku, Tokyo, Japan
[2] Division Manager of Implantation Research and Endoscopy, Center for Reproductive Medicine and Implantation Research, Sugiyama Clinic Shinjuku, Tokyo, Japan
[3] CEO, Center for Reproductive Medicine and Implantation Research, Sugiyama Clinic Shinjuku, Tokyo, Japan

1 辅助性 T 细胞在生殖医学中的作用

辅助性 T 细胞（Th 细胞）通过分泌激活免疫系统内其他细胞的多种因子，在免疫反应中发挥重要作用。这些细胞包括 B 细胞、细胞毒性 T 细胞、巨噬细胞等。Th 细胞表面表达 CD4，该蛋白通过结合人白细胞抗原（HLA）Ⅱ类分子在 Th 细胞激活中发挥关键作用，帮助免疫系统识别外来物质。Th 细胞可以分为两个具有不同特征和功能的亚群：Th1 和 Th2 细胞。这些亚群可通过细胞因子（化学信使）分泌的模式加以区分。Th1 细胞主要合成干扰素-γ（INF-γ）、肿瘤坏死因子-β（TNF-β）和白细胞介素-2（IL-2）等细胞因子。Th2 细胞主要分泌白细胞介素-4（IL-4）、IL-5、IL-6、IL-9、IL-10 和 IL-13。Th1 细胞的主要作用是刺激细胞毒性 T 细胞和巨噬细胞等介导的免疫反应，而 Th2 细胞主要协助刺激 B 细胞产生抗体。

Th 细胞激活需要几个步骤。第一步由抗原递呈细胞（如巨噬细胞）启动。这些细胞吞噬感染因子或外来颗粒，并将它们的片段（即抗原）呈现在细胞表面。Th 细胞的表面受体与 HLA 复合物结合。下一步，Th 细胞激活通过细胞因子刺激或共刺激信号蛋白 B7 的反应发生。B7 位于抗原递呈细胞的表面[1]，与 Th 细胞表面的 CD28 结合[2]。Th 细胞激活的结果是识别抗原的 Th 细胞数量增加，并且分泌 Th 细胞细胞因子。Th 细胞不像细胞毒性 T 细胞那样直接杀死被感染细胞或攻击其他细胞（外来细胞或已孵化的囊胚）。Th 细胞激活细胞毒性 T 细胞，帮助巨噬细胞攻击被感染或外来细胞，或刺激 B 细胞分泌抗体。

胚胎实现植入的第一步是形成一个被蜕膜化子宫内膜接受的孵化囊胚。当母体 Th 细胞识别已孵化的囊胚时，它们不会直接攻击它，而是会分泌各种细胞因子，例如 INF-γ、TNF-β 或 IL-2。在植入部位，母体-胎儿免疫相互作用既涉及排斥免疫的抑制，也涉及免疫耐受的诱导。这种现象在器官移植和癌细胞生物学领域也得到证明[3-6]。

妊娠期间的免疫反应与器官移植存在相似性，胎儿被视为移植的器官。然而，妊娠期间树突状细胞（DC）对 T 细胞的激活弱于器官移植。正常妊娠的免疫机制尚未完全阐明，但免疫耐受在胚胎种植前后都很关键。因此，抑制免疫排斥反应对于成功建立和维持妊娠至关重要。妊娠期间，必须抑制母体固有免疫的排斥反应。绒毛膜滋养层细胞来源于植入的胚胎，不表达组织相容性抗原 HLA-A、HLA-B 和 HLA-D[7]。因此，绒毛膜滋养层细胞可以成为自然杀伤细胞（NK）攻击的目标，但不会被细胞毒性 T 细胞攻击。然而，绒毛膜滋养层细胞表达 HLA-C、HLA-E 和 HLA-G[8-10]。尽管胎儿-母体 HLA-C 不匹配可能引发母体 NK 细胞激活，但母体免疫反应可以通过绒毛膜滋养层细胞上的

HLA-G表达而被抑制,从而避免NK细胞的攻击并抑制巨噬细胞的激活[8-10]。

免疫耐受的建立必须是有组织且方便的。尽管胎儿-母体HLA不匹配会引发母体NK和T细胞激活,但在精液预处理、充足的孕酮水平或HLA-G表达等条件下,母体免疫反应会转变为免疫耐受[10-13]。这种反应将耐受性DC与未成熟DC区分开,随后通过调节性T细胞诱导免疫耐受[14]。基于这一连锁反应,可以建立免疫耐受来维持妊娠。此外,抑制NK和NKT细胞功能、下调Ⅰ型细胞因子产生和抑制Th1细胞分化,都在对抗免疫排斥方面发挥作用。

Th细胞被认为机体防御系统的指挥者。当Th细胞通过DC接收来自外来物质(如细菌、病毒或孵化的囊胚)的信号时,Th1细胞会分泌细胞因子,包括INF-γ和TNF-α,以响应外来物质的入侵。细胞因子随后增强局部炎症反应,并刺激具有吞噬作用的巨噬细胞激活。众所周知,促炎细胞因子会抑制滋养层生长,并在母体子宫内膜的胚胎附着区域促进炎症反应,并对胚胎植入产生不利影响。相比之下,由Th2细胞分泌的IL-4、IL-6和IL-10可以通过单核细胞抑制Th1细胞诱导的组织因子产生。事实上,反复种植失败(RIF)患者的外周血样本中TNF-α/IL-4较高[15]。

2 Th细胞免疫病理学与反复种植失败

RIF的普遍定义是指在冷冻胚胎移植或新鲜胚胎移植周期中,3次移植高质量胚胎均失败[16]。众所周知,胚胎植入需要3个条件:优质胚胎、充分蜕膜化和适度的母体反应。RIF的病因在文献中已得到深入评估[17]。表18.1根据上述3个胚胎植入因素,总结了文献中关于RIF的病因。针对表18.1中每种病因的治疗策略见图18.1。

表18.1 反复种植失败的三个潜在病因分类

子宫环境	胚胎因素	母体因素
宫腔异常 子宫内膜息肉 子宫肌瘤 薄型子宫内膜 子宫内膜蜕膜化不良 输卵管积液 剖宫产瘢痕综合征 慢性子宫内膜炎	遗传异常 透明带硬化 不理想的培养 黏附分子表达的改变	子宫内膜异位症 免疫学因素 不理想的卵巢刺激 血栓形成倾向 生活方式

注:改编自Margalioth(2006,p.17)。

T淋巴细胞通常根据其分泌细胞因子的能力分为Th1或Th2细胞[18,19]。Th1和Th2细胞是决定排斥或耐受的免疫过程的主要角色[20]。通常认为,妊娠的建立是一种Th2优于Th1的免疫状态。相反,当Th1优于Th2时,结果是免疫排斥。因此,Th1优势会排斥移植的胚胎[20,21]。基于这一理论,胚胎种植失败被认为是同种异体移植排斥的一种情况[22]。

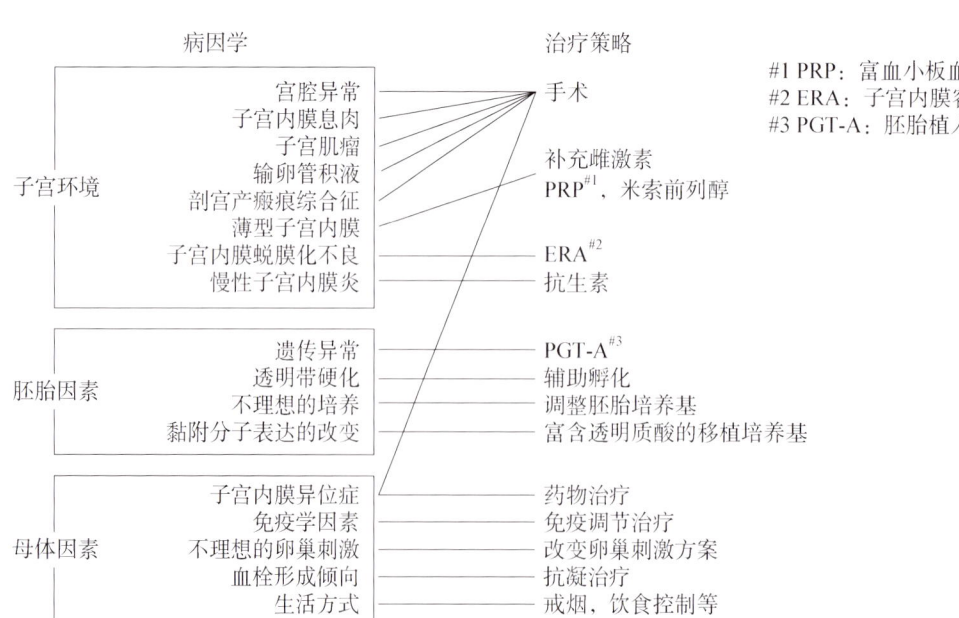

图18.1 列举应对反复种植失败潜在病因的各种策略。

Th 细胞介导的 RIF 被定义为 Th1/Th2 细胞比例升高,因为 Th1 升高、Th2 降低,或者两者同时升高和降低,都可导致 Th1/Th2 细胞比例升高。Th1 细胞升高会引发细胞介导的免疫和吞噬细胞依赖性炎症。相反,Th2 细胞降低会削弱对吞噬细胞多种功能的抑制作用[23]。Th1 和 Th2 细胞根据其细胞因子谱分类。已报道了几种 Th1/Th2 细胞比例的组合以及它们的截断值,如 TNF-α/IL-10(>30.6),INF-γ/IL-10(>20.5)[24] 以及 INF-γ/IL-4(≥10.3)[25]。

3 患病率

根据上述 RIF 的定义,10% 接受体外受精(IVF)治疗的夫妇会经历 RIF。不幸的是,一些胚胎成功植入的患者仍可能会面临早期妊娠丢失的打击[26]。对于反复接受高质量胚胎移植仍无法妊娠的患者,需要评估其不孕的潜在原因。

根据分泌 INF-γ/IL-4 的 Th 细胞比例的截断值[20],在 RIF 组中,Th1/Th2 细胞比例≥10.3 的女性患病率为 37.7%,明显高于对照组(包括 28 名既往有正常妊娠史的女性,见图 18.2)[25]。相比之下,189 名 RPL 患者中有 111 名(58.7%)存在细胞免疫异常(分泌 TNF-α/IL-10 的 Th1/Th2 细胞比例升高)[26]。因此,38%~59% 的 RIF 或 RPL 女性表现出 Th 细胞免疫异常。

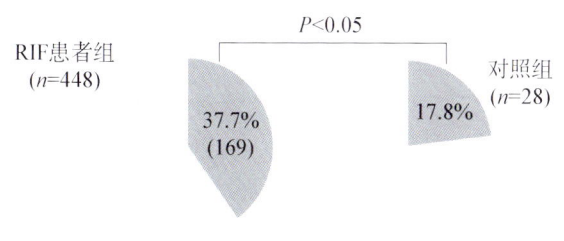

图 18.2 反复种植失败组与对照组中 Th1/Th2 细胞比值升高的患病率。

约 37.7% 的反复种植失败患者表现出 Th1/Th2 细胞比值升高,显著高于对照组。

4 反复种植失败免疫调节治疗的理论基础

胚胎的成功植入可解释为孵化的囊胚附着于子宫内膜表面,然后侵入蜕膜化内膜的过程。在囊胚侵入过程中,孵化的囊胚周围发生螺旋动脉的血管化和重塑,建立母胎循环。母体免疫效应器在响应囊胚侵入方面发挥重要作用。许多研究强调平衡的细胞因子环境的重要性,特别是 Th1 和 Th2 细胞分泌的Ⅰ型和Ⅱ型细胞因子之间的平衡。Th1 和 Th2 细胞比例有助于评估免疫应答是排斥反应强烈或是耐受性降低。向 Th1 细胞偏移会导致促炎细胞因子如 TNF-α、INF-γ 和 IL-2 的增加,这些细胞因子都对细胞毒性免疫反应起重要作用,包括吞噬作用和炎症。另一方面,Th2 细胞分泌多种白细胞介素,激活体液免疫反应并抑制吞噬细胞功能,其中之一就是抗炎反应[15]。许多观察性研究已经证明了一些理论机制,可以解释为什么有 RPL 史的女性会出现促炎细胞因子表达增加的现象[27]。

自然杀伤细胞(NK)是负责固有免疫的免疫细胞之一,当外周血中的 NK 细胞水平增加时,促炎细胞因子如 INF-γ 也会升高。炎症性免疫反应与心血管、退化性疾病、神经内分泌疾病和生殖障碍等多种全身炎症性疾病密切相关[28]。据报道,RIF 和 RPL 女性的 NK 细胞水平、细胞毒性以及 Th1 免疫反应均增加[29,30]。因此,母胎界面处的全身性和局部炎症性免疫反应被认为在 RIF 女性中发挥重要作用。炎症性免疫反应会引起微环境中的血栓形成,导致孵化囊胚种植失败。

关于容受性子宫内膜中由多种细胞因子诱导的促炎和抗炎平衡的观点存在分歧,减少母胎界面抗炎细胞因子的观点已被视为一种简单化的想法[31-33]。对 210 名女性在胚胎移植前提取宫腔液进行细胞因子浓度分析显示,在植入和早期妊娠期间,IL-10 和 TNF-α 呈正相关。相比之下,在同一时期,IL-1β 和单核细胞趋化蛋白 1(MCP-1)的水平呈负相关[34]。

5 评估

对于经历 3 次或 3 次以上新鲜或冷冻胚胎移植后均植入失败的女性,建议进行免疫学检查,例如 Th1/Th2 细胞比例。外周血 Th1/Th2 细胞比例可通过流式细胞术进行检测。淋巴细胞的特异性染色是通过将全血与抗 CD4-APC5 或抗 CD8-APC5 偶联单克隆抗体(mAb)孵育而进行的。表面染色后,再使用 FastImmune™ IFN-γ-FITC/IL-4-PE 进行特异性胞内染色。Th1 细胞定义为细胞内表达 IFN-γ 但不表达 IL-4 的 CD4+ 淋巴细胞。

Th2 细胞则为细胞内表达 IL-4 但不表达 IFN-γ 的 CD4[+] 淋巴细胞。IFN-γ 阳性 Th 细胞与 IL-4 阳性 Th 细胞的比值表示为 Th1/Th2[20]。

多项研究表明，外周血 NK 细胞增加与 RIF 或 RPL 女性的 Th1/Th2 细胞比值之间存在关联[15,35-37]。这些研究促使我们检测外周血 NK 细胞，但外周血 NK 细胞与子宫 NK（uNK）细胞之间的关系似乎并不明显[33,38]。相反，Tuckerman 等[39] 发现 RIF 患者的子宫内膜中 uNK 细胞数量更高。来自外周血或子宫内膜的 NK 细胞评估已成为探索母体方面 RIF 或 RPL 潜在病因的有用工具。这些实验室检查有助于临床医生为 RIF 或 RPL 患者选择适当的特定免疫调节治疗或药物。对于 RIF 患者，免疫调节治疗已被用来增强或抑制免疫反应，从而抑制排斥反应或增强耐受性，并最终增强子宫内膜接受囊胚的能力而不发生排斥反应。

6 针对辅助性 T 细胞病理的免疫调节治疗

当存在免疫紊乱时，糖皮质激素、他克莫司、静脉注射免疫球蛋白 G、抗肿瘤坏死因子-α 和脂质乳剂输注等免疫调节治疗已被用于改善 RIF 患者的生殖结局（表 18.2）[40-43]。本部分将讨论糖皮质激素和他克莫司治疗。

6.1 糖皮质激素

皮质类固醇是一种强效抗炎药物，在植入和早期妊娠期间使用时，能够抑制免疫细胞数量和活性。

表 18.2 反复种植失败和反复妊娠丢失患者异常细胞免疫应答的各种免疫调节治疗

项目	IVIG[a]	抗 TNF-α	脂肪乳剂	他克莫司
给药途径	静脉	静脉	静脉	口服
剂量	每天 400~500 mg/kg	每 2 周 40 mg	每天 10% 250 mL	每天 1~4 mg
起始用药时间	FET 周期前 2~4 周或 ET 当日	ET 前 90~120 天	取卵后	ET 前 2 天
妊娠试验阳性后[b]	持续，每 3~4 周	—	持续，每 2 周	持续
监测	外周血 NK 细胞计数、NK 细胞毒性、Th1/Th2	Th1/Th2	外周血 NK 细胞计数	Th1/Th2、Th1 水平
副作用	大多数副作用是短暂和轻微的[40] 罕见的副作用包括： -肾功能损害 -血栓形成 -心律失常 -无菌性脑膜炎 -溶血性贫血 -与输血相关的急性肺损伤	最常见的副作用是注射部位反应[41] 严重的副作用很少见，包括： -淋巴瘤 -严重感染 -潜伏性肺结核的再激活 -充血性心力衰竭	常见的副作用[42]是由于： -试管婴儿导管污染，引起败血症 -血栓性静脉炎 -较少的副作用与脂肪乳剂有更直接关系 -呼吸困难 -发绀 -过敏反应（大豆过敏） -高脂血症 -高凝状态 -延迟不良反应：肝肿大、黄疸、脾肿大 -血小板减少 -白细胞减少症 -肝酶升高 -超载综合征	大多数副作用并不严重[43] 严重的副作用是： -感染 -血镁含量降低 -血钾增加 -贫血 -中性粒细胞减少症 -对中枢神经系统的毒性作用 -胸膜炎 -肾功能下降 -癫痫发作 -失眠 -糖尿病变化

注：[a]IVIG，静脉注射免疫球蛋白。
[b]PT，妊娠试验。

皮质类固醇通常分为糖皮质激素和盐皮质激素两类。由于其起效迅速，而且在生殖和早期妊娠期间相对安全，因此糖皮质激素常被用于治疗 RIF。相比地塞米松（盐皮质激素），强的松（糖皮质激素）更常用于治疗 RIF，因为地塞米松的血管收缩作用大约是强的松的 10 倍，这种强效作用可能会干扰胚胎植入过程。

6.1.1 适应证

对于经辅助生殖技术（ART）治疗后出现与子宫胎盘血栓和血管收缩相关的自身抗体阳性的女性，糖皮质激素可作为治疗选择[44,45]。NK 细胞过度活跃的 RIF 患者也适合接受糖皮质激素治疗。有人提出，使用糖皮质激素可使 NK 细胞活性、细胞因子分泌恢复正常，并抑制炎症介质的过度产生，从而改善子宫内膜容受性[46]。糖皮质激素已被用于治疗类风湿关节炎，后者常与 Th1/Th2 细胞比例升高有关。文献表明，糖皮质激素可抑制 Th1 细胞的分泌 IFN-γ、TNF-α 等，同时上调 Th2 细胞分泌的 IL-4、IL-10 和 IL-13[47]。因此，糖皮质激素可以发挥抗炎作用，调节 Th1/Th2 细胞比值。Th1/Th2 细胞比值升高的 RIF 女性也是糖皮质激素治疗的获益人群。

6.1.2 用药剂量

由于强的松是一种口服药物，因此给药方式相对简单。与其他免疫调节药物相比，其成本也较为合理。然而，由于其强大的抗炎作用，该药物的用药时间和疗程非常重要。对于 RIF 患者，强的松应定期持续服用。根据既往的报道[48]，15～60 mg 的强的松用于治疗具有自身抗体的女性。在 Han 等[49]进行的一项研究中，对不明原因不孕且自身抗体水平升高、NK 细胞活性或 Th1/Th2 升高的女性，采用每天 10 mg 强的松治疗，从自然周期排卵后 48 小时或在 ART 周期前 2 周开始，必要时联合静脉注射免疫球蛋白 G 治疗。强的松的治疗剂量根据 Th1/Th2、NK 细胞水平或细胞毒性进行调整，并在妊娠 12～14 周开始逐渐减量[49]。

6.1.3 副作用

糖皮质激素会导致免疫抑制，减少淋巴细胞（包括 T 细胞和 B 细胞）和其他免疫活性细胞的数量和功能。因此，长期使用可能会增加感染的易感性。此外，糖皮质激素还会诱发多种全身性变化，例如高血糖、骨质疏松改变和消化性溃疡。

由于糖皮质激素是一种强效抗炎药物，当在围植入期使用时，可能会对没有 T 细胞免疫异常的女性造成植入障碍。因此，对于强的松治疗，应选择具有免疫异常的患者，例如存在自身免疫、NK 细胞数量和细胞毒性增加，或 Th1 或 Th1/Th2 升高。此外，在使用糖皮质激素治疗期间定期监测免疫和其他相关参数对于确定适当剂量并避免药物可能产生的副作用至关重要。

6.2 他克莫司（tacrolimus）

6.2.1 作用机制

近年来，新型免疫抑制药物的快速发展使得器官移植的存活率大幅提升[50]。他克莫司是一种免疫抑制剂，最早在日本研制成功，现已成为同种异体器官移植的标准治疗方案。其作用机制为抑制受者的免疫反应，有效降低移植器官的排斥反应[51]。

他克莫司是一种钙调磷酸酶抑制剂，其作用机制是抑制对同种异体抗原产生反应的淋巴细胞分化，减少细胞毒性 T 细胞的增殖，并促进 IL-2 受体的发育以及 T 细胞来源的可溶性介质 IL-2 和 IFN-γ 的产生[52]。他克莫司对于器官移植和其他免疫异常疾病（例如由 T 细胞激活引起的类风湿关节炎）患者的有效性是众所周知的[53,54]。

6.2.2 适应证

Th1/Th2 比值升高的 RIF 患者可能受益于他克莫司治疗[20]。我们近期发表了两项使用他克莫司治疗 RPL 和 RIF 的前瞻性队列研究[25,55,56]。在这些研究中，共有 124 名 Th1/Th2 升高（≥10.3）的 RIF 患者接受了他克莫司免疫调节治疗。患者在胚胎移植日前 1 或 2 天开始使用他克莫司，直至妊娠试验。在这 124 名患者中，有 58 名妊娠（妊娠率为 46.8%）[55]。最初，根据 Th1/Th2 细胞比值，他克莫司的每日使用剂量为 1～3 mg，但与接受 3 mg 剂量的患者相比，1 mg 治疗组临床妊娠率明显较低[57]。我们的研究还发现，仅 Th1 细胞百分比就可预测 ART 的结局，特别是持续妊娠率。对于高 Th1 细胞百分比（>28.8%）的患者，即使他们的 Th1/Th2 正常，他克莫司的剂量额外增加了 1 mg（每日 2～4 mg）[56]。根据他克莫司剂量的调整，高 Th1 细胞百分比患者的临床妊娠率得到改善（从 21.4% 提高至 44.4%）[57]。因此，用于 RIF 患者，他克莫司的每日剂量可根据 Th1 细胞水平来确定。

他克莫司的血药浓度被用来确定器官移植时的最佳剂量。与他克莫司的疗效依赖于浓度的预期不同,每日 2 mg 剂量组的初步结果与每日 3 mg 剂量组相似,因此怀疑低剂量他克莫司(1~3 mg/d)可能不如更高剂量(≥4 mg/d)在预防 RIF 中有效。据报道,在移植案例中,他克莫司的最佳浓度为每天 5~15 ng/mL。在我们的研究中,当考虑±2 SD 范围时,≥4 mg/天的剂量已达到了 5 ng/mL 以上的浓度(图 18.3)。对于 Th1/Th2 细胞比值升高的 RIF 患者,他克莫司的治疗效果非常显著。此外,他克莫司对于 RPL 患者也十分有效[58]。RCT 试验有望进一步证实他克莫司在 RIF 患者中的有效性,将增强对该治疗方法的信心。

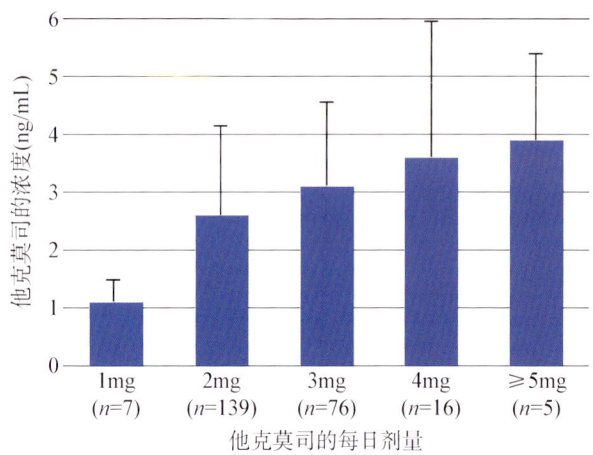

图 18.3 他克莫司不同每日剂量(ng/mL)的血药浓度。

他克莫司每日服用剂量为 1 mg、2 mg、3 mg、4 mg 和 ≥5 mg 的女性血清中他克莫司浓度分别为 1.1±0.4 ng/mL、2.6±1.6 ng/mL、3.1±1.5 ng/mL、3.6±2.3 ng/mL 和 3.9±1.4 ng/mL(均值±标准差)。

7 生殖结局

他克莫司对 Th1/Th2 细胞比值升高的 RIF 患者的疗效已得到证实。我们的研究指出,Th1/Th2 细胞比值升高的 RIF 患者在接受他克莫司治疗后,有 40%~50% 妊娠,而那些没有接受他克莫司治疗的 RIF 患者妊娠机会很小[25,57]。很少有报道评估使用糖皮质激素治疗具有异常 Th 细胞免疫的 RIF 患者与对照组之间的生殖结局。目前正在进行的一项随机对照试验评估强的松治疗 RIF 的临床效果[59],将为强的松对 RIF 患者生殖结局的影响提供更多证据。

8 总结和建议

Th 细胞对于保护自身免受病原体或外来细胞侵袭是不可或缺的,但抑制免疫排斥反应对于成功妊娠的建立和维持同样重要。表现出较高 Th1 细胞免疫水平的女性患有 RIF 的风险增加。Th 细胞免疫反应失调(如 Th1 细胞增加和 Th1/Th2 细胞比值升高)与 RIF 有关。针对这些炎症性 T 细胞的免疫调节治疗已被报道可以改善 RIF 患者的生殖结局。

糖皮质激素因其在生殖和早期妊娠中的快速作用和安全性而常被用于 RIF 治疗。他克莫司是另一种有效的免疫调节药物,可抑制 T 细胞来源的可溶性介质 IL-2 和 IFN-γ。由于在植入期需要适当的炎症反应,因此这些药物适用于 Th1/Th2 细胞比例失衡或 Th1 免疫增强的 RIF 患者,而不应该盲目给予其他 RIF 患者。

- 相当比例患有 RIF 的女性(37.7%)存在 Th1/Th2 细胞比例失衡。
- 可以考虑为具有自身免疫和细胞免疫异常证据的 RIF 患者提供糖皮质激素治疗。
- 钙调磷酸酶抑制剂他克莫司已被报道在具有细胞免疫异常尤其是 T 细胞异常的 RIF 患者中是有效的。
- 不应盲目给予 RIF 患者免疫抑制治疗。
- 在 RIF 患者接受免疫抑制治疗期间,需要定期监测免疫和其他相关参数,以确保充足的剂量和预防可能的副作用。

参考文献

[1] McAdam AJ, Schweitzer AN, Sharpe AH. The role of B7 co-stimulation in activation and differentiation of CD4+ and CD8+ T cells. Immunol Rev 1988;165:231-47.

[2] Linterman MA, Denton AE, Divekar DP, et al. CD28 expression is required after T cell priming for helper T cell responses and protective immunity to infection. ELife. 2014. Available from: https://doi.org/10.7554/eLife.03180.

[3] Colf LA, Bankovich AJ, Hanick NA, et al. How a single T cell receptor recognizes both self and foreign. Cell. 2007;129:135-46.

[4] Borbulevych OY, Piepenbrick KH, Gloor BE, et al. T cell receptor cross-reactivity directed by antigen-dependent tuning of peptide-MHC molecular flexibility. Immunity 2009;31:885-96.

[5] Borst J, Ahrends T, Bąbała N. CD4+ T cell help in cancer immunology and immunotherapy. Nat Rev Immunol 2018;18: 635-47.

[6] Ahrends T, Brost J. The opposing roles of CD4+ T cells in anti-tumor immunity. Immunology 2018;154:582-92.

[7] Loke YW, King A. Human implantation: Cell Biology and Immunology. Cambridge, UK: Cambridge University Press; 1995.

[8] Kovates S, Main EK, Librach C. A class I antigen, HLA-G, expressed human trophoblasts. Science 1990;248:220-3.

[9] Hiby SE, King A, Sharkey A. Molecular studies of trophoblast HLA-G: polymorphism, isoforms, imprinting and expression in preimplantation embryo. Tissue Antigens 1999; 53:1-13.

[10] King A, Burrows TD, Hiby SE, et al. Surface expression of HLA-C antigen by human extravillous trophoblast. Placenta 2000;21:376-87.

[11] Kahn DA, Baltimore D. Pregnancy induces a fetal antigen-specific maternal T regulatory cell response that contributes to tolerance. Proc Natl Acad Sci USA 2000;18:9299-304.

[12] Triburgs T, Scherjon SA, van der Mast BJ, et al. Fetal-maternal HLA-C mismatch is associated with decidual T cell activation and induction of functional T regulatory cells. J Reprod Immunol 2009;82:148-57.

[13] Shakwat A, Shaikly V, Elzatma E. Interaction between HLA-G and monocyte/macrophage in human preg-nancy. J Reprod Immunol 2010;85:40-6.

[14] Maldonado RA, von Andrian UH. How tolegenic dendtric cells induce regulatory T cell. Adv Immunol 2010;108:111-65.

[15] Kwak-Kim JYH, Chung-Bang HS, Ng SC, et al. Increased T helper 1 cytokine responses by circulating T cells are present in women with recurrent pregnancy losses and in infertile women with multiple implantation failures after IVF. Hum Reprod 2003;18:767-73.

[16] Coughlan C, Ledger W, Wang Q, et al. Recurrent implantation failure: definition and management. Reprod Biomed Online 2014;28:14-38.

[17] Margalioth EJ, Ben-Chetrit A, Gal M. Investigation and treatment of repeated implantation failure following IVF-ET. Hum Reprod 2006;21:3036-46.

[18] Hviid MM, Macklon N. Immune modulation treatments — where is the evidence? Fertil Steril 2017;107:1284-93.

[19] Chaouat G, Ledee-Bataille N. Th1/Th2 paradigm in pregnancy: paradigm last? Int Arch Immunol. 2004;134:93-119.

[20] Saito S, Nakashima A. Th1/Th2/Th17 and regulatory T-cell paradigm in pregnancy. Am J Reprod Immunol 2010;63: 601-10.

[21] Ng SC, Gilman-Sachs A, Thakar P. Expression of intracellular Th1 and Th2 cytokines in women with recurrent spontaneous abortion, implantation failures after IVF-ET or normal pregnancy. Am J Reprod Immunol 2002;48;77-86.

[22] Riley JK. Trophoblast immune receptors in maternal-fetal tolerance. Immunol Invest 2008;37:395-426.

[23] Mosmann J, Moore K. The role of IL-10 in crossregulation of TH1 and TH2 response. Immunol Today 1991;12:A49.

[24] Winger EE, Reed JL, Ashoush S. Elevated preconception CD56+16+ and/or Th1:Th2 levels predict benefit from IVIG therapy in subfertile women undergoing IVF. Am J Reprod Immunol 2011;66:394-403.

[25] Nakagawa K, Kwak-Kim J, Ota K. Immunosuppression with Tacrolimus improved reproductive outcome of women with repeated implantation failure and elevated peripheral blood Th1/Th2 cell ratios. Am J Reprod Immunol 2015;73:353-61.

[26] Lee SK, Kim JY, Han AR, et al. Intravenous immunoglobulin improves pregnancy outcome in women with recurrent pregnancy losses with cellular immune abnormalities. Am J Reprod Immunol 2016;75:59-68.

[27] Raghupathy R, Makhseed M, Azizich F. Maternal Th1-and Th2-type reactivity to placental antigens in normal human pregnancy and unexplained recurrent spontaneous abortions. Cell Immunol 1999;196:122-30.

[28] Kawk-Kim J, Bao S, Lee SK. Immunological modes of pregnancy loss: inflammation, immune effectors, and stress. Am J Reprod Immunol 2014;72:129-40.

[29] Kwak-Kim JY, Beaman KD, Gilman-Sachs A. Up-regulated expression of CD56+, CD56+/CD16+, and CD19+ cells in peripheral blood lymphocytes in pregnant women with recurrent pregnancy losses. Am J Reprod Immunol 1995;34: 93-9.

[30] Lee SK, Na BJ, Kim JY, et al. Determination of clinical cellular immune markers in women with recurrent pregnancy loss. Am J Reprod Immunol 2013;70:398-411.

[31] Chaouat G, Zourbas S, et al. New insights into maternal-fetal interactions at implantation. Reprod Biomed Online 2001;2: 198-203.

[32] Mekinian A, Cohen J, Alijotas-Reig J, et al. Unexplained recurrent miscarriage and recurrent implantation failure: is there a place for immunomodulation? Am J Reprod Immunol 2016;76:8-28.

[33] Robertson SA, Jin M, Yu D, et al. Corticosteroid therapy in assisted reproduction-immune suppression is a faulty premise. Hum Reprod 2016;31:2164-73.

[34] Boomsma CM, Kavelaars A, Eijkemans MJC, et al. Endometrial secretion analysis identifies a cytokine profile predictive of pregnancy in IVF. Hum Reprod 2009;24:1427-35.

[35] Matsubayashi H, Hosaka T, Sugiyama Y, et al. Increased natural killer-cell activity is associated with infertile women. Am J Reprod Immunol 2001;46:318-22.

[36] Emmer PM, Nelen WL, Steegers EA. Peripheral natural killer cytotoxicity and CD56(pos)CD16(pos) cells increase during early pregnancy in women with a history of recurrent spontaneous abortion. Hum Reprod 2000;15:1163-9.

[37] King K, Smith S, Chapman M. Detailed analysis of peripheral blood natural killer (NK) cells in women with recurrent miscarriage. Hum Reprod 2010;25:52-8.

[38] Moffett A, Shreeve N. First do no harm: uterine natural killer (NK) cells in assisted reproduction. Hum Reprod 2015; 30:1519-25.

[39] Tuckerman E, Mariee N, Prakash A. Uterine natural killer cells in peri-implantation endometrium from women with repeated implantation failure after IVF. J Reprod Immunol 2010;87:60-6.

[40] Guo Y, Tian X, Wang X. Adverse effects of immunoglobulin therapy. Front Immunol 2018;9:1299. Available from: https://doi.org/10.3389/fimmu.2018.01299.

[41] Scheinfeld N. Adalimumab: a review of side effects. Expert Opin Drug Saf 2005;4:637-41. Available from: https://doi.org/10.1517/14740338.4.4.637. PMID:16011443.

[42] https://www.drugs.com/pro/intralipid.html.

[43] Kim YH, Shin HY, Kim SM. Long-term safety and efficacy

of tacrolimus in *Myasthenia gravis*. Yonsei Med J 2019;60:633-9. Available from: https://doi.org/10.3349/ymj.2019.60.7.633.

[44] Geva E, Amit A, Lerner-Geva L, et al. Prednisone and aspirin improve pregnancy rate in patients with repro-ductive failure and autoimmune antibodies: a prospective study. Am J Reprod Imunol. 2000;43:36-40.

[45] Hasegawa I, Yamamoto Y, Suzuki M, et al. Prednisolone plus low-dose aspirin improves the implantation rate in women with autoimmune conditions who are undergoing in vitro fertilization. Fertil Steril 1998;70:1044-8.

[46] Boomsma CM, Keay SD, Macklon NS. Peri-implantation glucocorticoid administration for assisted reproductive technology cycles. Cochrane Database Syst Rev 2012;Cd005996.

[47] Elenkov IJ. Glucocorticoids and the Th1/Th2 balance. Ann N Y Acad Sci 2004;1024:138-46.

[48] Taniguchi F. Results of prednisolone given to improve the outcome of in vitro fertilization-embryo transfer in women with antinuclear antibodies. J Reprod Med 2005;50:383-8.

[49] Han AR, Ahn H, Vu P, et al. Obstetrical outcome of anti-inflammatory and anticoagulation therapy in women with recurrent pregnancy loss or unexplained infertility. Am J Reprod Immunol 2012;68:418-27.

[50] Goring SM, Lew AR, Ghement I. A network meta-analysis of the efficacy of belatacept, cyclosporine and tacrolimus for immunosuppression therapy in adult renal transplant recipients. Curr Ned Res Opin. 2014;30:1473-87.

[51] Uchida K. Long-term Prograf multicenter retrospective study in kidney transplantation: seven-year follow-up. Transplant Now. 2006;19:380-9.

[52] Kino T, Hatanaka H, Miyata S. FK-506, a novel immunosuppressant isolated from a *Streptomyces*. II. Immunosuppressive effect of FK-506 in vitro. J Antibiot. 1987;40:1256-65.

[53] Ram R, Gafter-Gvili A, Yeshuru M. Prophylaxis regimens for GVHD: systematic review and meta-analysis. Bone Marrow Transplant 2009;43:643-53.

[54] Ramiro S, Gaujoux-Viala C, Nam JL, et al. Safety of synthetic and biological DMARDs: a systematic literature review informing the 2013 update of the EULAR recommendations for management of rheumatoid arthritis. Ann Rheum Dis 2014;73:529-35.

[55] Nakagawa K, Kwak-Kim J, Kuroda K. Immunosuppressive treatment using tacrolimus promotes pregnancy outcome in infertile women with repeated implantation failures. Am J Reprod Immunol 2017. Available from: https://doi.org/10.1111/aji.12682.

[56] Nakagawa K, Kwak-Kim J, Hisano M, et al. Obstetrical and perinatal outcome of the women with repeated implantation failures or recurrent pregnancy losses who received pre-and post-conception tacrolimus treatment. Am J Reprod Immunol 2019;82:e13142.

[57] Nakagawa K, Sugiyama R. Immunomodulating treatment for the patients with repeated implantation failures caused by immunological rejection. In: Kuroda K, Brosens J, Quenby S, Takeda S, editors. Treatment Strategy for Unexplained Infertility and Recurrent Miscarriage. Singapore: Springer; 2018. p.460.

[58] Nakagawa K, Kuroda K, Sugiyama R. After 12 consecutive miscarriages, a patient received immunosuppressive treatment and delivered an infant. Reprod Med Biol. 2017. Available from: https://doi.org/10.1002/rmb2.12040.

[59] Wei D, Chen ZJ, Sun Y. Prednisone for patients with recurrent implantation failure: study protocol for a double-blind, multicenter, randomized, placebo-controlled trial. Trials 2020;21:719.

第 19 章

B 细胞病理学与反复种植失败

B-cell pathology and repeated implantation failures

Shihua Bao, Mengyang Du and Xiao Wang

Department of Reproductive Immunology, Shanghai First Maternity and Infant Hospital, Tongji University School of Medicine, Shanghai, P.R. China

1 引言

反复种植失败（RIF）对于受影响夫妇和临床医生都是一个极具挑战性的问题，其治疗也是体外受精（IVF）和胚胎移植（ET）领域中最棘手的难题之一。据报道，高龄、父母双方吸烟史、高体重指数、压力、卵子质量差（特别是在高龄女性中）、血栓性疾病、子宫因素（如先天性子宫畸形、子宫内膜息肉、子宫黏膜下肌瘤、宫腔粘连）以及附件病变（如输卵管积液）都是 RIF 的可能原因[1-3]。然而，在绝大多数病例中，病因仍不清楚。

开创性的研究表明，免疫系统在胚胎成功植入中起着至关重要的作用，而该系统的紊乱会导致种植失败。为了成功妊娠，母体免疫系统需要执行看似矛盾的功能。它必须对不断生长的半同种异体胎儿具有免疫耐受性，同时保持识别和应对外来抗原的能力。支持健康妊娠所需的免疫特征变化已在固有和适应性免疫细胞中得到充分记录，包括抑制胎儿抗原的特异性效应 T 细胞，产生调节性 T 细胞（Tregs），以及改变自然杀伤（NK）细胞、巨噬细胞、单核细胞和树突状细胞（DC）的比例和功能[4,5]。

然而，从历史上看，相较于适应性免疫中其他免疫细胞，B 细胞在妊娠中的作用并未得到同等关注。早期的研究主要探索了 B 细胞的传统功能，即产生抗体，并仅暗示 B 细胞可从多方面对妊娠产生影响。然而，对其他疾病的研究拓宽了对 B 细胞功能的理解。现在人们普遍认为，B 细胞表现出功能上的多样性，既能作为适应性免疫的效应细胞，又能执行类似固有免疫的抑制功能[6,7]。了解 B 细胞调控免疫的机制对于设计免疫介导的妊娠病理的创新疗法至关重要，因为许多研究已反复表明，免疫功能失调与妊娠疾病（如 RPL，子痫前期和免疫性不孕症）相关[8-11]。

尽管在妊娠背景下，对调节性 B 细胞（Breg）的性质和作用机制的了解仍然有限，但使用早期流产小鼠模型的开创性研究揭示了它们的重要性，表明 Breg 细胞能够恢复母体的免疫耐受性并支持健康的妊娠[12-15]。此外，临床研究已确立了 Breg 损伤与不良妊娠结局（如 RIF 和反复流产）之间的关联[10,16-18]。迄今为止，有越来越多的证据表明，在妊娠免疫网络中，Breg 发挥着关键作用，这种作用可被开发成治疗妊娠病理的一种免疫治疗形式。当前针对不明原因 RPL 的免疫疗法，如淋巴细胞免疫治疗、滋养层膜免疫治疗和静脉注射免疫球蛋白 G（IVIgG）等，已被证实能改善产科结局[19]。然而，开发有效的靶向免疫疗法以进一步改善妊娠结局仍是一个有待探索的研究领域。在本章中，我们将回顾探索 B 细胞病理学的最新研究，以阐明其与 RIF 的联系。此外，我们还强调了 B 细胞亚群的潜在功能，以作为免疫治疗手段，用于预防或治疗妊娠病理和并发症。

2 B 细胞免疫病理学与生殖

2.1 B 细胞亚群

长期以来，B 细胞被视为免疫效应器，专门负责适应性免疫。最近，B细胞亚群在固有免疫和适应性免疫之间架起的桥梁作用也得到了认可。B1和B2细胞的正常协调在维持保护性免疫和预防自身免疫性疾病中发挥着至关重要的作用[20]。因此，值得认真研究妊娠期间B细胞亚群的作用。

小鼠的B细胞亚群已得到广泛研究，这有助于从功能和发生学上区分B1和B2亚群[6]。与小鼠不同，基于表型的人类B细胞亚群的划分仍不明确，一直是持续争论的问题[21-25]。尽管存在争议，近期已将$CD20^+CD27^+CD43^+CD38^{lo/int}$细胞定义为人类B-1细胞亚群[26,27]。在小鼠中，B1细胞从胎儿肝脏的造血干细胞（HSC）发育而来，并根据CD5的表达分为B-1a或B-1b。然而，人类B-1细胞中的CD5表达并不明显。人类B-1细胞还表达CD20、CD27和CD43[28]。与小鼠不同，在人类中，B1和B2细胞是从$Lin^-CD34^+CD38^{lo}$干细胞群发育而来的。在小鼠中，B1细胞主要存在于腹腔，并分布于胸腔、脾脏和肠道[29]，而在人类中，它们主要存在于外周循环中[30]。

B2细胞自出生后就从它们的骨髓（BM）前体细胞分化而来，产生表达表面免疫球蛋白M（sIgM）的细胞[31]。这些细胞离开BM并迁移到脾脏。在脾脏中，它们成熟为边缘区或滤泡B细胞[32]。B细胞的体细胞超突变及其Ig类别转换是通过暴露于抗原并得到辅助性T细胞（Th）的信号而实现的[33]。在小鼠中，已报道了在没有任何免疫应答的情况下，生发中心外的T细胞发生非依赖性体细胞超突变[34-36]。此外，Toll样受体介导的人类和小鼠B细胞刺激可以诱导T细胞非依赖的激活和Ig类别转换[37]。激活的B细胞随后分化为浆细胞和记忆细胞[33]。

2.2 妊娠期产生抗体的B细胞

B细胞的功能在传统上主要与体液免疫相关，因此，B细胞被认为通过产生抗体在妊娠中发挥作用。20世纪70年代进行的实验显示，母体血清的IgG部分可以阻止母体效应T细胞对同种异体滋养组织产生功能性细胞毒性反应[38]。此外，妊娠期间自发性体液免疫反应的激活，如子宫引流淋巴结中分泌IgG和IgM的细胞水平增加，早期被报道为妊娠期间可能存在的抑制性机制之一[39]。最近，小鼠和临床研究提供了支持证据，其特征在于与非妊娠对照组相比，妊娠个体的IgM和IgA血清水平显著增加[14,18,40]。一项关于妊娠期间人类记忆B细胞表型的研究同样显示，记忆标志物CD27在妊娠期间的表达水平显著增加，这直接影响了所产生的免疫球蛋白亚型的特征。在该研究中，CD27表达上调与IgG和IgA同种型产生增加相关[41]。另有报道称，与具有良好妊娠结局的小鼠相比，不良妊娠结局的小鼠模型的脾脏B细胞产生更高滴度的IgG同种型、IgA和IgM[42]。因此，激活B细胞的体液免疫应答以产生抗体对于实现健康妊娠是必需的。

2.3 非沉淀性不对称抗体

在20世纪70年代，人们发现了一类名为"不对称抗体"的IgG亚型。不对称抗体是一种IgG，具有与一个Fab区域结合的富含甘露糖的寡糖残基，因此使它们无法激活免疫效应功能，如补体结合、吞噬作用和细胞毒性[43]。在妊娠期间，孕妇血清中含有比非妊娠女性更高滴度的不对称抗体，其中大部分具有父源抗原特异性[44,45]。相反，经历反复自然流产的女性血清中不对称抗体的比例显著低于健康孕妇[45,46]。因此推测不对称抗体在妊娠期间具有保护作用，并称之为保护性母体抗体；然而，在随后的临床前和临床研究中尚未进一步证实这种应答的机制。

2.4 自身抗体

与妊娠期的保护性抗体相反，自身抗体的存在被认为与妊娠失败有关。其中大部分研究探讨了抗磷脂抗体（aPL）和肾素-血管紧张素转换酶Ⅱ型受体的激动性自身抗体对妊娠的影响[47-49]。高水平的aPL被认为是aPL综合征的病因，这是一种以高凝状态为特征的自身免疫性疾病，导致全身性的血液凝固（血栓形成）。在妊娠期间，aPL综合征会损害生殖结局，如流产、胎儿死亡和严重的子痫前期[47,50,51]。β2糖蛋白Ⅰ是抗心磷脂抗体的辅因子。研究表明，30%的RIF患者标准或非标准aPL抗体检测呈阳性，如抗磷脂酰肌醇（aPI）、抗磷脂酰乙醇胺（aPE）和抗磷脂酰丝氨酸（aPS）抗体，而健康对照组中只有16%呈阳性（$P=0.019$）[52,53]。由于APS和RIF均存在特异性抗体，因此有必要考虑是否应将RIF添加到aPL综合征的临床诊断标准中[54]。

此外，肾素-血管紧张素转换酶Ⅱ型受体自身抗体可能在子痫前期的启动和免疫病理学中起着重要作用。这些激动性自身抗体模仿肾素-血管紧张素转换酶Ⅰ型受体的天然配体，诱导产生下游抗血管生成因子(如 s-Flt1 和 Endoglin),导致子痫前期症状的发生,包括高血压、蛋白尿、肾小球内皮细胞增生,从而引起胎盘和胚胎异常[55,56]。

2.5 妊娠期的调节性 B 细胞(Breg 细胞)

近年来,一类名为 Breg 的 B 细胞亚群已成为免疫耐受中潜在的关键角色。Breg 细胞因其调节其他类型免疫细胞的能力而得名,在自身免疫、移植、免疫耐受和癌症等领域得到广泛研究。尽管其数量较少,但一致认为 Breg 细胞能够有效调节免疫反应[7]。Breg 细胞通过抑制 DC 的分化、抑制 Th1 和 Th17 细胞的增殖,并诱导转录因子叉头蛋白 P3(FoxP3)阳性调节性 T 细胞(FoxP3+ Treg)的分化来抑制免疫反应(图 19.1)[57]。Breg 细胞的明确表型和特征标记尚未确定。B 细胞表型的分子结构和功能很大程度上受外部环境和外来抗原存在的影响[6]。因此,在妊娠的动态情况下,随着父源抗原的表达逐渐增加,可以合理预期 B 细胞结构发生相应的变化,以支持母体免疫反应对妊娠的适应性调整[58]。

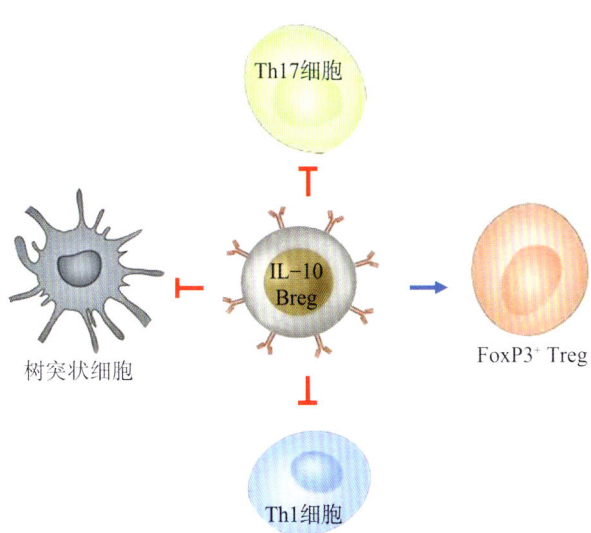

图 19.1　调节性 B 细胞(Breg 细胞)抑制辅助性 T 细胞(Th)1 和 Th17 细胞的增殖,抑制树突状细胞的分化,并诱导转录因子叉头蛋白 P3(FoxP3)阳性调节性 T 细胞(FoxP3+ Treg)的分化。

已在小鼠妊娠时认定为 Breg 的 B 细胞亚群包括 IL-10+、CD5+CD1d+、CD80+CD86+、CD80+CD86+CD27+IL-10+、IL-35+ B 细胞和 PIBF1+ 绒毛蜕膜 B 细胞。在人类妊娠时鉴定的 Breg 亚群包括 IL-10+ 和 CD24hiCD27+ B 细胞、CD24hiCD38hi 过渡性 B 细胞、CD27+ IgM+ 记忆 B 细胞、CD38hiCD27hi 浆母细胞、边缘区 B 细胞和 IL-35+ B 细胞。无论是在小鼠还是在人类中,分泌 IL-10 和较少 TGF-β 的能力仍然是识别 Breg 的标志。然而,据报道,其他标志物如 IL-35 和 PIBF1 可以在妊娠期间赋予 B 细胞调节能力[15,59,60]。由于通过细胞因子分泌来精确识别 Breg 存在困难,因此可采用替代标记,例如在小鼠中用 CD5+ CD1d+ 标记分泌 IL-10 的 B 细胞(B10 细胞),而在人类中则采用 CD24hiCD27+ 标记[61,62]。

Breg 在妊娠期间的调节作用尚未完全阐明。然而,在迄今为止进行的研究中,出现了几个重复出现的主题:①循环中 Breg 水平降低和(或)功能障碍可能提示不良产科结局。②Breg 可能参与营造胚胎种植所必需的适当条件。③Breg 可在免疫介导的妊娠并发症中恢复胎儿耐受性。

在小鼠中的开创性研究明确表明,早期妊娠期间 Breg 细胞比例的降低与自发性流产有关[13,17]。通过被动转移脾脏 CD5+ CD1dhi B10 细胞以重建 Breg 细胞,从而抑制 DC 成熟和扩增 Treg 细胞群以挽救妊娠失败[13]。同样,过继转移 B10 细胞,而不是 IL-10 阴性的 B 效应细胞或来自 IL-10 缺陷小鼠的 B 细胞,通过减少 T 细胞分泌的 IL-17A 和 IL-6 并扩增 Treg 细胞群,可预防由 LPS 驱动的炎症所引起的胎儿死亡[12]。正常妊娠女性外周血中分泌 IL-10 的 CD19+CD24hiCD27+ B 细胞显著高于非妊娠或自发性流产女性[17,60]。此外,从早期妊娠女性采集的外周血中分离的 CD19+CD24hiCD27+ Breg 细胞可成功地在体外抑制活化 T 效应细胞分泌的 TNF[17](图 19.2)。

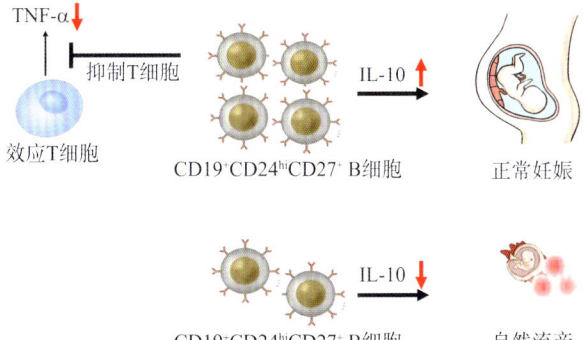

图 19.2　正常妊娠外周血中分泌 IL-10 的 CD19+CD24hiCD27+ B 细胞比例显著高于自然流产,从正常妊娠女性中分离的 CD19+ CD24hiCD27- B 细胞可通过体外激活效应 T 细胞抑制肿瘤坏死因子的分泌。

近期的小鼠研究表明，Breg 在胚胎植入前期参与其中。受孕后 3.5 天，脾脏 B 细胞上调了与 Breg 相关的标志物 TLR9 和 CD86，同时在受孕后 2.5～8.5 天观察到子宫 B 细胞的显著扩增和 B 细胞表型的变化[63,64]。此外，这些富含 CD80$^+$、CD86$^+$ 和 IL-10$^+$ B 细胞亚群的子宫 B 细胞可以有效抑制同源 CD4$^+$ 效应 T 细胞的增殖和活化[64]。B 细胞表型的改变可能发生于妊娠早期，这很可能是滋养细胞驯化的结果[61]。有报道称，B 细胞分泌 IL-10 受损是 RIF 的关键病理机制之一，因为有 RIF 病史的女性外周血 B 细胞在体外重新刺激后表达的 IL-10 mRNA 水平较低，并且分泌的 IL-10 水平显著低于健康对照组[16]。这些研究表明，在妊娠早期，Breg 对于胚胎适当植入发挥有益作用。尽管数量有限，但这些研究突显了 Breg 在妊娠中的关键调节作用，这与在自身免疫性疾病、移植耐受和癌症中观察到的结果相似。在所有情况下，Breg 通过诱导和维持 Treg、改变 Th 细胞反应以及通过细胞毒性 T 细胞、NK 细胞和 DC 抑制效应细胞反应，有助于控制组织环境。

3 反复种植失败与 B 细胞失调

有关 B 细胞及其亚群在生育障碍女性中的研究已有报道。经历流产和 RIF 的女性外周血中 CD19$^+$ B 细胞水平显著低于随后成功生育的女性[65,66]。多次 IVF 失败且卵巢低反应(POR)和维生素 D(VD)低水平的女性，CD19$^+$ B 细胞和 CD19$^+$/5$^+$ B1 细胞水平显著高于正常卵巢反应和 VD 低水平以及 POR 和 VD 正常水平的女性($P<0.05$)[67]。此外，在一例有 RPL 和不孕病史的女性病例报告中，外周血 CD19$^+$ B 细胞数量的增加与记忆 B 细胞亚群水平持续下降相关[10]。检测外周血 CD19$^+$ B 细胞亚群可能有助于预测 RIF 患者的妊娠结局。

在 IVF 周期中，具有高水平 VD 女性的成熟卵母细胞数和囊胚形成率明显更高。采用孕激素促排卵方案的低水平 VD 女性，其外周血 B 细胞和 NK 细胞比例以及 Th/Tc 细胞比例显著高于具有高水平 VD 女性($P<0.05$)。同样，在采用激动剂方案的患者中，低水平 VD 女性的外周血 B 细胞比例和 Th/Tc 细胞比例也高于具有高水平 VD 女性($P<0.05$)[68]。据报道，在多发性硬化症患者中，低水平 VD 通过富集经历过抗原类别转换的记忆 B 细胞和分泌抗体的浆细胞，诱导过度的 B 细胞反应[69]。因此，B 细胞的 VD 缺乏可能会加剧母体生长卵泡和子宫内膜的促炎环境。

在患有 aPL 综合征的患者中，循环 CD5$^+$ B 细胞的数量增加与高水平 aPL 相关，并与 RPL 女性的免疫紊乱有关。这种独特的天然样 B 细胞亚群的特点是产生能与氧化磷脂表位相互作用的多特异性抗体[70]。有趣的是，在人类和小鼠的研究中，针对 B 细胞的治疗似乎具有临床和血清学上的双重益处，包括降低 aPL 滴度[71,72]。因此，aPL 中的 B 细胞免疫病理可能具有比我们目前所认识的更为广泛的临床和免疫学表现[73]。没有同型转换的持续性 IgM aPL 可能是一种罕见的 aPL 表现形式，与 B 细胞亚群失调相关[66]。

4 临床转化视角下的 B 细胞免疫病理

4.1 强的松

强的松因其具有抗炎和免疫抑制作用，常用于炎症性和自身免疫性疾病。多种药理学机制已经解释了强的松在 RIF 和 RPL 患者中的疗效。自然杀伤细胞(uNK 细胞)数量过多、毒性增强以及 Th1 免疫占主导与 RIF 和妊娠丢失有关。据报道，强的松可显著减少 uNK 细胞数量(从 14% 降至 9%)。此外，强的松还可通过抑制 Th1 细胞因子的分泌，增加调节性 T 细胞数量以及抑制 NK 细胞的细胞毒性以调节免疫系统[74-76]。在一项非随机临床试验中，联合使用低分子肝素和强的松提高了反复 IVF 失败患者的妊娠率和活产率[77]。中国目前正在进行一项前瞻性多中心、随机、双盲、安慰剂对照临床试验(强的松与安慰剂的 1∶1 比例，注册号 ChiCTR1800018783)，旨在确定强的松是否能在 RIF 患者中提高作为主要结局指标的活产率[78](译者注：该研究已于 2023 年 5 月发表于 JAMA 杂志)。

4.2 羟氯喹

羟氯喹是一种抗疟药物，广泛用于多种自身免疫性疾病患者，尤其是系统性红斑狼疮(SLE)。除了具有抗血栓作用外，羟氯喹还具有免疫调节特性，可以抑制促炎细胞因子的产生[79]。一些体外研究显示，在 aPL 综合征中，羟氯喹可能有助于早期滋养细胞迁移和胚胎植入。羟氯喹可以恢复被 aPL

抗体抑制的滋养细胞融合和分化,降低 TLR4 的表达[80]。羟氯喹还可减少 aPL 抗体与合体滋养层细胞的结合,并恢复膜联蛋白 A5 的表达[81]。目前尚缺乏生理病理研究以证明羟氯喹在不明原因 RPL 和 RIF 患者中的效果。

目前,有限的临床数据显示羟氯喹对不明原因 RPL 和 RIF 患者有效。对难治性产科 aPL 综合征的一项小型回顾性研究(30 名患者,共 35 次妊娠)显示,与常规妊娠治疗相比,添加羟氯喹治疗后妊娠丢失率从 81% 下降到 19%($P<0.05$)[82]。一些慢性绒毛间质炎患者在使用羟氯喹后成功妊娠[83]。羟氯喹的免疫调节效应在不明原因 RPL 和免疫紊乱相关的 RIF 患者中值得进一步探索。

4.3 静脉注射免疫球蛋白

已有研究阐述了 IVIG 改善妊娠的机制,包括:①抑制 B 细胞自身抗体产生。②降低 Th1/Th2 细胞因子平衡。③降低外周血 NK 细胞百分比。④抑制 NK 细胞毒性。⑤增加 RPL 和 RIF 患者 T 细胞抑制活性[84-86]。Heilmann 等(2010 年)[87]对 188 名 ET 前 7 天接受 0.2g/kg 免疫球蛋白 G 治疗的 RIF 患者(3 次或更多次 RIF)进行回顾性研究,结果显示研究组的种植率和活产率分别为 21.0% 和 42.0%。而对照组的种植率和活产率分别为 9.3% 和 16.1%。2017 年的一项研究还报道,RIF 患者在接受 IVIG 治疗后,调节性 T 细胞表达的 Foxp3 mRNA 增加,外周血 Th17 细胞比例降低[88]。一项系统回顾也报道了 IVIG 在 IVF/ICSI 周期中对这些患者的益处[89]。使用 IVIG 与种植率提高显著相关,与安慰剂相比,RR 为 2.708(95% CI 1.302~5.629)。随机接受 IVIG 治疗的患者临床妊娠率和活产率显著增加,临床妊娠率的 RR 为 1.475(95% CI 1.191~1.825),活产率的 RR 为 1.616(95% CI 1.243~2.101)。总体而言,最近的荟萃分析支持 IVIG 治疗;然而,由于研究人群存在显著异质性,推荐 IVIG 治疗的证据还不充分[86]。

4.4 利妥昔单抗

利妥昔单抗是一种人鼠嵌合单克隆抗体,靶向前 B 细胞、未成熟 B 细胞和成熟 B 细胞上表达的 CD20 抗原,已被用于治疗 B 细胞数量过多、B 细胞过度活跃或功能失调的疾病,包括多种自身免疫性疾病、B 细胞恶性肿瘤和移植排异反应[90]。当利妥昔单抗用于正常妊娠的大鼠中时,观察到 B 细胞耗竭和子宫灌注压降低(RUPP)[91]。接受利妥昔单抗治疗的 RUPP 大鼠,在诱导的胎盘缺血反应中血压增加较少[92]。这些数据为人类不良妊娠结局提供了潜在的见解,从而为治疗妊娠失败提供了新的治疗方法。因此,最近的一份病例报告描述了一名历经两次 IVF 失败和抗心磷脂抗体(ACA)阳性的患者在接受利妥昔单抗治疗后成功妊娠。该患者经过一段时间的利妥昔单抗治疗,ACA 转为阴性,通过 IVF 治疗成功受孕[93]。利妥昔单抗破坏了表面具有 CD20 的 B 细胞,无论是正常还是恶性的 B 细胞。然而,CD20 并不在干细胞和大多数浆细胞上表达。因此,在接受抗 CD20 抗体治疗后,B 细胞仍可能再生,并且浆细胞合成免疫球蛋白亦不受影响[94,95]。

4.5 基于 Breg 的治疗

从临床角度来看,Breg 作为临床免疫稳态重要组成部分的作用已被认可和重视,尤其是在自身免疫领域,首次证明了利妥昔单抗全面耗竭 B 细胞的疗效在一定程度上受限于其同时去除了有益的 Breg 细胞[96]。然而,由于 Breg 领域仍然未被充分探索,创新性的临床转化研究非常有限。过去 10 年涉及 Breg 的临床研究主要集中在确定 Breg 作为疾病的预后或诊断标志物的潜力[58]。此外,这些研究仅限于自身免疫性疾病,如慢性免疫性血小板减少症、炎性风湿性疾病和 SLE(clinicaltrials.gov)。在知识产权方面,2018 年授予的一项专利涵盖了分泌 IL-10 的 B 细胞作为操纵自身免疫性或炎症性疾病以及治疗传染病和(或)癌症的工具[97]。此外还有一项制备分泌 IL-10 的 B 细胞的方法获得专利[97]。但除此之外,尚无将基于 Breg 的疗法作为任何一种疾病的干预措施以进行临床应用。

5 总结和建议

总之,B 细胞在妊娠过程中除了产生抗体外,还在免疫调节中发挥着作用。目前,关于 Breg 及其在正常妊娠中的作用的研究仍处于起步阶段。尽管取得了进展,但仍有许多问题尚未解决,特别是围绕这种免疫细胞群体与其他已有深入研究的细胞群体之间的相互作用,以及它们如何协同诱导和维持母体免疫耐受。此外,由于许多妊娠病理的基础在于胚胎植入不理想,而植入又是妊娠期的关键阶段,受免疫的高度调控,对植入事件的认识不足成为临床转化的障碍。然而,我们预测,随着对母体耐受背后基础免疫机制的进一步探索,再加上癌症领域细胞免疫治疗的快速且令人兴奋的进展,可以利用这些发现,设计和应用创新性免疫干预措施来治疗许多病理妊娠。毫无疑问,Breg 细胞具有作为这种治疗干预基础的理想特征,这也是目前正在研究的一种方法。

- B 细胞及其亚群的异常与生殖障碍有关。
- 激活 B 细胞体液反应以产生抗体是实现正常妊娠的必要步骤。
- 自身抗体的存在与妊娠失败有关。
- aPL 综合征能导致不良妊娠结局,如流产、胎儿死亡和重度子痫前期。
- 检测外周血 CD19$^+$ B 细胞亚群可能有助于预测 RIF 患者的妊娠结局。
- 循环 Breg 水平降低和(或)功能障碍可能预测生殖障碍和不良产科结局。
- Breg 细胞可能参与促进胚胎植入所需的适当条件。
- 在免疫介导的妊娠并发症中,Breg 可以恢复胎儿的耐受性。
- 强的松和羟氯喹在 RPL 和 RIF 患者中的效果令人期待,需要进一步评估。
- IVIG 治疗在 IVF/ICSI 周期中的应用对于 RIF 患者是有益的。

参考文献

[1] Somigliana E, Vigano P, Busnelli A, Paffoni A, Vegetti W, Vercellini P. Repeated implantation failure at the crossroad between statistics, clinics and over-diagnosis. Reprod Biomed Online 2018;36(1):32-8. Available from: https://doi.org/10.1016/j.rbmo.2017.09.012 (In eng).

[2] Cakiroglu Y, Tiras B. Determining diagnostic criteria and cause of recurrent implantation failure. Curr Opin Obstet Gynecol 2020;32(3):198-204. Available from: https://doi.org/10.1097/gco.0000000000000620 (In eng).

[3] Sheikhansari G, Pourmoghadam Z, Danaii S, Mehdizadeh A, Yousefi M. Etiology and management of recurrent implantation failure: a focus on intra-uterine PBMC-therapy for RIF. J Reprod Immunol 2020;139:103121. Available from: https://doi.org/10.1016/j.jri.2020.103121 (In eng).

[4] Arck PC, Hecher K. Fetomaternal immune cross-talk and its consequences for maternal and offspring's health. Nat Med 2013;19(5):548-56. Available from: https://doi.org/10.1038/nm.3160 (In eng).

[5] Mor G, Cardenas I. The immune system in pregnancy: a unique complexity. Am J Reprod Immunol 2010;63(6):425-33. Available from: https://doi.org/10.1111/j.1600-0897.2010.00836.x (In eng).

[6] LeBien TW, Tedder TF. B lymphocytes: how they develop and function. Blood 2008;112(5):1570-80. Available from: https://doi.org/10.1182/blood-2008-02-078071 (In eng).

[7] Boothby MR, Hodges E, Thomas JW. Molecular regulation of peripheral B cells and their progeny in immunity. Genes Dev 2019;33(1-2):26-18. Available from: https://doi.org/10.1101/gad.320192.118 (In eng).

[8] Ghaebi M, Nouri M, Ghasemzadeh A, et al. Immune regulatory network in successful pregnancy and reproductive failures. Biomed Pharmacother 2017;88:61-73. Available from: https://doi.org/10.1016/j.biopha.2017.01.016 (In eng).

[9] Marron K, Walsh D, Harrity C. Detailed endometrial immune assessment of both normal and adverse reproductive outcome populations. J Assist Reprod Genet 2019;36(2): 199-210. Available from: https://doi.org/10.1007/s10815-018-1300-8 (In eng).

[10] Sung N, Byeon HJ, Garcia MDS, et al. Deficiency in memory B cell compartment in a patient with infertility and recurrent pregnancy losses. J Reprod Immunol 2016;118:70-5. Available from: https://doi.org/10.1016/j.jri.2016.09.003 (In eng).

[11] Yang F, Zheng Q, Jin L. Dynamic function and composition changes of immune cells during normal and pathological pregnancy at the maternal-fetal interface. Front Immunol 2019;10:2317. Available from: https://doi.org/10.3389/fimmu.2019.02317 (In eng).

[12] Busse M, Campe KJ, Nowak D, et al. IL-10 producing B cells rescue mouse fetuses from inflammation-driven fetal death and are able to modulate T cell immune responses. Sci Rep 2019;9(1):9335. Available from: https://doi.org/10.1038/s41598-019-45860-2 (In eng).

[13] Jensen F, Muzzio D, Soldati R, Fest S, Zenclussen AC. Regulatory B10 cells restore pregnancy tolerance in a mouse model. Biol Reprod 2013;89(4):90. Available from: https://doi.org/10.1095/biolreprod.113.110791 (In eng).

[14] Muzzio DO, Ziegler KB, Ehrhardt J, Zygmunt M, Jensen F. Marginal zone B cells emerge as a critical component of pregnancy well-being. Reproduction 2016;151(1):29-37. Available from: https://doi.org/10.1530/rep-15-0274 (In eng).

[15] Slawek A, Lorek D, Kedzierska AE, Chelmonska-Soyta A. Regulatory B cells with IL-35 and IL-10 expression in a normal and abortion-prone murine pregnancy model. Am J Reprod Immunol (New York, NY: 1989) 2020;83(3):e13217. Available from: https://doi.org/10.1111/aji.13217 (In eng).

[16] Koushaeian L, Ghorbani F, Ahmadi M, et al. The role of IL-10-producing B cells in repeated implantation failure patients with cellular immune abnormalities. Immunol Lett 2019;214:16-22. Available from: https://doi.org/10.1016/j.imlet.2019.08.002 (In eng).

[17] Rolle L, Memarzadeh Tehran M, Morell-García A, et al. Cutting edge: IL-10-producing regulatory B cells in early human pregnancy. Am J Reprod Immunol 2013;70(6):448-53. Available from: https://doi.org/10.1111/aji.12157 (In eng).

[18] Ziegler KB, Muzzio DO, Matzner F, et al. Human pregnancy is accompanied by modifications in B cell development and immunoglobulin profile. J Reprod Immunol 2018;129:40-7. Available from: https://doi.org/10.1016/j.jri.2018.07.003 (In eng).

[19] Wong LF, Porter TF, Scott JR. Immunotherapy for recurrent miscarriage. Cochrane Database Syst Rev 2014; 2014(10):Cd000112. Available from: https://doi.org/10.1002/14651858.CD000112.pub3 (In eng).

[20] Quách TD, Hopkins TJ, Holodick NE, et al. Human B-1 and B-2 B cells develop from Lin-CD34+ CD38lo stem cells. J Immunol 2016;197(10):3950-8. Available from: https://doi.org/10.4049/jimmunol.1600630 (In eng).

[21] Perez-Andres M, Grosserichter-Wagener C, Teodosio C, van Dongen JJ, Orfao A, van Zelm MC. The nature of circulating CD27+ CD43+ B cells. J Exp Med 2011;208(13):2565-6. Available from: https://doi.org/10.1084/jem.20112203 (In eng).

[22] Descatoire M, Weill JC, Reynaud CA, Weller S. A human equivalent of mouse B-1 cells? J Exp Med 2011;208(13):2563-4. Available from: https://doi.org/10.1084/jem.20112232 (In eng).

[23] Griffin DO, Holodick NE, Rothstein TL. Human B1 cells are CD3-: a reply to "a human equivalent of mouse B-1 cells?" and "the nature of circulating CD27+ CD43+ B cells.". J Exp Med 2011;208(13):2566-9. Available from: https://doi.org/10.1084/jem.20111761 (In eng).

[24] Reynaud CA, Weill JC. Gene profiling of CD11b$^+$ and CD11b$^-$ B1 cell subsets reveals potential cell sorting artifacts. J Exp Med 2012;209(3):433-4. Available from: https://doi.org/10.1084/jem.20120402 (In eng).

[25] Rothstein TL, Griffin DO, Holodick NE, Quach TD, Kaku H. Human B-1 cells take the stage. Ann N Y Acad Sci 2013; 1285:97-114. Available from: https://doi.org/10.1111/nyas.12137 (In eng).

[26] Quách TD, Rodríguez-Zhurbenko N, Hopkins TJ, et al. Distinctions among circulating antibody-secreting cell populations, including B-1 cells, in human adult peripheral blood. J Immunol 2016;196(3):1060-9. Available from: https://doi.org/10.4049/jimmunol.1501843 (In eng).

[27] Engelbertsen D, Vallejo J, Quách TD, et al. Low levels of IgM antibodies against an advanced glycation endproduct-modified apolipoprotein B100 peptide predict cardiovascular events in nondiabetic subjects. J Immunol 2015;195(7):3020-5. Available from: https://doi.org/10.4049/jimmunol.1402869 (In eng).

[28] Griffin DO, Holodick NE, Rothstein TL. Human B1 cells in umbilical cord and adult peripheral blood express the novel phenotype CD20+ CD27+ CD43+ CD70. J Exp Med 2011; 208(1):67-80. Available from: https://doi.org/10.1084/jem.20101499 (In eng).

[29] Montecino-Rodriguez E, Dorshkind K. New perspectives in B-1 B cell development and function. Trends Immunol 2006; 27(9):428-33. Available from: https://doi.org/10.1016/j.it.2006.07.005 (In eng).

[30] Griffin DO, Rothstein TL. A small CD11b(+) human B1 cell subpopulation stimulates T cells and is expanded in lupus. J Exp Med 2011;208(13):2591-8. Available from: https://doi.org/10.1084/jem.20110978 (In eng).

[31] Fettke F, Schumacher A, Costa SD, Zenclussen AC. B cells: the old new players in reproductive immunology. Front Immunol 2014;5:285. Available from: https://doi.org/10.3389/fimmu.2014.00285 (In eng).

[32] Monroe JG, Dorshkind K. Fate decisions regulating bone marrow and peripheral B lymphocyte development. Adv Immunol 2007;95:1-50. Available from: https://doi.org/10.1016/s0065-2776(07)95001-4 (In eng).

[33] Pillai S, Cariappa A, Moran ST. Marginal zone B cells. Annu Rev Immunol 2005;23:161-96. Available from: https://doi.org/10.1146/annurev.immunol.23.021704.115728 (In eng).

[34] William J, Euler C, Christensen S, Shlomchik MJ. Evolution of autoantibody responses via somatic hypermutation outside of germinal centers. Science 2002;297(5589):2066-70. Available from: https://doi.org/10.1126/science.1073924 (In eng).

[35] Weller S, Braun MC, Tan BK, et al. Human blood IgM "memory" B cells are circulating splenic marginal zone B cells harboring a prediversified immunoglobulin repertoire. Blood 2004;104(12):3647-54. Available from: https://doi.org/10.1182/blood-2004-01-0346 (In eng).

[36] Toellner KM, Jenkinson WE, Taylor DR, et al. Low-level hypermutation in T cell-independent germinal centers compared with high mutation rates associated with T cell-dependent germinal centers. J Exp Med 2002;195(3):383-9. Available from: https://doi.org/10.1084/jem.20011112 (In eng).

[37] He B, Qiao X, Cerutti A. CpG DNA induces IgG class switch DNA recombination by activating human B cells through an innate pathway that requires TLR9 and cooperates with IL-10. J Immunol 2004;173(7):4479-91. Available from: https://doi.org/10.4049/jimmunol.173.7.4479 (In eng).

[38] Taylor PV, Hancock KW. Antigenicity of trophoblast and possible antigen-masking effects during pregnancy. Immunology 1975;28(5):973-82 (In eng).

[39] Carter J, Dresser DW. Pregnancy induces an increase in the number of immunoglobulin-secreting cells. Immunology 1983; 49(3):481-90 (In eng).

[40] Muzzio DO, Soldati R, Ehrhardt J, et al. B cell development undergoes profound modifications and adaptations during pregnancy in mice. Biol Reprod 2014;91(5):115. Available from: https://doi.org/10.1095/biolreprod.114.122366 (In eng).

[41] Grimsholm O, Piano Mortari E, Davydov AN, et al. The interplay between CD27(dull) and CD27(bright) B cells ensures the flexibility, stability, and resilience of human B cell memory. Cell Rep 2020;30(9):2963-77. Available from: https://doi.org/10.1016/j.celrep.2020.02.022 e6. (In eng).

[42] Fröhlich C, Ehrhardt J, Krüger D, Trojnarska D, Zygmunt M, Muzzio DO. Pregnancy status alters IL-21-mediated effects on murine B lymphocytes. Reproduction 2020;159(3):351-9. Available from: https://doi.org/10.1530/rep-19-0407 (In eng).

[43] Margni RA, Paz CB, Cordal ME. Immunochemical behavior of sheep non-precipitating antibodies isolated by immunoadsorption. Immunochemistry 1976;13(3):209-14. Available from: https://doi.org/10.1016/0019-2791(76)90217-2 (In eng).

[44] Malan Borel I, Gentile T, Angelucci J, et al. IgG asymmetric molecules with antipaternal activity isolated from sera and placenta of pregnant human. J Reprod Immunol 1991;20(2):129-40. Available from: https://doi.org/10.1016/0165-0378(91)90029-p (In eng).

[45] Zenclussen AC, Gentile T, Kortebani G, Mazzolli A, Margni R. Asymmetric antibodies and pregnancy. Am J Reprod Immunol 2001;45(5):289-94. Available from: https://doi.org/10.1111/j.8755-8920.2001.450504.x (In eng).

[46] Barrientos G, Fuchs D, Schröcksnadel K, et al. Low levels of serum asymmetric antibodies as a marker of threatened pregnancy. J Reprod Immunol 2009;79(2):201-10. Available from: https://doi.org/10.1016/j.jri.2008.11.002 (In eng).

[47] Di Prima FA, Valenti O, Hyseni E, et al. Antiphospholipid syndrome during pregnancy: the state of the art. J Prenatal Med 2011;5(2):41-53 (In eng).

[48] Herse F, LaMarca B. Angiotensin II type 1 receptor autoantibody (AT1-AA)-mediated pregnancy hypertension. Am J Reprod Immunol 2013;69(4):413-18. Available from: https://doi.org/10.1111/aji.12072 (In eng).

[49] Salmon JE, Girardi G. Antiphospholipid antibodies and pregnancy loss: a disorder of inflammation. J Reprod Immunol 2008;77(1):51-6. Available from: https://doi.org/10.1016/j.jri.2007.02.007 (In eng).

[50] Heilmann L, Schorsch M, Hahn T, Fareed J. Antiphospholipid syndrome and preeclampsia. Semin Thromb Hemost 2011;37(2):141-5. Available from: https://doi.org/10.1055/s-0030-1270341 (In eng).

[51] Vinatier D, Dufour P, Cosson M, Houpeau JL. Antiphospholipid syndrome and recurrent miscarriages. Eur J Obstet Gynecol Reprod Biol 2001;96(1):37-50. Available from: https://doi.org/10.1016/s0301-2115(00)00404-8 (In eng).

[52] Stern C, Chamley L, Hale L, Kloss M, Speirs A, Baker HW. Antibodies to beta2 glycoprotein I are associated with in vitro fertilization implantation failure as well as recurrent miscarriage: results of a prevalence study. Fertil Steril 1998;70(5):938-44. Available from: https://doi.org/10.1016/s0015-0282(98)00312-4 (In eng).

[53] Kwak-Kim J, Skariah A, Wu L, Salazar D, Sung N, Ota K. Humoral and cellular autoimmunity in women with recurrent pregnancy losses and repeated implantation failures: a possible role of vitamin D. Autoimmun Rev 2016;15(10):943-7. Available from: https://doi.org/10.1016/j.autrev.2016.07.015 (In eng).

[54] Bashiri A, Halper KI, Orvieto R. Recurrent implantation failure-update overview on etiology, diagnosis, treatment and future directions. Reprod Biol Endocrinol 2018;16(1):121. Available from: https://doi.org/10.1186/s12958-018-0414-2 (In eng).

[55] Robinson CJ, Johnson DD, Chang EY, Armstrong DM, Wang W. Evaluation of placenta growth factor and soluble Fms-like tyrosine kinase 1 receptor levels in mild and severe preeclampsia. Am J Obstet Gynecol 2006;195(1):255-9. Available from: https://doi.org/10.1016/j.ajog.2005.12.049.

[56] Zhou CC, Zhang Y, Irani RA, et al. Angiotensin receptor agonistic autoantibodies induce preeclampsia in pregnant mice. Nat Med 2008;14(8):855-62. Available from: https://doi.org/10.1038/nm.1856 (In eng).

[57] Cai X, Zhang L, Wei W. Regulatory B cells in inflammatory diseases and tumor. Int Immunopharmacol 2019;67:281-6. Available from: https://doi.org/10.1016/j.intimp.2018.12.007 (In eng).

[58] Guzman-Genuino RM, Hayball JD, Diener KR. Regulatory B cells: dark horse in pregnancy immunotherapy? J Mol Biol 2021;433(1):166596. Available from: https://doi.org/10.1016/j.jmb.2020.07.008 (In eng).

[59] Huang B, Faucette AN, Pawlitz MD, et al. Interleukin-33-induced expression of PIBF1 by decidual B cells protects against preterm labor. Nat Med 2017;23(1):128-35. Available from: https://doi.org/10.1038/nm.4244 (In eng).

[60] Liu J, Chen X, Hao S, et al. Human chorionic gonadotropin and IL-35 contribute to the maintenance of peripheral immune tolerance during pregnancy through mediating the generation of IL-10(+) or IL-35(+) Breg cells. Exp Cell Res 2019;383(2):111513. Available from: https://doi.org/10.1016/j.yexcr.2019.111513 (In eng).

[61] Iwata Y, Matsushita T, Horikawa M, et al. Characterization of a rare IL-10-competent B-cell subset in humans that parallels mouse regulatory B10 cells. Blood 2011;117(2):530-41. Available from: https://doi.org/10.1182/blood-2010-07-294249 (In eng).

[62] Yanaba K, Bouaziz JD, Haas KM, Poe JC, Fujimoto M, Tedder TF. A regulatory B cell subset with a unique CD1dhiCD5+ phenotype controls T cell-dependent inflammatory responses. Immunity 2008;28(5):639-50. Available from: https://doi.org/10.1016/j.immuni.2008.03.017 (In eng).

[63] Lorek D, Kedzierska AE, Slawek A, Chelmonska-Soyta A. Expression of Toll-like receptors and costimulatory molecules in splenic B cells in a normal and abortion-prone murine pregnancy model. Am J Reprod Immunol (New York, NY: 1989)2019;82(2):e13148. Available from: https://doi.org/10.1111/aji.13148 (In eng).

[64] Guzman-Genuino RM, Eldi P, Garcia-Valtanen P, Hayball JD, Diener KR. Uterine B cells exhibit regulatory properties during the peri-implantation stage of murine pregnancy. Front Immunol 2019;10:2899. Available from: https://doi.org/10.3389/fimmu.2019.02899 (In eng).

[65] Tu W, Li Y, Ding Q, et al. Association between peripheral CD19+ B cells and reproductive outcome in women with recurrent implantation failure. Clin Lab 2020;66(1). Available from: https://doi.org/10.7754/Clin.Lab.2019.190510 (In eng).

[66] Ota K, Dambaeva S, Lee J, Gilman-Sachs A, Beaman K, Kwak-Kim J. Persistent high levels of IgM antipho-spholipid antibodies in a patient with recurrent pregnancy losses and rheumatoid arthritis. Am J Reprod Immunol 2014;71(3):286-92. Available from: https://doi.org/10.1111/aji.12196 (In eng).

[67] Wu L, Vendiola JA, Salazar Garcia MD, et al. Poor ovarian response is associated with serum vitamin D levels and pro-inflammatory immune responses in women undergoing in-vitro fertilization. J Reprod Immunol 2019;136:102617. Available from: https://doi.org/10.1016/j.jri.2019.102617 (In eng) (In eng).

[68] Wu L, Kwak-Kim J, Zhang R, et al. Vitamin D level affects IVF outcome partially mediated via Th/Tc cell ratio. Am J Reprod Immunol 2018;80(6):e13050. Available from: https://doi.org/10.1111/aji.13050 (In eng).

[69] Haas J, Schwarz A, Korporal-Kuhnke M, Faller S, Jarius S,

Wildemann B. Hypovitaminosis D upscales B-cell immunoreactivity in multiple sclerosis. J Neuroimmunol 2016;294:18 – 26. Available from: https://doi.org/10.1016/j.jneuroim.2016.03.011 (In eng).

[70] Youinou P, Renaudineau Y. The antiphospholipid syndrome as a model for B cell-induced autoimmune diseases. Thromb Res 2004;114(5 – 6):363 – 9. Available from: https://doi.org/10.1016/j.thromres.2004.06.019 (In eng).

[71] Binder CJ, Silverman GJ. Natural antibodies and the autoimmunity of atherosclerosis. Springer Semin Immunopathol 2005;26(4):385 – 404. Available from: https://doi.org/10.1007/s00281-004-0185-z (In eng).

[72] Hörkkö S, Binder CJ, Shaw PX, et al. Immunological responses to oxidized LDL. Free Radic Biol Med 2000;28(12):1771 – 9. Available from: https://doi.org/10.1016/s0891-5849(00)00333-6 (In eng).

[73] Khattri S, Zandman-Goddard G, Peeva E. B-cell directed therapies in antiphospholipid antibody syndrome new directions based on murine and human data. Autoimmun Rev 2012;11(10):717 – 22. Available from: https://doi.org/10.1016/j.autrev.2011.12.011 (In eng).

[74] Quenby S, Kalumbi C, Bates M, Farquharson R, Vince G. Prednisolone reduces preconceptual endometrial natural killer cells in women with recurrent miscarriage. Fertil Steril 2005;84(4):980 – 4. Available from: https://doi.org/10.1016/j.fertnstert.2005.05.012 (In eng).

[75] Schiessl B, Innes BA, Bulmer JN, et al. Localization of angiogenic growth factors and their receptors in the human placental bed throughout normal human pregnancy. Placenta 2009;30(1):79 – 87. Available from: https://doi.org/10.1016/j.placenta.2008.10.004 (In eng).

[76] Huang Q, Wu H, Li M, Yang Y, Fu X. Prednisone improves pregnancy outcome in repeated implantation failure by enhance regulatory T cells bias. J Reprod Immunol 2021;143:103245. Available from: https://doi.org/10.1016/j.jri.2020.103245 (In eng).

[77] Siristatidis C, Chrelias C, Creatsa M, et al. Addition of prednisolone and heparin in patients with failed IVF/ICSI cycles: a preliminary report of a clinical trial. Hum Fertil (Camb) 2013;16(3):207 – 10. Available from: https://doi.org/10.3109/14647273.2013.803608 (In eng).

[78] Lu Y, Yan J, Liu J, et al. Prednisone for patients with recurrent implantation failure: study protocol for a double-blind, multicenter, randomized, placebo-controlled trial. Trials 2020;21(1):719. Available from: https://doi.org/10.1186/s13063-020-04630-6 (In eng).

[79] Mekinian A, Costedoat-Chalumeau N, Masseau A, et al. Obstetrical APS: is there a place for hydroxychloroquine to improve the pregnancy outcome? Autoimmun Rev 2015;14(1):23 – 9. Available from: https://doi.org/10.1016/j.autrev.2014.08.040 (In eng).

[80] Marchetti T, Ruffatti A, Wuillemin C, de Moerloose P, Cohen M. Hydroxychloroquine restores trophoblast fusion affected by antiphospholipid antibodies. J Thromb Haemost 2014;12(6):910 – 20. Available from: https://doi.org/10.1111/jth.12570 (In eng).

[81] Wu XX, Guller S, Rand JH. Hydroxychloroquine reduces binding of antiphospholipid antibodies to syncytiotrophoblasts and restores annexin A5 expression. Am J Obstet Gynecol 2011;205(6):576. Available from: https://doi.org/10.1016/j.ajog.2011.06.064 e7 – 14. (In eng).

[82] Mekinian A, Lazzaroni MG, Kuzenko A, et al. The efficacy of hydroxychloroquine for obstetrical outcome in anti-phospholipid syndrome: Data from a European multicenter retrospective study. Autoimmun Rev 2015;14(6):498 – 502. Available from: https://doi.org/10.1016/j.autrev.2015.01.012 (In eng).

[83] Mekinian A, Costedoat-Chalumeau N, Masseau A, et al. Chronic histiocytic intervillositis: outcome, associated diseases and treatment in a multicenter prospective study. Autoimmunity 2015;48(1):40 – 5. Available from: https://doi.org/10.3109/08916934.2014.939267 (In eng).

[84] Coulam CB, Acacio B. Does immunotherapy for treatment of reproductive failure enhance live births? Am J Reprod Immunol (New York, NY: 1989) 2012;67(4):296 – 304. Available from: https://doi.org/10.1111/j.1600-0897.2012.01111.x (In eng).

[85] Yamada H, Morikawa M, Furuta I, et al. Intravenous immunoglobulin treatment in women with recurrent abortions: increased cytokine levels and reduced Th1/Th2 lymphocyte ratio in peripheral blood. Am J Reprod Immunol 2003;49(2):84 – 9. Available from: https://doi.org/10.1034/j.1600-0897.2003.01184.x (In eng).

[86] Saab W, Seshadri S, Huang C, Alsubki L, Sung N, Kwak-Kim J. A systemic review of intravenous immunoglobulin G treatment in women with recurrent implantation failures and recurrent pregnancy losses. Am J Reprod Immunol 2021;85(4):e13395. Available from: https://doi.org/10.1111/aji.13395 (In eng).

[87] Heilmann L, Schorsch M, Hahn T. CD3 – CD56+ CD16+ natural killer cells and improvement of pregnancy outcome in IVF/ICSI failure after additional IVIG-treatment. Am J Reprod Immunol 2010;63(3):263 – 5. Available from: https://doi.org/10.1111/j.1600-0897.2009.00790.x (In eng).

[88] Ahmadi M, Abdolmohammadi-Vahid S, Ghaebi M, et al. Regulatory T cells improve pregnancy rate in RIF patients after additional IVIG treatment. Syst Biol Reprod Med 2017;63(6):350 – 9. Available from: https://doi.org/10.1080/19396368.2017.1390007 (In eng).

[89] Li J, Chen Y, Liu C, Hu Y, Li L. Intravenous immunoglobulin treatment for repeated IVF/ICSI failure and unexplained infertility: a systematic review and a meta-analysis. Am J Reprod Immunol 2013;70(6):434 – 47. Available from: https://doi.org/10.1111/aji.12170 (In eng).

[90] Chambers SA, Isenberg D. Anti-B cell therapy (rituximab) in the treatment of autoimmune diseases. Lupus 2005;14(3):210 – 14. Available from: https://doi.org/10.1191/0961203305lu2138oa (In eng).

[91] Parrish MR, Murphy SR, Rutland S, et al. The effect of immune factors, tumor necrosis factor-alpha, and agonistic autoantibodies to the angiotensin II type I receptor on soluble fms-like tyrosine-1 and soluble endoglin production in response to hypertension during pregnancy. Am J Hypertens 2010;23(8):911 – 16. Available from: https://doi.org/10.1038/ajh.2010.70 (In eng).

[92] LaMarca B, Wallace K, Herse F, et al. Hypertension in response to placental ischemia during pregnancy: role of B lymphocytes. Hypertension 2011;57(4):865 – 71. Available from: https://doi.org/10.1161/hypertensiona-ha.110.167569 (In eng).

[93] Ng CT, O'Neil M, Walsh D, Walsh T, Veale DJ. Successful pregnancy after rituximab in a women with recurrent in vitro

fertilisation failures and anti-phospholipid antibody positive. Ir J Med Sci 2009;178(4):531-3. Available from: https://doi.org/10.1007/s11845-008-0265-5 (In eng).

[94] Cianchini G, Corona R, Frezzolini A, Ruffelli M, Didona B, Puddu P. Treatment of severe pemphigus with rituximab: report of 12 cases and a review of the literature. Arch Dermatol 2007;143(8):1033-8. Available from: https://doi.org/10.1001/archderm.143.8.1033 (In eng).

[95] Fatourechi MM, el-Azhary RA, Gibson LE. Rituximab: applications in dermatology. Int J Dermatol 2006;45(10): 1143-55. Available from: https://doi.org/10.1111/j.1365-4632.2006.03007.x quiz 1155. (In eng).

[96] Jamin C, Morva A, Lemoine S, Daridon C, de Mendoza AR, Youinou P. Regulatory B lymphocytes in humans: a potential role in autoimmunity. Arthritis Rheum 2008;58(7):1900-6. Available from: https://doi.org/10.1002/art.23187 (In eng).

[97] Thomas F. Tedder, Ayumi Yoshizaki, Tomomitsu Miyagaki, Evgueni Kountikov, Jonathan C. Poe. Methods of expanding and assessing B cells and using expanded B cells to treat disease. U.S. Patent 10611999B2.2018-6-5.

第 20 章

子宫内膜病理学和反复种植失败
Endometrial pathology and repeated implantation failures

Maud Lansiaux[1], Virginie Vaucoret[1] and Nathalie Lédée[1,2]

[1] Hôpital des Bluets, Centre de PMA, Paris, France
[2] MatriceLab Innove, Pépinière Paris-Santé-Cochin, Paris, France

1 引言

人类子宫内膜是我们这个物种独特的组织。它是一种动态组织,在长达 45 年的时间里,月经周期循环往复,经历着连续的增殖、分化、脱落和再生的过程。这种复杂的周期性转化是卵巢来源的雌激素和孕激素共同作用的结果。雌激素诱导子宫内膜增殖,而排卵后孕激素水平升高又触发了一个协调的分化程序,其特征是上皮细胞的增殖停滞和分泌转化、子宫自然杀伤细胞(uNK)的涌入、血管重塑以及基质成纤维细胞分化为专门的蜕膜细胞。这种协调的子宫内膜重塑的一个功能结果是,它能短暂接纳胚胎植入。这种现象被称为"种植窗(WOI)"。

WOI 可能是辅助生殖技术(ART)中最关键的事件之一。在过去的 30 年里,为了提高 ART 周期的成功率,已进行了许多改进,包括更好的胚胎培养条件和选择标准,将胚胎培养延长至囊胚阶段,并允许最优质的胚胎移植。然而,尽管在全球范围内 ART 的经验不断丰富,但仍有很多体外受精(IVF)尝试未获得成功妊娠,其中最重要的是种植失败。事实上,试管婴儿的成功率依旧不高,每个启动周期的活产率为 25%～30%[1]。

胚胎植入过程包括两个主要部分:①具有植入潜力的合格胚胎。②能够植入的容受性子宫内膜[2]。胚胎和子宫内膜之间的"交互对话"最终引起胚胎的定位、黏附和侵入,这对于成功植入和随后的正常胎盘形成是必需的。这些过程正在被深入的研究,涉及来自胚胎、子宫内膜和母体免疫系统的许多介质[3-5]。因此,胚胎、子宫内膜或母体免疫系统的任何异常都会导致植入失败,这解释了评估反复种植失败(RIF)原因的复杂性。

在本章中,我们将专注于子宫内膜及其免疫环境。此外,我们还讨论了可能导致胚胎植入失败的子宫内膜病理学,并回顾了修复不易接受胚胎植入的子宫内膜的潜在治疗方法。

2 子宫内膜病理学

2.1 解剖学异常

各种与 RIF 相关的子宫内膜结构异常可以被识别。事实上,无论是先天性还是获得性子宫解剖结构畸形,都可能干扰正常胚胎植入[6-8]。若有可能,应纠正这些异常[9],并清除输卵管积液以促进植入[6]。

纵隔子宫是最常见的先天性子宫异常,可能导致 RIF。Lavergne 等[10]报道,与在 IVF 治疗前接受子宫成形术的女性相比,未经治疗的纵隔子宫女性 IVF 结局较差。Ban-Frangež 等[11]的另一项研究还显示,有纵隔子宫的女性在 IVF/ICSI 后流产率更高(80%),手术治疗后流产率降至 30%。

黏膜下肌瘤和肌壁间肌瘤会使子宫内膜变形,与试图自然受孕或进行试管婴儿治疗的女性妊娠率和种植率降低有关[12,13]。一些研究表明,切除这些肌瘤后,妊娠率会有所提高[14,15]。Pritts 等[15]在对文献进行系统回顾并对现有对照研究进行荟萃分析后得出结论,切除黏膜下肌瘤可提高临床妊娠率和种植率。肌壁间肌瘤可能会降低生育能力,但肌瘤剔除术的效果尚不明确。相反,浆膜下肌瘤不会影响生育,切除肌瘤也不会带来益处。子宫肌瘤对胚胎植入产生不利影响有多种机制,包括子宫收缩力增强、细胞因子谱紊乱、血管形成异常和慢性子宫内膜炎[16,17]。总的来说,对于黏膜下肌瘤(FIGO 0型、1型、2型和3型,与子宫内膜相邻)和>5 cm的肌壁间肌瘤(FIGO 4型),大多会使宫腔变形,应在ART之前行肌瘤切除术[18],而浆膜下肌瘤(FIGO 5型、6型、7型)则无须治疗。

子宫内膜息肉也可能干扰胚胎植入。三项非随机研究发现,切除子宫内膜息肉可提高自然妊娠率[13,19,20]。最近的一项系统综述表明,宫腔镜切除子宫内膜息肉可使接受宫腔内人工授精治疗的患者临床妊娠率增加1倍[21]。因此,子宫内膜息肉很可能导致RIF。

宫腔粘连的存在可能会干扰胚胎成功植入。宫腔粘连通常发生于为终止意外妊娠而行刮宫术后,或在分娩及流产后残留妊娠物的情况下。非妊娠子宫的宫腔手术或宫内感染也可能导致宫腔粘连的形成。Demirol和Gurgan报道称,8.5%的RIF患者存在宫腔粘连[9]。到目前为止,已有的证据表明,宫腔镜下去除宫腔粘连可改善生育结局[22,23]。

2.2 种植窗移位

无论胚胎质量如何,胚胎只能在很短的时间内植入,从排卵后4～5天开始,持续4天[24]。多年来,人们一直认为所有女性的WOI都是恒定的。因此,根据对植入时间的经典研究,体外受精后囊胚移植通常在取卵后第5天或孕酮给药后第5～6天进行[25]。然而,研究人员最近证明了存在"WOI移位"[2,26,27],这被认为是导致RIF的一个重要因素[28]。为了确定子宫内膜周期中与WOI开始时间相对应的时刻,已开发了一些诊断工具(窗口种植试验和子宫内膜容受性分析),旨在根据结果进行个性化的胚胎移植(ET)。

2.2.1 窗口种植试验

窗口种植试验(WIN)由法国蒙彼利埃大学开发。Haouzi等[29]采用转录组学方法鉴定了11个基因,与分泌期容受前状态的子宫内膜(LH+2)相比,这些基因在容受状态的子宫内膜(LH+7)中强表达。当这11个基因的平均表达≥70%时,子宫内膜被定义为"容受";当平均表达为50%～70%时,被定义为"部分容受";而当平均表达量低于阳性对照表达水平的50%时,则被定义为"非容受"。

子宫内膜活检必须在种植窗口期采集:自然周期中为自发LH升高后的6～9天(LH+6至LH+9),或激素替代治疗周期中孕酮给药后的5～9天(Pg+5至Pg+9)。当子宫内膜处于容受状态时,移植囊胚。在容受前48～72小时移植第2天或第3天的胚胎。2021年,Haouzi等[30]报道,在接受WIN试验的RIF患者($n=217$)中,个性化ET组的种植率(22.7% vs 7.2%)和每位患者的活产率(31.8% vs 8.3%)均显著高于传统ET组。

2.2.2 子宫内膜容受性分析

子宫内膜容受性分析(ERA)是西班牙开发的一种诊断工具,2009年Igenomix研发部门获得专利。它分析了248个与子宫内膜容受性相关的基因。ERA将子宫内膜活检的结果分为容受性和非容受性,并进一步分为容受前或容受后。在激素替代治疗周期中,孕酮给药后5天活检。在2013年发表的一项研究中,Ruiz-Alonso等[31]报道,每10位种植失败患者中就有3位存在WOI移位。22位RIF患者($n=22/85$;25.9%)的子宫内膜为非容受,其中15位的第二次ERA验证了WOI移位。她们中的8位在ERA指定的日期进行个性化ET,妊娠率为50.0%,种植率为38.5%。有必要进行更多人群的队列研究和随机对照研究,以证明ERA的意义。

3 子宫内膜免疫病理学

3.1 如何检测子宫内膜免疫病理

子宫免疫图谱(UtimPro)检测是一个创新概念,它依赖于对种植窗口期子宫内膜局部免疫反应的分析。关键的免疫子宫内膜转换应发生于种植窗口期,不仅可以避免半同种异体胚胎的排斥反应,还可以促进其生长和营养[32]。由于胚胎植入是辅助生殖的关键,因此需要了解局部免疫环境以及子宫内膜和胚胎之间的相互作用。在此期间,重要的免疫细胞离开子宫(如B淋巴细胞和一些$CD8^+$淋巴细胞),而其他免疫细胞则进入子宫内膜。在种植窗口期,几乎所有属于适应性免疫的免疫细胞从子宫内膜逃逸,而固有免疫细胞(如巨噬细胞、uNK和树突状细胞)则进入子宫内膜[33]。新形成的免疫环境在胚胎植入中起着关键作用[33]。uNK细胞与循环 NK 细胞的不同之处在于其表型、激活性和抑制性受体谱、分泌的细胞因子以及低细胞毒性潜能。调节性 T 细胞是适应性免疫和局部免疫之间的纽带。缺乏活性的免疫细胞无法产生必要的植入反应；相反，过度活跃的免疫细胞会导致子宫内膜破坏，最终引起胚胎排斥。这种独特的免疫反应对促进胚胎黏附至关重要，而这种反应的破坏很可能会阻碍胚胎植入。

早期研究认为，种植窗口期的理想环境主要含有 Th2（而非 Th1）细胞因子，这将选择性允许促进免疫趋向性和血管生成的局部机制形成，同时下调炎症和细胞毒性通路[34]。随着时间的推移，妊娠作为 Th2 现象的概念已经演变成 Th1/Th2 平衡的概念，因为 Th1 细胞因子的缺乏和过剩都被认为对胚胎植入和胎盘形成有害，Th2 细胞因子的缺乏亦如此[35]。一过性的 Th2 免疫转换以及充分的 uNK 细胞激活似乎是建立母体局部耐受性和胎儿存活的基础。白细胞介素（IL）-15 直接参与排卵后子宫内 uNK 细胞的招募和成熟[36]，在 IL-15 的控制下，对 Th2 细胞因子的充分产生至关重要。IL-15 对血液 NK 细胞的作用与对 uNK 细胞的作用不同，不会将它们转化为强大的细胞溶解细胞，而是直接参与它们的成熟过程[37]。IL-18 是一种促 Th2 的细胞因子，通过血管生成素-2 的作用影响螺旋动脉的关键性失稳[38,39]。在人类子宫内膜中，IL-18 的表达在种植窗口期增加。其主要作用是重塑母体侧血管。然而，由子宫内膜上皮或基质细胞产生的 IL-15 和 IL-18 都是二价的：在高水平和不受免疫调节时，它们表现为促炎性的 Th1 细胞因子，反映了局部产生的 IFN-γ 和 TNF-α，而 IFN-γ 和 TNF-α 则可激活 uNK 细胞，使其具有细胞毒性[40]。我们重点研究了 TNF 弱凋亡诱导因子（TWEAK）及其配体成纤维细胞生长因子诱导分子 14（Fn-14）作为局部免疫平衡的免疫调节因子的作用。利用动物模型观察到，TWEAK 在胚胎植入过程中可保护胚胎免受 Th1 主导（富含 TNF）环境的有害影响，从而提高胚胎存活率[41]，提示 TWEAK 及其配体 Fn-14 是人类子宫内膜 Th1/Th2 细胞因子平衡的免疫调节因子[42]。

3.2 UtimPro 检测

UtimPro 检测适用于种植失败或不明原因的反复流产（RM）患者。在辅助生殖治疗前的黄体中期抽吸采集子宫内膜，UtimPro 通过定量实时 PCR 对靶向生物标志物（IL-18、IL-15、TWEAK、Fn-14、CD56）进行量化，以记录胚胎移植时的免疫性子宫内膜环境。该子宫内膜免疫特征法（专利号：PCT/EP2013/065355）是一种用于提高辅助生殖治疗时胚胎种植成功率的技术。这些生物标志物在正常生育队列中的表达已被记录在案，如果在此期间没有手术或妊娠，免疫图谱可在 6 个月内从一个周期复制到另一个周期。根据免疫检查结果，为后续的 ET 提出一些个性化建议，目的是重新平衡免疫环境。

3.3 UtimPro 检测结果

UtimPro 可诊断四种类型的子宫内膜免疫谱。

（1）平衡的子宫内膜免疫激活，特征是 IL-18/TWEAK 和 IL15/Fn-14 mRNA 比值以及 CD56$^+$ 细胞计数与既往在正常生育队列中定义的范围相同。

（2）低水平的子宫内膜免疫激活，特征是 IL-15/Fn-14（反映未成熟的 uNK 细胞）和（或）IL-18/TWEAK 的 mRNA 比值降低，或缺乏 uNK 募集。

（3）过度的子宫内膜免疫激活，特征是 IL-18/TWEAK 和（或）IL-15/Fn-14 的 mRNA 比值升高，和（或）CD56$^+$ 细胞计数增加。

（4）混合型子宫内膜免疫谱，特征是 IL-18/TWEAK 的 mRNA 比值升高（Th1 细胞因子过多），同时 IL-15/Fn-14 降低（反映未成熟的 NK）。

3.4 UtimPro 检测异常的发生率

每次宫内事件（包括任何宫内手术或妊娠）发生时，子宫内膜免疫谱都易发生改变。2020 年，Lédée 等[43]发表了一项包含 1 738 名不孕患者的队列研究，结果显示 83.5% 的患者存在子宫内膜免疫失调（45% 的患者存在过度免疫局部激活，28% 的患者存在低水平免疫局部激活，10.5% 的患者为混合型）。基于免疫特征，提出了个性化的 IVF 治疗方案，以控制 uNK 细胞的激活或促进胚胎黏附的局部机制。与未接受个体化治疗的患者相比，有 RIF 或 RM 病史的患者在经过诊断和个体化治疗后，妊娠率明显更高（分别为 37.7% 和 56% vs 26.9% 和 24%，$P<0.001$）。

4 针对免疫异常女性的免疫治疗

4.1 个性化及其原理

辅助疗法旨在根据子宫内膜的免疫特征以形成"理想"的免疫环境,具体内容见表20.1。没有一种方法是适用于所有人的。因此,精准医学显然是生殖医学的未来。然而,尽管使用了经典分子(与妊娠相容),但关于其适应证和确切的作用机制仍有待进一步研究。

表20.1 根据子宫内膜免疫特征建议的疗法

子宫内膜免疫特征	糖皮质激素	脂肪乳剂	黄体期hCG	LMWH	子宫内膜搔刮	补充孕酮	ET后暴露于精浆
免疫未失调	—	—	—	—	—	—	—
低水平免疫激活	—	—	X	—	X	—	X
过度免疫激活	X	X	—	X	—	X	—
混合型	X	X	X	X	X	X	—

注:LMWH,低分子肝素;hCG,人绒毛膜促性腺激素;ET,胚胎移植。

4.2 糖皮质激素

根据UtimPro检测,糖皮质激素被推荐作为过度或混合型子宫内膜免疫激活女性的一线治疗药物。2018年,Lédée等[44]在RIF人群中记录了强的松对子宫内膜容受时免疫生物标志物表达的影响。有趣的是,54.5%的病例中两种免疫生物标志物(IL-18/TWEAK和IL-15/Fn-14的mRNA比值)均恢复正常,只有16.5%的病例在强的松治疗后其中一种恢复正常。在强的松治疗后妊娠的患者中,反映Th1/Th2局部平衡的IL-18/TWEAK mRNA比值因TWEAK表达的显著增加而明显降低。TWEAK的显著增加似乎是一种潜在的免疫机制,能够解释对局部细胞毒性的控制。值得注意的是,先前有文献表明,IL-18/TWEAK在子宫内膜局部的高表达反映了一种有害的Th1优势环境,并与固有免疫细胞的细胞毒性激活有关[40]。此外,Mas等[41]发现,TWEAK可保护胚胎免受植入过程中Th1主导(富含TNF)环境的有害影响,从而提高胚胎存活率[42]。

治疗包括每日口服皮质类固醇(即,若为免疫过度激活,强的松每天20 mg;若为混合型,则每天10 mg)。治疗从ET前一个周期的第3天开始,然后持续到妊娠的前3个月。需要在皮质类固醇的作用下进行周期性检测,以评估皮质类固醇是否能够使免疫环境正常化。事实上,根据我们的经验,有30%过度免疫激活的RIF患者对皮质类固醇耐药。治疗时需逐渐降低剂量,以避免肾上腺功能不全。已发表的使用皮质类固醇治疗的数据令人欣慰,但仍应提醒患者注意骨密度下降的风险(在治疗期间补充维生素D可预防骨密度下降)。

4.3 脂肪乳剂

脂肪乳剂治疗(ILT)是免疫过度激活的二线治疗方法,这些患者在使用糖皮质激素后仍未妊娠,或免疫功能依旧失调。尽管实现免疫调节的确切机制尚不清楚,但一些学者认为ILT可抑制促炎介质,特别是Th1细胞[45],并对NK细胞具有免疫抑制特性[46,47]。

ILT是一种20%的脂肪乳剂,通常包含20%大豆油、1.2%蛋黄磷脂、2.25%甘油和水。在住院条件下,将100 mL的脂肪乳剂稀释在400 mL盐水中,以缓慢静脉输注(IV)的方式给药,90分钟完成。ILT在ET周期的第8天进行。如果妊娠,则在停经的第5周和第9周重复进行治疗。ILT输注均应在医院内进行,并接受医疗监督。据报道,患者对ILT输注的耐受性非常好。在Lédée等[47]发表的一项研究中,94例接受慢速ILT的女性没有一例报告在输注过程中或输注后出现副作用。值得注意的是,这些女性没有观察到任何未稀释的脂肪乳剂输注所描述的过敏反应或偶发症状,如头痛、头晕、潮红、嗜睡、恶心或出汗。另一方面,脂肪乳剂在胚胎植入初期和妊娠期间的安全性也已得到间接评估,因为脂肪乳剂是用丙泊酚稀释的,而丙泊酚是取卵麻醉和妊娠期间手术使用的主要麻醉药物[48]。

4.4 补充人绒毛膜促性腺激素

对于局部子宫内膜免疫活性较低的女性,建议在种植窗口期补充人绒毛膜促性腺激素(hCG)。胚胎在妊娠期间会生理性产生 hCG。它直接参与局部反应,引起免疫耐受,并在母胎界面诱导充分血管生成和 uNK 细胞激活[49-52]。Kane 等[53]在 2008 年报道称,hCG 是一种通过激活甘露糖受体触发 uNK 细胞增殖和成熟的激素。因此,补充 hCG 可纠正观察到的 uNK 失调,如募集不足和(或)不成熟。在 ET 后的黄体中期给予低剂量的 hCG(1 500 U 皮下注射):新鲜 ET,在取卵后第 4、6 和 8 天注射 3 次;冷冻 ET,在孕酮给药后的+4、+6 和 8 天注射 3 次。

4.5 低分子肝素

如果对皮质类固醇和 ILT 耐药,可将低分子量肝素(LMWH)作为过度或混合型子宫内膜免疫活女性的三线治疗方法。LMWH 用于预防与血栓性疾病相关的妊娠并发症(尤其是抗磷脂综合征)。最近的研究表明,肝素可能会直接影响胎盘滋养细胞,而不依赖于其抗凝活性。此外,有证据表明,肝素还具有抗补体作用[54,55]。

建议在取卵当天或从 ET 周期的种植窗开始时使用预防性剂量的 LMWH(即依诺肝素每天 40 mg)。女性自行皮下注射 LMWH,若 ET 后 14 天的妊娠试验呈阳性,则低分子肝素持续至妊娠 12 周;若为阴性,则停用 LMWH。应在取卵当天监测血小板计数,每周监测两次。

4.6 子宫内膜搔刮

如果出现局部低水平的子宫内膜免疫激活,或具有低 IL-15/Fn-14 mRNA 比值的混合型特征,可解释为 uNK 细胞不成熟,建议进行子宫内膜搔刮。

子宫内膜搔刮可增强 uNK 细胞的成熟,这在很大程度上取决于 IL-15 的充分表达。在月经周期的黄体中期进行任何形式的局部损伤(如子宫内膜活检)都会在下一个黄体期通过 Toll 样受体途径激活并刺激黏附分子、趋化因子和 IL-15 的表达[56]。2015 年,Gnainsky 等[57]证明子宫内膜搔刮可上调促炎细胞因子的表达,这些细胞因子参与了单核细胞的募集及向巨噬细胞和树突状细胞的分化。虽然它们在胚胎植入时的人类子宫内膜中的作用尚不清楚,但似乎在组织重塑和血管生成中发挥重要作用,而这是子宫内膜蜕膜化和滋养层侵袭调节所必需的。同样,Yu Liang 等[58]也证实了这些发现,并报道子宫内膜搔刮可诱导血管内皮生长因子增加,它是一种参与局部血管生成和胎盘形成的核心生长因子。

因此,子宫内膜搔刮必须在新鲜或冷冻 ET 之前的黄体中期进行。子宫内膜搔刮术是指用一根 3 mm 宽的小导管(称为吸管)获取子宫内膜活检样本。通常,在不钩住宫颈的情况下,将导管通过宫颈向前推至宫底,然后以环形运动的方式缩回,以刺激子宫内膜。这种手术风险低,并发症发生率低,可在门诊进行,无须麻醉,大多数患者会感到轻微疼痛。

4.7 补充孕酮

在局部过度免疫激活或具有混合型特征的女性,适用于黄体支持。孕酮除了具有内分泌作用外,还是成功妊娠所需的局部免疫耐受的重要介质。孕酮通过不同的途径影响母体免疫系统[56]:①产生孕酮诱导的阻断因子(PIBF),抑制 NK 细胞活性,导致母体淋巴细胞产生 Th2 主导的细胞因子。②诱导 Galectin-1(一种孕酮诱导的分子,对于诱导耐受性树突状细胞至关重要),进而促进分泌 IL-10 的 Treg 细胞在体内扩增。

当观察到局部免疫过度激活时,鉴于孕酮的免疫抑制特性,建议每天使用大剂量的阴道孕酮给药(1 200 mg),或阴道联合肌内或皮下注射孕酮。从取卵当天,或从 ET 周期的种植窗开始,每日阴道微粒化孕酮或双重给药(阴道和皮下)。若妊娠,则 ET 后 8 周内继续服用。监测血浆孕酮水平是确保阴道组织正确吸收的关键。应在开始摄入孕酮后至少 48 小时采集血样。

与口服给药相比,阴道使用孕酮绕过了肝脏首过效应,因此具有更好的生物利用度。它没有副作用,如嗜睡、疲劳和头痛[59]。与肌内注射相比,阴道使用孕酮后,子宫内膜的生物利用度也更高,这是因为孕酮直接从阴道输送到子宫,即所谓的"子宫首过效应"。肌内注射的副作用轻微,一般仅限于注射部位[60,61]。阴道孕酮制剂的一个主要缺点是它可能会比较脏,与阴道分泌物和刺激有关。

5 总结与建议

(1)由于胚胎发育和植入过程中涉及不同的因素,接受 ART 周期的不孕患者的反复种植失败是一个复杂的问题。

（2）尽管全球在ART方面的经验不断丰富，但很多试管婴儿尝试都未成功妊娠，主要原因是种植失败。

（3）免疫性子宫内膜容受性被描述为胚胎植入的"最后一道屏障"。

（4）所有免疫相关探索都应在对解剖学异常进行精确检查并确认子宫内膜充分增生后开始。

（5）子宫内膜免疫谱是规划个性化IVF/ICSI治疗的关键因素。

（6）个性化的目标是实现"理想"的免疫环境，以提高胚胎植入的可能性。

（7）在低水平子宫内膜免疫激活的情况下，建议在ET周期前的黄体中期进行局部损伤（搔刮），在黄体期补充人类绒毛膜促性腺激素，并在ET后进行性交。

（8）在子宫内膜免疫过度激活的情况下，建议从试管周期的第1天开始使用皮质类固醇作为一线治疗，或缓慢输注脂肪乳剂作为二线治疗（之前使用皮质类固醇治疗失败或使用皮质类固醇后宫腔检查未恢复正常者），在黄体期使用大剂量黄体酮（1 200 mg阴道用药），移植后禁止性交。

（9）只有在辅助治疗下免疫谱恢复正常，才能证明其疗效。

参考文献

[1] Toftager M, Bogstad J, Løssl K, Prætorius L, Zedeler A, Bryndorf T, et al. Cumulative live birth rates after one ART cycle including all subsequent frozen-thaw cycles in 1050 women: secondary outcome of an RCT comparing GnRH-antagonist and GnRH-agonist protocols. Hum Reprod Oxf Engl 2017;32(3):556 – 67 Mar 1.

[2] Lessey BA. Assessment of endometrial receptivity. Fertil Steril 2011;96(3):522 – 9 Sep 1.

[3] Achache H, Revel A. Endometrial receptivity markers, the journey to successful embryo implantation. Hum Reprod Update 2006;12(6):731 – 46 Dec.

[4] Fukui A, Funamizu A, Yokota M, Yamada K, Nakamua R, Fukuhara R, et al. Uterine and circulating natural killer cells and their roles in women with recurrent pregnancy loss, implantation failure and preeclampsia. J Reprod Immunol 2011;90(1):105 – 10 Jun.

[5] Gonen-Gross T, Goldman-Wohl D, Huppertz B, Lankry D, Greenfield C, Natanson-Yaron S, et al. Inhibitory NK receptor recognition of HLA-G: regulation by contact residues and by cell specific expression at the fetal-maternal interface. PLoS One 2010;5(1):e8941 Jan 28.

[6] Practice Committee of American Society for Reproductive Medicine in Collaboration with Society of Reproductive Surgeons. Myomas and reproductive function. Fertil Steril 2008;90(5 Suppl):S125 – 30 Nov.

[7] Sanders B. Uterine factors and infertility. J Reprod Med 2006;51(3):169 – 76 Mar.

[8] Strandell A. The influence of hydrosalpinx on IVF and embryo transfer: a review. Hum Reprod Update 2000;6(4):387 – 95 Aug.

[9] Demirol A, Gurgan T. Effect of treatment of intrauterine pathologies with office hysteroscopy in patients with recurrent IVF failure. Reprod Biomed Online 2004;8(5):590 – 4 Jan.

[10] Lavergne N, Aristizabal J, Zarka V, Erny R, Hedon B. Uterine anomalies and in vitro fertilization: what are the results? Eur J Obstet Gynecol Reprod Biol 1996;68(12):29 – 34 Sep.

[11] Ban-Frangez H, Tomazevic T, Virant-Klun I, Verdenik I, Ribic-Pucelj M, Bokal EV. The outcome of singleton pregnancies after IVF/ICSI in women before and after hysteroscopic resection of a uterine septum compared to normal controls. Eur J Obstet Gynecol Reprod Biol 2009;146(2):184 – 7 Oct.

[12] Bernard G, Darai E, Poncelet C, Benifla J-L, Madelenat P. Fertility after hysteroscopic myomectomy: effect of intramural myomas associated. Eur J Obstet Gynecol Reprod Biol 2000;88(1):85 – 90 Jan 1.

[13] Varasteh NN, Neuwirth RS, Levin B, Keltz MD. Pregnancy rates after hysteroscopic polypectomy and myomectomy in infertile women. Obstet Gynecol 1999;94(2):168 – 71 Aug.

[14] Fernandez H. Hysteroscopic resection of submucosal myomas in patients with infertility. Hum Reprod 2001;16(7):1489 – 92 Jul 1.

[15] Pritts EA, Parker WH, Olive DL. Fibroids and infertility: an updated systematic review of the evidence. Fertil Steril 2009;91(4):1215 – 23 Apr.

[16] Donnez J, Jadoul P. What are the implications of myomas on fertility? A need for a debate? Hum Reprod Oxf Engl 2002;17(6):1424 – 30 Jun.

[17] Taylor E, Gomel V. The uterus and fertility. Fertil Steril 2008;89(1):1 – 16 Jan.

[18] Hart R, Khalaf Y, Yeong CT, Seed P, Taylor A, Braude P. A prospective controlled study of the effect of intramural uterine fibroids on the outcome of assisted conception. Hum Reprod Oxf Engl 2001;16(11):2411 – 17 Nov.

[19] Shokeir TA, Shalan HM, El-Shafei MM. Significance of endometrial polyps detected hysteroscopically in eumenorrheic infertile women. J Obstet Gynaecol Res 2004;30(2):84 – 9.

[20] Spiewankiewicz B, Stelmachów J, Sawicki W, Cendrowski K, Wypych P, Swiderska K. The effectiveness of hysteroscopic polypectomy in cases of female infertility. Clin Exp Obstet Gynecol 2003;30(1):23 – 5.

[21] Bosteels J, Weyers S, Puttemans P, Panayotidis C, Van Herendael B, Gomel V, et al. The effectiveness of hysteroscopy in improving pregnancy rates in subfertile women without other gynaecological symptoms: a systematic review. Hum Reprod Update 2010;16(1):1 – 11 Feb.

[22] Yasmin H, Nasir A, Noorani K. Hystroscopic management of

Ashermans Syndrome. JPMA J Pak Med Assoc 2007;57:553-5 Dec 1.

[23] Zikopoulos KA, Kolibianakis EM, Platteau P, de Munck L, Tournaye H, Devroey P, et al. Live delivery rates in subfertile women with Asherman's syndrome after hysteroscopic adhesiolysis using the resectoscope or the Versapoint system. Reprod Biomed Online 2004;8(6):720-5 Jan 1.

[24] Psychoyos A. From Lataste to the "window of implantation": 100 years of fascinating discoveries. Contracept Fertil Sex 1992;21(4):333-8.

[25] Wilcox AJ, Baird DD, Weinberg CR. Time of implantation of the conceptus and loss of pregnancy. N Engl J Med 1999;340(23):1796-9 Jun 10.

[26] Galliano D, Bellver J, Díaz-García C, Simón C, Pellicer A. ART and uterine pathology: how relevant is the maternal side for implantation? Hum Reprod Update 2015;21(1):13-38 Feb.

[27] Kliman HJ, Frankfurter D. Clinical approach to recurrent implantation failure: evidence-based evaluation of the endometrium. Fertil Steril 2019;111(4):618-28 Apr.

[28] Valdes CT, Schutt A, Simon C. Implantation failure of endometrial origin: it is not pathology, but our failure to synchronize the developing embryo with a receptive endometrium. Fertil Steril 2017;108(1):15-18 Jul.

[29] Haouzi D, Mahmoud K, Fourar M, Bendhaou K, Dechaud H, De Vos J, et al. Identification of new biomarkers of human endometrial receptivity in the natural cycle. Hum Reprod 2009;24(1):198-205 Jan 1.

[30] Haouzi D, Entezami F, Torre A, Innocenti C, Antoine Y, Mauries C, et al. Customized frozen embryo transfer after identification of the receptivity window with a transcriptomic approach improves the implantation and live birth rates in patients with repeated implantation failure. Reprod Sci Thousand Oaks Calif 2021;28(1):69-78 Jan.

[31] Ruiz-Alonso M, Blesa D, Díaz-Gimeno P, Gómez E, Fernández-Sánchez M, Carranza F, et al. The endometrial receptivity array for diagnosis and personalized embryo transfer as a treatment for patients with repeated implantation failure. Fertil Steril 2013;100(3):818-24 Sep.

[32] Liu S, Diao L, Huang C, Li Y, Zeng Y, Kwak-Kim JYH. The role of decidual immune cells on human pregnancy. J Reprod Immunol 2017;124:44-53 Nov.

[33] Lee JY, Lee M, Lee SK. Role of endometrial immune cells in implantation. Clin Exp Reprod Med 2011;38(3):119-25 Sep.

[34] Wegmann TG, Lin H, Guilbert L, Mosmann TR. Bidirectional cytokine interactions in the maternal-fetal relationship: is successful pregnancy a TH2 phenomenon? Immunol Today 1993;14(7):353-6 Jul.

[35] Chaouat G. The Th1/Th2 paradigm: still important in pregnancy? Semin Immunopathol 2007;29(2):95-113 Jun.

[36] Kitaya K, Yamaguchi T, Honjo H. Central role of interleukin-15 in post-ovulatory recruitment of peripheral blood CD16(-) natural killer cells into human endometrium. J Clin Endocrinol Metab 2005;90(5):2932-40 May.

[37] Verma S, Hiby SE, Loke YW, King A. Human decidual natural killer cells express the receptor for and respond to the cytokine interleukin 15. Biol Reprod 2000;62(4):959-68 Apr.

[38] Croy BA, Esadeg S, Chantakru S, van den Heuvel M, Paffaro VA, He H, et al. Update on pathways regulating the activation of uterine natural killer cells, their interactions with decidual spiral arteries and homing of their precursors to the uterus. J Reprod Immunol 2003;59(2):175-91 Aug.

[39] Goldman-Wohl DS, Ariel I, Greenfield C, Lavy Y, Yagel S. Tie-2 and angiopoietin-2 expression at the fetal-maternal interface: a receptor ligand model for vascular remodelling. Mol Hum Reprod 2000;6(1):81-7 Jan.

[40] Petitbarat M, Rahmati M, Sérazin V, Dubanchet S, Morvan C, Wainer R, et al. TWEAK appears as a modulator of endometrial IL-18 related cytotoxic activity of uterine natural killers. PLoS One 2011;6(1):e14497 Jan 7.

[41] Mas AE, Petitbarat M, Dubanchet S, Fay S, Ledée N, Chaouat G. Immune regulation at the interface during early steps of murine implantation: involvement of two new cytokines of the IL-12 family (IL-23 and IL-27) and of TWEAK. Am J Reprod Immunol N Y N 1989 2008;59(4):323-38 Apr.

[42] Petitbarat M, Serazin V, Dubanchet S, Wayner R, de Mazancourt P, Chaouat G, et al. Tumor necrosis factor-like weak inducer of apoptosis (TWEAK)/fibroblast growth factor inducible-14 might regulate the effects of interleukin 18 and 15 in the human endometrium. Fertil Steril 2010;94(3):1141-3 Aug.

[43] Lédée N, Petitbarat M, Chevrier L, Vitoux D, Vezmar K, Rahmati M, et al. The uterine immune profile may help women with repeated unexplained embryo implantation failure after in vitro fertilization. Am J Reprod Immunol N Y N 1989 2016;75(3):388-401.

[44] Lédée N, Prat-Ellenberg L, Petitbarat M, Chevrier L, Simon C, Irani EE, et al. Impact of prednisone in patients with repeated embryo implantation failures: beneficial or deleterious? J Reprod Immunol 2018;127:11-15 Jun.

[45] Granato D, Blum S, Rössle C, Boucher JL, Malnoë A, Dutot G. Effects of parenteral lipid emulsions with different fatty acid composition on immune cell functions in vitro. J Parenter Enter Nutr 2000;24(2):113-18.

[46] Roussev RG, Acacio B, Ng SC, Coulam CB. Duration of intralipid's suppressive effect on NK cell's functional activity. Am J Reprod Immunol N Y N 1989 2008;60(3):258-63.

[47] Lédée N, Vasseur C, Petitbarat M, Chevrier L, Vezmar K, Dray G, et al. Intralipid ® may represent a new hope for patients with reproductive failures and simultaneously an over-immune endometrial activation. J Reprod Immunol 2018;130:18-22 Nov.

[48] Jarahzadeh MH, Jouya R, Mousavi FS, Dehghan-Tezerjani M, Behdad S, Soltani HR. Propofol or Thiopental sodium in patients undergoing reproductive assisted technologies: Differences in hemodynamic recovery and outcome of oocyte retrieval: a randomized clinical trial. Iran J Reprod Med 2014;12(1):77-82 Jan.

[49] Perrier d'Hauterive S, Berndt S, Tsampalas M, Charlet-Renard C, Dubois M, Bourgain C, et al. Dialogue between blastocyst hCG and endometrial LH/hCG receptor: which role in implantation? Gynecol Obstet Invest 2007;64(3):156-60.

[50] Bansal AS, Bora SA, Saso S, Smith JR, Johnson MR, Thum M-Y. Mechanism of human chorionic gonadotrophin-mediated immunomodulation in pregnancy. Expert Rev Clin Immunol 2012;8(8):747-53 Nov.

[51] Berndt S, Blacher S, d'Hauterive S, Thiry M, Tsampalas M, Cruz A, et al. Chorionic gonadotropin stimulation of angiogenesis and pericyte recruitment. J Clin Endocrinol

Metab 2009;94:4567-74 Nov 1.

[52] Tsampalas M, Gridelet V, Berndt S, Foidart J-M, Geenen V, Perrier d'Hauterive S. Human chorionic gonado-tropin: a hormone with immunological and angiogenic properties. J Reprod Immunol 2010;85(1):93-8 May.

[53] Kane N, Kelly R, Saunders PTK, Critchley HOD. Proliferation of uterine natural killer cells is induced by human chorionic gonadotropin and mediated via the mannose receptor. Endocrinology 2009;150(6):2882-8 Jun.

[54] Oberkersch R, Attorresi AI, Calabrese GC. Low-molecular-weight heparin inhibition in classical complement activation pathway during pregnancy. Thromb Res 2010;125(5):e240-5 May.

[55] Girardi G, Redecha P, Salmon JE. Heparin prevents antiphospholipid antibody-induced fetal loss by inhibiting complement activation. Nat Med 2004;10(11):1222-6 Nov.

[56] Lédée N, Petitbarat M, Prat-Ellenberg L, Dray G, Cassuto GN, Chevrier L, et al. Endometrial immune profiling: a method to design personalized care in assisted reproductive medicine Front Immunol [Internet] 2020; [cited 2021 Apr 27]; 11. Available from: https://www.frontiersin.org/articles/10.3389/fimmu.2020.01032/full.

[57] Gnainsky Y, Granot I, Aldo P, Barash A, Or Y, Mor G, et al. Biopsy-induced inflammatory conditions improve endometrial receptivity: the mechanism of action. Reprod Camb Engl 2015;149(1):75-85 Jan.

[58] Liang Y., Han J., Jia C., Ma Y., Lan Y., Li Y., et al. Effect of endometrial injury on secretion of endometrial cytokines and ivf outcomes in women with unexplained subfertility. Mediators Inflamm [Internet]. 2015 [cited 2021 Apr 27]; 2015. Available from: <https://www.ncbi.nlm.nih.gov/pmc/articles/PMC4637501/>.

[59] Friedler S, Raziel A, Schachter M, Strassburger D, Bukovsky I, Ron-El R. Luteal support with micronized progesterone following in-vitro fertilization using a down-regulation protocol with gonadotrophin-releasing hor-mone agonist: a comparative study between vaginal and oral administration. Hum Reprod Oxf Engl 1999;14(8):1944-8 Aug.

[60] Miles RA, Paulson RJ, Lobo RA, Press MF, Dahmoush L, Sauer MV. Pharmacokinetics and endometrial tissue levels of progesterone after administration by intramuscular and vaginal routes: a comparative study. Fertil Steril 1994;62(3):485-90 Sep.

[61] Cicinelli E, de Ziegler D, Bulletti C, Matteo MG, Schonauer LM, Galantino P. Direct transport of progesterone from vagina to uterus. Obstet Gynecol 2000;95(3):403-6 Mar.

第 21 章

易栓症、抗磷脂抗体和抗凝治疗与反复种植失败

Thrombophilia, antiphospholipid antibodies, and anticoagulation in recurrent implantation failure

Marcelo Borges Cavalcante[1,2] and Ricardo Barini[3]

[1] Postgraduate Program in Medical Sciences, Universidade de Fortaleza (UNIFOR), Fortaleza, Ceará, Brazil
[2] CONCEPTUS — Reproductive Medicine, Fortaleza, Ceará, Brazil
[3] Department of Obstetrics and Gynecology, Campinas University (UNICAMP), Campinas, São Paulo, Brazil

1 引言

在有限的种植窗口期，囊胚和容受性子宫内膜之间发生了密切的相互作用，其中许多细胞和分子事件尚未完全揭示。在自然受孕过程中，约有30%的胚胎无法植入子宫内膜，其中10%的胚胎以生化妊娠告终[在没有临床妊娠诊断的情况下可检测到人绒毛膜促性腺激素（hCG）升高][1,2]。种植失败发生于早期植入阶段，如胚胎附着或黏附，妊娠试验为阴性。也可发生于胚胎成功侵入子宫内膜后，对于该种情况，可在血液或尿液中检测到β-hCG，但在看到宫内孕囊之前妊娠失败，这被定义为生化妊娠。当超声检测到宫内孕囊（约妊娠5周）时，即可诊断为临床妊娠。

"胚胎种植失败"一词可用于试图自然受孕或接受辅助生殖技术（ART）周期的患者。然而，术语"反复种植失败（RIF）"仅适用于接受ART周期的患者。目前对于RIF存在多个定义。最流行的RIF定义是在40岁以下女性的至少3个新鲜或冷冻周期内移植至少4个优质胚胎（基于形态学评估）后未能实现临床妊娠[2,3]。RIF是生殖医学领域专家面临的一项挑战。即使近年来ART技术不断取得进步，仍有相当多的夫妇在多次尝试体外受精（IVF）、胚胎移植（ET）和冷冻胚胎移植（FET）后仍无法受孕。此外，由于对RIF的病因知之甚少，缺乏对RIF的合理解释也让他们更加沮丧。RIF的根本原因可分为胚胎因素和母体因素。整倍体胚胎的植入潜力取决于精子和卵母细胞的质量，以及配子显微操作和胚胎培养所涉及的实验室因素。年龄是影响女性生育力的另一个主要因素，它反映了胚胎质量、子宫内膜容受性和妊娠成功率。导致种植失败的其他因素包括子宫因素（先天性畸形、子宫肌瘤、子宫腺肌病、子宫内膜炎、子宫内膜息肉、宫腔粘连和输卵管积液）、子宫内膜异位症、全身性感染、超重/肥胖、压力、睡眠障碍、生活方式、环境因素、激素状况、免疫因素（自身免疫和同种免疫）以及易栓症（获得性和遗传性）[4-6]。

2 易栓症的定义

子宫（尤其是子宫内膜/蜕膜）和胎盘的最佳血流似乎对胚胎植入和顺利分娩至关重要。从历史上看，Virchow三联征，包括高凝状态、血液动力学变化（瘀血和湍流）以及内皮损伤/功能障碍，描述了可引起血流变化的因素[7]。易栓症可定义为一组会增加静脉或动脉血栓形成（异常"凝血"）风险的疾病。易栓症可以是遗传性的，也可以是获得性的（非遗传性）。遗传性易栓症是由于产生凝血因子的基因发生了突变（称为基因突变）。导致血栓形成的获得性

易栓症是由于血液中促凝物、抗凝物和纤维蛋白溶解物失衡、不良血管状况或存在特定抗体（如抗磷脂抗体）[6]。

几十年来，人们一直在描述易栓症[遗传性和（或）获得性]与生殖障碍之间的关系，特别是关于抗磷脂综合征（APS）与产科并发症之间的关系。产科并发症包括反复流产、胎儿宫内死亡、子痫前期和胎盘功能不全。然而，易栓症与RIF之间的关系尚未得到很好的阐明[8-10]。患有易栓症的女性发生不良生殖结局的可能机制包括蜕膜微血管闭塞和母体血管血栓形成。这将引起绒毛间隙灌注减少，导致胚胎种植失败。

2.1 获得性易栓症

APS是一种获得性易栓症，1983年Hughes首次将其描述为系统性红斑狼疮和狼疮抗凝物阳性合并血栓形成、反复妊娠丢失和（或）血小板减少症[11]。它是一种与自身抗体相关的自身免疫性疾病。标准抗磷脂抗体（APA）包括抗心磷脂抗体（aCL）、抗β2-糖蛋白Ⅰ抗体（抗β2GPⅠ）和狼疮抗凝物抗体（LAC）。非标准APA包括磷脂酸、磷脂酰乙醇胺、磷脂酰肌醇、磷脂酰丝氨酸、磷脂酰甘油和磷脂酰胆碱，但未将其用于APS诊断[8,12-15]。

APS与反复妊娠丢失之间的关系在文献中得到充分证实。大量研究报道了APS和APA与RIF相关。有研究发现，在IVF周期有胚胎种植失败史的女性中，APA的患病率更高。然而，其他研究没有发现这种关联[13,14]。需进一步的研究以探索APA与种植失败之间的关系，并进一步关注APA的实验室检测方法和诊断标准的标准化，最好遵循札幌标准，以及评估接受ART的不同患者群体，如种植失败和RIF[8,12-15]。

2.2 遗传性易栓症

遗传性易栓症是一种异质性的遗传性疾病，会增加携带者血栓形成的风险。遗传多态性可以表现为杂合突变（仅1个等位基因突变）或纯合突变（2个等位基因突变）。血栓栓塞事件的风险可能因遗传性易栓症和变异等位基因的数量而异。纯合突变或2个及2个以上杂合突变组合可在早期导致临床上明显的血栓性疾病。遗传性易栓症增加了母体静脉血栓栓塞症（VTE）的风险和母胎界面血栓形成的风险，引起产科并发症，如妊娠丢失、子痫前期、宫内生长受限和胎盘早剥[16-18]。

凝血因子Ⅴ莱顿突变（FVL）、凝血酶原（PT）G20210A突变、亚甲基四氢叶酸还原酶（MTHFR）突变、蛋白C（PC）和蛋白S（PS）缺乏、抗凝血酶（AT）和纤溶酶原激活物抑制物-1（PAI-1）4G/5G多态性是与不良产科结局相关的遗传性易栓症。遗传性易栓症可分为VTE高风险或低风险。导致VTE的高风险易栓症包括AT缺乏、FVL基因纯合突变、PT基因纯合突变以及FVL和PT基因杂合突变的组合。导致VTE的低风险遗传性易栓症包括FVL和PT基因杂合突变以及PC和PS基因缺乏[16-18]。

2.2.1 凝血因子Ⅴ莱顿突变

FⅤ是活化因子Ⅹ（FⅩa）的辅因子，是凝血的重要调节因子。活化因子Ⅴ（FⅤa）和FⅩa形成凝血酶原复合物，将凝血酶原转化为活性凝血酶。1994年，Bertina等首次报道了位于1号染色体（1q24.2）上的FⅤ基因缺陷，该缺陷使其不易被活化PC（APC）灭活。FⅤL是一种不易被APC在第506位核苷酸切割的基因变体。外显子10第1691位核苷酸处的鸟嘌呤（G）转变为腺嘌呤（A）后，会形成一种FⅤ分子变体（FⅤL、FⅤR506Q或FⅤ:Q506），在氨基酸的第506位，鸟嘌呤取代了精氨酸。这种突变赋予FⅤa对活化PC的部分抗性，并减少因子Ⅷa的降解。因此，有缺陷的FⅤa仍具有促凝活性，因为它不会自然阻断PC，从而易于形成异常的和潜在的有害血栓[16-18]。

2.2.2 凝血酶原基因突变

凝血酶原，即凝血因子Ⅱ，被激活后（凝血酶）可促进纤维蛋白原转化为纤维蛋白，并积极参与血小板的血栓形成。Poort等于1996年首次报道了G20210A突变，该突变由位于11号染色体（11p11.2）上凝血酶原基因第20210位核苷酸G到A的转变。单个基因突变可能涉及2个等位基因的纯合突变，也可能是涉及1个等位基因的杂合突变。G等位基因是非突变的，而A等位基因相当于突变等位基因。携带该突变的个体具有高凝血酶原水平，因此表现出凝血状态恶化，血栓栓塞事件的风险增加[16-18]。

2.2.3 亚甲基四氢叶酸还原酶突变

MTHFR由位于1号染色体（1p36.3）上的一个基因编码。在文献中描述的数十种MTHFR基因多态性中，最常研究的两种变异是C677T和

A1298C:在第一种变异中,第 677 位的胞嘧啶被胸腺嘧啶取代(C677T);在第二种变体中,第 1 298 位的腺苷被胞嘧啶取代(A1298C)。发生这两种变异,MTHFR 酶的活性都会下降[18]。

MTHFR 的作用是调节细胞甲基化反应,催化 5-10 亚甲基四氢叶酸酯转化为 5-甲基四氢叶酸,其中的甲基自由基被用于将同型半胱氨酸再甲基化为甲硫氨酸(图 21.1)。MTHFR 活性降低会引起对叶酸的需求增加,而叶酸可维持正常的同型半胱氨酸到甲硫氨酸的再甲基化。在缺乏足够叶酸的情况下,细胞内同型半胱氨酸积累,甲硫氨酸的再合成减少,从而影响主要的甲基化反应[16-18]。MTHFR 酶活性降低导致同型半胱氨酸水平升高。高同型半胱氨酸血症是血栓栓塞事件的风险因素,由多种机制引起,如血管氧化应激增加、局部炎症反应和内皮细胞损伤[16-18]。

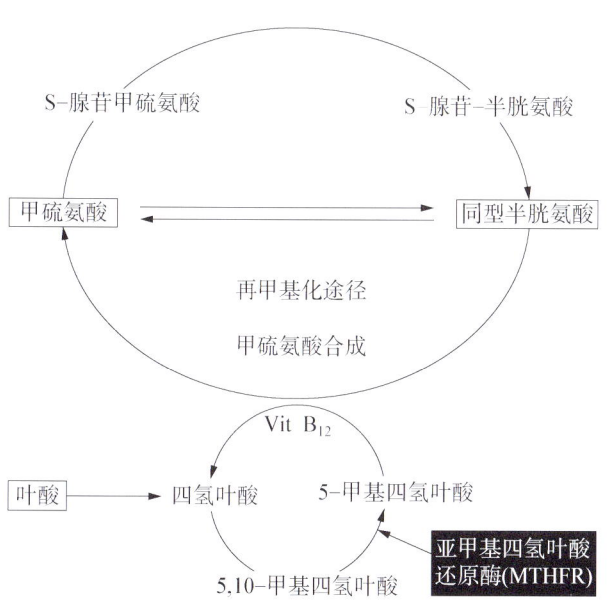

图 21.1 亚甲基四氢叶酸还原酶(MTHFR)在同型半胱氨酸代谢中的作用(再甲基化途径)。

由于甲硫氨酸再合成失败,MTHFR 突变增加了高同型半胱氨酸血症的风险。

2.2.4 蛋白 S、蛋白 C 和抗凝血酶缺乏

需要天然抗凝物来帮助阻止凝血过程。因此,这些物质的缺乏会改变平衡,导致血栓形成状态。PC、PS 和 AT 是参与这一过程的主要天然抗凝物。PC、PS 和 AT 的缺陷通常由位于 2 号染色体[*PROC* 基因(2q13-q14)]、3 号染色体[*PROS* 基因(3q11-q11.2)]和 1 号染色体[*SERPINC1* 基因(1q23-25)]上的基因突变引起。这三种疾病均为常染色体隐性遗传[16-18]。

2.2.5 纤溶酶原激活物抑制剂-1 4G/5G 多态性

纤维蛋白溶解是纤维蛋白凝块(凝血产物)溶解的过程。纤溶系统或纤溶酶原/纤溶酶系统由多种蛋白质(血清蛋白酶和抑制剂)组成,可调节纤溶酶原生成纤溶酶。纤溶酶原具有降解纤维蛋白和激活细胞外基质金属蛋白酶的功能。目前已知有两种生理性纤溶酶原激活剂:组织型纤溶酶原激活剂(tPA)和尿激酶型纤溶酶原激活剂(u-PA)。纤维蛋白溶解由纤维蛋白溶解系统的抑制剂如 PAI-1 控制。PAI-1 是纤溶酶原生理性激活剂(tPA)的主要抑制剂(图 21.2)。血浆中 PAI-1 水平升高可损害纤溶系统并促进持续性纤维蛋白凝块[6,16,17]。

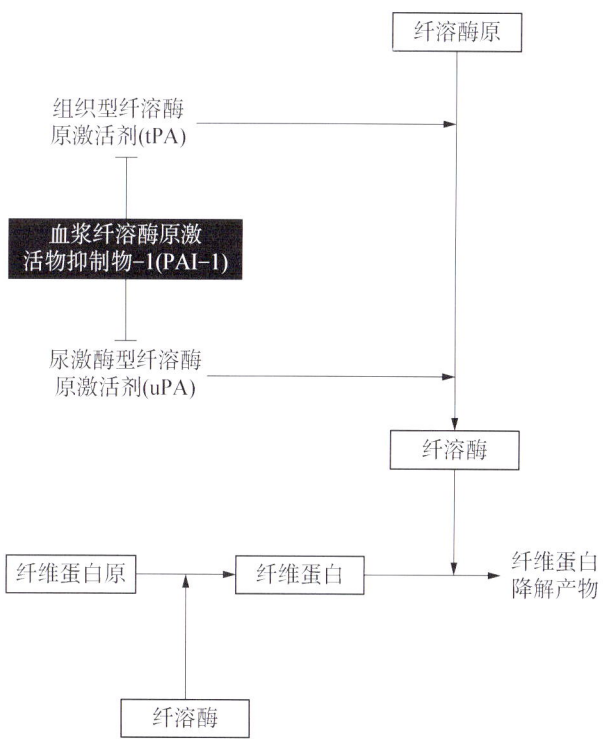

图 21.2 尿激酶型纤溶酶原激活剂(uPA)和组织型纤溶酶原激活剂(tPA)是纤溶酶原激活剂。

血浆纤溶酶原激活物抑制剂-1(PAI-1)水平升高可损害纤溶系统,促进持续性纤维蛋白凝块。

PAI-1 在血管内皮、肝脏和脂肪等不同组织中分泌。PAI-1 4G/5G 多态性,也称为 *SERPINE1* 基因的 675 多态性,位于 7 号染色体(7q21.3-22),由翻译起始位点 675 bp 的鸟苷插入或缺失组成,影响该基因的转录,导致 PAI-1 的血浆浓度改变。4G 等位基因具有转录激活剂的结合位点,反映了更

高浓度的PAI-1,而5G等位基因则具有转录抑制剂的额外结合位点,导致循环PAI-1水平降低。4G等位基因纯合子的PAI-1浓度比5G纯合子高25%。4G等位基因的存在与血栓栓塞事件和心血管疾病的风险增加有关。此外,不明原因早期流产患者体内存在高浓度PAI-1,这是由于纤维蛋白溶解功能受损促进纤维蛋白在胎盘循环中沉积[6,16-18]。

3 患病率

3.1 抗磷脂抗体

APS和遗传性易栓症在普通人群中的患病率尚不清楚。除了种族和环境因素外,非标准化的诊断标准,特别是定义APS病例的标准(基于2006年悉尼标准),是确定准确患病率的最大限制。Duarte García等观察到,在18岁以下的普通人群中,APS的年发病率为每10万人2.1例[95%置信区间(CI):1.4~2.8],男女发病率相似。此外,据报道,APS的估计患病率为50/100 000(95% CI:42~58)[19]。在这项研究中,APS最常见的自身抗体是LAC(75%的病例),其次是aCL-IgM(42%)、aCL-IgG(39%)、抗β2-GPI-IgG(22%)和抗β2-GPI-IgM(11%)[19]。

通常情况下,有不孕和种植失败病史的女性并不符合APS的临床标准。因此,大多数研究仅限于评估APA在这一人群中的发生频率。Buckingham和Chamley收集了27项研究的数据,评估了APA与女性不孕症的关系,并报道称APA在这一人群中的患病率为22.2%(范围为0%~66%)。此外,在患有RIF的女性中,APA的患病率更高(14项研究,29.7%,范围为4%~66%)[12]。也有人描述了非标准APA与生殖障碍的关系。Varla-Leftherioti等观察到,在反复流产(2次自然流产)和患者RIF的女性中,APA的发生率增加。共有26.9%的女性至少有一种APA阳性。aCL抗体更为常见(56.1%),其次是抗β2-GPI(52.6%)、抗PS(28.9%)、抗PI(13.1%)、抗PA(10.8%)和LAC(8.6%)[12]。

3.2 遗传性易栓症

遗传性易栓症的患病率在健康人群和特定患者群体之间差异很大,尤其是有VTE病史的患者。全球高加索人群中易栓症的患病率约为每100 000人中有10~7 000人。在健康的高加索人群中,FVL是最常见的遗传性易栓症(FVL杂合子:2%~7%;FVL纯合子:0.06%~0.25%),其次是G20210A突变(杂合子:1%~2%;纯合子:罕见)、高同型半胱氨酸血症(<5%)、PC缺乏症(0.2%~0.5%)、PS缺乏症(0.1%~0.7%)、FVL和G20210A联合突变杂合子(0.1%),以及AT缺乏症(0.02%)[20,21]。在有VTE发病史和复发史的人群中,易栓症的发病率要高得多。在这一组中,FVL也更为普遍(12%~50%),其次是G20210A突变(3%~20%)、高同型半胱氨酸血症(<10%)、PC缺乏症(2%~10%)、PS缺乏症(1%~10%)和AT缺乏症(1%~5%)[20-22]。

已报道了遗传性易栓症与RIF之间的关系。Safdarian等评估了有RIF病史的女性中FVL、MTHFR C677T突变、凝血酶原20210A突变、同型半胱氨酸水平、PAI-1突变、PS/PC和AT缺乏的频率。至少有一种易栓症的患病率为61.5%(59/96),其中FVL的患病率最高(16.7%),其次是MTHFR C677T突变(纯合:6.3%;杂合:11.5%)、凝血酶原20210A突变(9.4%)、高同型半胱氨酸血症(7.3%)、PC缺乏症(4.2%)、PS缺乏症(4.2%)、AT缺乏症(2.1%)和PAI-1突变(纯合:2.1%;杂合:10.4%)。至少存在一种易栓症(95% CI=1.74~5.70,OR=3.15,P=0.00)、FVL(95% CI=1.26~10.27,OR=3.06,P=0.01)和MTHFR C677T突变(95% CI=1.55~97.86,OR=12.33,P=0.05)与胚胎种植失败具有显著的统计学相关性[23]。多项研究证实了这些结果,但仍有一些研究未能证实[6,24-26]。

4 与生殖相关的潜在病理生理学

母胎界面的凝血和随之而来的血栓事件可导致APS患者的妊娠丢失。然而,绒毛间隙的发育发生在妊娠10周后,因此很难仅仅用蜕膜血管中的微血栓形成来解释种植失败。据推测,遗传性/获得性易栓症或两者兼有的患者种植失败的病理生理学机制还涉及其他因素[8,13,27]。APA的促炎作用可能会破坏卵母细胞发育或子宫内膜蜕膜化,从而影响生育能力[13,28,29]。研究表明,APA可减少滋养细胞的增殖、侵袭和合胞化以及hCG的产生。此外,由于血管细胞(包括内皮细胞、血小板和单核细胞)的激活,诱发细胞外囊泡的促凝血作用和细胞表面抗凝物

Annexin A5 屏蔽的破坏，可能会导致生殖障碍[13,29,30]。APA 还与补体激活有关，因为补体和凝血途径紧密相连[31,32]。补体系统的激活也与生殖障碍密切相关[33]。

凝血酶原 20210A 突变与种植失败之间的关系尚未明确。可溶性 fms 样酪氨酸激酶-1(sFlt-1 或 sVEGFR-1)是一种具有抗血管生成特性的蛋白质，能与血管内皮生长因子(VEGF)和胎盘生长因子等血管生成因子结合，减少新生血管生成。蜕膜细胞中高水平的凝血酶可诱导产生大量 sFlt-1，从而抑制与绒毛外滋养细胞侵袭相关的酶[34,35]。

最近，有研究证实了叶酸代谢与胚胎植入过程之间的联系。叶酸和同型半胱氨酸存在于卵泡液中。卵泡液中同型半胱氨酸水平升高与卵母细胞质量差有关[36]。此外，MTHFR 677TT（纯合突变，TT）女性的同型半胱氨酸和 NK 细胞的细胞毒性显著高于患有 MTHFR-677CC 和 677-CT 的女性[37]，而据报道，NK 细胞的细胞毒性增加与 RIF 有关[38]。组织病理学研究发现，患有高同型半胱氨酸血症的孕妇除了血管形成不良外，绒毛总面积也减少[39]。这些机制加强了 MTHFR 基因突变与高同型半胱氨酸血症或不与 RIF 之间的可能联系。

纤维蛋白溶解对植入过程至关重要。纤溶酶原的激活通过蛋白水解和基底膜的溶解促进细胞迁移。增加的纤溶酶原激活物抑制剂如 PAI-1 对纤维蛋白溶解的抑制可能会损害滋养细胞充分侵袭的深度[40,41]。因此，4G/5G 多态性引起的低纤维蛋白溶解可能是种植失败的一个危险因素。

5 诊断

5.1 抗磷脂综合征

APS 的第一个诊断标准——札幌标准于 1999 年提出。随后，2006 年在悉尼举行的国际会议对札幌标准进行了修订。目前，APS 的诊断需要至少有 1 个临床和 1 个实验室标准（表 21.1）[42]。

表 21.1 抗磷脂综合征的诊断标准（悉尼，2006）

临床标准
（1）血管血栓
任何组织或器官中的动脉、静脉或小血管血栓形成，一次或多次临床发作。血栓形成必须经客观有效的标准（即适当的影像学或组织病理学检查有明确发现）证实。如需组织病理学确认，血栓应在血管壁无明显炎症证据的情况下存在
（2）妊娠并发症
a. 在妊娠第 10 周或 10 周以后，形态正常的胎儿出现一次或多次不明原因的死亡，超声或直接检查证实胎儿形态正常，或 b. 因(i)根据标准定义的子痫或重度子痫前期，或(ii)公认的胎盘功能不全特征，在妊娠 34 周前发生一次或多次形态正常的新生儿早产，或 c. 在妊娠 10 周前连续发生 3 次或 3 次以上不明原因的自然流产，且排除母体解剖或激素异常以及双方染色体原因
实验室标准
（1）根据国际血栓与止血学会[狼疮抗凝物(LA)/磷脂依赖性抗体科学小组委员会]的指导意见，血浆中出现 LA 2 次或 2 次以上，间隔至少 12 周 （2）用标准化 ELISA 检测，血清或血浆中 IgG 和（或）IgM 同种型的 aCL 抗体，出现中高滴度(即 >40 GPL 或 MPL，或 >第 99 百分位数)，2 次或 2 次以上，间隔至少 12 周 （3）根据推荐程序，用标准化 ELISA 检测，血清或血浆中 IgG 和（或）IgM 同种型的抗 β2 糖蛋白-I 抗体（滴度 >第 99 百分位数），出现 2 次或更多次，间隔至少 12 周

注：引自 Miyakis et al.（2006）。

5.2 遗传性易栓症

遗传性易栓症（FVL、MTHFR C677T 突变、凝血酶原 20210A 突变和 PAI-1 4G/5G 多态性）的诊断是通过分子遗传技术寻找多态性，确定突变等位基因的存在和数量[9,18]。

PC 缺乏症的诊断依据是通过酶联免疫吸附试验（ELISA）、放射免疫测定法或电免疫测定法测得的 PC 含量。PC 活性水平在严重缺乏时为 0%~30%，在部分缺乏时为 30%~70%。PC 缺乏症有两种生物学形式。Ⅰ型缺乏症的特点是 PC 和抗原活性持续降低。在Ⅱ型缺乏症中，PC 活性降低，但 PC 抗原正常。可以进行分子检测，但并非诊断的必要条件[43]。

PS 缺乏症的诊断基于抗原水平（总蛋白 S 或游离蛋白 S）和抗凝血活性的量化。游离 PS 和总 PS 是通过 ELISA 测定，包括三种生物形式。Ⅰ型和Ⅲ型是最常见的类型，存在定量缺陷和低水平的游离抗原（Ⅲ型的总 PS 水平正常，而Ⅰ型的总 PS 水平降低）。Ⅱ型（罕见型）为定性缺陷，总 PS 和游离 PS 水平正常。可进行分子检测，但并非诊断的必要条件[43]。

AT 缺乏症分为以下两种类型：Ⅰ型（定量型，以血浆抗原水平和 AT 功能活性降低为特征）和Ⅱ型（定性型，以在血浆中存在变异 AT 为特征，抗原水平正常，活性降低）。Ⅱ型可进一步细分为反应位点、肝素结合位点和多效性缺陷（突变聚集在一个称为 s1C-s4B 的区域）。AT 缺乏症的诊断和分类是通过使用功能和免疫学方法对抗原活性和浓度进行血浆测定来进行的[44]。

PC、PS 和 AT 缺乏症的异常结果应在 1 个或多个单独样本中重复检测加以确认。单个异常结果不足以诊断这些缺乏症。妊娠期摄入维生素 K、使用肝素、血栓事件急性期或存在肝脏疾病时，实验室检查结果并不可靠[43,44]。

血浆中约 70% 的同型半胱氨酸与白蛋白和其他蛋白质结合，一小部分以同型半胱氨酸和同型半胱氨酸二硫化物的形式游离。用于测量游离氨基酸的方法无法检测少量游离同型半胱氨酸。因此，需要在样本中加入还原剂，如二硫苏糖醇或 β-巯基乙醇，使同型半胱氨酸从血浆蛋白中释放出来，从而测定血浆总同型半胱氨酸（tHcy）。所有检测 tHcy 的方法都能得到相似的生理水平（$5\sim15~\mu mol/L$ 或 μM）。目前，大多数实验室使用基于高效液相色谱或稳定同位素稀释气相色谱-质谱的方法。其他检测 tHcy 的方法包括荧光偏振免疫测定法、化学发光免疫酶法和荧光检测色谱法[45]。

6 治疗

鉴于文献中的数据存在争议，对于有流产、子痫前期、胎儿生长受限、胎盘早剥、不孕症或胚胎种植失败等妊娠并发症史的女性，筛查和治疗遗传性易栓症以改善妊娠结局，目前国际上尚未达成共识。尽管在这些人群中已积累了易栓症的证据，但只有具有 VTE 个人史或一级亲属（例如父母或兄弟姐妹）罹患高危遗传性易栓症病史的女性才适合进行遗传性易栓症筛查[46]。

传统上，APS 治疗以抗血小板和抗凝治疗为基础，严重病例则使用免疫抑制或调节药物，如强的松、羟氯喹、静脉注射免疫球蛋白、利妥昔单抗和依库珠单抗。目前，对于诊断为单纯产科 APS（定义为至少存在 1 种临床产科标准和 1 种实验室标准）的患者，治疗方案是低剂量阿司匹林（LDA，$75\sim100~mg/d$）和预防剂量的肝素［普通肝素（UFH）或低分子肝素（LMWH）］的组合[47]。这一建议基于两项随机对照研究，在这两项试验中，将反复妊娠丢失和 APA 阳性患者随机分为 LDA 组或阿司匹林联合 UFH 组[48,49]。与单独使用 LDA 相比，LDA 联合 UFH 治疗组的活产率明显更高（71% vs 42%，OR 3.37，95% $CI=1.40\sim8.10$）[48]。在治疗与 APA 相关的反复妊娠丢失时，LDA 联合低剂量肝素（每 12 小时 1 万 U 的 UFH）与 LDA 联合大剂量肝素（每 2 小时 2 万 U 的 UFH）疗效相同[49]。

尽管易栓症（获得性和遗传性）与胚胎种植失败之间相关性的证据相互矛盾，但肝素（UFH 或 LMWH）单独或与 LDA 联用已被作为接受 ART 治疗患者的辅助疗法。Cochrane 循证医学研究显示，无论是否诊断易栓症，使用肝素对 ART 周期的临床结局都有益处。与安慰剂组（OR 1.77，95% $CI=1.07\sim2.90$，三项研究，386 名女性，$I^2=51\%$，低质量证据）或未进行任何干预组（OR 1.61，95% $CI=1.053\sim2.53$，三项试验，386 名女性，$I^2=29\%$，低质量证据）相比，治疗组具有更高的活产率（LBR），临床妊娠率也有所提高[50]。Potdar 等的另一项荟萃分析证实了这些结果。有 RIF 和肝素治疗史（有或无易栓症）的女性 LBR 得到改善（RR 1.79，95% $CI=1.10\sim2.90$，$P=0.02$），流产率降低（RR 0.22，95% $CI=0.06\sim0.78$，$P=0.02$）[51]。与此相反，其他研究（包括 Cochrane 之前报道的一项荟萃分析）并没有观察到接受 IVF/ICSI（有或无种植失败史）和肝素治疗（有或无 LDA）的患者临床结局有所改善[52-54]。

肝素在改善胚胎种植过程中的有益作用不仅被解释为具有抗凝活性，还可解释为具有抗炎作用，以改善绒毛外滋养细胞的侵袭，减少滋养细胞凋亡[55,56]。此外，肝素在体内抑制补体激活（在经典、旁路和终末途径的不同点），并在小鼠模型中保护母体免受 APA 诱导的妊娠并发症[57,58]。肝素是妊娠期广泛使用的药物，尤其是用于预防和治疗血栓栓塞事件[21]，其在 APS 治疗中的应用已得到证实[8]。美国食品药品监督管理局将肝素列为 B 类。由于其分子量大，它不会穿过胎盘，也不会从母乳中排出。在妊娠和哺乳期间使用肝素（最好是低分子肝素）被认为是安全的。应认识到患者在妊娠期和产后，使用 LMWH 的预防剂量（分别为 0.5% 和 1%）或治疗剂量（分别为 1.5% 和 2%）都有出血风险，以及使用肝素时的其他并发症，如血小板减少症和骨质疏松症[56]。

7 总结和建议

研究表明，易栓症引起的微血栓形成可导致子宫内膜/蜕膜血流量变化影响胚胎植入。其他机制包括炎症性子宫环境加剧、滋养细胞侵袭减少和补体系统激活，似乎也降低了易栓症患者的种植率。

目前，APS、APA 和遗传性易栓症与 RIF 之间的关系尚不清楚。因此，不建议对有胚胎种植失败史的女性进行常规筛查。然而，尽管对这些患者的评估缺乏共识，但最近的荟萃分析表明，当单独给予肝素或肝素联合 LDA 辅助治疗时，RIF 患者在 IVF/ET 和 FET 周期中的生殖结局有所改善。需要进行设计严谨的随机双盲临床试验，并制定严格的临床和实验室诊断标准。

- 易栓症可分为获得性（如 APS）和遗传性。
- 易栓症引起的微血栓导致子宫内膜/蜕膜血流量减少似乎会损害胚胎植入。
- 炎症性子宫环境、补体激活和滋养细胞侵袭受损是易栓症导致种植失败的潜在机制。
- 对于患有 RIF 的女性是否具有更高水平的 APS、APA 和遗传性易栓症，尚未达成普遍共识。
- 抗血小板（低剂量阿司匹林）和抗凝剂（肝素）可作为 ART 的辅助治疗，以改善有种植失败史的女性的临床结局。

参考文献

[1] Ashary N, Tiwari A, Modi D. Embryo implantation: war in times of love. Endocrinology 2018;159:1188–98.

[2] Coughlan C, Ledger W, Wang Q, et al. Recurrent implantation failure: definition and management. Reprod Biomed Online 2014;28:14–38.

[3] Kolte AM, Bernardi LA, Christiansen OB, et al. Terminology for pregnancy loss prior to viability: a consensus statement from the ESHRE early pregnancy special interest group. Hum Reprod 2015;30:495–8.

[4] Shaulov T, Sierra S, Sylvestre C. Recurrent implantation failure in IVF: a Canadian fertility and andrology society clinical practice guideline. Reprod Biomed Online 2020;41: 819–33.

[5] Bashiri A, Halper KI, Orvieto R. Recurrent implantation failure-update overview on etiology, diagnosis, treatment and future directions. Reprod Biol Endocrinol 2018;16;121.

[6] Ivanov P, Tsvyatkovska T, Konova E, Komsa-Penkova R. Inherited thrombophilia and IVF failure: the impact of coagulation disorders on implantation process. Am J Reprod Immunol 2012;68:189–98.

[7] Devis P, Knuttinen MG. Deep venous thrombosis in pregnancy: incidence, pathogenesis and endovascular management. Cardiovasc Diagn Ther. 2017;7;S309–19.

[8] Garcia D, Erkan D. Diagnosis and management of the antiphospholipid syndrome. N Engl J Med 2018;378:2010–21.

[9] Arachchillage DRJ, Makris M. Inherited thrombophilia and pregnancy complications: should we test? Semin Thromb Hemost 2019;45;50–60.

[10] Simcox LE, Ormesher L, Tower C, Greer IA. Thrombophilia and pregnancy complications. Int J Mol Sci. 2015;16;28418–28.

[11] Hughes GR. Thrombosis, abortion, cerebral disease, and the lupus anticoagulant. Br Med J 1983;287:1088–9.

[12] Varla-Leftherioti M, Keramitsoglou T, Gourniezaki G, et al. Retrospective analysis on the incidence of the types and isotypes of antiphospholipid antibodies in subfertile women. J Reprod Immunol 2014;101–102;59.

[13] Ata B, Urman B. Thrombophilia and assisted reproduction technology-any detrimental impact or unnecessary overuse? J Assist Reprod Genet 2016;33;1305–10.

[14] Stern C, Chamley L. Antiphospholipid antibodies and coagulation defects in women with implantation failure after IVF and recurrent miscarriage. Reprod Biomed Online 2006; 13;29–37.

[15] Kwak-Kim J, Park JC, Ahn HK, Kim JW, Gilman-Sachs A. Immunological modes of pregnancy loss. Am J Reprod Immunol 2010;63;611–23.

[16] Middeldorp S. Inherited thrombophilia: a double-edged sword. Hematology Am Soc Hematol Educ Program 2016; 2016;1–9.

[17] Phillippe HM, Hornsby LB, Treadway S, Armstrong EM, Bellone JM. Inherited thrombophilia. J Pharm Pract. 2014; 27;227–323.

[18] Dautaj A, Krasi G, Bushati V, et al. Hereditary thrombophilia. Acta Biomed 2019;90;44–6.

[19] Duarte-García A, Pham MM, Crowson CS, et al. The epidemiology of antiphospholipid syndrome: a population-

based study. Arthritis Rheumatol. 2019;71:1545-52.
[20] Seligsohn U, Lubetsky A. Genetic susceptibility to venous thrombosis. N Engl J Med 2001;344:1222-31.
[21] Stevens SM, Woller SC, Bauer KA, et al. Guidance for the evaluation and treatment of hereditary and acquired thrombophilia. J Thromb Thrombolysis 2016;41:154-64.
[22] Cohoon KP, Heit JA. Inherited and secondary thrombophilia. Circulation 2014;129:254-7.
[23] Safdarian L, Najmi Z, Aleyasin A, Aghahosseini M, Rashidi M, Asadollah S. Recurrent IVF failure and hereditary thrombophilia. Iran J Reprod Med. 2014;12:467-70.
[24] Qublan HS, Eid SS, Ababneh HA, et al. Acquired and inherited thrombophilia: implication in recurrent IVF and embryo transfer failure. Hum Reprod 2006;21:2694-8.
[25] Steinvil A, Raz R, Berliner S, et al. Association of common thrombophilias and antiphospholipid antibodies with success rate of in vitro fertilisation. Thromb Haemost 2012;108:1192-7.
[26] Han AR, Han JW, Lee SK. Inherited thrombophilia and anticoagulant therapy for women with reproductive failure. Am J Reprod Immunol 2021;85:e13378.
[27] Rey E, Kahn SR, David M, Shrier I. Thrombophilic disorders and fetal loss: a meta-analysis. Lancet 2003;361:901-8.
[28] Tomassetti C, Meuleman C, Pexsters A, et al. Endometriosis, recurrent miscarriage and implantation failure: is there an immunological link? Reprod Biomed Online 2006;13:58-64.
[29] Kwak-Kim J, Agcaoili MS, Aleta L, et al. Management of women with recurrent pregnancy losses and anti-phospholipid antibody syndrome. Am J Reprod Immunol 2013;69:596-607.
[30] de Laat B, Mertens K, de Groot PG. Mechanisms of disease: antiphospholipid antibodies-from clinical association to pathologic mechanism. Nat Clin Pract Rheumatol 2008;4:192-9.
[31] Chaturvedi S, Brodsky RA, McCrae KR. Complement in the pathophysiology of the antiphospholipid syndrome. Front Immunol 2019;10:449.
[32] Foley JH, Conway EM. Cross talk pathways between coagulation and inflammation. Circ Res 2016;118:1392-408.
[33] Tincani A, Cavazzana I, Ziglioli T, Lojacono A, De Angelis V, Meroni P. Complement activation and pregnancy failure. Clin Rev Allergy Immunol 2010;39:153-9.
[34] Lockwood CJ, Krikun G, Rahman M, Caze R, Buchwalder L, Schatz F. The role of decidualization in regulating endometrial hemostasis during the menstrual cycle, gestation, and in pathological states. Semin Thromb Hemost 2007;33:111-17.
[35] Lockwood CJ, Toti P, Arcuri F, et al. Thrombin regulates soluble fms-like tyrosine kinase-1 (sFlt-1) expression in first trimester decidua: implications for preeclampsia. Am J Pathol 2007;170:1398-405.
[36] Szymański W, Kazdepka-Ziemińska A. Wpływ stezenia homocysteiny w płynie pecherzykowym na stopień dojrzałości komórki jajowej [effect of homocysteine concentration in follicular fluid on a degree of oocyte maturity]. Ginekol Pol 2003;74:1392-6.
[37] Ota K, Takahashi T, Han A, Damvaeba S, Mizunuma H, Kwak-Kim J. Effects of MTHFR C677T polymorphism on vitamin D, homocysteine and natural killer cell cytotoxicity in women with recurrent pregnancy losses. Hum Reprod 2020;35:1276-87.

[38] Sung N, Khan SA, Yiu ME, Jubiz G, Salazar MD, Skariah A, et al. Reproductive outcomes of women with recurrent pregnancy losses and repeated implantation failures are significantly improved with immunomodulatory treatment. J Reprod Immunol 2021;148:103369.
[39] Nelen WL, Bulten J, Steegers EA, Blom HJ, Hanselaar AG, Eskes TK. Maternal homocysteine and chorionic vascularization in recurrent early pregnancy loss. Hum Reprod 2000;15:954-60.
[40] Lang IM, Moser KM, Schleef RR. Elevated expression of urokinase-like plasminogen activator and plasminogen activator inhibitor type 1 during the vascular remodeling associated with pulmonary thromboembolism. Arterioscler Thromb Vasc Biol 1998;18:808-15.
[41] Gris JC, Ripart-Neveu S, Maugard C, et al. Respective evaluation of the prevalence of haemostasis abnormalities in unexplained primary early recurrent miscarriages. The Nimes Obstetricians and Haematologists (NOHA) study. Thromb Haemost 1997;77:1096-103.
[42] Miyakis S, Lockshin MD, Atsumi T, et al. International consensus statement on an update of the classification criteria for definite antiphospholipid syndrome (APS). J Thromb Haemost 2006;4:295-306.
[43] Wypasek E, Undas A. Protein C and protein S deficiency — practical diagnostic issues. Adv Clin Exp Med. 2013;22:459-67.
[44] Khor B, Van Cott EM. Laboratory tests for antithrombin deficiency. Am J Hematol 2010;85:947-50.
[45] American Society of Human Genetics/American College of Medical Genetics Test and Transfer Committee Working Group. Measurement and use of total plasma homocysteine. Am J Hum Genet 1998;63:1541-3.
[46] American College of Obstetricians and Gynecologists' Committee on Practice Bulletins-Obstetrics. ACOG practice bulletin No. 197: inherited thrombophilias in pregnancy. Obstet Gynecol 2018;132:e18-34.
[47] Ghembaza A, Saadoun D. Management of antiphospholipid syndrome. Biomedicines. 2020;8:508.
[48] Rai R, Cohen H, Dave M, Regan L. Randomised controlled trial of aspirin and aspirin plus heparin in pregnant women with recurrent miscarriage associated with phospholipid antibodies (or antiphospholipid antibodies). BMJ 1997;314:253-7.
[49] Kutteh WH, Ermel LD. A clinical trial for the treatment of antiphospholipid antibody-associated recurrent pregnancy loss with lower dose heparin and aspirin. Am J Reprod Immunol 1996;35:402-7.
[50] Akhtar MA, Sur S, Raine-Fenning N, Jayaprakasan K, Thornton JG, Quenby S. Heparin for assisted reproduction. Cochrane Database Syst Rev 2013;8:CD009452.
[51] Potdar N, Gelbaya TA, Konje JC, Nardo LG. Adjunct low-molecular-weight heparin to improve live birth rate after recurrent implantation failure: a systematic review and meta-analysis. Hum Reprod Update 2013;19:674-84.
[52] Akhtar MA, Eljabu H, Hopkisson J, Raine-Fenning N, Quenby S, Jayaprakasan K. Aspirin and heparin as adjuvants during IVF do not improve live birth rates in unexplained implantation failure. Reprod Biomed Online 2013;26:586-94.
[53] Siristatidis C, Dafopoulos K, Salamalekis G, et al. Administration of low-molecular-weight heparin in patients with two or more unsuccessful IVF/ICSI cycles: a multicenter cohort study. Gynecol Endocrinol 2018;34:747-51.

[54] Seshadri S, Sunkara SK, Khalaf Y, El-Toukhy T, Hamoda H. Effect of heparin on the outcome of IVF treatment: a systematic review and meta-analysis. Reprod Biomed Online 2012;25:572-84.

[55] Tersigni C, Marana R, Santamarìa A, Castellani R, Scambia G, Simone ND. In vitro evidences of heparin's effects on embryo implantation and trophoblast development. Reprod Sci 2012;19:454-62.

[56] Mulloy B, Hogwood J, Gray E, Lever R, Page CP. Pharmacology of heparin and related drugs. Pharmacol Rev 2016;68:76-141.

[57] Girardi G, Redecha P, Salmon JE. Heparin prevents antiphospholipid antibody-induced fetal loss by inhibiting complement activation. Nat Med 2004;10:1222-6.

[58] Ninomiya H, Kawashima Y, Nagasawa T. Inhibition of complement-mediated haemolysis in paroxysmal nocturnal haemoglobinuria by heparin or low-molecular weight heparin. Br J Haematol 2000;109:875-81.

第 4 篇

生殖障碍中的神经-免疫-内分泌网络失调

Dysregulated neuroimmune-endocrine network in reproductive failures

第 22 章

卵巢免疫病理学与生殖功能障碍

The ovarian immune pathology and reproductive failures

Li Wu[1], Xuhui Fang[1], Yanshi Wang[1] and Joanne Kwak-Kim[2]

[1] Reproductive Medicine Center, Department of Obstetrics and Gynecology, The First Affiliated Hospital of USTC, Division of Life Sciences and Medicine, University of Science and Technology of China, Hefei, Anhui, P.R. China

[2] Reproductive Medicine and Immunology, Obstetrics and Gynecology, Clinical Sciences Department, Chicago Medical School, Rosalind Franklin University of Medicine and Science, Vernon Hills, IL, United States

1 引言

人类卵巢是自身免疫攻击的常见靶点，会导致免疫性炎症，引起卵巢功能障碍，如卵泡发育异常、排卵障碍、黄体功能不足、不孕甚至妊娠失败。体液和细胞自身免疫反应均可参与卵巢自身免疫的发生。抗卵巢抗体（AOA）主要与早发性卵巢功能不全（POI）、卵巢早衰（POF）和不明原因不孕症（UI）相关[1]。事实上，有3.0%~66.6%的POF病例与自身免疫机制有关[2-6]。卵巢淋巴细胞浸润，即"淋巴细胞性卵巢炎"是一种典型的POF病理，通常与卵巢中的单核细胞浸润、卵巢抗原自身抗体的存在以及其他自身免疫性疾病有关[7]。值得注意的是，在自身免疫性病因导致的POF女性中，自身免疫状态缓解后，卵巢功能常常可以恢复[8]。

根据临床表现或实验室检查结果，卵巢自身免疫可能被诊断为不同的临床疾病，如POI、POF、卵巢储备功能低下（POR）、卵巢储备功能减退（DOR）、自身免疫性卵巢炎和UI[9]。卵巢自身免疫常常与其他基础疾病相关，包括多囊卵巢综合征（PCOS）和子宫内膜异位症（EMS），其中自身免疫是常见的基础病因[9,10]。有趣的是，患有自身免疫性卵巢炎的女性可能出现多囊样卵巢和血清LH水平升高，会被误认为是PCOS，但她们并没有表现出高雄激素血症。值得注意的是，自身免疫机制一直被认为是PCOS的潜在病因之一。相反，PCOS患者由于稀发排卵或无排卵和相对高雌激素引起的低孕酮水平，会过度刺激免疫系统，从而产生自身抗体[12]。

通过建立母体对胎儿的免疫耐受，及时转换和平衡促炎与抗炎免疫反应对胚胎成功种植和维持妊娠至关重要，而不平衡的免疫反应则会导致炎症过程和病理变化，引起不孕症，尤其是不明原因不孕症和反复种植失败（RIF）[13]。例如，患有卵巢子宫内膜异位症的女性血清和腹腔液中炎症细胞因子和自身抗体水平升高，与不孕症及妊娠丢失有关[14]。此外，自身免疫性疾病，包括自身免疫性卵巢炎、抗磷脂综合征（APS）和自身免疫性甲状腺疾病，主要影响育龄期女性，并对人类生殖的各个阶段产生影响，导致卵巢功能衰竭、种植失败和妊娠丢失。因此，本章将全面回顾与卵巢自身免疫相关的免疫病理、临床表现和管理。

2 卵巢免疫学

卵巢周期包括卵泡发生、排卵、月经或胚胎植入。神经内分泌激素、免疫效应因子和相关因素控制着卵巢周期的生理变化。因此，了解人类生殖过程中卵巢和子宫内膜在卵巢周期内的免疫反应至关重要。在卵巢周期中，外周血免疫效应因子被招募到卵巢基质、卵泡和子宫内膜，并积极参与卵泡发生、排卵、黄体（CL）形成、黄体溶解和即将进行的胚胎植入[14]。因此，卵巢和子宫内膜的异常免疫反应常常导致生殖障碍，例如卵泡发育不良、卵巢反应不良、卵子质量差、RIF 和反复妊娠丢失（RPL）[14]。

卵巢周期中的两个非概念事件，如排卵和月经，与炎症过程有相似之处[15]。据报道，卵泡较多的女性血清 C 反应蛋白（CRP）水平较高。事实上，较高的 CRP 水平与孕酮水平升高相关，这表明，正常的卵巢周期可能与炎症有关[12,15]。然而，这些"生理性"炎症不同于病理性炎症，后者往往以自身免疫为结局。此外，月经和胚胎种植具有相似的炎症特征，如组织水肿和大量炎性细胞浸润。排卵后，子宫内膜通过免疫增强和血管生成为胚胎成功植入做好准备[16]。在胚胎植入前，子宫内膜中就出现了多种免疫效应物，它们通过参与组织重塑和血管生成来促进植入，而如果胚胎没有植入，月经就会开始。有研究认为，孕酮水平的降低会诱导子宫内膜组织的破坏、再生和修复，提示孕酮可抑制炎症反应。此外，雌激素具有促炎和抗炎作用，这取决于免疫刺激和随后的抗原特异性免疫反应、细胞类型、具有特定微环境的靶器官、生殖状态、雌激素浓度、雌激素受体表达和雌激素的细胞内代谢[17]。因此，排卵失败或失调和卵巢过度刺激可能诱发卵巢自身免疫和全身促炎反应，导致潜在的产科并发症，包括 RIF、RPL 和子痫前期[18]。

3 卵巢自身免疫

3.1 自身免疫性淋巴细胞性卵巢炎

自身免疫性淋巴细胞性卵巢炎是 POI 和 POF 的一种已知的特殊病因，首次在罹患 Addison 病和肾上腺自身免疫性疾病的患者中被描述。其特征是在生长卵泡和黄体的卵泡膜细胞层中有单核炎性细胞浸润，而保留原始卵泡和初级卵泡[19]。卵巢活检标本中的组织炎症特征以及循环卵巢和肾上腺自身抗体是自身免疫性 POI 的诊断特征[20]。细胞免疫和体液免疫可能在自身免疫性淋巴细胞性卵巢炎中发挥重要作用。浸润的炎性细胞主要是 T（CD4$^+$、CD8$^+$）细胞、自然杀伤细胞（NK）、B 细胞和主要产生 IgG 抗体的浆细胞[21]。炎症通常存在于血管周围和神经周围区域，影响排卵前卵泡中的类固醇生成细胞，尤其是卵泡膜、黄体的内/外层，偶尔也会影响颗粒细胞[22]。这些独特的免疫病理学发现为免

疫抑制治疗可能恢复自身免疫性 POI 患者的生育能力提供了理论上的可能性。此外，调节性 T 细胞（Treg）在卵巢抗原的系统耐受中起关键作用，在小鼠模型中诱导小鼠透明带（ZP）蛋白 3 特异性 Treg 细胞可改善自身免疫性卵巢疾病[23]。

此外，在患有自身免疫性卵巢炎的女性中，卵巢多囊样表现并伴有血清 LH 水平升高会被误认为是 PCOS[24]。然而，与 PCOS 患者相比，自身免疫性卵巢炎患者不会出现雄激素过多的迹象。相反，由于自身免疫性卵巢炎而发生 POI 的女性可能有雄激素缺乏的临床和实验室证据，可能与卵泡膜细胞和肾上腺雄激素的产生受损有关。在大多数情况下，任何有关自身免疫性卵巢炎和 PCOS 鉴别诊断的问题都可通过检测循环肾上腺皮质自身抗体及测定 FSH 和血清雄激素水平来解决。

3.2 卵巢自身免疫的分子和细胞靶点

血清 AOA 在卵巢病理中的作用仍有争议。据报道，在 24%～73% 的 POI 女性中发现 AOA[24]。AOA 阳性与 1/3 的女性不明原因不孕症相关。各种自身抗体参与卵巢功能不全，已报道卵巢中存在多种靶点（图 22.1）。这些自身抗体结合到产生类固醇激素的细胞，包括颗粒细胞、卵母细胞、促性腺激素、促性腺激素受体、卵母细胞的透明带以及黄体[3]。最常见的靶点是促性腺激素及其受体，尤其是 FSH 的 β 亚基[25]。

大多数自身免疫性 POI 通常与临床或临床前自身免疫性 Addison 病相关。受累女性的体内总是存在针对类固醇生成酶的自身抗体，如 21-羟化酶（21OH）、17-羟化酶（17OH）、侧链裂解酶（P450scc）等类固醇生成细胞色素 P450 酶[11,25]，针对这些分子的自身抗体可识别由类固醇生成细胞自身免疫（SCA-POI）引起的 POI。AOA 的其他分子靶点包括胚胎所需的母体抗原（MATER）、乙醛脱氢酶-1A1（ALDH1A1）、硒结合蛋白 1（SBP1）、人热休克蛋白 90-β（HSP90β）、3β-羟类固醇脱氢酶（3b HSD）和 α-烯醇化酶[22,26]。此外，还有报道称抗心磷脂抗体和抗核抗体等多种自身抗体可作为卵巢自身免疫的标志物。可疑自身抗原和相关抗体的多样性表明，导致卵巢损伤的病理过程具有多重性[3]。

据报道，在受精失败和获卵失败的病例中，抗卵母细胞胞浆抗体的检出率较高[27,28]。这些抗体能识别 MATER，MATER 主要在甲状旁腺组织中表达，

淋巴细胞性卵巢炎	（1）抗类固醇生成细胞抗体：21-羟化酶抗体，17-羟化酶抗体和抗侧链裂解酶抗体（P450scc抗体）。 （2）抗甲状腺抗体（抗TPO和抗TG抗体）。 （3）抗核抗体（ANA）和抗心磷脂抗体。 （4）针对促性腺激素及其受体、MATER、醛缩酶1A1、硒结合蛋白1、人热休克蛋白90-β、3β-羟类固醇脱氢酶和α-烯醇化酶的自身抗体
自身免疫性疾病	（1）器官特异性自身免疫性疾病：桥本甲状腺炎、Graves病、重症肌无力、类风湿关节炎、恶性贫血、白癜风、克罗恩病、乳糜泻和多发性硬化病。 （2）非器官特异性（系统性）自身免疫性疾病：系统性红斑狼疮和特发性血小板减少症
自身免疫性多内分泌综合征	（1）Ⅰ型：自身免疫性多内分泌腺病-念珠菌病-外胚层营养不良症。 （2）Ⅱ型：以下3种中至少2种。Addisons病、自身免疫性甲状腺疾病引起的Graves病或甲状腺功能减退症和Ⅰ型糖尿病。Schmidt Carpenter综合征，包括肾上腺和甲状腺自身免疫以及1型糖尿病。 （3）Ⅲ型：自身免疫性甲状腺炎伴有另一种器官特异性自身免疫性疾病，如糖尿病、恶性贫血、白癜风、脱发、重症肌无力和Sjögren综合征，不包括Addison病

图 22.1 自身免疫性 POI 的免疫病理基础。

在卵母细胞中表达较少，并持续到囊胚阶段[29]。基因敲除小鼠模型表明，该基因失活会导致雌性小鼠不育[30]。在人类中，58%的自身免疫性多内分泌腺病综合征（APES）1 型患者、7%的 Addison 病患者、12%类固醇生成细胞自身免疫性 POI（SCA - POI）患者、0%的特发性 POI 患者和<1%的健康对照者检测到 MATER（人类同源物 NALP5）自身抗体。因此，NALP5 自身抗体是对卵泡膜细胞进行自身免疫攻击的女性亚群中卵巢自身免疫的间接标志物。基于上述原因，抗 21OH 抗体仍是诊断自身免疫性 POI 最准确的标志物。相反，缺乏抗 NALP5 抗体可能表明为特发性 POI[31]。

透明带是卵母细胞周围的一种细胞外物质，由糖蛋白组成，具有潜在的抗原性。透明带在精子附着、受精、支持卵母细胞与卵泡之间的通信等过程中起着不可或缺的作用。基于这些功能，推测抗透明带抗体可能破坏卵母细胞与颗粒细胞之间的通信[32]。抗透明带抗体在 IVF 反应差和受精率低的女性中一直都有报道[33]。然而，存在抗透明带抗体的女性并没有一致的模式，表明存在针对卵母细胞胞质或卵巢类固醇产生细胞的抗体[32]。为了澄清这些争议，已开发了高灵敏度的检测方法，但抗透明带抗体与不明原因不孕症之间尚未建立显著关联。

抗黄体抗体也被报道与 POI 相关。在 40 岁以下女性系统性红斑狼疮（SLE）患者血清中发现一种 67kDa 抗原，该抗原与抗黄体抗体相互作用。存在抗黄体抗体的 SLE 患者血清 FSH 水平较高，代表卵巢功能障碍的早期阶段[34]。因此，SLE 患者，特别是育龄期女性，应仔细评估自身免疫性 POI 的存在。

AOA 可能是自身免疫性 POI 的原因或结果。相反，其滴度与疾病的临床严重程度相关性很低[32]。此外，据报道，AOA 的假阳性率很高，在正常对照组中也存在显著阳性[32]，其部分原因可能是天然存在的抗白蛋白抗体[35]。在卵巢功能正常但患有各种器官特异性或系统性自身免疫性疾病或不明原因反复生殖失败的患者中，确定 AOA 的意义更具挑战性，原因如下：①AOA 可识别卵巢中的多个抗原靶点。②AOA 反应可能是一过性的或随时间变化的。③AOA 的存在并不意味着其在疾病表现中的致病作用[34]。需要进一步研究以确定 AOA 的具体分子靶点。

4 原发性卵巢功能不全

4.1 定义

POI 通常表现为 POF 或过早绝经，是导致女性不孕的常见原因。POI/POF 的定义是 40 岁前卵巢功能丧失，影响约 1%的育龄期女性[36]。主要症状是缺乏规律的月经周期、不孕症，以及与健康相关的生活质量下降[36]。根据欧洲人类生殖与胚胎学会

(ESHRE)指南,如果女性出现以下情况,即可诊断为POI/POF:①闭经或月经稀发至少4个月。②卵泡刺激素(FSH)水平升高,2次间隔至少4周,每次>25 U/L[36,37]。术语"不全"比"丧失"更可取,因为"不全"包括在卵泡完全衰竭之前仍有卵泡活动的低生育状态。相比之下,DOR的特征是月经规律,但反应卵巢储备功能的抗苗勒管激素(AMH)和窦卵泡计数(AFC)发生了改变[38]。

4.2 临床表现

POI的临床症状主要是雌激素缺乏所致,可能包括闭经、月经量少、血管运动障碍(潮热、盗汗)、睡眠障碍、外阴阴道萎缩、尿频变化和反复泌尿生殖道感染。情绪障碍包括易怒和情绪不稳定。其他内分泌失调,如雄激素缺乏,也会显著影响POI的症状。雄激素缺乏的特点是性欲低下、性交困难和缺乏活力[39]。POI女性患心血管疾病、痴呆症、认知能力下降、帕金森病和骨质疏松症的风险也会增加[37]。值得注意的是,这些患者会经历生殖障碍,如种植失败和RPL[37]。

4.3 原发性卵巢功能不全的组织病理学类型

POI可根据组织病理类型分为无卵泡型和有卵泡型。无卵泡型的特点是卵泡的耗竭和卵巢功能的丧失。性腺发育不全、混合性腺母细胞瘤及两性畸形等潜在疾病,都是卵泡完全耗竭的主要原因。与此相反,有卵泡型在组织学上表现为卵巢功能自发或诱导恢复,与以下三种卵巢情况有关:①卵巢炎(卵泡炎症)。②卵巢中卵泡数量减少。③大量原始卵泡(即抗性卵巢综合征)[40]。POI既不是不可逆的,也不是永久性的,因为卵巢中残留的卵母细胞可以补充、排卵和受精。据报道,POI/POF患者的自然妊娠率为2.17%[41]。随着疾病的进展,有卵泡型可能转变为无卵泡型。

4.4 原发性卵巢功能不全的病因

POI的病因很多。潜在的病因可分为不同组:遗传性、自身免疫性、环境性、医源性和特发性[42]。然而,在大多数情况下,无法确定确切的病因,因此仍属于特发性。

4.4.1 原发性卵巢功能不全的自身免疫病因学

约有4%的自发性原发POI女性患有自身免疫性卵巢炎[11]。POI的自身免疫病因可通过存在淋巴细胞性卵巢炎、卵巢抗原自身抗体和其他以血清卵巢、肾上腺皮质或类固醇细胞自身抗体为特征的自身免疫性疾病来确定(图22.1)。源于自身免疫的POI可分为肾上腺自身免疫、非肾上腺自身免疫和孤立性自身免疫。其中,特异性抗肾上腺抗体最为常见,占60%～80%。另外10%～30%的自身免疫性POI患者伴有自身免疫性疾病,尤其是自身免疫性甲状腺炎和1型糖尿病[43]。10%～20%的Addison病患者患有POI,2.5%～20%的POI女性表现出肾上腺自身免疫的迹象,包括血清中存在高水平针对类固醇生成细胞的抗体[44]。

自身免疫性疾病通常发生在育龄期女性,这将增加POI的风险。自身免疫性疾病的特点是存在器官特异性和非器官特异性自身抗体。器官特异性自身免疫性疾病,如桥本甲状腺炎、Graves病、肌无力、类风湿关节炎、恶性贫血、白癜风、克罗恩病、乳糜泻、多发性硬化症等,以及一些非器官特异性疾病,如SLE、特发性血小板减少症等,均与POI相关[45]。

POI通常与同一患者的多种自身免疫性疾病相关,即所谓的APES[46-48]。目前已描述了三种不同类型的APES:①APES-Ⅰ,又称自身免疫性多内分泌腺病-念珠菌病-外胚层营养不良症(APECED),包括肾上腺和甲状旁腺自身免疫[49]。它是由自身免疫调节基因突变引起的,具有T细胞介导的自身免疫特征。45%～60%的Ⅰ型APES患者会发展为POF。②APES-Ⅱ,又称为Schmidt Carpenter综合征,包括肾上腺和甲状腺自身免疫以及1型糖尿病。这些患者由于特定的HLA等位基因决定了自身反应性T细胞的靶组织,从而产生自身免疫[47],其中5%～50%的患者卵巢早衰。③APES-Ⅲ,包括恶性贫血或白癜风等自身免疫性疾病,但无Addison病。POI患者中APES-Ⅲ型的患病率为33.7%[48]。

4.4.2 其他病因

POI可为家族性,亦可为散发性。约有7%的病例属于纯遗传性的。遗传机制包括卵母细胞、酶或激素受体中的特定基因突变、减数分裂抑制对染色体的非特异性影响、原始卵泡池减少以及由于颗粒细胞凋亡或卵泡不完全成熟而导致的卵泡闭锁增加等[50]。

相当一部分POI是由环境因素引起的。最常见的相关环境因素是吸烟,是导致未来 POI 的重要风险因素[51]。此外,报道最多的物质是邻苯二甲酸酯、双酚 A 和杀虫剂,它们通过增加卵泡耗竭而降低卵巢功能,引起更年期提前开始。暴露发生在生命中的任何时间,都会产生这些影响,其主要机制似乎是窦前卵泡闭锁增加[52]。

如上所述,POI 可与局限性或系统性非肾上腺疾病相关,如甲状腺疾病、甲状旁腺功能减退症、垂体炎、1 型糖尿病和非内分泌自身免疫性疾病。

医源性 POI 常见于恶性肿瘤患者。常见的原因包括卵巢手术、化疗和(或)盆腔放疗[53]。

5 卵巢自身免疫性疾病

5.1 多囊卵巢综合征

PCOS 是一种代谢综合征,其特征为慢性稀发排卵/无排卵,临床和(或)生化高雄激素血症,阴道超声表现为多囊卵巢。PCOS 常见于育龄期女性,患病率为 6%~10%[54]。PCOS 的临床症状包括月经过少、不孕、痤疮、多毛、肥胖和黑棘皮病。此外,PCOS 患者可能合并其他内分泌和代谢性疾病,罹患乳腺癌或子宫内膜癌、糖耐量受损、胰岛素抵抗(IR)、维生素 D 缺乏、糖尿病和心血管疾病的风险增加[55,56]。据报道,长期使用雌激素而不添加孕酮可能会增加 PCOS 患者罹患乳腺癌或子宫内膜癌的风险[57]。

PCOS 发病机制的研究主要集中在 IR 和高雄激素血症两个相互关联的代谢因素上[58]。PCOS 与 IR 和甲状腺疾病密切相关,炎症和自身免疫因子在其发病机制中起重要作用。据报道,PCOS 患者甲状腺自身免疫的患病率高于一般女性人群。抗甲状腺过氧化物酶抗体(抗 TPO)和抗甲状腺球蛋白抗体(抗 TG)是甲状腺自身免疫、桥本甲状腺炎(HT)的主要生物标志物[59]。许多研究表明,甲状腺抗体与不孕症的特定原因(如 PCOS、子宫内膜异位症和卵巢储备功能减退)之间存在显著相关性[60]。例如,PCOS 和 HT 与育龄期女性的生殖问题相关,如不孕症、自然流产以及妊娠高血压、子痫前期、早产、低出生体重和产后出血等产科并发症[61],表明导致甲状腺功能减退和甲状腺功能亢进的功能性自身抗体可能会对卵巢造成类似的损害。引起甲状腺功能亢进的自身抗体可能诱发 PCOS,而甲状腺功能减退的自身抗体则可能导致 POI[9,62]。PCOS 和 HT 的共同存在与 AMH 水平降低有关,表明这些女性的卵巢储备功能减退可能比单纯 PCOS 患者更快、更严重[9,62]。然而,自身免疫性甲状腺炎和自身抗体暴露导致卵巢储备功能降低的持续时间尚未得到很好的阐明。

5.2 卵巢子宫内膜异位症

EMS 是一种雌激素依赖的慢性炎症性疾病,影响 5%~10% 的育龄期女性[10]。EMS 的定义是子宫内膜腺体和间质出现在子宫外部位[63]。月经逆行理论已被广泛接受为 EMS 的潜在病因。超过 1/3 的 EMS 患者伴有盆腔疼痛、排便困难和痛经,导致妊娠失败或不孕[10,64]。生殖障碍的潜在机制包括盆腔粘连扭曲、输卵管阻塞和卵泡生成减少。另一种解释 EMS 与不孕症关系的机制是慢性腹腔内炎症和促炎细胞因子增加。炎症状态可影响卵母细胞与精子的相互作用、胚胎发育和种植。近年来的研究报道,内分泌因素通过自分泌方式和免疫相关因子,特别是固有免疫,参与 EMS 相关不孕症的病理生理过程。此外,EMS 与自身抗体的存在有关。在不孕症患者的腹腔液和血清中,各种自身抗体,如抗核抗体(ANA)、抗 SSA/Ro、抗 SSB/la 和抗磷脂抗体(aPL)在 EMS 组中的检出率高于对照组[10]。

5.3 反复妊娠丢失

据推测,卵母细胞特异性遗传因素可能在 RPL 的发病机制中发挥作用。事实上,妊娠丢失的风险随着母亲年龄的增长而增加[65]。同样,也有报道称母亲年龄与卵母细胞染色体异常之间存在指数关系。由于卵巢的生理年龄决定妊娠结局,患有 POI 的女性卵巢功能衰退会导致卵母细胞质量和数量下降,减数分裂增加,胚胎非整倍体增加,继而导致流产[66,67]。研究发现,40%~50% 的早孕流产是由胎儿染色体异常引起的[68]。在接受辅助生殖技术(ART)的高龄女性中,供卵通常比其自身卵子具有更好的生殖结局,因为这些女性的生育能力下降主要与卵子的质量和数量有关,而不是与子宫环境有关[69]。在生理性(正常衰老)和病理性 POI 女性中,卵母细胞质量与 RPL 之间存在相关性,提示它们可能有共同的致病途径。探索与影响卵母细胞质量的生理衰老和病理性疾病相关的分子途径,有助于研究者和临床医生改善患者生育能力和妊娠结局。

卵巢储备的整个过程,包括建立、青春期激活、年龄依赖性或病理性耗竭,在很大程度上受遗传倾向的影响。涉及这些过程的基因缺陷可能引起一系列卵巢功能异常,包括 POI。迄今为止,已报道多个卵母细胞特异性基因的致病突变与 POI 相关,如 *BMP15* 和 *GDF9*,这些基因与人类卵母细胞成熟、受精、胚胎质量和妊娠结局呈正相关[70,71]。因此,卵巢内 BMP/GDF 系统在调节卵巢功能,发育为合格的卵母细胞以形成胚胎方面极其重要,而该系统的失调可能导致不孕、低生育力和流产[72]。由于 POI 与不孕症有关,导致 POI 的因素也可能与 RPL 有关。事实上,不孕症患者的流产风险增加,反之亦然[73]。此外,亦报道了 ART 治疗后的高流产率[74]。

FOXO3 和 FOXL2 属于 FOXO(叉头盒 O)家族转录因子,负调节卵泡成熟,维持正常卵巢功能。因此,这些蛋白的激活可能会阻止原始卵泡的生长并导致不孕[75]。研究还证明,包括 FOXO1 和 FOXL2 在内的 FOX 因子在子宫内膜蜕膜化过程中起着核心作用,子宫内膜蜕膜化通过维持胚胎植入和生长所需的适当微环境,对于胚胎植入和胎盘形成不可或缺[75]。由于这些 FOX 蛋白在子宫组织中的高水平表达且具有多种功能,推测这些基因的突变可能在 RPL 中具有重要意义,并可能在 POI 中发挥作用[76,77]。

5.4 不明原因不孕症

不明原因不孕症占不孕女性的 10%~17%[78]。不明原因或特发性不孕症是指夫妇在没有明确原因的情况下无法受孕。68% 的不明原因不孕症患者 AOA 阳性,ALDH1A1 和 SBP1 是不明原因不孕症患者卵巢自身免疫的独特抗原[8]。ALDH1A1 是乙醛脱氢酶的胞质形式,参与维甲酸代谢[79]。由于维甲酸参与类固醇生成[80]、卵母细胞成熟[81]、早期胚胎发育[82]、FSH 诱导的 FSH 和 LH 受体表达降低[83],以及颗粒细胞成熟[84],ALDH1A1 表达改变可能会影响生殖过程。SBP1 是一种胞质蛋白,在卵巢表面的上皮细胞中表达。在不明原因不孕女性中,卵泡液中的硒含量降低[86],而 SP56(SBP1 的结合肽)会降低小鼠模型的生育能力[87]。基于这些发现,推测 SBP1 自身抗体对不孕症有不利影响。自身抗体如 AOA、抗磷脂抗体、抗甲状腺抗体、失调的细胞因子和趋化因子可能导致不明原因不孕症。因此,获得性免疫反应的改变可能导致不孕,尤其是不明原因不孕症[88,89]。

6 原发性卵巢功能不全的诊断

POI 的诊断可通过详细的病史记录、激素检查和超声评估来完成(图 22.2)。目前对于 POI 的最佳诊断标准尚无共识。ESHRE 指南建议以下诊断标准:①月经过少或闭经至少 4 个月。②FSH 水平升高>25 U/L,至少间隔 4 周重复一次[36]。美国妇产科学会建议诊断标准为:①月经不规律至少连续 3 个月。②FSH 和雌二醇水平(通常以 FSH 水平升高>30~40 U/L 和雌激素水平降低≤50 pg/mL 或根据实验室标准确认)至少每隔 1 个月重复一次。③泌乳素和甲状腺功能检测[90,91]。虽然抗苗勒管激素(AMH)也被提出作为诊断标准,但只有当与 FSH 和雌激素水平一起解释时才具有重要意义[92]。抑制素 B 不适合作为诊断指标,因为它随月经周期天数的变化而变化[93]。盆腔超声检查有助于诊断。典型的发现是卵巢小,腔内卵泡少,卵泡无生长[94]。

6.1 诊断方法

尽管对 POI 的潜在病因进行了许多探索,但仍缺乏确凿证据证明 POI 与相关因素之间存在因果关系。因此,建议采用以下筛查方法以诊断 POI。

(1) 染色体异常。

a. 对患有 POI 的女性进行脆性 X 检测。

b. 应考虑筛查 Turner 综合征、X 三体综合征、*FMR1* 和位于 X 染色体上的 *BMP15* 突变,因为这些情况是与 POI 相关的常见染色体和基因异常。

c. 一旦在女性中检测到 Y 染色体,建议进行性腺切除术,因为这些女性罹患性腺肿瘤的风险很高。

(2) 自身免疫异常。

a. 建议筛查肾上腺自身抗体、21-羟化酶抗体(21OH-Ab)或肾上腺皮质抗体(ACA),以识别可能患有 Addison 病的患者。

b. 筛查甲状腺抗体(如 TPO-Ab)似乎是合理的,因为 POI 通常与甲状腺功能减退有关。

c. 建议 POI 患者筛查其他自身免疫性疾病,如自身免疫性多内分泌腺病综合征(APS)、Sjögren 综合征和 1 型糖尿病。

(3) 由于与 POI 可能存在因果关系,因此应筛查医疗或手术干预史[36]。例如,卵巢肿瘤患者可能接受过化疗、放疗和卵巢手术操作,导致性腺供血减少。

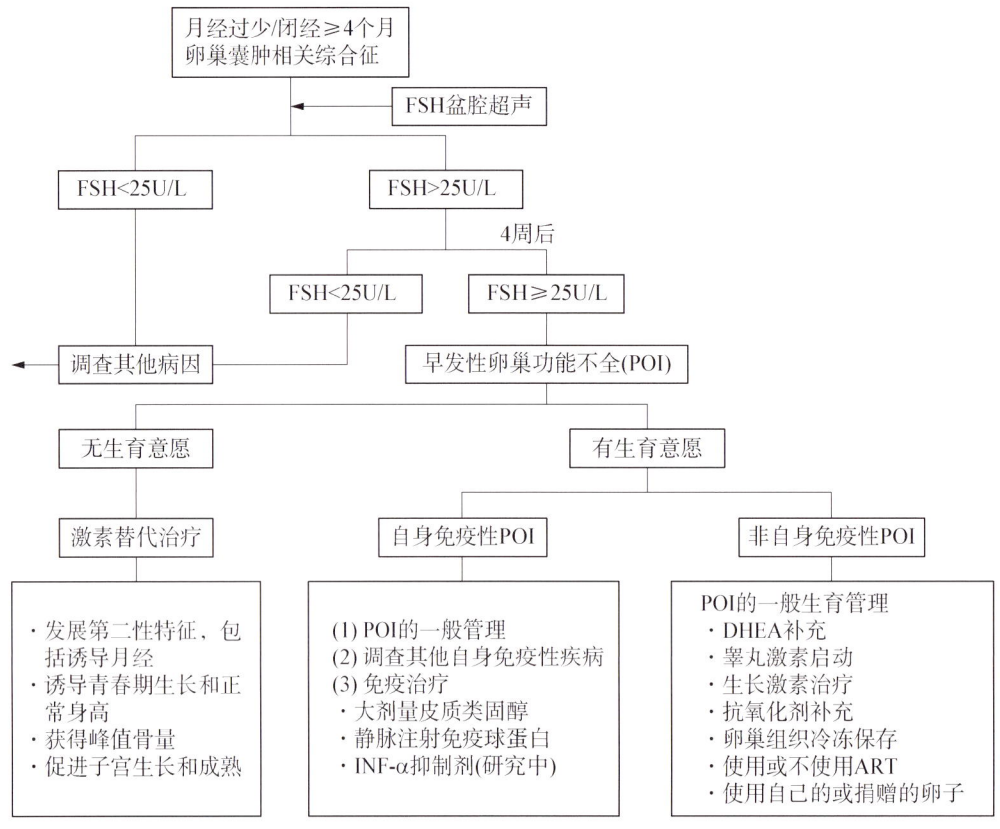

图 22.2　POI 的诊断策略和管理。

（4）可考虑进行感染筛查，包括流行性腮腺炎和人类免疫缺陷病毒。然而，目前的证据还不足以进行常规筛查[36,95]。

（5）可考虑筛选污染物和毒素，因为它们可能影响卵巢。

6.2　自身免疫性卵巢炎的诊断

自身免疫性卵巢炎的诊断通常具有挑战性，因为没有一种单一的检测方法可以诊断自身免疫性卵巢炎，而且临床症状可能因其预后和其他基础疾病而异。POI 患者应检测抗肾上腺抗体（最常见的抗 21-羟化酶，CYP21）和抗甲状腺抗体（抗 TPO 和抗 TG 抗体）。这些抗体的存在可能提示 POI 的自身免疫原因。此外，必要时还应考虑对肾上腺和甲状腺异常进行进一步评估和治疗，以改善女性的生育能力[96]。

7　自身免疫性原发性卵巢功能不全的治疗

7.1　有生育意愿的女性

大多数自身免疫性卵巢炎患者可能仍有一定程度的卵巢功能，但在接受 ART 周期治疗前已诊断为 POI、POF、卵巢低反应（POR）和 DOR。免疫抑制疗法是保留初级和原始卵泡的自身免疫性卵巢炎女性恢复卵巢功能的一种可行方法。据报道，使用大剂量皮质类固醇和静脉注射免疫球蛋白治疗可使 POI 女性的卵巢功能恢复正常[97,98]。在治疗伴有自身免疫性卵巢损伤的 POI 时，其他不常用的实验性免疫治疗方法可能是单克隆抗体[如肿瘤坏死因子（TNF）-α 抑制剂]，以恢复免疫反应，尤其是 Th2 占优势的状态[99]。然而，关于免疫疗法在接受 ART 周期治疗的自身免疫性卵巢炎女性中可能发挥的作用，目前还没有系统的研究报告。不过，考虑到其潜在的病因，对这一人群应用免疫疗法有可能改善生殖结局。

肾上腺网状带的自身免疫攻击会减少肾上腺雄激素的产生而影响卵巢功能，从而导致低雄激素水平。雄激素水平低对卵巢功能有不利影响。因此，补充 DHEA 对这些患有肾上腺和甲状腺自身免疫以及合并低睾酮和低 DHEAS 的女性应该有益处[100]。在过去的几十年中，各种研究评估了在控制性卵巢过度刺激前或期间补充睾酮对 POR 女性的作用,但结果并不一致[101]。最近一项随机对照试验的荟萃分析显示,补充睾酮可显著增加卵母细胞、胚胎和MII卵母细胞的数量,对POR有益[102]。大量证据证实了睾酮在早期卵泡生长发育和颗粒细胞增殖中的关键作用,如促进早期卵泡发育、增加窦前卵泡和窦卵泡的数量和易感性、刺激初级卵泡发育为次级卵泡等[102,103]。

据报道,在小鼠模型中,GH治疗可通过激活卵巢组织中的Notch-1信号通路促进卵巢组织修复、雌激素释放和卵母细胞成熟[104]。此外,GH治疗联合促性腺激素可上调卵巢内IGF-I,增强FSH对卵泡发生的刺激作用[105,106]。然而,GH治疗的生殖结局在POR患者中一直是有争议的,目前仅推荐给GH缺乏(生长激素激发试验阴性)的POR患者[106,107]。

最后,对于需要保留生育能力的POI女性,有报道称采用玻璃化技术冷冻卵巢组织,然后体外激活休眠/抑制的卵泡[108]。

7.2 无生育意愿的女性

由于卵巢自身免疫具有广泛的临床表现和生殖问题,因此根据患者的年龄、临床症状和生殖愿望了解患者的需求非常重要。对于化疗或放疗引起的青春期延迟患者,诱导青春期的治疗目标是:①发展第二性特征,包括诱导月经。②诱导青春期生长和正常身高。③获得峰值骨量。④促进子宫生长和成熟[91]。建议采用激素替代疗法(HRT)来缓解POI患者的低雌激素症状。然而,由于HRT可导致包括乳腺癌在内的不良风险,且POI患者有各种潜在病因,因此需要定期随访。例如:①建议在Turner综合征女性的正常生育期使用HRT。②有乳腺癌病史的女性,禁止使用HRT。③HRT对EMS患者可能有效。④对于高血压、肥胖或有静脉血栓栓塞史的女性,经皮雌二醇是首选的给药方法[109-112]。⑤患有偏头痛或肌瘤的女性,HRT不是禁忌证。关于雄激素治疗,只有有限的数据支持,长期健康影响尚不清楚。还鼓励保持积极的生活方式,避免或停止吸烟,保持适当的体重,以优化骨骼健康[36,37]。目前还没有关于免疫治疗在这一人群中可能作用的系统研究报道。

8 生殖结局

POI患者的生殖结局可能因诊断时残留的卵泡而异。如果POI患者保留了初级和原始卵泡并立即开始治疗,则其生殖结局比未保留初级和原始卵泡或延迟治疗的女性更为有利。一些POI患者可通过激素和免疫治疗(无论是否ART)生育自己的孩子。晚期POI患者通常没有机会获得自己的卵子,只能接受捐卵周期治疗。

9 总结和建议

- 自身免疫,包括抗磷脂综合征(APS)、甲状腺和卵巢自身免疫,主要影响育龄期女性。
- POI的诊断可根据月经紊乱、激素水平和生化证实,包括血清AMH和AFC的超声评估。
- POI的潜在病因包括遗传、环境、医源性、自身免疫和特发性因素。
- POI的自身免疫病因可通过淋巴细胞性卵巢炎、卵巢抗原自身抗体和其他以血清卵巢、肾上腺皮质或类固醇细胞自身抗体为特征的自身免疫性疾病的存在来确定。
- 在患有自身免疫性卵巢炎的女性中,可能出现多囊样卵巢和血清LH水平升高,会被误认为是多囊卵巢综合征。
- 治疗POI前,应检测抗肾上腺和抗甲状腺抗体。
- 自身免疫性卵巢炎中可疑自身抗原和相关抗体的多样性表明,导致卵巢损伤的自身免疫性病理具有多样性。
- 大剂量皮质类固醇和静脉注射免疫球蛋白治疗可使自身免疫性POI患者的卵巢功能恢复正常。
- 关于免疫治疗在接受ART周期的自身免疫性卵巢炎患者中可能发挥的作用,尚无系统研究报告。
- 考虑到自身免疫的病因,对患有自身免疫性POI的女性应用免疫治疗有可能改善生殖结局。

参考文献

[1] Luborsky J. Ovarian autoimmune disease and ovarian autoantibodies. J Womens Health Gend Based Med 2002;11(7):585-99.

[2] Falorni A, Laureti S, Candeloro P, et al. Steroid-cell autoantibodies are preferentially expressed in women with premature ovarian failure who have adrenal autoimmunity. Fertil Steril 2002;78(2):270-9.

[3] Forges T, Monnier-Barbarino P, Faure GC, Bene MC. Autoimmunity and antigenic targets in ovarian pathology. Hum Reprod Update 2004;10(2):163-75.

[4] Kelkar RL, Meherji PK, Kadam SS, Gupta SK, Nandedkar TD. Circulating auto-antibodies against the zona pellucida and thyroid microsomal antigen in women with premature ovarian failure. J Reprod Immunol 2005;66(1):53-67.

[5] Luborsky J, Llanes B, Davies S, Binor Z, Radwanska E, Pong R. Ovarian autoimmunity: greater frequency of autoantibodies in premature menopause and unexplained infertility than in the general population. Clin Immunol 1999;90(3):368-74.

[6] Yan G, Schoenfeld D, Penney C, Hurxthal K, Taylor AE, Faustman D. Identification of premature ovarian failure patients with underlying autoimmunity. J Women's Health Gend Based Med 2000;9(3):275-87.

[7] Mande PV, Parikh FR, Hinduja I, et al. Identification and validation of candidate biomarkers involved in human ovarian autoimmunity. Reprod Biomed Online 2011;23(4):471-83.

[8] Edassery SL, Shatavi SV, Kunkel JP, et al. Autoantigens in ovarian autoimmunity associated with unexplained infertility and premature ovarian failure. Fertil Steril 2010;94(7):2636-41.

[9] Serin AN, Birge O, Uysal A, Gorar S, Tekeli F. Hashimoto's thyroiditis worsens ovaries in polycystic ovary syndrome patients compared to anti-Mullerian hormone levels. BMC Endocr Disord 2021;21(1):44.

[10] de Ziegler D, Borghese B, Chapron C. Endometriosis and infertility: pathophysiology and management. Lancet. 2010;376(9742):730-8.

[11] Bakalov VK, Anasti JN, Calis KA, et al. Autoimmune oophoritis as a mechanism of follicular dysfunction in women with 46, XX spontaneous premature ovarian failure. Fertil Steril 2005;84(4):958-65.

[12] Jilma B, Dirnberger E, Loscher I, et al. Menstrual cycle-associated changes in blood levels of interleukin-6, alpha1 acid glycoprotein, and C-reactive protein. J Lab Clin Med 1997;130(1):69-75.

[13] Wang W, Sung N, Gilman-Sachs A, Kwak-Kim JT. Helper (Th) cell profiles in pregnancy and recurrent pregnancy losses: Th1/Th2/Th9/Th17/Th22/Tfh Cells. Front Immunol 2020;11:2025.

[14] Yang X, Gilman-Sachs A, Kwak-Kim J. Ovarian and endometrial immunity during the ovarian cycle. J Reprod Immunol 2019;133:7-14.

[15] Clancy KB, Baerwald AR, Pierson RA. Systemic inflammation is associated with ovarian follicular dynamics during the human menstrual cycle. PLoS One 2013;8(5):e64807.

[16] Ledee N, Petitbarat M, Chevrier L, et al. The uterine immune profile may help women with repeated unexplained embryo implantation failure after in vitro fertilization. Am J Reprod Immunol 2016;75(3):388-401.

[17] Straub RH. The complex role of estrogens in inflammation. Endocr Rev 2007;28(5):521-74.

[18] Kwak-Kim JY, Chung-Bang HS, Ng SC, et al. Increased T helper 1 cytokine responses by circulating T cells are present in women with recurrent pregnancy losses and in infertile women with multiple implantation failures after IVF. Hum Reprod 2003;18(4):767-73.

[19] Welt CK. Autoimmune oophoritis in the adolescent. Ann N Y Acad Sci 2008;1135:118-22.

[20] La Marca A, Brozzetti A, Sighinolfi G, Marzotti S, Volpe A, Falorni A. Primary ovarian insufficiency: autoimmune causes. Curr Opin Obstet Gynecol 2010;22(4):277-82.

[21] Kalantaridou SN, Braddock DT, Patronas NJ, Nelson LM. Treatment of autoimmune premature ovarian failure. Hum Reprod 1999;14(7):1777-82.

[22] Ebrahimi M, Akbari Asbagh F. The role of autoimmunity in premature ovarian failure. Iran J Reprod Med 2015;13(8):461-72.

[23] Li J, Jin H, Zhang F, et al. Treatment of autoimmune ovarian disease by co-administration with mouse zona pellucida protein 3 and DNA vaccine through induction of adaptive regulatory T cells. J Gene Med 2008;10(7):810-20.

[24] Xiong J, Tan R, Wang W, Wang H, Pu D, Wu J. Evaluation of CD4(+)CD25(+)FOXP3(+) regulatory T cells and FOXP3 mRNA in premature ovarian insufficiency. Climacteric. 2020;23(3):267-72.

[25] Bakalov VK, Vanderhoof VH, Bondy CA, Nelson LM. Adrenal antibodies detect asymptomatic auto-immune adrenal insufficiency in young women with spontaneous premature ovarian failure. Hum Reprod 2002;17(8):2096-100.

[26] Kobayashi M, Nakashima A, Yoshino O, et al. Decreased effector regulatory T cells and increased activated CD4(1) T cells in premature ovarian insufficiency. Am J Reprod Immunol 2019;81(6):e13125.

[27] Luborsky JL, Visintin I, Boyers S, Asari T, Caldwell B, DeCherney A. Ovarian antibodies detected by immobilized antigen immunoassay in patients with premature ovarian failure. J Clin Endocrinol Metab 1990;70(1):69-75.

[28] Pires ES. Multiplicity of molecular and cellular targets in human ovarian autoimmunity: an update. J Assist Reprod Genet 2010;27(9-10):519-24.

[29] Tong ZB, Nelson LM. A mouse gene encoding an oocyte antigen associated with autoimmune premature ovarian failure. Endocrinology. 1999;140(8):3720-6.

[30] Nelson LM. Autoimmune ovarian failure: comparing the mouse model and the human disease. J Soc Gynecol Investig 2001;8(1 Suppl Proceedings):S55-7.

[31] Brozzetti A, Alimohammadi M, Morelli S, et al. Autoantibody response against NALP5/MATER in primary ovarian insufficiency and in autoimmune'Addison's disease. J Clin Endocrinol Metab 2015;100(5):1941-8.

[32] Novosad JA, Kalantaridou SN, Tong ZB, Nelson LM. Ovarian antibodies as detected by indirect immunofluorescence are unreliable in the diagnosis of autoimmune premature ovarian failure: a controlled evaluation. BMC Women's Health 2003;3(1):2.

[33] Mardesic T, Ulcova-Gallova Z, Huttelova R, et al. The influence of different types of antibodies on in vitro fertilization results. Am J Reprod Immunol 2000;43(1):1-5.

[34] Pasoto SG, Viana VS, Mendonca BB, Yoshinari NH, Bonfa E. Anti-corpus luteum antibody: a novel serological marker for ovarian dysfunction in systemic lupus erythematosus? J Rheumatol 1999;26(5):1087-93.

[35] Pires ES, Parte PP, Meherji PK, Khan SA, Khole VV. Naturally occurring anti-albumin antibodies are responsible for false positivity in diagnosis of autoimmune premature ovarian failure. J Histochem Cytochem 2006;54(4):397-405.

[36] European Society for Human R, Embryology Guideline Group on POI, Webber L, et al. ESHRE guideline: management of women with premature ovarian insufficiency. Hum Reprod 2016;31(5):926-37.

[37] Faubion SS, Kuhle CL, Shuster LT, Rocca WA. Long-term health consequences of premature or early menopause and considerations for management. Climacteric. 2015;18(4):483-91.

[38] Practice Committee of the American Society for Reproductive M. Testing and interpreting measures of ovarian reserve: a committee opinion. Fertil Steril 2012;98(6):1407-15.

[39] Domniz N, Meirow D. Premature ovarian insufficiency and autoimmune diseases. Best Pract Res Clin Obstet Gynaecol 2019;60:42-55.

[40] Hoek A, Schoemaker J, Drexhage HA. Premature ovarian failure and ovarian autoimmunity. Endocr Rev 1997;18(1):107-34.

[41] Gargus E, Deans R, Anazodo A, Woodruff TK. Management of primary ovarian insufficiency symptoms in survivors of childhood and adolescent cancer. J Natl Compr Canc Netw 2018;16(9):1137-49.

[42] Laven JS. Primary ovarian insufficiency. Semin Reprod Med 2016;34(4):230-4.

[43] Ellis JS, Wan X, Braley-Mullen H. Transient depletion of CD4 + CD25 + regulatory T cells results in multiple autoimmune diseases in wild-type and B-cell-deficient NOD mice. Immunology. 2013;139(2):179-86.

[44] Irvine WJ, Chan MM, Scarth L, et al. Immunological aspects of premature ovarian failure associated with idiopathic Addison's disease. Lancet. 1968;2(7574):883-7.

[45] Aikawa NE, Sallum AM, Pereira RM, et al. Subclinical impairment of ovarian reserve in juvenile systemic lupus erythematosus after cyclophosphamide therapy. Clin Exp Rheumatol 2012;30(3):445-9.

[46] Ahonen P, Myllarniemi S, Sipila I, Perheentupa J. Clinical variation of autoimmune polyendocrinopathy-candidiasis-ectodermal dystrophy (APECED) in a series of 68 patients. N Engl J Med 1990;322(26):1829-36.

[47] Michels AW, Gottlieb PA. Autoimmune polyglandular syndromes. Nat Rev Endocrinol 2010;6(5):270-7.

[48] Szlendak-Sauer K, Jakubik D, Kunicki M, Skorska J, Smolarczyk R. Autoimmune polyglandular syndrome type 3 (APS - 3) among patients with premature ovarian insufficiency (POI). Eur J Obstet Gynecol Reprod Biol 2016;203:61-5.

[49] Perheentupa J. APS-I/APECED: the clinical disease and therapy. Endocrinol Metab Clin North Am 2002;31(2):295-320 vi.

[50] Vujovic S. Aetiology of premature ovarian failure. Menopause Int 2009;15(2):72-5.

[51] Jin M, Yu Y, Huang H. An update on primary ovarian insufficiency. Sci China Life Sci 2012;55(8):677-86.

[52] Hassold T, Hall H, Hunt P. The origin of human aneuploidy: where we have been, where we are going. Hum Mol Genet 2007;R203-8 16 Spec No. 2.

[53] Bricaire L, Laroche E, Bourcigaux N, Donadille B, Christin-Maitre S. Premature ovarian failures. Presse Med 2013;42(11):1500-7.

[54] Azziz R, Woods KS, Reyna R, Key TJ, Knochenhauer ES, Yildiz BO. The prevalence and features of the polycystic ovary syndrome in an unselected population. J Clin Endocrinol Metab 2004;89(6):2745-9.

[55] Wild RA, Carmina E, Diamanti-Kandarakis E, et al. Assessment of cardiovascular risk and prevention of cardiovascular disease in women with the polycystic ovary syndrome: a consensus statement by the androgen excess and polycystic ovary syndrome (AE-PCOS) society. J Clin Endocrinol Metab 2010;95(5):2038-49.

[56] Fux Otta C, Fiol de Cuneo M, Szafryk de Mereshian P. Polycystic ovary syndrome: physiopathology review. Rev Fac Cien Med Univ Nac Cordoba 2013;70(1):27-30.

[57] Hardiman P, Pillay OC, Atiomo W. Polycystic ovary syndrome and endometrial carcinoma. Lancet. 2003;361(9371):1810-12.

[58] Buccola JM, Reynolds EE. Polycystic ovary syndrome: a review for primary providers. Prim Care 2003;30(4):697-710.

[59] Hepsen S, Karakose M, Cakal E, et al. The assessment of thyroid autoantibody levels in euthyroid patients with polycystic ovary syndrome. J Turk Ger Gynecol Assoc 2018;19(4):215-19.

[60] Ho CW, Chen HH, Hsieh MC, et al. Increased risk of polycystic ovary syndrome and it's comorbidities in women with autoimmune thyroid disease. Int J Env Res Public Health 2020;17(7).

[61] Medenica S, Nedeljkovic O, Radojevic N, Stojkovic M, Trbojevic B, Pajovic B. Thyroid dysfunction and thyroid autoimmunity in euthyroid women in achieving fertility. Eur Rev Med Pharmacol Sci 2015;19(6):977-87.

[62] Gleicher N, Barad D, Weghofer A. Functional autoantibodies, a new paradigm in autoimmunity? Autoimmun Rev 2007;7(1):42-5.

[63] Bulun SE. Endometriosis. N Engl J Med 2009;360(3):268-79.

[64] Tanbo T, Fedorcsak P. Endometriosis-associated infertility: aspects of pathophysiological mechanisms and treatment options. Acta Obstet Gynecol Scand 2017;96(6):659-67.

[65] Nybo Andersen AM, Wohlfahrt J, Christens P, Olsen J, Melbye M. Maternal age and fetal loss: population based register linkage study. BMJ. 2000;320(7251):1708-12.

[66] El-Toukhy T, Khalaf Y, Hart R, Taylor A, Braude P. Young age does not protect against the adverse effects of reduced ovarian reserve-an eight year study. Hum Reprod 2002;17(6):1519-24.

[67] Dean DD, Agarwal S, Tripathi P. Connecting links between genetic factors defining ovarian reserve and recurrent miscarriages. J Assist Reprod Genet 2018;35(12):2121-8.

[68] Choi TY, Lee HM, Park WK, Jeong SY, Moon HS. Spontaneous abortion and recurrent miscarriage: a comparison of cytogenetic diagnosis in 250 cases. Obstet Gynecol Sci 2014;57(6):518-25.

[69] Wang YA, Farquhar C, Sullivan EA. Donor age is a major determinant of success of oocyte donation/recipient programme. Hum Reprod 2012;27(1):118-25.

[70] Gode F, Gulekli B, Dogan E, et al. Influence of follicular fluid GDF9 and BMP15 on embryo quality. Fertil Steril 2011;95(7):2274-8.

[71] Wu YT, Tang L, Cai J, et al. High bone morphogenetic protein-15 level in follicular fluid is associated with high quality oocyte and subsequent embryonic development. Hum Reprod 2007;22(6):1526-31.

[72] Li Y, Li RQ, Ou SB, et al. Increased GDF9 and BMP15 mRNA levels in cumulus granulosa cells correlate with oocyte maturation, fertilization, and embryo quality in humans. Reprod Biol Endocrinol 2014;12:81.

[73] Coulam CB. Association between infertility and spontaneous abortion. Am J Reprod Immunol 1992;27(3-4):128-9.

[74] Torrealday S, Kodaman P, Pal L. Premature ovarian insufficiency — an update on recent advances in understanding and management. F1000Res. 2017;6:2069.

[75] Liu L, Rajareddy S, Reddy P, et al. Infertility caused by retardation of follicular development in mice with oocyte-specific expression of Foxo3a. Development. 2007;134(1):199-209.

[76] Elbaz M, Hadas R, Bilezikjian LM, Gershon E. Uterine Foxl2 regulates the adherence of the trophectoderm cells to the endometrial epithelium. Reprod Biol Endocrinol 2018;16(1):12.

[77] Popovici RM, Betzler NK, Krause MS, et al. Gene expression profiling of human endometrial-trophoblast interaction in a coculture model. Endocrinology. 2006;147(12):5662-75.

[78] Gelbaya TA, Potdar N, Jeve YB, Nardo LG. Definition and epidemiology of unexplained infertility. Obstet Gynecol Surv 2014;69(2):109-15.

[79] Marchitti SA, Brocker C, Stagos D, Vasiliou V. Non-P450 aldehyde oxidizing enzymes: the aldehyde dehy-drogenase superfamily. Expert Opin Drug Metab Toxicol 2008;4(6):697-720.

[80] Clagett-Dame M, DeLuca HF. The role of vitamin A in mammalian reproduction and embryonic develop-ment. Annu Rev Nutr 2002;22:347-81.

[81] Mohan M, Thirumalapura NR, Malayer J. Bovine cumulus-granulosa cells contain biologically active retinoid receptors that can respond to retinoic acid. Reprod Biol Endocrinol 2003;1:104.

[82] Mark M, Ghyselinck NB, Chambon P. Function of retinoic acid receptors during embryonic development. Nucl Recept Signal 2009;7:e002.

[83] Minegishi T, Hirakawa T, Kishi H, et al. The mechanisms of retinoic acid-induced regulation on the follicle-stimulating hormone receptor in rat granulosa cells. Biochim Biophys Acta 2000;1495(3):203-11.

[84] Hattori M, Takesue K, Nishida N, Kato Y, Fujihara N. Inhibitory effect of retinoic acid on the development of immature porcine granulosa cells to mature cells. J Mol Endocrinol 2000;25(1):53-61.

[85] Huang KC, Park DC, Ng SK, et al. Selenium binding protein 1 in ovarian cancer. Int J Cancer 2006;118(10):2433-40.

[86] Paszkowski T, Traub AI, Robinson SY, McMaster D. Selenium dependent glutathione peroxidase activity in human follicular fluid. Clin Chim Acta 1995;236(2):173-80.

[87] Hardy CM, Clydesdale G, Mobbs KJ. Development of mouse-specific contraceptive vaccines: infertility in mice immunized with peptide and polyepitope antigens. Reproduction. 2004;128(4):395-407.

[88] An LF, Zhang XH, Sun XT, Zhao LH, Li S, Wang WH. Unexplained infertility patients have increased serum IL-2, IL-4, IL-6, IL-8, IL-21, TNFalpha, IFNgamma and increased Tfh/CD4 T cell ratio: increased Tfh and IL-21 strongly correlate with presence of autoantibodies. Immunol Invest 2015;44(2):164-73.

[89] Sauer R, Roussev R, Jeyendran RS, Coulam CB. Prevalence of antiphospholipid antibodies among women experiencing unexplained infertility and recurrent implantation failure. Fertil Steril 2010;93(7):2441-3.

[90] Nelson LM. Clinical practice. Primary ovarian insufficiency. N Engl J Med 2009;360(6):606-14.

[91] Collins G, Patel B, Thakore S, Liu J. Primary ovarian insufficiency: current concepts. South Med J 2017;110(3):147-53.

[92] Rudnicka E, Kruszewska J, Klicka K, et al. Premature ovarian insufficiency-aetiopathology, epidemiology, and diagnostic evaluation. Prz Menopauzalny 2018; 17 (3):105-8.

[93] Nelson SM. Biomarkers of ovarian response: current and future applications. Fertil Steril 2013;99(4):963-9.

[94] Beck-Peccoz P, Persani L. Premature ovarian failure. Orphanet J Rare Dis 2006;1:9.

[95] Kokcu A. Premature ovarian failure from current perspective. Gynecol Endocrinol 2010;26(8):555-62.

[96] Tsigkou A, Marzotti S, Borges L, et al. High serum inhibin concentration discriminates autoimmune oophoritis from other forms of primary ovarian insufficiency. J Clin Endocrinol Metab 2008;93(4):1263-9.

[97] Corenblum B, Rowe T, Taylor PJ. High-dose, short-term glucocorticoids for the treatment of infertility resulting from premature ovarian failure. Fertil Steril 1993;59(5):988-91.

[98] Cowchock FS, McCabe JL, Montgomery BB. Pregnancy after corticosteroid administration in premature ovarian failure (polyglandular endocrinopathy syndrome). Am J Obstet Gynecol 1988;158(1):118-19.

[99] Simon A, Laufer N. Repeated implantation failure: clinical approach. Fertil Steril 2012;97(5):1039-43.

[100] Gleicher N, Kushnir VA, Darmon SK, et al. New PCOS-like phenotype in older infertile women of likely autoimmune adrenal etiology with high AMH but low androgens. J Steroid Biochem Mol Biol 2017;167:144-52.

[101] Bosdou JK, Venetis CA, Dafopoulos K, et al. Transdermal testosterone pretreatment in poor responders undergoing ICSI: a randomized clinical trial. Hum Reprod 2016;31(5):977-85.

[102] Noventa M, Vitagliano A, Andrisani A, et al. Testosterone therapy for women with poor ovarian response undergoing IVF: a meta-analysis of randomized controlled trials. J Assist Reprod Genet 2019;36(4):673-83.

[103] Montoya-Botero P, Rodriguez-Purata J, Polyzos NP. Androgen supplementation in assisted reproduction: where are we in 2019? Curr Opin Obstet Gynecol 2019;31(3):188-94.

[104] Liu TE, Wang S, Zhang L, et al. Growth hormone treatment of premature ovarian failure in a mouse model via stimulation of the Notch-1 signaling pathway. Exp Ther Med 2016;12(1):215-21.

[105] Adashi EY, Resnick CE, D'Ercole AJ, Svoboda ME, Van Wyk JJ. Insulin-like growth factors as intraovarian regulators of granulosa cell growth and function. Endocr Rev 1985;6

(3):400-20.

[106] Blumenfeld Z, Dirnfeld M, Gonen Y, Abramovici H. Growth hormone co-treatment for ovulation induction may enhance conception in the co-treatment and succeeding cycles, in clonidine negative but not clonidine positive patients. Hum Reprod 1994;9(2):209-13.

[107] Albu D, Albu A. Is growth hormone administration essential for in vitro fertilization treatment of female patients with growth hormone deficiency? Syst Biol Reprod Med 2019;65(1):71-4.

[108] Suzuki N, Yoshioka N, Takae S, et al. Successful fertility preservation following ovarian tissue vitrification in patients with primary ovarian insufficiency. Hum Reprod 2015;30(3):608-15.

[109] Canonico M, Oger E, Conard J, et al. Obesity and risk of venous thromboembolism among postmenopausal women: differential impact of hormone therapy by route of estrogen administration. The ESTHER Study. J Thromb Haemost 2006;4(6):1259-65.

[110] Canonico M, Plu-Bureau G, Lowe GD, Scarabin PY. Hormone replacement therapy and risk of venous thromboembolism in postmenopausal women: systematic review and meta-analysis. BMJ. 2008;336(7655):1227-31.

[111] Langrish JP, Mills NL, Bath LE, et al. Cardiovascular effects of physiological and standard sex steroid replacement regimens in premature ovarian failure. Hypertension. 2009;53(5):805-11.

[112] White WB. Drospirenone with 17beta-estradiol in the postmenopausal woman with hypertension. Climacteric. 2007;10(Suppl 1):25-31.

第 23 章

多囊卵巢综合征与生殖障碍

Polycystic ovarian syndrome and reproductive failure

Joseph Duero and Reshef Tal

Department of Obstetrics, Gynecology and Reproductive Sciences, Yale School of Medicine, New Haven, CT, United States

1 引言

多囊卵巢综合征（PCOS）是一种复杂的内分泌疾病，影响约 10% 的育龄期女性[1]。1935 年 Stein 和 Leventhal 首次描述了 PCOS[2]，其具有 3 个主要特征：临床或生化高雄激素血症、排卵功能障碍和多囊卵巢。根据鹿特丹标准[3,4]，其中 2 个特征必须同时存在才能确诊。PCOS 的临床表现因人而异[5]。高雄激素血症常导致痤疮、脱发和（或）多毛症[6]。慢性稀发排卵或无排卵可引起闭经或少经[7]。PCOS 患者通常卵巢增大，间质体积增大，卵泡发育停滞引起卵泡数量增加[8]。超过半数的 PCOS 患者肥胖[9]，这既可归因于胰岛素抵抗特征，也可加剧胰岛素抵抗特征，65%～70% 的 PCOS 患者存在胰岛素抵抗特征，包括 70%～80% 的肥胖患者和 20%～25% 的瘦型患者[10]。

虽然 PCOS 的病理生理学尚不清楚，但雄激素过多是 PCOS 的一个标志性特征，60%～80% 的 PCOS 女性会出现这一症状[11-15]。高雄激素血症通常以临床表现诊断，最常见的是多毛症，和（或）循环雄激素水平异常，包括总睾酮、游离睾酮、性激素结合球蛋白（SHBG）、雄烯二酮和脱氢表雄酮（DHEA）[16]。健康女性的肾上腺和卵巢产生的雄激素水平相似。卵巢中雄激素分泌过多被认为是 PCOS 的一个标志，会对卵泡发育产生负面影响，导致排卵功能障碍[18]。然而，20%～30% 的 PCOS 患者也表现出肾上腺雄激素分泌升高[19]。雄激素分泌过多可能是由于下丘脑-垂体-性腺轴/肾上腺轴功能失调，以及胰岛素抵抗和代偿性高胰岛素血症的副产物[20]。PCOS 患者在尝试妊娠时面临的最大障碍是排卵，主要是由于卵巢功能障碍，高雄激素血症也会对子宫内膜和胎盘产生负面影响。过量雄激素通过多种机制导致子宫内膜容受性降低[21]和胎盘功能障碍[22]。即使受孕成功，PCOS 患者也面临更高的早期妊娠丢失和流产风险[23-25]。

除高雄激素血症外，胰岛素抵抗在 PCOS 的病理生理过程中起重要作用。胰岛素抵抗与肥胖、糖尿病和心血管疾病的高风险相关[26,27]。对于已经患有肥胖症的女性来说，这些风险更高。超过半数的 PCOS 患者是肥胖者[9]。虽然 PCOS 患者的胰岛素抵抗与肥胖无关，但肥胖患者增加的内脏脂肪组织进一步降低了机体对胰岛素的反应[28]。胰岛素抵抗和代偿性高胰岛素血症导致不孕的主要机制是高雄激素血症[29]。胰岛素已被证明具有通过多种机制刺激卵巢类固醇生成的能力[30,31]。胰岛素还抑制 SHBG[32] 和胰岛素生长因子结合蛋白-1（IGFBP-1）的分泌[33]，从而分别导致更多的游离雄激素和胰岛素。PCOS 患者的胰岛素作用异常，与肥胖无关[34]。然而，在肥胖的 PCOS 患者中，肥胖和 PCOS 相关的胰岛素抵抗协同作用，对糖代谢产生负面影响[35]，形成恶性循环。具体而言，在卵巢功能方面，高胰岛素血症导致卵泡发育停滞，阻碍窦卵泡完全成熟[36]。胰岛素抵抗还通过影响子宫内膜容受性[21]，降低种植率[37]，并能引起胎盘异常[22]。

越来越多的证据表明，PCOS 是一种促炎症状态，并且生殖障碍中的慢性炎症与这种状态有关。PCOS 患者的促炎细胞因子水平升高，进而导致胰岛素抵抗和雄激素分泌[38]。PCOS患者的脂肪组织、卵巢和子宫内膜中的多种炎性基因也发生改变[39-42]。虽然脂肪组织中的基因表达异常可通过雄激素相关途径导致不孕症,但炎症也直接影响卵巢、子宫内膜和胎盘的生殖功能。卵巢中炎症基因表达的改变会引起卵泡发育停滞[43]。PCOS与氧化应激增加和抗氧化能力降低有关[44]。活性氧(ROS)是排卵所必需的,但过量的ROS具有细胞毒性,在PCOS中经常出现,会降低卵母细胞质量[45,46]。炎性基因在多种细胞类型中上调,炎性细胞因子通过多种机制降低子宫内膜容受性[21]。同样,慢性炎症会导致胎盘功能障碍[47]。虽然PCOS相关的慢性低度炎症与肥胖无关[48],但PCOS肥胖患者的脂肪增加会通过NF-κB途径加剧炎症状态[49,50]。

PCOS对卵巢、子宫和胎盘的影响会导致生殖障碍,表现为排卵能力降低、子宫内膜容受性下降、种植失败、胎盘功能障碍、反复妊娠丢失和各种妊娠并发症。对比较PCOS和对照组之间妊娠结局的研究进行meta分析发现,PCOS导致不良妊娠结局的风险显著增加,包括妊娠期糖尿病、妊娠期高血压综合征、子痫前期和早产[51,52]。由于诊断标准和研究设计的差异,PCOS与流产率之间存在联系的报道并不一致[53]。然而,几项荟萃分析已经建立了PCOS与接受IVF的患者流产率升高之间的相关性[53-55]。本章回顾了高雄激素血症、胰岛素抵抗和炎症在PCOS与生殖障碍相关的病理生理学中各自的作用以及相互作用。

2 多囊卵巢综合征的高雄激素血症与生殖障碍

高雄激素症的诊断是通过临床表现和(或)生化证据,通常以血清雄激素水平升高来确定。睾酮以游离睾酮的形式存在于血清中,或与SHBG和白蛋白等蛋白质结合[56]。在正常情况下,80%的睾酮与SHBG结合,19%与白蛋白结合,1%在循环中保持游离[57,58]。然而,PCOS患者的SHBG浓度较低,雄激素分泌增加,导致具有生物活性的游离睾酮浓度较高[59]。因此,循环游离睾酮是诊断高雄激素血症的一个参数。其他参数包括游离雄激素指数、雄烯二酮和DHEAS[3]。除雄激素水平升高外,PCOS患者的黄体生成素(LH)与卵泡刺激素(FSH)比值(LH:FSH)升高[60]。雄激素分泌过多和LH:FSH升高被认为是通过干扰卵巢和子宫内膜功能而导致不孕症[18,21,60]。高雄激素血症影响生殖功能的具体机制将在下文中讨论。

2.1 高雄激素血症的原因

导致PCOS雄激素分泌过多有三种机制。第一种是下丘脑-垂体-卵巢(HPO)轴功能障碍。在正常的HPO轴中,下丘脑释放促性腺激素释放激素(GnRH),刺激垂体释放LH和FSH[61]。"两种细胞,两种促性腺激素"的概念,建立了卵巢雌激素的产生模型,包括以下内容:LH刺激卵泡膜细胞的LH受体,然后激活cAMP介导的途径表达胆固醇侧链裂解酶,包括细胞色素P450(CYP11A),3β-羟类固醇脱氢酶(3β-HSD)和17α-羟化酶/C17-20裂解酶细胞色素P450(CYP17)。有了这三种酶,卵泡膜细胞可以将胆固醇转化为雄烯二酮。雄烯二酮随后通过基底膜扩散到相邻的颗粒细胞。FSH刺激颗粒细胞,并通过cAMP介导的机制,表达芳香化酶细胞色素P450(CYP19)和17β-羟基类固醇脱氢酶(17β-HSD)。CYP19将雄烯二酮转化为雌酮,随后由17β-HSD介导转化为雌二醇[62]。PCOS患者由于LH升高和FSH不足,通常表现出不恰当的高LH:FSH比值[63,64]。一种可能发生这种情况的机制是GnRH脉冲性增强,这使得LH脉冲频率高于FSH,并导致卵泡膜细胞相对于颗粒细胞的过度刺激[65]。卵泡膜细胞过度刺激加上颗粒细胞由于FSH刺激不足而无法将卵泡膜细胞来源的雄激素转化为雌激素,引起高雄激素血症[66]。

雄激素过度产生的第二种机制与关键的雄激素合成酶的表达有关。编码CYP11a基因的过度活跃等位基因变异与血清睾酮水平升高相关,CYP11a负责卵泡膜细胞内雄烯二酮合成途径的侧链裂解[67-72]。同样,CYP17表达失调,也参与雄烯二酮的产生,很可能是PCOS卵巢高雄激素症的一个原因[73-81]。负责催化雄激素向雌激素转化的CYP19下调,也会由于转化不足而导致产生过多的雄激素[82-86]。

雄激素过度产生的第三种机制是通过胰岛素介导的卵泡膜细胞中睾酮的生物合成[87-89]。在正常生理功能下,胰岛素对卵巢的类固醇生成作用维持在健康水平。然而,在表现出胰岛素抵抗的PCOS患者中,代偿性高胰岛素血症会导致高浓度的胰岛素,从而刺激卵泡膜细胞产生过多的雄激素[90,91]。为了刺激雄激素的产生,胰岛素与其自身受体结合,激活由肌醇-聚糖信使驱动的信号级联反应,以传递刺激信号[92]。该途径的一个重要方面是,它仍然独立于胰岛素介导的葡萄糖摄取途径。这意味着,在葡萄糖摄取途径受损并因此产生胰岛素抵抗的PCOS患者中[93],胰岛素刺激类固醇生成的机制保持完整,并因代偿性高胰岛素血症而变得过度活跃[94]。

2.2 高雄激素血症与卵巢

高雄激素血症通过干扰卵泡发育而对卵巢功能产生不利影响。卵泡发育受颗粒细胞调节,PCOS患者颗粒细胞功能失调且数量较少,导致卵泡发育异常[95]。PCOS患者的窦卵泡数量增多;然而,它们在发育的早期阶段就发生停滞[96-98]。雄激素刺激窦前卵泡生长[99]。雄激素进一步刺激小卵泡,使卵泡膜细胞来源的雄激素转化为雌激素。但在窦卵泡阶段,雄激素抑制颗粒细胞内FSH介导的雄激素向雌激素的转化,导致激素失衡和卵泡发育停滞[100]。卵巢中过量雄激素的存在也被证明会引起卵泡发育不良[99,101,102]。

雄激素水平与卵泡发育相关,低水平促进卵泡发育[103],而高水平则会导致卵泡过度募集。卵泡过度募集与颗粒细胞分泌抗苗勒管激素(AMH)过多有关,AMH是颗粒细胞的专属产物,与PCOS卵巢功能障碍有关[104]。多项研究表明,PCOS患者血清AMH与LH和雄激素水平相关[105-108]。LH可使PCOS卵巢颗粒细胞产生的AMH增加4倍,但对正常卵巢没有影响[109]。此外,雄激素在刺激卵泡生长的早期阶段(FSH非依赖性)发挥作用,因此可能有助于增加 AMH 的分泌[110,111]。然而,Carlsen等[112]研究发现,使用地塞米松抑制雄激素6个月并不会改变AMH水平,表明其他机制可能与PCOS诱导和维持AMH的产生有关。事实上,PCOS的卵泡停滞发生在颗粒细胞AMH分泌最多的时候(窦前和小窦卵泡)。这就解释了为什么PCOS患者的血清AMH浓度高于卵巢功能正常的女性[113-115]。AMH可能与PCOS无排卵的发病机制有关[104];它除了抑制芳香化酶的表达外,还抑制FSH诱导的卵泡生长,通过抑制生长直接导致卵泡发育停滞,并可通过抑制雄激素-雌激素的转换间接引起雄激素分泌过多和雌激素缺乏,而雌激素是卵泡成熟所必需的[116,117]。稀发排卵/无排卵是由于长期的卵泡发育停滞和长时间的优势卵泡选择障碍[118],阻碍自然受孕。

2.3 高雄激素血症与子宫内膜

雄激素过多会导致无排卵和卵巢功能障碍,从而对妊娠构成重大挑战,同时,它也会通过子宫内膜直接作用而阻碍受孕。在PCOS患者中,高雄激素血症通过多种机制降低子宫内膜容受性。雄激素过多会抑制胚胎种植所必需的蜕膜化[119],导致蜕膜化延迟,影响种植窗口期[120]。在种植窗口期,子宫内膜基质细胞通常会表达Wilms抑癌基因(WT1)[121]。然而,雄激素受体(AR)在高雄激素血症时上调,而AR反过来下调WT1[122]。Bcl2常被WT1抑制,上调并激活p27,阻断细胞周期并干扰子宫内膜基质细胞的功能[122]。此外,表皮生长因子(EGFR)在月经后子宫内膜再生中发挥作用[123],直接受WT1调节[124],而AR介导的WT1抑制则会下调EGFR。EGFR下调导致子宫内膜再生能力受损,导致子宫内膜容受性降低[21]。

HOXA 基因对子宫内膜容受性和胚胎种植也至关重要[125-127]。多项研究表明,PCOS与子宫内膜 *HOXA-10* 和 *HOXA-11* 下调有关[128,129]。雌激素和孕激素刺激 *HOXA-10* 的上调,而雄激素则具有相反的作用[128,130]。高雄激素血症还直接影响子宫内膜内各种蛋白的表达。细胞周期蛋白依赖性抑制剂CDKN2A对胚胎种植很重要,在雄激素过量时下调[131]。L-选择素配体的表达在种植窗口期表达,也受睾酮的抑制[132]。多种类型的细胞-细胞黏附蛋白,包括αvβ3-整合素、E-Cadherin、Mucin-1、claudin-4、occludin等,在雄激素过量时下调,影响子宫内膜的通透性和选择性,并直接影响容受性[133-135]。由于多种机制导致子宫内膜容受性受损,高雄激素性PCOS患者流产的风险更高[23-25,131,136]。

2.4 高雄激素血症与胎盘

与非PCOS的孕妇相比,不论胎儿性别,PCOS孕妇的循环雄激素水平均升高[137,138]。由于母体的雄激素不会穿过胎盘[139],且胎儿通过胎盘芳香酶介导的雄激素向雌激素转化而免受过量雄激素的影响,因此母体高雄激素血症影响胎儿发育的一个潜在机制是通过改变胎盘和(或)胎儿类固醇生成导致胎儿胎盘雄激素过量[22,140-143]。这一概念得到了一项研究的支持,该研究显示,与非PCOS妇女相比,PCOS孕妇胎盘组织中3β-羟基类固醇脱氢酶1活性上调,芳香化酶活性降低,意味着雄激素分泌上调,雄激素向雌激素的转化减少[142]。

多种动物模型显示高雄激素血症和胎盘异常之间存在关联。母亲服用睾酮会导致妊娠期高雄激素血症[144-146]。对大鼠和绵羊给予睾酮处理也有助于了解雄激素在胎盘功能中的作用，显示了对胎盘的多种影响，包括胎儿和胎盘重量下降、胎盘氨基酸转运减少、胎盘 AR 表达增加、子宫动脉血流减少和胎盘分化提前[139,141,147-153]。动物模型也证明了产前雄激素水平与胎盘血管病变之间的相关性[154-156]。雄激素过多会降低胎盘促血管生成因子的表达[157,158]，增加子宫动脉的血管张力，进而对子宫的主要血液供应产生负面影响[147]。子痫前期是母体和胎儿发病的主要原因，被认为是胎盘发育异常的结果，也与雄激素过多有关[159-161]。

3　多囊卵巢综合征的胰岛素抵抗与生殖障碍

胰岛素在胰腺的 β 细胞中合成，介导细胞摄取葡萄糖，对代谢调节至关重要[162]。在健康人体内，胰岛素与其细胞表面的受体结合，诱导活化信号级联，激活依赖胰岛素的跨膜蛋白 GLUT4，促进葡萄糖进入细胞[163]。胰岛素抵抗时，细胞摄取葡萄糖能力下降的代偿反应会产生更多的胰岛素，从而导致高胰岛素血症[164]。65%～70%的 PCOS 患者存在胰岛素抵抗和代偿性高胰岛素血症，包括 70%～80%的肥胖患者和 20%～25%的瘦型患者[10]。此外，胰岛素抵抗还可通过间接和直接机制影响女性的生育能力，下文将对此进行讨论。

3.1　胰岛素抵抗的分子基础

PCOS 的胰岛素抵抗是由于胰岛素与其受体结合后的下游信号通路存在多种缺陷所致[93]。胰岛素受体(IR)是一种异四聚体，由两对相同的二聚体组成，IRα 含有配体结合位点，IRβ 含有酪氨酸磷酸化位点[165,166]。在正常情况下，一旦胰岛素与 IRα 结合，受体就会发生构象变化，导致 IRβ 的酪氨酸磷酸化，然后与多种细胞内蛋白相互作用，传递胰岛素信号[167]。然而，与其酪氨酸磷酸化位点相反，IRβ 还包含一个丝氨酸磷酸化位点，该位点在磷酸化时终止胰岛素信号传导[168-170]。在 PCOS 患者中，该丝氨酸位点过度磷酸化，阻断胰岛素的信号转导，而不影响胰岛素与其受体结合的能力[93]。超过 50%的 PCOS 患者存在这种异常[171]。

另一种结合后缺陷被认为是 PCOS 患者胰岛素抵抗的原因，涉及与酪氨酸磷酸化的 IRβ 相互作用的信号转导分子。胰岛素受体底物(IRS)蛋白是胞质蛋白，在与酪氨酸磷酸化 IRβ 结合时传递胰岛素信号[172]。一旦 IRβ 被激活，就会招募 IRS-1，在酪氨酸残基上将其磷酸化，这对信号的持续转导至关重要。随后，IRS-1 激活磷脂酰肌醇 3-激酶(PI3K)，这是 GLUT4 介导的葡萄糖摄取所必需的[173]。酪氨酸磷酸化的 IRS-1 开始信号转导，而丝氨酸磷酸化的 IRS-1 根据磷酸化模式可增强或终止信号转导[172]。PCOS 患者 PI3K 活性降低，支持 IRS-1 丝氨酸磷酸化是 PCOS 相关胰岛素抵抗的潜在原因[93]。

多项研究报道了 IRS-1 基因多态性在胰岛素抵抗和 PCOS 中的潜在作用。最初的一项研究发现，IRS-1 基因单核苷酸多态性 G972R 与 PCOS 之间可能存在联系，引起了人们的关注[171]，但随后的多项研究却报道了相互矛盾的结果[173,175-181]。然而，在对 IRS-1 基因多态性与 PCOS 之间潜在联系的研究进行荟萃分析后发现，IRS-1 G972R 变异与胰岛素抵抗和代偿性高胰岛素血症导致的 PCOS 发病风险之间存在显著相关性[182]。

3.2　胰岛素抵抗与肥胖

在 PCOS 患者中，胰岛素抵抗与肥胖无关[31]，但肥胖会加剧胰岛素抵抗[35]。肥胖患者有更多的脂肪组织，这些脂肪组织会释放多种影响胰岛素分泌的代谢物[183]。因此，虽然瘦型 PCOS 患者仍会出现胰岛素抵抗，但肥胖型 PCOS 患者的胰岛素抵抗和代偿性高胰岛素血症更为严重[9,184]。下文将解释高胰岛素血症如何影响卵巢、子宫内膜和胎盘，从而导致生殖障碍。

3.3　胰岛素抵抗与卵巢

胰岛素以多种方式影响卵巢功能。第一种途径是促进高雄激素血症及其对卵巢的影响。胰岛素可以直接刺激卵巢的类固醇生成[30,31,185]。胰岛素受体存在于卵巢基质细胞、卵泡膜细胞和颗粒细胞上[185]。通过与受体结合，胰岛素可刺激 P450c17 的活性，最终产生过量的睾酮[92]。此外，胰岛素还可增加垂体分泌的 LH，进而刺激卵泡膜细胞雄激素的产生[31,186-190]。胰岛素加剧高雄激素血症的第 3 个机制是通过抑制 SHBG 的合成[32]，使更多的循环睾酮保持游离，从而干扰卵巢功能。

胰岛素除了通过高雄激素发挥作用外,还可直接作用于卵巢。在正常月经周期中,优势卵泡的颗粒细胞在卵泡直径约为 20 mm 时对 LH 敏感,而较小的和未成熟的卵泡则不敏感[191,192]。一旦受到 LH 刺激,对 LH 敏感的颗粒细胞开始终末分化,只经历两轮细胞分裂[193]。对于 PCOS 患者,卵巢环境中存在的过量胰岛素会导致颗粒细胞对 LH 过早致敏,引起颗粒细胞提前终末分化,进而导致卵泡在最后两轮细胞分裂后停滞,使得 PCOS 患者出现更多的小窦卵泡[36,194,195]。

3.4 胰岛素抵抗与子宫内膜

体外受精研究结果表明,胰岛素抵抗的 PCOS 患者的卵母细胞能够正常发育。然而,这些患者的妊娠率明显低于对照组,表明胰岛素抵抗在子宫内膜容受性和胚胎种植中发挥作用[37,196]。

胰岛素抵抗和代偿性高胰岛素血症影响子宫内膜的主要机制是干扰蜕膜化过程。糖代谢对子宫内膜蜕膜化至关重要[197-200]。没有适当的蜕膜化,胚胎种植就不能发生[201]。有胰岛素抵抗的 PCOS 患者存在糖代谢异常,因此其子宫内膜无法正常蜕膜化的风险更大;PCOS 患者子宫内膜中胰岛素依赖的跨膜葡萄糖转运蛋白 GLUT4 mRNA 表达较低,这种变化进一步导致 PCOS 患者感知葡萄糖的能力受损,使其糖代谢发生改变[202]。最后,胰岛素生长因子结合蛋白-1(IGFBP-1)是蜕膜化和子宫内膜容受性的成熟生物标志物之一[203],在 PCOS 患者体内下调,表明蜕膜化和子宫内膜容受性存在缺陷[204]。

3.5 胰岛素抵抗与胎盘

胰岛素抵抗与多胎妊娠并发症有关,包括流产、妊娠期高血压综合征和胎儿生长受限[205]。这些关联的存在,加上对胎盘胰岛素受体表达的深入研究[206],提示胎盘在胰岛素抵抗介导的妊娠并发症中发挥作用[207,208]。在妊娠早期,高血糖可能会增加流产和子痫前期的发生率,这很可能是由于滋养细胞侵袭受损所致[22,209]。一项研究表明,胰岛素抵抗导致胎盘组织中胰岛素生长因子 1(IGF-1)信号受损。受损的 IGF-1 信号会减少滋养细胞向母体螺旋动脉的迁移和侵入[207],这对胎盘发育和胎儿正常生长至关重要[210]。与 PCOS 相关的胰岛素抵抗一致,PCOS 患者妊娠早期 IGF-1 水平低于非 PCOS 对照组[211,212]。PCOS 患者由于胰岛素抵抗,患妊娠期糖尿病的风险也更高[213-215]。妊娠期糖尿病可能对胎盘功能有多种影响,包括血管生成受损、胎盘凋亡减少和缺血增加[216-220]。

4 多囊卵巢综合征的慢性炎症和生殖障碍

炎症过程包括趋化因子、促炎细胞因子和炎症标志物的上调和释放。研究发现,与 BMI 和年龄匹配的对照组相比,PCOS 患者的炎症标志物,如 C 反应蛋白(CRP)、白细胞介素 18(IL-18)、肿瘤坏死因子(TNF-α)和白细胞介素 6(IL-6)水平显著升高[221-224]。在评估 PCOS 慢性低度炎症的研究中,对 CRP 进行了深入研究。大量研究表明,与对照组相比,PCOS 患者血清 CRP 水平升高[223,225-228]。两项荟萃分析得出结论,与对照组相比,PCOS 患者的 CRP 平均升高 96%[229,230]。研究还表明,IL-18 血清水平与 PCOS 之间存在相关性[231-233]。IL-18 是一种促炎性细胞因子,与胰岛素抵抗和心血管疾病风险相关[221]。CRP 和 IL-18 升高均表明 PCOS 存在促炎症状态,炎症已被认为是影响 PCOS 病理生理的一般因素[234-237]。

PCOS 的慢性炎症以多种方式影响卵巢、子宫内膜和胎盘。炎症是三联征的一个组成部分(还包括高雄激素血症和胰岛素抵抗),使 PCOS 患者的激素和代谢功能持续异常,并导致不孕[238](图 23.1)。慢性炎症导致生殖障碍的具体机制将在下文中讨论。

4.1 多囊卵巢综合征的炎症机制及其与胰岛素抵抗和高雄激素血症的相互作用

PCOS 患者的炎症主要由以下几个原因引起。首先是卵巢和子宫内膜中存在多种促炎细胞因子的基因表达改变,这些细胞因子促进炎症反应,导致 PCOS 相关的慢性、低度炎症状态[40-43]。其次是炎症标志物和胰岛素抵抗之间相互作用的结果。由于葡萄糖摄取受损,PCOS 胰岛素抵抗患者在摄入葡萄糖时诱发炎症反应[239]。循环单核细胞(MNC)利用葡萄糖进行糖酵解并合成烟酰胺腺嘌呤二核苷酸磷酸(NADPH)[240]。NADPH 氧化酶氧化 NADPH 后,产生超氧化物形式的 ROS,诱导氧化应激[241]。氧化应激激活核因子 κB(NF-κB),进而上调 MNC 表达和分泌 TNF-α 和 IL-6,从而使 NF-κB 触发的炎症反应持续存在[242]。TNF-α 除了在炎症中

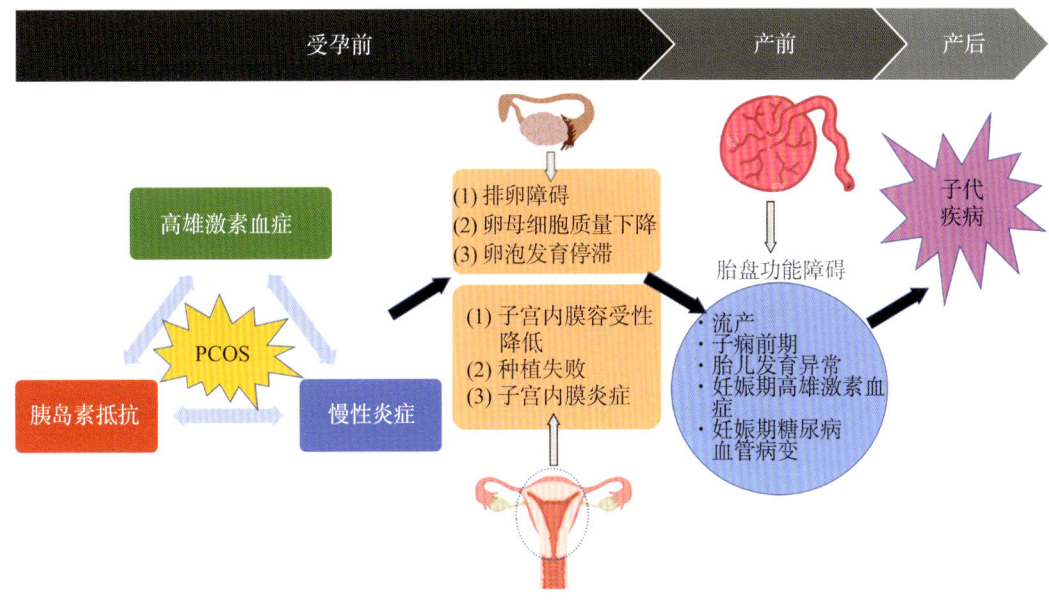

图 23.1　多囊卵巢综合征 (PCOS) 与生殖功能障碍。
PCOS 卵巢和子宫内膜中多种促炎细胞因子发生改变，引起慢性、低度炎症状态。PCOS 的三个主要特征，即高雄激素血症、胰岛素抵抗和低度慢性炎症，相互作用形成恶性循环，导致生殖功能障碍。在受孕前，对卵巢的影响包括排卵障碍、卵母细胞质量下降和卵泡发育停滞；对子宫内膜的影响包括子宫内膜容受性降低、炎症和种植失败。在产前，胎盘功能障碍则会引起流产、子痫前期、胎儿发育异常、妊娠期高雄激素血症、妊娠期糖尿病和血管病变，进而导致子代疾病。

的作用外，还参与胰岛素抵抗。TNF-α 与其受体结合后，激活 c-Jun 氨基末端激酶 (JNK)，导致 IRS-1 的 307 位丝氨酸磷酸化，阻止酪氨酸磷酸化及随后的 IRS-1 激活[243,244]。通过这种机制，胰岛素抵抗和炎症发生循环往复激活，形成恶性循环。

导致 PCOS 患者炎症的第 3 个机制是肥胖和腹部脂肪过多。超半数 PCOS 患者为肥胖者，所有 PCOS 患者因 PCOS 而出现腹部脂肪过多和（或）肥胖的风险更大[9]。脂肪组织扩张导致的脂肪细胞缺氧相关死亡会引起 MNC 和 MNC 衍生的巨噬细胞大量涌入，而后者是 TNF-α 和 IL-6 的主要来源[245]。在脂肪组织中，TNF-α 进一步刺激促炎细胞因子释放，引起 PCOS 肥胖患者的炎症状态[246]。尽管在 PCOS 患者中观察到的慢性、低度炎症状态与肥胖无关，但过多的腹部脂肪会加剧与该疾病相关的激素和代谢异常[239]。

高雄激素血症本身是促进 PCOS 炎症的另一个潜在机制。当正常体重有排卵的女性通过口服雄激素急性诱发高雄激素血症至 PCOS 的程度时，MNC 衍生的 ROS 生成、磷酸化 p47 蛋白含量、活化的 NF-κB、TNF-α mRNA 表达和 TNF-α 分泌在空腹状态和摄入葡萄糖时都会增加[247-249]。这表明，MNC 中的 AR 依赖性机制是造成这种促氧化和促炎症效应的原因[250]。另一方面，PCOS 的炎症反应可能直接促进高雄激素血症和卵巢功能障碍，而不依赖于胰岛素抵抗。这是因为 MNC 衍生的巨噬细胞浸润卵巢[251]。抗炎药物（他汀类药物和白藜芦醇）能抑制大鼠和人多囊卵巢中分泌雄激素的卵泡膜细胞增殖，而 TNF-α 则发挥刺激作用[252,253]。此外，体外证据表明，卵泡膜细胞内的雄激素合成酶 CYP17 在促炎刺激后上调，而在白藜芦醇和他汀类药物治疗后下调[254]。因此，被招募到多囊卵巢的 MNC 可能会促进局部炎症反应，增加卵泡膜细胞的数量并诱导其类固醇生成能力，从而直接刺激 PCOS 患者的卵巢雄激素分泌[236]。

4.2　慢性炎症与卵巢

如前所述，炎症是高雄激素血症和胰岛素抵抗恶性循环中的第 3 个主要因素。慢性炎症影响卵巢的第 1 个途径是促进胰岛素抵抗和高雄激素血症。然而，炎症也直接影响卵巢功能。多种炎症基因在 PCOS 卵巢中上调，包括 TNF-α 和 IL-6[39-42]。在接受 IVF 治疗的 PCOS 患者中，卵巢中 TNF-α 的升高与卵母细胞发育不良和妊娠结局有关[255-257]。另一项对寻求 IVF 的 PCOS 患者进行的研究发现，其血清和卵泡液中 TNF-α 和 IL-6 的水平显著升高[258]。研究表明,TNF-α会影响卵泡成熟[259-261],并抑制颗粒细胞分化[262],表明 TNF-α 过量会对卵泡发育产生负面影响。具体而言,在 PCOS 患者的颗粒细胞中,其他在卵泡发生中起作用的炎症基因表达上调。IL-1β 和 IL-8 通常在排卵期间招募和激活白细胞[263],引起白细胞过早侵入并破坏卵泡的最终成熟[43]。此外,PCOS 患者的卵巢微环境中存在多种血管生成细胞因子的失调[264],其中包括血管内皮生长因子[265-267]、血管生成素[268,269]、转化生长因子-β(TGF-β)[270,271]、血小板衍生生长因子[269]和碱性成纤维细胞生长因子[266]。这种血管生成失调被认为是导致卵泡发育异常、基质血管增多和卵巢过度刺激综合征倾向的原因之一[264]。血管生成和炎症在许多慢性炎症性疾病中长期相互关联,包括银屑病、类风湿关节炎、克罗恩病、糖尿病、肥胖和癌症[272]。PCOS 患者对克罗米芬的抵抗与循环中血管生成素-2 水平降低以及炎症标志物 CRP 和 CXCL16(已知的单核细胞趋化因子)水平升高有关,表明血管生成和炎症之间可能存在相互作用,从而改变卵巢对克罗米芬的反应[273]。阐明将这两个过程联系在一起的潜在细胞和分子机制对于理解它们的协同作用和开发治疗 PCOS 的新方法至关重要。综上所述,PCOS 患者的卵巢细胞因子表达谱异常,各种促炎细胞因子对卵泡发育和卵母细胞质量都有不利影响。

4.3 慢性炎症与子宫内膜

与卵巢相似,促炎细胞因子的基因表达改变也会干扰子宫内膜功能。与对照组相比,IL-18 在 PCOS 患者的子宫内膜中上调[274]。PCOS 患者未蜕膜化的基质细胞中 IL-6、IL-8 和其他促炎标志物的水平也升高,其条件培养基对免疫细胞(T 细胞、单核细胞)具有更强的趋化活性,表明正常的蜕膜化和子宫内膜容受性受到了干扰[275]。IL-6 和 TNF-α 能下调胰岛素增敏分子脂联素的表达,引起子宫内膜的胰岛素信号转导和糖代谢受损,干扰子宫内膜容受性[239,276,277]。TNF-α 还通过激活 NF-κB 途径加剧子宫内膜的炎症反应[278,279]。其他细胞因子,包括 IL-1α,在 PCOS 患者中显著下调[280]。同样,PCOS 大鼠模型显示,IL-1 mRNA 表达降低与子宫内膜变薄和胚胎种植率降低有关[280,281]。PCOS 患者体内亦存在 STC-1 水平下降,STC-1 是一种防止炎症的促生存因子,可能对胚胎种植微环境产生负面影响[21,282]。

4.4 慢性炎症与胎盘

尽管 PCOS 患者卵泡发育和子宫内膜容受性受损,但如果受孕,炎症是否仍可能对妊娠产生负面影响? 低度慢性炎症在妊娠期间持续存在,并且会因妊娠而加剧。妊娠的 PCOS 患者在基线和孕期的白细胞计数、CRP 和铁蛋白水平均高于对照组,且这些炎症标志物与不良妊娠和新生儿结局相关[283]。此外,PCOS 患者胎盘中磷酸化 STAT-3 增加[284]。胎盘 STAT-3 增加的临床影响仍有待确定,但可能反映出类似于在肥胖孕妇中观察到的促炎状态[284]。肥胖孕妇的胎盘中有更多促炎巨噬细胞浸润,这些细胞表达高水平的 IL-1、TNF-α 和 IL-6,同时母体间隙和胎盘血管肌层中趋化细胞因子和中性粒细胞表达增加[285]。这些异常的炎症通路随后可能与胎盘/蜕膜相互作用中的免疫和血管功能障碍相关,从而导致蜕膜血管内滋养细胞的侵袭能力严重受损[286]。事实上,多项研究已经证明 PCOS 中炎症标志物上调与妊娠并发症之间存在联系,包括妊娠糖尿病、早产、子痫前期、胎儿生长受限和产前出血[283,287-289]。

5 结论

PCOS 是一种以高雄激素血症、稀发排卵和多囊样卵巢为特征的异质性激素和代谢疾病,是影响育龄期女性最常见的内分泌疾病。患有 PCOS 的女性罹患 2 型糖尿病、心血管疾病、代谢综合征、肥胖、生殖功能障碍和不良妊娠结局的风险更高。PCOS 的三个主要特征,即高雄激素血症、胰岛素抵抗和低度慢性炎症,形成一个恶性循环,每一种特征都与另外两种特征相互作用,导致生殖功能障碍。PCOS 患者由于这种恶性循环而导致卵巢和子宫内膜功能异常,通过多种机制引起不孕。同样明显的是,高雄激素血症、胰岛素抵抗和低度慢性炎症导致一系列子宫内膜和胎盘改变,也是这些患者不良妊娠和产科结局的基础。虽然 PCOS 与肥胖无关,但肥胖会导致炎症、PCOS 相关的胰岛素抵抗、代偿性高胰岛素血症以及高雄激素血症,从而加重 PCOS。了解导致 PCOS 相关不孕症、种植失败和产科并发症发生率增加的炎症、内分泌和代谢机制之间的相互作用,对于开发新的治疗方法至关重要。

6　总结和建议

- PCOS 影响约 10% 的育龄期女性，其具有三个标志性特征：高雄激素血症、稀发排卵/无排卵和多囊样卵巢。
- 高雄激素血症、胰岛素抵抗和慢性炎症形成恶性循环，通过对卵巢、子宫和胎盘产生负面影响而导致生殖功能障碍。
- PCOS 患者的卵巢异常包括卵泡发育异常、稀发排卵/无排卵以及卵子质量下降。
- 子宫异常包括子宫内膜基因表达改变、炎症增加和子宫内膜容受性降低。
- PCOS 对卵巢、子宫和胎盘的影响最终会导致生殖功能障碍，包括排卵能力降低、子宫内膜容受性降低、胚胎种植失败、胎盘功能障碍、反复妊娠丢失和各种产科并发症，包括早产和子痫前期。
- 越来越多的证据表明，PCOS 是一种促炎症状态，并且慢性炎症与生殖障碍相关。
- 虽然 PCOS 与肥胖无关，但肥胖可通过引起炎症、PCOS 相关的胰岛素抵抗、代偿性高胰岛素血症以及高雄激素血症而加重 PCOS 的生殖和内分泌功能障碍。
- PCOS 患者除了生殖功能障碍外，还面临更大的心血管和代谢紊乱风险。

参考文献

[1] Deswal R, Narwal V, Dang A, Pundir CS. The prevalence of polycystic ovary syndrome: a brief systematic review. J Hum Reprod Sci 2020;13(4):261–71. Available from: https://doi.org/10.4103/jhrs.JHRS_95_18.

[2] Stein I, Leventhal ML. Amenorrhea associated with bilateral polycystic ovaries. Am J Obstet Gynecol 1935;29:181–91.

[3] Rotterdam EA-SPcwg. Revised 2003 consensus on diagnostic criteria and long-term health risks related to polycystic ovary syndrome (PCOS). Hum Reprod 2004;19(1):41–7. Available from: https://doi.org/10.1093/humrep/deh098.

[4] Teede HJ, Misso ML, Costello MF, et al. Recommendations from the international evidence-based guideline for the assessment and management of polycystic ovary syndrome. Clin Endocrinol (Oxf) 2018;89(3):251–68. Available from: https://doi.org/10.1111/cen.13795.

[5] Acien P, Quereda F, Matallin P, et al. Insulin, androgens, and obesity in women with and without polycystic ovary syndrome: a heterogeneous group of disorders. Fertil Steril 1999;72(1):32–40. Available from: https://doi.org/10.1016/s0015-0282(99)00184-3.

[6] Witchel SF, Oberfield SE, Peña AS. Polycystic ovary syndrome: pathophysiology, presentation, and treatment with emphasis on adolescent girls. J Endocr Soc 2019;3(8):1545–73. Available from: https://doi.org/10.1210/js.2019-00078.

[7] van Hooff MH, Voorhorst FJ, Kaptein MB, Hirasing RA, Koppenaal C, Schoemaker J. Polycystic ovaries in adolescents and the relationship with menstrual cycle patterns, luteinizing hormone, androgens, and insulin. Fertil Steril 2000;74(1):49–58. Available from: https://doi.org/10.1016/s0015-0282(00)00584-7.

[8] Silfen ME, Denburg MR, Manibo AM, et al. Early endocrine, metabolic, and sonographic characteristics of polycystic ovary syndrome (PCOS): comparison between nonobese and obese adolescents. J Clin Endocrinol Metab 2003;88(10):4682–8. Available from: https://doi.org/10.1210/jc.2003-030617.

[9] Pasquali R. The impact of obesity on hyperandrogenism and polycystic ovary syndrome in premenopausal women. Clin Endocrinol (Oxf) 1993;39(1):1–16. Available from: https://doi.org/10.1111/j.1365-2265.1993.tb01744.x 1993.

[10] DeUgarte CM, Bartolucci AA, Azziz R. Prevalence of insulin resistance in the polycystic ovary syndrome using the homeostasis model assessment. Fertil Steril 2005;83(5):1454–60. Available from: https://doi.org/10.1016/j.fertnstert.2004.11.070.

[11] Balen AH, Conway GS, Kaltsas G, et al. Polycystic ovary syndrome: the spectrum of the disorder in 1741 patients. Hum Reprod 1995;10(8):2107–11. Available from: https://doi.org/10.1093/oxfordjournals.humrep.a136243.

[12] Chang WY, Knochenhauer ES, Bartolucci AA, Azziz R. Phenotypic spectrum of polycystic ovary syndrome: clinical and biochemical characterization of the three major clinical subgroups. Fertil Steril 2005;83(6):1717–23. Available from: https://doi.org/10.1016/j.fertnstert.2005.01.096.

[13] Conway GS, Honour JW, Jacobs HS. Heterogeneity of the polycystic ovary syndrome: clinical, endocrine and ultrasound features in 556 patients. Clin Endocrinol (Oxf) 1989;30(4):459–70. Available from: https://doi.org/10.1111/j.1365-2265.1989.tb00446.x.

[14] Hahn S, Tan S, Elsenbruch S, et al. Clinical and biochemical characterization of women with polycystic ovary syndrome in North Rhine-Westphalia. Horm Metab Res 2005;37(7):438–44. Available from: https://doi.org/10.1055/s-2005-870236.

[15] Orio Jr. F, Matarese G, Di Biase S, et al. Exon 6 and 2 peroxisome proliferator-activated receptor-gamma polymorphisms in polycystic ovary syndrome. J Clin Endocrinol Metab 2003;88(12):5887–92. Available from: https://doi.org/10.1210/jc.2002-021816.

[16] De Leo V, Musacchio MC, Cappelli V, Massaro MG, Morgante G, Petraglia F. Genetic, hormonal and metabolic aspects of PCOS: an update. Reprod Biol Endocrinol 2016;14(1):38. Available from: https://doi.org/10.1186/s12958-

016-0173-x.

[17] Carmina E, Rosato F, Janni A, Rizzo M, Longo RA. Extensive clinical experience: relative prevalence of different androgen excess disorders in 950 women referred because of clinical hyperandrogenism. J Clin Endocrinol Metab 2006;91(1):2-6. Available from: https://doi.org/10.1210/jc.2005-1457.

[18] Abinaya S, Siva D, Sabitha R, Achiraman S. An overview of hyperandrogenism in PCOS and the prospective underlying factors. Res J Life Sci Bioinform Pharm Chem Sci 2019;1(5):179-86.

[19] Kumar A, Woods KS, Bartolucci AA, Azziz R. Prevalence of adrenal androgen excess in patients with the polycystic ovary syndrome (PCOS). Clin Endocrinol (Oxf) 2005;62(6):644-9. Available from: https://doi.org/10.1111/j.1365-2265.2005.02256.x.

[20] Diamanti-Kandarakis E, Dunaif A. Insulin resistance and the polycystic ovary syndrome revisited: an update on mechanisms and implications. Endocr Rev 2012; 33(6); 981-1030. Available from: https://doi.org/10.1210/er.2011-1034.

[21] Jiang N-X, Li X-L. The disorders of endometrial receptivity in PCOS and its mechanisms. Reprod Sci 2021; Available from: https://doi.org/10.1007/s43032-021-00629-9 2021/05/27.

[22] Kelley AS, Smith YR, Padmanabhan V. A narrative review of placental contribution to adverse pregnancy outcomes in women with polycystic ovary syndrome. J Clin Endocrinol Metab 2019;104(11):5299-315. Available from: https://doi.org/10.1210/jc.2019-00383.

[23] Balen AH, Tan SL, MacDougall J, Jacobs HS. Miscarriage rates following in-vitro fertilization are increased in women with polycystic ovaries and reduced by pituitary desensitization with buserelin. Hum Reprod 1993;8(6):959-64. Available from: https://doi.org/10.1093/oxfordjournals.humrep.a138174.

[24] Boomsma CM, Fauser BC, Macklon NS. Pregnancy complications in women with polycystic ovary syndrome. © Thieme Medical Publishers; 2008, p.072-84.

[25] Sagle M, Bishop K, Ridley N, et al. Recurrent early miscarriage and polycystic ovaries. BMJ 1988; 297 (6655): 1027-8. Available from: https://doi.org/10.1136/bmj.297.6655.1027.

[26] Teede HJ, Hutchison S, Zoungas S, Meyer C. Insulin resistance, the metabolic syndrome, diabetes, and cardiovascular disease risk in women with PCOS. Endocrine. 2006;30(1):45-53.

[27] Zhao L, Zhu Z, Lou H, et al. Polycystic ovary syndrome (PCOS) and the risk of coronary heart disease (CHD): a meta-analysis. Oncotarget 2016;7(23):33715-21. Available from: https://doi.org/10.18632/oncotarget.9553.

[28] Gambineri A, Pelusi C, Vicennati V, Pagotto U, Pasquali R. Obesity and the polycystic ovary syndrome. Int J Obes 2002; 26(7):883-96. Available from: https://doi.org/10.1038/sj.ijo.0801994 2002/07/01.

[29] Toprak S, Yonem A, Cakir B, et al. Insulin resistance in nonobese patients with polycystic ovary syndrome. Horm Res 2001;55(2):65-70. Available from: https://doi.org/10.1159/000049972.

[30] McGee E, Sawetawan C, Bird I, Rainey WE, Carr BR. The effects of insulin on 3β-hydroxysteroid dehydroge-nase expression in human luteinized granulosa cells. J Soc Gynecol Investig: JSGI 1995;2(3):535-41.

[31] Nestler JE, Jakubowicz DJ. Decreases in ovarian cytochrome P450c17α activity and serum free testosterone after reduction of insulin secretion in polycystic ovary syndrome. N Engl J Med 1996;335(9):617-23.

[32] Plymate SR, Matej LA, Jones RE, Friedl KE. Inhibition of sex hormone-binding globulin production in the human hepatoma (Hep G2) cell line by insulin and prolactin. J Clin Endocrinol Metab 1988;67(3):460-4.

[33] Poretsky L, Chandrasekher Y, Bai C, Liu H, Rosenwaks Z, Giudice L. Insulin receptor mediates inhibitory effect of insulin, but not of insulin-like growth factor (IGF)-I, on IGF binding protein 1 (IGFBP-1) production in human granulosa cells. J Clin Endocrinol Metab 1996;81(2):493-6.

[34] Dunaif A, Segal KR, Futterweit W, Dobrjansky A. Profound peripheral insulin resistance, independent of obesity, in polycystic ovary syndrome. Diabetes 1989;38(9):1165-74. Available from: https://doi.org/10.2337/diab.38.9.1165.

[35] Dunaif A, Segal KR, Shelley DR, Green G, Dobrjansky A, Licholai T. Evidence for distinctive and intrinsic defects in insulin action in polycystic ovary syndrome. Diabetes 1992;41(10):1257-66. Available from: https://doi.org/10.2337/diab.41.10.1257.

[36] Jonard S, Robert Y, Cortet-Rudelli C, Pigny P, Decanter C, Dewailly D. Ultrasound examination of polycystic ovaries: is it worth counting the follicles? Hum Reprod 2003;18(3):598-603. Available from: https://doi.org/10.1093/humrep/deg115.

[37] Chang EM, Han JE, Seok HH, Lee DR, Yoon TK, Lee WS. Insulin resistance does not affect early embryo development but lowers implantation rate in in vitro maturation-in vitro fertilization-embryo transfer cycle. Clin Endocrinol 2013; 79(1):93-9.

[38] Samy N, Hashim M, Sayed M, Said M. Clinical significance of inflammatory markers in polycystic ovary syndrome: their relationship to insulin resistance and body mass index. Dis Markers 2009;26(4):163-70. Available from: https://doi.org/10.3233/DMA-2009-0627.

[39] Escobar-Morreale HF, Calvo RM, Sancho J, San Millan JL. TNF-alpha and hyperandrogenism: a clinical, biochemical, and molecular genetic study. J Clin Endocrinol Metab 2001;86(8):3761-7. Available from: https://doi.org/10.1210/jcem.86.8.7770.

[40] Escobar-Morreale HF, Calvo RM, Villuendas G, Sancho J, San Millán JL. Association of polymorphisms in the interleukin 6 receptor complex with obesity and hyperandrogenism. Obes Res 2003;11(8):987-96.

[41] Peral B, San Millan JL, Castello R, Moghetti P, Escobar-Morreale HF. Comment: the methionine 196 arginine polymorphism in exon 6 of the TNF receptor 2 gene (TNFRSF1B) is associated with the polycystic ovary syndrome and hyperandrogenism. J Clin Endocrinol Metab 2002;87(8):3977-83. Available from: https://doi.org/10.1210/jcem.87.8.8715.

[42] Villuendas G, San Millan JL, Sancho J, Escobar-Morreale HF. The-597 G-> A and-174 G-> C polymorphisms in the promoter of the IL-6 gene are associated with hyperandrogenism. J Clin Endocrinol Metab 2002;87(3):1134-41. Available from: https://doi.org/10.1210/jcem.87.3.8309.

[43] Schmidt J, Weijdegård B, Mikkelsen AL, Lindenberg S, Nilsson L, Brännström M. Differential expression of inflammation-related genes in the ovarian stroma and

[44] Fenkci V, Fenkci S, Yilmazer M, Serteser M. Decreased total antioxidant status and increased oxidative stress in women with polycystic ovary syndrome may contribute to the risk of cardiovascular disease. Fertil Steril 2003;80(1):123-7. Available from: https://doi.org/10.1016/s0015-0282(03)00571-5.

[45] Shkolnik K, Tadmor A, Ben-Dor S, Nevo N, Galiani D, Dekel N. Reactive oxygen species are indispensable in ovulation. Proc Natl Acad Sci USA 2011;108(4):1462-7. Available from: https://doi.org/10.1073/pnas.1017213108.

[46] Wu LL, Norman RJ, Robker RL. The impact of obesity on oocytes: evidence for lipotoxicity mechanisms. Reprod Fertil Dev 2011;24(1):29-34. Available from: https://doi.org/10.1071/RD11904.

[47] Palomba S, Russo T, Falbo A, et al. Macroscopic and microscopic findings of the placenta in women with polycystic ovary syndrome. Hum Reprod 2013;28(10):2838-47. Available from: https://doi.org/10.1093/humrep/det250.

[48] Çakıroğlu Y, Vural F, Vural B. The inflammatory markers in polycystic ovary syndrome: association with obesity and IVF outcomes. J Endocrinol Investigation 2016;39(8):899-907. Available from: https://doi.org/10.1007/s40618-016-0446-4 2016/08/01.

[49] Baldwin Jr. AS. Series introduction: the transcription factor NF-kappaB and human disease. J Clin Invest 2001;107(1):3-6. Available from: https://doi.org/10.1172/JCI11891.

[50] Wisse BE. The inflammatory syndrome: the role of adipose tissue cytokines in metabolic disorders linked to obesity. J Am Soc Nephrol 2004;15(11):2792-800. Available from: https://doi.org/10.1097/01.ASN.0000141966.69934.21.

[51] Boomsma CM, Eijkemans MJC, Hughes EG, Visser GHA, Fauser BCJM, Macklon NS. A meta-analysis of pregnancy outcomes in women with polycystic ovary syndrome. Hum Reprod Update 2006;12(6):673-83. Available from: https://doi.org/10.1093/humupd/dml036.

[52] Kjerulff LE, Sanchez-Ramos L, Duffy D. Pregnancy outcomes in women with polycystic ovary syndrome: a metaanalysis. Am J Obstet Gynecol 2011;204(6):558.e1-6. Available from: https://doi.org/10.1016/j.ajog.2011.03.021 2011/06/01.

[53] Yu HF, Chen HS, Rao DP, Gong J. Association between polycystic ovary syndrome and the risk of pregnancy complications: a PRISMA-compliant systematic review and meta-analysis. Med (Baltim) 2016;95(51):e4863. Available from: https://doi.org/10.1097/MD.0000000000004863.

[54] Bahri Khomami M, Joham AE, Boyle JA, et al. Increased maternal pregnancy complications in polycystic ovary syndrome appear to be independent of obesity—a systematic review, meta-analysis, and meta-regression. Obes Rev 2019;20(5):659-74. Available from: https://doi.org/10.1111/obr.12829.

[55] Sha T, Wang X, Cheng W, Yan Y. A meta-analysis of pregnancy-related outcomes and complications in women with polycystic ovary syndrome undergoing IVF. Reprod Biomed Online 2019;39(2):281-93. Available from: https://doi.org/10.1016/j.rbmo.2019.03.203.

[56] Ashraf S, Nabi M, Rasool SUA, Rashid F, Amin S. Hyperandrogenism in polycystic ovarian syndrome and role of CYP gene variants: a review. Egypt J Med Hum Genet 2019;20(1):25. Available from: https://doi.org/10.1186/s43042-019-0031-4 2019/11/20.

[57] Chen MJ, Yang WS, Yang JH, Hsiao CK, Yang YS, Ho HN. Low sex hormone-binding globulin is associated with low high-density lipoprotein cholesterol and metabolic syndrome in women with PCOS. Hum Reprod 2006;21(9):2266-71. Available from: https://doi.org/10.1093/humrep/del175.

[58] Parker Jr. CR, Slayden SM, Azziz R, et al. Effects of aging on adrenal function in the human: responsiveness and sensitivity of adrenal androgens and cortisol to adrenocorticotropin in premenopausal and postmenopausal women. J Clin Endocrinol Metab 2000;85(1):48-54. Available from: https://doi.org/10.1210/jcem.85.1.6265.

[59] Deswal R, Yadav A, Dang AS. Sex hormone binding globulin-an important biomarker for predicting PCOS risk: a systematic review and meta-analysis. Syst Biol Reprod Med 2018;64(1):12-24. Available from: https://doi.org/10.1080/19396368.2017.1410591 2018/01/02.

[60] Malini NA, Roy George K. Evaluation of different ranges of LH: FSH ratios in polycystic ovarian syndrome (PCOS) — clinical based case control study. Gen Comp Endocrinol 2018;260:51-7. Available from: https://doi.org/10.1016/j.ygcen.2017.12.007 2018/05/01/.

[61] Conn PM, Huckle WR, Andrews WV, McArdle CA. The molecular mechanism of action of gonadotropin releasing hormone (GnRH) in the pituitary. In: Clark JH, editor. Proceedings of the 1986 Laurentian Hormone Conference. Academic Press; 1987, p. 29-68.

[62] Magoffin DA. Ovarian theca cell. Int J Biochem Cell Biol 2005;37(7):1344-9.

[63] Rebar R, Judd HL, Yen SS, Rakoff J, Vandenberg G, Naftolin F. Characterization of the inappropriate gonadotropin secretion in polycystic ovary syndrome. J Clin Invest 1976;57(5):1320-9. Available from: https://doi.org/10.1172/JCI108400.

[64] Yen SS, Vela P, Rankin J. Inappropriate secretion of follicle-stimulating hormone and luteinizing hormone in polycystic ovarian disease. J Clin Endocrinol Metab 1970;30(4):435-42. Available from: https://doi.org/10.1210/jcem-30-4-435.

[65] Waldstreicher J, Santoro NF, Hall JE, Filicori M, Crowley Jr. WF. Hyperfunction of the hypothalamic-pituitary axis in women with polycystic ovarian disease: indirect evidence for partial gonadotroph desensitization. J Clin Endocrinol Metab 1988;66(1):165-72. Available from: https://doi.org/10.1210/jcem-66-1-165.

[66] Wood JR, Nelson VL, Ho C, et al. The molecular phenotype of polycystic ovary syndrome (PCOS) theca cells and new candidate PCOS genes defined by microarray analysis. J Biol Chem 2003;278(29):26380-90.

[67] Daneshmand S, Weitsman SR, Navab A, Jakimiuk AJ, Magoffin DA. Overexpression of theca-cell messenger RNA in polycystic ovary syndrome does not correlate with polymorphisms in the cholesterol side-chain cleavage and 17alpha-hydroxylase/C(17-20) lyase promoters. Fertil Steril 2002;77(2):274-80. Available from: https://doi.org/10.1016/s0015-0282(01)02999-5.

[68] Diamanti-Kandarakis E, Bartzis MI, Bergiele AT, Tsianateli TC, Kouli CR. Microsatellite polymorphism (tttta)(n) at-528 base pairs of gene CYP11alpha influences hyperandrogenemia in patients with polycystic ovary syndrome. Fertil Steril 2000;73(4):735-41. Available from: https://doi.org/10.1016/s0015-0282(99)00628-7.

[69] Gharani N, Waterworth DM, Batty S, et al. Association of the steroid synthesis gene Cyp11a with polycystic ovary syndrome and hyperandrogenism. Hum Mol Genet 1997; 6(3): 397-402. Available from: https://doi.org/10.1093/hmg/6.3.397.

[70] Pusalkar M, Meherji P, Gokral J, Chinnaraj S, Maitra A. CYP11A1 and CYP17 promoter polymorphisms associate with hyperandrogenemia in polycystic ovary syndrome. Fertil Steril 2009; 92(2): 653-9. Available from: https://doi.org/10.1016/j.fertnstert.2008.07.016.

[71] Reddy KR, Deepika ML, Supriya K, et al. CYP11A1 microsatellite (tttta)n polymorphism in PCOS women from South India. J Assist Reprod Genet 2014; 31(7): 857-63. Available from: https://doi.org/10.1007/s10815-014-0236-x.

[72] Wang Y, Wu XK, Cao YX, et al. Microsatellite polymorphism of (tttta)n in the promoter of CYP11a gene in Chinese women with polycystic ovary syndrome. Zhonghua Yi Xue Za Zhi 2005; 85(48): 3396-400.

[73] Carey AH, Waterworth D, Patel K, et al. Polycystic ovaries and premature male pattern baldness are associated with one allele of the steroid metabolism gene CYP17. Hum Mol Genet 1994; 3(10): 1873-6. Available from: https://doi.org/10.1093/hmg/3.10.1873.

[74] Crocitto LE, Feigelson HS, Yu MC, Kolonel LN, Henderson BE, Coetzee GA. A polymorphism in intron 6 of the CYP17 gene. Clin Genet 1997; 52(1): 68-9. Available from: https://doi.org/10.1111/j.1399-0004.1997.tb02519.x.

[75] Diamanti-Kandarakis E, Bartzis MI, Zapanti ED, et al. Polymorphism T->C (-34 bp) of gene CYP17 promoter in Greek patients with polycystic ovary syndrome. Fertil Steril 1999; 71(3): 431-5. Available from: https://doi.org/10.1016/s0015-0282(98)00512-3.

[76] Ehrmann DA, Rosenfield RL, Barnes RB, Brigell DF, Sheikh Z. Detection of functional ovarian hyperandrogenism in women with androgen excess. N Engl J Med 1992; 327(3): 157-62. Available from: https://doi.org/10.1056/NEJM199207163270304.

[77] Escobar-Morreale H, Serrano-Gotarredona J, Garcia-Robles R, Sancho J, Varela C. Mild adrenal and ovarian steroidogenic abnormalities in hirsute women without hyperandrogenemia: does idiopathic hirsutism exist? Metabolism. 1997; 46(8): 902-7.

[78] Gilling-Smith C, Willis DS, Beard RW, Franks S. Hypersecretion of androstenedione by isolated thecal cells from polycystic ovaries. J Clin Endocrinol Metab 1994; 79(4): 1158-65. Available from: https://doi.org/10.1210/jcem.79.4.7962289.

[79] Miyoshi Y, Iwao K, Ikeda N, Egawa C, Noguchi S. Genetic polymorphism in CYP17 and breast cancer risk in Japanese women. Eur J Cancer 2000; 36(18): 2375-9. Available from: https://doi.org/10.1016/s0959-8049(00)00334-8.

[80] Wickenheisser JK, Nelson-DeGrave VL, McAllister JM. Dysregulation of cytochrome P450 17α-hydroxylase messenger ribonucleic acid stability in theca cells isolated from women with polycystic ovary syndrome. J Clin Endocrinol Metab 2005; 90(3): 1720-7.

[81] Wickenheisser JK, Nelson-DeGrave VL, Quinn PG, McAllister JM. Increased cytochrome P450 17alpha-hydroxylase promoter function in theca cells isolated from patients with polycystic ovary syndrome involves nuclear factor-1. Mol Endocrinol 2004; 18(3): 588-605. Available from: https://doi.org/10.1210/me.2003-0090.

[82] Erickson GF, Hsueh AJ, Quigley ME, Rebar RW, Yen SS. Functional studies of aromatase activity in human granulosa cells from normal and polycystic ovaries. J Clin Endocrinol Metab 1979; 49(4): 514-19. Available from: https://doi.org/10.1210/jcem-49-4-514.

[83] Ito Y, Fisher CR, Conte FA, Grumbach MM, Simpson ER. Molecular basis of aromatase deficiency in an adult female with sexual infantilism and polycystic ovaries. Proc Natl Acad Sci USA 1993; 90(24): 11673-7. Available from: https://doi.org/10.1073/pnas.90.24.11673.

[84] Jakimiuk AJ, Weitsman SR, Brzechffa PR, Magoffin DA. Aromatase mRNA expression in individual follicles from polycystic ovaries. Mol Hum Reprod 1998; 4(1): 1-8. Available from: https://doi.org/10.1093/molehr/4.1.1.

[85] Mostafa RA, Al-Sherbeeny MM, Abdelazim IA, et al. Relation between aromatase gene CYP19 variation and hyperandrogenism in polycystic ovary syndrome Egyptian women. J Infertility Reprod Biol 2016; 4(1): 1-5.

[86] Zhang X-L, Zhang C-W, Xu P, et al. SNP rs2470152 in CYP19 is correlated to aromatase activity in Chinese polycystic ovary syndrome patients. Mol Med Rep 2012; 5(1): 245-9.

[87] Nahum R, Thong KJ, Hillier SG. Metabolic regulation of androgen production by human thecal cells in vitro. Hum Reprod 1995; 10(1): 75-81. Available from: https://doi.org/10.1093/humrep/10.1.75.

[88] Romero G, Gamez G, Huang LC, Lilley K, Luttrell L. Anti-inositolglycan antibodies selectively block some of the actions of insulin in intact BC3H1 cells. Proc Natl Acad Sci USA 1990; 87(4): 1476-80. Available from: https://doi.org/10.1073/pnas.87.4.1476.

[89] Romero G, Luttrell L, Rogol A, Zeller K, Hewlett E, Larner J. Phosphatidylinositol-glycan anchors of membrane proteins: potential precursors of insulin mediators. Science 1988; 240(4851): 509-11. Available from: https://doi.org/10.1126/science.3282305.

[90] Barbieri RL, Makris A, Randall RW, Daniels G, Kistner RW, Ryan KJ. Insulin stimulates androgen accumulation in incubations of ovarian stroma obtained from women with hyperandrogenism. J Clin Endocrinol Metab 1986; 62(5): 904-10. Available from: https://doi.org/10.1210/jcem-62-5-904.

[91] Jakubowicz DJ, Nestler JE. 17 Alpha-fydroxyprogesterone responses to leuprolide and serum androgens in obese women with and without polycystic ovary syndrome offer dietary weight loss. J Clin Endocrinol Metab 1997; 82(2): 556-60. Available from: https://doi.org/10.1210/jcem.82.2.3753.

[92] Nestler JE, Jakubowicz DJ, de Vargas AF, Brik C, Quintero N, Medina F. Insulin stimulates testosterone biosynthesis by human thecal cells from women with polycystic ovary syndrome by activating its own receptor and using inositolglycan mediators as the signal transduction system. J Clin Endocrinol Metab 1998; 83(6): 2001-5. Available from: https://doi.org/10.1210/jcem.83.6.4886.

[93] Corbould A, Kim YB, Youngren JF, et al. Insulin resistance in the skeletal muscle of women with PCOS involves intrinsic and acquired defects in insulin signaling. Am J Physiol Endocrinol Metab 2005; 288(5): E1047-54. Available from: https://doi.org/10.1152/ajpendo.00361.2004.

[94] Nestler JE. Insulin regulation of human ovarian androgens. Hum Reprod 1997; 12(Suppl 1): 53-62. Available from: https://doi.org/10.1093/humrep/12.suppl_1.53.

[95] Wang M, Liu M, Sun J, et al. MicroRNA-27a-3p affects estradiol and androgen imbalance by targeting Creb1 in the granulosa cells in mouse polycystic ovary syndrome model. Reprod Biol 2017;17(4):295-304.

[96] Erickson GF, Magoffin DA, Garzo VG, Cheung AP, Chang RJ. Granulosa cells of polycystic ovaries: are they normal or abnormal? Hum Reprod 1992;7(3):293-9.

[97] Hsueh AJ. 6 Paracrine mechanisms involved in granulosa cell differentiation. Clin Endocrinol Metab 1986;15(1):117-34.

[98] Mason HD, Willis DS, Beard RW, Winston R, Margara R, Franks S. Estradiol production by granulosa cells of normal and polycystic ovaries: relationship to menstrual cycle history and concentrations of gonadotropins and sex steroids in follicular fluid. J Clin Endocrinol Metab 1994;79(5):1355-60.

[99] Rodrigues J, Navarro P, Zelinski M, Stouffer R, Xu J. Direct actions of androgens on the survival, growth and secretion of steroids and anti-Müllerian hormone by individual macaque follicles during three-dimensional culture. Hum Reprod 2015;30(3):664-74.

[100] Harlow C, Shaw H, Hillier S, Hodges J. Factors influencing follicle-stimulating hormone-responsive steroidogenesis in marmoset granulosa cells: effects of androgens and the stage of follicular maturity. Endocrinology. 1988;122(6):2780-7.

[101] Pierre A, Taieb J, Giton F, et al. Dysregulation of the anti-Müllerian hormone system by steroids in women with polycystic ovary syndrome. J Clin Endocrinol Metab 2017;102(11):3970-8.

[102] Xu F, Liu R, Cao X. Hyperandrogenism stimulates inflammation and promote apoptosis of cumulus cells. Cell Mol Biol 2017;63(10):64-8.

[103] Ware VC. The role of androgens in follicular development in the ovary. I. A quantitative analysis of oocyte ovulation. J Exp Zool 1982;222(2):155-67.

[104] Garg D, Tal R. The role of AMH in the pathophysiology of polycystic ovarian syndrome. Reprod BioMed Online 2016;33(1):15-28. Available from: https://doi.org/10.1016/j.rbmo.2016.04.007.

[105] Eldar-Geva T, Margalioth EJ, Gal M, et al. Serum anti-Mullerian hormone levels during controlled ovarian hyperstimulation in women with polycystic ovaries with and without hyperandrogenism. Hum Reprod 2005;20(7):1814-19. Available from: https://doi.org/10.1093/humrep/deh873.

[106] Homburg R, Ray A, Bhide P, et al. The relationship of serum anti-Mullerian hormone with polycystic ovarian morphology and polycystic ovary syndrome: a prospective cohort study. Hum Reprod 2013;28(4):1077-83. Available from: https://doi.org/10.1093/humrep/det015.

[107] Pigny P, Merlen E, Robert Y, et al. Elevated serum level of anti-mullerian hormone in patients with polycystic ovary syndrome: relationship to the ovarian follicle excess and to the follicular arrest. J Clin Endocrinol Metab 2003;88(12):5957-62. Available from: https://doi.org/10.1210/jc.2003-030727.

[108] Tal R, Seifer DB, Khanimov M, Malter HE, Grazi RV, Leader B. Characterization of women with elevated antimüllerian hormone levels (AMH): correlation of AMH with polycystic ovarian syndrome phenotypes and assisted reproductive technology outcomes. Am J Obstet Gynecol 2014;211(1):59.e1-8. Available from: https://doi.org/10.1016/j.ajog.2014.02.026 2014/07/01/.

[109] Pellatt L, Hanna L, Brincat M, et al. Granulosa cell production of anti-Mullerian hormone is increased in polycystic ovaries. J Clin Endocrinol Metab 2007;92(1):240-5. Available from: https://doi.org/10.1210/jc.2006-1582.

[110] Vendola KA, Zhou J, Adesanya OO, Weil SJ, Bondy CA. Androgens stimulate early stages of follicular growth in the primate ovary. J Clin Invest 1998;101(12):2622-9. Available from: https://doi.org/10.1172/JCI2081.

[111] Weil S, Vendola K, Zhou J, Bondy CA. Androgen and follicle-stimulating hormone interactions in primate ovarian follicle development. J Clin Endocrinol Metab 1999;84(8):2951-6. Available from: https://doi.org/10.1210/jcem.84.8.5929.

[112] Carlsen SM, Vanky E, Fleming R. Anti-Mullerian hormone concentrations in androgen-suppressed women with polycystic ovary syndrome. Hum Reprod 2009;24(7):1732-8. Available from: https://doi.org/10.1093/humrep/dep074.

[113] Fallat ME, Siow Y, Marra M, Cook C, Carrillo A. Mullerian-inhibiting substance in follicular fluid and serum: a comparison of patients with tubal factor infertility, polycystic ovary syndrome, and endometriosis. Fertil Steril 1997;67(5):962-5. Available from: https://doi.org/10.1016/s0015-0282(97)81417-3.

[114] Laven JS, Mulders AG, Visser JA, Themmen AP, De Jong FH, Fauser BC. Anti-Mullerian hormone serum concentrations in normoovulatory and anovulatory women of reproductive age. J Clin Endocrinol Metab 2004;89(1):318-23. Available from: https://doi.org/10.1210/jc.2003-030932.

[115] Mulders AG, Laven JS, Eijkemans MJ, de Jong FH, Themmen AP, Fauser BC. Changes in anti-Mullerian hormone serum concentrations over time suggest delayed ovarian ageing in normogonado-trophic anovulatory infertility. Hum Reprod 2004;19(9):2036-42. Available from: https://doi.org/10.1093/humrep/deh373.

[116] Hayes E, Kushnir V, Ma X, et al. Intra-cellular mechanism of anti-Müllerian hormone (AMH) in regulation of follicular development. Mol Cell Endocrinol 2016;433:56-65. Available from: https://doi.org/10.1016/j.mce.2016.05.019 2016/09/15/.

[117] Visser JA, Durlinger AL, Peters IJ, et al. Increased oocyte degeneration and follicular atresia during the estrous cycle in anti-Mullerian hormone null mice. Endocrinology 2007;148(5):2301-8.

[118] Franks S, Stark J, Hardy K. Follicle dynamics and anovulation in polycystic ovary syndrome. Hum Reprod Update 2008;14(4):367-78. Available from: https://doi.org/10.1093/humupd/dmn015.

[119] Lee MH, Yoon JA, Kim HR, et al. Hyperandrogenic milieu dysregulates the expression of insulin signaling factors and glucose transporters in the endometrium of patients with polycystic ovary syndrome. Reprod Sci 2020;27(8):1637-47. Available from: https://doi.org/10.1007/s43032-020-00194-7.

[120] Younas K, Quintela M, Thomas S, et al. Delayed endometrial decidualisation in polycystic ovary syndrome; the role of AR-MAGEA11. J Mol Med 2019;97(9):1315-27.

[121] Barcena C, Oliva E. WT1 expression in the female genital tract. Adv Anat Pathol 2011;18(6):454-65. Available from: https://doi.org/10.1097/PAP.0b013e318234aaed.

[122] Gonzalez D, Thackeray H, Lewis PD, et al. Loss of WT1 Expression in the endometrium of infertile PCOS patients: a

[123] Ejskjaer K, Sorensen BS, Poulsen SS, Mogensen O, Forman A, Nexo E. Expression of the epidermal growth factor system in human endometrium during the menstrual cycle. Mol Hum Reprod 2005;11(8):543-51. Available from: https://doi.org/10.1093/molehr/gah207.

[124] Jafferji I, Bain M, King C, Sinclair JH. Inhibition of epidermal growth factor receptor (EGFR) expression by human cytomegalovirus correlates with an increase in the expression and binding of Wilms' tumour 1 protein to the EGFR promoter. J Gen Virol 2009;90(Pt 7):1569-74. Available from: https://doi.org/10.1099/vir.0.009670-0.

[125] Akbas GE, Taylor HS. HOXC and HOXD gene expression in human endometrium: lack of redundancy with HOXA paralogs. Biol Reprod 2004;70(1):39-45.

[126] McGinnis W, Krumlauf R. Homeobox genes and axial patterning. Cell 1992;68(2):283-302. Available from: https://doi.org/10.1016/0092-8674(92)90471-n.

[127] Taylor HS. Transcriptional regulation of implantation by HOX genes. Rev Endocr Metab Disord 2002;3(2):127-32. Available from: https://doi.org/10.1023/a:1015454828489.

[128] Cermik D, Selam B, Taylor HS. Regulation of HOXA-10 expression by testosterone in vitro and in the endo-metrium of patients with polycystic ovary syndrome. J Clin Endocrinol Metab 2003;88(1):238-43.

[129] Kara M, Ozcan SS, Aran T, Kara O, Yilmaz N. Evaluation of endometrial receptivity by measuring HOXA-10, HOXA-11, and leukemia inhibitory factor expression in patients with polycystic ovary syndrome. Gynecol Minim Invasive Ther 2019;8(3):118.

[130] He H, Li T, Yin D, et al. HOXA10 expression is decreased by testosterone in luteinized granulosa cells in vitro. Mol Med Rep 2012;6(1):51-6.

[131] Rahman TU, Ullah K, Guo M-X, et al. Androgen-induced alterations in endometrial proteins crucial in recurrent miscarriages. Oncotarget 2018;9(37):24627.

[132] Mokhtar MH, Giribabu N, Salleh N. Testosterone decreases the number of implanting embryos, expression of pinopode and L-selectin ligand (MECA-79) in the endometrium of early pregnant rats. Int J Env Res Public Health 2020;17(7). Available from: https://doi.org/10.3390/ijerph17072293.

[133] Mokhtar M, Giribabu N, Salleh N. Testosterone down-regulates expression of αVβ3-integrin, E-cadherin and mucin-1 during uterine receptivity period in rats. Sains Malaysiana 2018;47(10):2509-17.

[134] Mokhtar MH, Giribabu N, Salleh N. Testosterone reduces tight junction complexity and down-regulates expression of claudin-4 and occludin in the endometrium in ovariectomized, sex-steroid replacement rats. vivo 2020;34(1):225-31.

[135] Quezada S, Avellaira C, Johnson MC, Gabler F, Fuentes A, Vega M. Evaluation of steroid receptors, coregulators, and molecules associated with uterine receptivity in secretory endometria from untreated women with polycystic ovary syndrome. Fertil Steril 2006;85(4):1017-26.

[136] Su Y, Shi H. High androgen level causes recurrent miscarriage and impairs endometrial receptivity. Tropical J Pharm Res 2019;18(7):1547-52.

[137] Glintborg D, Jensen RC, Bentsen K, et al. Testosterone levels in third trimester in polycystic ovary syndrome: odense child cohort. J Clin Endocrinol Metab 2018;103(10):3819-27. Available from: https://doi.org/10.1210/jc.2018-00889.

[138] Sir-Petermann T, Maliqueo M, Angel B, Lara HE, Perez-Bravo F, Recabarren SE. Maternal serum androgens in pregnant women with polycystic ovarian syndrome: possible implications in prenatal androgenization. Hum Reprod 2002;17(10):2573-9. Available from: https://doi.org/10.1093/humrep/17.10.2573.

[139] Sathishkumar K, Elkins R, Chinnathambi V, Gao H, Hankins GD, Yallampalli C. Prenatal testosterone-induced fetal growth restriction is associated with down-regulation of rat placental amino acid transport. Reprod Biol Endocrinol 2011;9:110. Available from: https://doi.org/10.1186/1477-7827-9-110.

[140] Barry JA, Hardiman PJ, Siddiqui MR, Thomas M. Meta-analysis of sex difference in testosterone levels in umbilical cord blood. J Obstet Gynaecol 2011;31(8):697-702. Available from: https://doi.org/10.3109/01443615.2011.614971.

[141] Beckett EM, Astapova O, Steckler TL, Veiga-Lopez A, Padmanabhan V. Developmental programing: impact of testosterone on placental differentiation. Reproduction 2014;148(2):199-209. Available from: https://doi.org/10.1530/REP-14-0055.

[142] Maliqueo M, Lara HE, Sanchez F, Echiburu B, Crisosto N, Sir-Petermann T. Placental steroidogenesis in pregnant women with polycystic ovary syndrome. Eur J Obstet Gynecol Reprod Biol 2013;166(2):151-5. Available from: https://doi.org/10.1016/j.ejogrb.2012.10.015.

[143] Palomba S, Falbo A, Russo T, Tolino A, Orio F, Zullo F. Pregnancy in women with polycystic ovary syndrome: the effect of different phenotypes and features on obstetric and neonatal outcomes. Fertil Steril 2010;94(5):1805-11. Available from: https://doi.org/10.1016/j.fertnstert.2009.10.043.

[144] Domonkos E, Borbelyova V, Kolatorova L, et al. Sex differences in the effect of prenatal testosterone exposure on steroid hormone production in adult rats. Physiol Res 2017;66(Suppl 3):S367-74. Available from: https://doi.org/10.33549/physiolres.933722.

[145] Padmanabhan V, Veiga-Lopez A. Sheep models of polycystic ovary syndrome phenotype. Mol Cell Endocrinol 2013;373(1-2):8-20. Available from: https://doi.org/10.1016/j.mce.2012.10.005.

[146] Shah AB, Nivar I, Speelman DL. Elevated androstenedione in young adult but not early adolescent prenatally androgenized female rats. PLoS One 2018;13(5):e0196862. Available from: https://doi.org/10.1371/journal.pone.0196862.

[147] Chinnathambi V, Blesson CS, Vincent KL, et al. Elevated testosterone levels during rat pregnancy cause hypersensitivity to angiotensin II and attenuation of endothelium-dependent vasodilation in uterine arteries. Hypertension 2014;64(2):405-14. Available from: https://doi.org/10.1161/HYPERTENSIONAHA.114.03283.

[148] Cleys ER, Halleran JL, Enriquez VA, et al. Androgen receptor and histone lysine demethylases in ovine placenta. PLoS One 2015;10(2):e0117472. Available from: https://doi.org/10.1371/journal.pone.0117472.

[149] Fornes R, Maliqueo M, Hu M, et al. The effect of androgen excess on maternal metabolism, placental function and fetal growth in obese dams. Sci Rep 2017;7(1):8066. Available

[150] Fornes R, Manti M, Qi X, et al. Mice exposed to maternal androgen excess and diet-induced obesity have altered phosphorylation of catechol-O-methyltransferase in the placenta and fetal liver. Int J Obes (Lond) 2019;43(11):2176-88. Available from: https://doi.org/10.1038/s41366-018-0314-8.

[151] Gopalakrishnan K, Mishra JS, Chinnathambi V, et al. Elevated testosterone reduces uterine blood flow, spiral artery elongation, and placental oxygenation in pregnant rats. Hypertension 2016;67(3):630-9. Available from: https://doi.org/10.1161/HYPERTENSIONAHA.115.06946.

[152] Hu M, Richard JE, Maliqueo M, et al. Maternal testosterone exposure increases anxiety-like behavior and impacts the limbic system in the offspring. Proc Natl Acad Sci USA 2015;112(46):14348-53. Available from: https://doi.org/10.1073/pnas.1507514112.

[153] Sun M, Maliqueo M, Benrick A, et al. Maternal androgen excess reduces placental and fetal weights, increases placental steroidogenesis, and leads to long-term health effects in their female offspring. Am J Physiol Endocrinol Metab 2012;303(11):E1373-85. Available from: https://doi.org/10.1152/ajpendo.00421.2012.

[154] Kumar S, Gordon GH, Abbott DH, Mishra JS. Androgens in maternal vascular and placental function: implications for preeclampsia pathogenesis. Reproduction 2018;156(5):R155-67. Available from: https://doi.org/10.1530/REP-18-0278.

[155] Metzler VM, de Brot S, Robinson RS, et al. Androgen dependent mechanisms of pro-angiogenic networks in placental and tumor development. Placenta 2017;56:79-85. Available from: https://doi.org/10.1016/j.placenta.2017.02.018.

[156] Williams CJ, Chu A, Jefferson WN, et al. Epithelial membrane protein 2 (EMP2) deficiency alters placental angiogenesis, mimicking features of human placental insufficiency. J Pathol 2017;242(2):246-59. Available from: https://doi.org/10.1002/path.4893.

[157] Fornes R, Hu M, Maliqueo M, et al. Maternal testosterone and placental function: effect of electroacupuncture on placental expression of angiogenic markers and fetal growth. Mol Cell Endocrinol 2016;433:1-11. Available from: https://doi.org/10.1016/j.mce.2016.05.014.

[158] Maliqueo M, Echiburu B, Crisosto N. Sex steroids modulate uterine-placental vasculature: implications for obstetrics and neonatal outcomes. Front Physiol 2016;7:152. Available from: https://doi.org/10.3389/fphys.2016.00152.

[159] Brown SH, Eather SR, Freeman DJ, Meyer BJ, Mitchell TW. A lipidomic analysis of placenta in preeclampsia: evidence for lipid storage. PLoS One 2016;11(9):e0163972. Available from: https://doi.org/10.1371/journal.pone.0163972.

[160] Mastrogiannis DS, Spiliopoulos M, Mulla W, Homko CJ. Insulin resistance: the possible link between gestational diabetes mellitus and hypertensive disorders of pregnancy. Curr Diab Rep 2009;9(4):296-302. Available from: https://doi.org/10.1007/s11892-009-0046-1.

[161] Scioscia M, Gumaa K, Rademacher TW. The link between insulin resistance and preeclampsia: new perspectives. J Reprod Immunol 2009;82(2):100-5. Available from: https://doi.org/10.1016/j.jri.2009.04.009.

[162] Fu Z, Gilbert ER, Liu D. Regulation of insulin synthesis and secretion and pancreatic Beta-cell dysfunction in diabetes. Curr Diab Rev 2013;9(1):25-53.

[163] Ducluzeau PH, Fletcher LM, Vidal H, Laville M, Tavare JM. Molecular mechanisms of insulin-stimulated glucose uptake in adipocytes. Diab Metab 2002;28(2):85-92.

[164] Crofts CAP, Zinn C, Wheldon M, Schofield G. Hyperinsulinemia: a unifying theory of chronic disease. Diabesity 2015;1(4):34-43.

[165] Goldfine ID. The insulin receptor: molecular biology and transmembrane signaling. Endocr Rev 1987;8(3):235-55.

[166] Ullrich A, Bell J, Chen EY, et al. Human insulin receptor and its relationship to the tyrosine kinase family of oncogenes. Nature. 1985;313(6005):756-61.

[167] Bremer AA, Miller WL. The serine phosphorylation hypothesis of polycystic ovary syndrome: a unifying mechanism for hyperandrogenemia and insulin resistance. Fertil Steril 2008;89(5):1039-48. Available from: https://doi.org/10.1016/j.fertnstert.2008.02.091 2008/05/01/.

[168] Bollage G, Roth R, Beaudoin J, Mochly-Rosen D, Doshland Jr. DE. Protein kinase C directly phosphorylates the insulin receptor in vitro and reduces its protein-tyrosine kinase activity. Proc Natl Acad Sci USA 1986;83:5822-4.

[169] Stadtmauer L, Rosen O. Increasing the cAMP content of IM-9 cells alters the phosphorylation state and protein kinase activity of the insulin receptor. J Biol Chem 1986;261(7):3402-7.

[170] Takayama S, White M, Kahn C. Phorbol ester-induced serine phosphorylation of the insulin receptor decreases its tyrosine kinase activity. J Biol Chem 1988;263(7):3440-7.

[171] Dunaif A, Xia J, Book C-B, Schenker E, Tang Z. Excessive insulin receptor serine phosphorylation in cultured fibroblasts and in skeletal muscle. A potential mechanism for insulin resistance in the polycystic ovary syndrome. J Clin Investig 1995;96(2):801-10.

[172] Gual P, Le Marchand-Brustel Y, Tanti J-F. Positive and negative regulation of insulin signaling through IRS-1 phosphorylation. Biochimie 2005;87(1):99-109. Available from: https://doi.org/10.1016/j.biochi.2004.10.019 2005/01/01/.

[173] Ertunc D, Tok EC, Aktas A, Erdal EM, Dilek S. The importance of IRS-1 Gly972Arg polymorphism in evaluating the response to metformin treatment in polycystic ovary syndrome. Hum Reprod 2005;20(5):1207-12. Available from: https://doi.org/10.1093/humrep/deh747.

[174] Sir-Petermann T, Perez-Bravo F, Angel B, Maliqueo M, Calvillan M, Palomino A. G972R polymorphism of IRS-1 in women with polycystic ovary syndrome. Diabetologia. 2001;44(9):1200-1.

[175] Dilek S, Ertunc D, Tok EC, Erdal EM, Aktas A. Association of Gly972Arg variant of insulin receptor substrate-1 with metabolic features in women with polycystic ovary syndrome. Fertil Steril 2005;84(2):407-12.

[176] Dravecká I, Lazúrová I, Habalová V. The prevalence of Gly972Arg and C825T polymorphisms in Slovak women with polycystic ovary syndrome and their relation to the metabolic syndrome. Gynecol Endocrinol 2010;26(5):356-60.

[177] El Mkadem SA, Lautier C, Macari F, et al. Role of allelic variants Gly972Arg of IRS-1 and Gly1057Asp of IRS-2 in moderate-to-severe insulin resistance of women with polycystic ovary syndrome. Diabetes. 2001;50(9):2164-8.

[178] Lin T-C, Yen J-M, Gong K-B, et al. Abnormal glucose tolerance and insulin resistance in polycystic ovary syndrome

amongst the Taiwanese population-not correlated with insulin receptor substrate-1 Gly972Arg/Ala513Pro polymorphism. BMC Med Genet 2006;7(1):1-8.

[179] Pappalardo M, Vita R, Di Bari F, Le Donne M, Trimarchi F, Benvenga S. Gly972Arg of IRS-1 and Lys121Gln of PC-1 polymorphisms act in opposite way in polycystic ovary syndrome. J Endocrinol Investig 2017;40(4):367-76.

[180] Sir-Petermann T, Angel B, Maliqueo M, et al. Insulin secretion in women who have polycystic ovary syndrome and carry the Gly972Arg variant of insulin receptor substrate-1 in response to a high-glycemic or low-glycemic carbohydrate load. Nutrition. 2004;20(10):905-10.

[181] Valdés P, Cerda A, Barrenechea C, Kehr M, Soto C, Salazar LA. No association between common Gly972Arg variant of the insulin receptor substrate-1 and polycystic ovary syndrome in Southern Chilean women. Clinica Chim Acta 2008;390(1-2):63-6.

[182] Ioannidis A, Ikonomi E, Dimou NL, Douma L, Bagos PG. Polymorphisms of the insulin receptor and the insulin receptor substrates genes in polycystic ovary syndrome: a Mendelian randomization meta-analysis. Mol Genet Metab 2010;99(2):174-83. Available from: https://doi.org/10.1016/j.ymgme.2009.10.013 2010/02/01/.

[183] Vettor R, Lombardi A, Fabris R, et al. Substrate competition and insulin action in animal models. Int J Obes 2000;24(2):S22-4.

[184] Ciaraldi TP, Morales AJ, Hickman MG, Odom-Ford R, Olefsky JM, Yen SS. Cellular insulin resistance in adipocytes from obese polycystic ovary syndrome subjects involves adenosine modulation of insulin sensitivity. J Clin Endocrinol Metab 1997;82(5):1421-5.

[185] Poretsky L, Cataldo NA, Rosenwaks Z, Giudice LC. The insulin-related ovarian regulatory system in health and disease. Endocr Rev 1999;20(4):535-82.

[186] Adashi EY, Hsueh AJ, Yen SS. Insulin enhancement of luteinizing hormone and follicle-stimulating hor-mone release by cultured pituitary cells. Endocrinology 1981;108(4):1441-9. Available from: https://doi.org/10.1210/endo-108-4-1441.

[187] Dunaif A, Scott D, Finegood D, Quintana B, Whitcomb R. The insulin-sensitizing agent troglitazone improves metabolic and reproductive abnormalities in the polycystic ovary syndrome. J Clin Endocrinol Metab 1996;81(9):3299-306. Available from: https://doi.org/10.1210/jcem.81.9.8784087.

[188] Nestler JE, Jakubowicz DJ. Lean women with polycystic ovary syndrome respond to insulin reduction with decreases in ovarian P450c17 alpha activity and serum androgens. J Clin Endocrinol Metab 1997;82(12):4075-9. Available from: https://doi.org/10.1210/jcem.82.12.4431.

[189] Soldani R, Cagnacci A, Yen SS. Insulin, insulin-like growth factor I (IGF-I) and IGF-II enhance basal and gonadotrophin-releasing hormone-stimulated luteinizing hormone release from rat anterior pituitary cells in vitro. Eur J Endocrinol 1994;131(6):641-5. Available from: https://doi.org/10.1530/eje.0.1310641.

[190] Velazquez EM, Mendoza S, Hamer T, Sosa F, Glueck CJ. Metformin therapy in polycystic ovary syndrome reduces hyperinsulinemia, insulin resistance, hyperandrogenemia, and systolic blood pressure, while facilitating normal menses and pregnancy. Metabolism 1994;43(5):647-54. Available from: https://doi.org/10.1016/0026-0495(94)90209-7.

[191] Hillier S. Current concepts of the roles of follicle stimulating hormone and luteinizing hormone in folliculo-genesis. Hum Reprod 1994;9(2):188-91.

[192] Willis DS, Watson H, Mason HD, Galea R, Brincat M, Franks S. Premature response to luteinizing hormone of granulosa cells from anovulatory women with polycystic ovary syndrome: relevance to mechanism of anovulation. J Clin Endocrinol Metab 1998;83(11):3984-91.

[193] McNatty K, Smith DM, Osathanondh R, Ryan K. The human antral follicle: functional correlates of growth and atresia. EDP Sciences; 1979. p.1547-58.

[194] Franks S, Gilling-Smith C, Watson H, Willis D. Insulin action in the normal and polycystic ovary. Endocrinol Metab Clin North Am 1999;28(2):361-78. Available from: https://doi.org/10.1016/S0889-8529(05)70074-8 1999/06/01/.

[195] Jonard S, Dewailly D. The follicular excess in polycystic ovaries, due to intra-ovarian hyperandrogenism, may be the main culprit for the follicular arrest. Hum Reprod Update 2004;10(2):107-17. Available from: https://doi.org/10.1093/humupd/dmh010.

[196] Qi J, Wang W, Zhu Q, et al. Local cortisol elevation contributes to endometrial insulin resistance in polycystic ovary syndrome. J Clin Endocrinol Metab 2018;103(7):2457-67. Available from: https://doi.org/10.1210/jc.2017-02459.

[197] Frolova AI, Moley KH. Glucose transporters in the uterus: an analysis of tissue distribution and proposed physiological roles. Reproduction 2011;142(2):211-20. Available from: https://doi.org/10.1530/REP-11-0114.

[198] Frolova AI, Moley KH. Quantitative analysis of glucose transporter mRNAs in endometrial stromal cells reveals critical role of GLUT1 in uterine receptivity. Endocrinology 2011;152(5):2123-8. Available from: https://doi.org/10.1210/en.2010-1266.

[199] Kim ST, Moley KH. Regulation of facilitative glucose transporters and AKT/MAPK/PRKAA signaling via estradiol and progesterone in the mouse uterine epithelium. Biol Reprod 2009;81(1):188-98. Available from: https://doi.org/10.1095/biolreprod.108.072629.

[200] von Wolff M, Ursel S, Hahn U, Steldinger R, Strowitzki T. Glucose transporter proteins (GLUT) in human endometrium: expression, regulation, and function throughout the menstrual cycle and in early pregnancy. J Clin Endocrinol Metab 2003;88(8):3885-92. Available from: https://doi.org/10.1210/jc.2002-021890.

[201] Okada H, Tsuzuki T, Murata H. Decidualization of the human endometrium. Reprod Med Biol 2018;17(3):220-7.

[202] Zhai J, Liu C-X, Tian Z-R, Jiang Q-H, Sun Y-P. Effects of metformin on the expression of GLUT4 in endome-trium of obese women with polycystic ovary syndrome. Biol Reprod 2012;87(2):29 1-5.

[203] Kim JJ, Fazleabas AT. Uterine receptivity and implantation: the regulation and action of insulin-like growth factor binding protein-1 (IGFBP-1), HOXA10 and forkhead transcription factor-1 (FOXO-1) in the baboon endometrium. Reprod Biol Endocrinol 2004;2(1):34. Available from: https://doi.org/10.1186/1477-7827-2-34 2004/06/16.

[204] Giudice LC, Dsupin BA, Irwin JC. Steroid and peptide regulation of insulin-like growth factor-binding proteins secreted by human endometrial stromal cells is dependent on stromal differentiation. J Clin Endocrinol Metab 1992;75

[205] Frasca F, Pandini G, Sciacca L, et al. The role of insulin receptors and IGF-I receptors in cancer and other diseases. Arch Physiol Biochem 2008;114(1):23-37. Available from: https://doi.org/10.1080/13813450801969715.

(5):1235-41. Available from: https://doi.org/10.1210/jcem.75.5.1385468.

[206] Westermeier F, Saez T, Arroyo P, et al. Insulin receptor isoforms: an integrated view focused on gestational diabetes mellitus. Diabetes Metab Res Rev 2016;32(4):350-65. Available from: https://doi.org/10.1002/dmrr.2729.

[207] Mayama R, Izawa T, Sakai K, Suciu N, Iwashita M. Improvement of insulin sensitivity promotes extravillous trophoblast cell migration stimulated by insulin-like growth factor-I. Endocr J 2013;60(3):359-68. Available from: https://doi.org/10.1507/endocrj.ej12-0241.

[208] Solomon CG, Seely EW. Brief review: hypertension in pregnancy: a manifestation of the insulin resistance syndrome? Hypertension 2001;37(2):232-9. Available from: https://doi.org/10.1161/01.hyp.37.2.232.

[209] Gabbay-Benziv R, Baschat AA. Gestational diabetes as one of the "great obstetrical syndromes"-the maternal, placental, and fetal dialog. Best Pract Res Clin Obstet Gynaecol 2015;29(2):150-5. Available from: https://doi.org/10.1016/j.bpobgyn.2014.04.025.

[210] Huppertz B. Traditional and new routes of trophoblast invasion and their implications for pregnancy diseases. Int J Mol Sci 2019;21(1). Available from: https://doi.org/10.3390/ijms21010289.

[211] Jakubowicz DJ, Essah PA, Seppala M, et al. Reduced serum glycodelin and insulin-like growth factor-binding protein-1 in women with polycystic ovary syndrome during first trimester of pregnancy. J Clin Endocrinol Metab 2004;89(2):833-9. Available from: https://doi.org/10.1210/jc.2003-030975.

[212] Morris DV, Falcone T. The relationship between insulin sensitivity and insulin-like growth factor-binding protein-1. Gynecol Endocrinol 1996;10(6):407-12. Available from: https://doi.org/10.3109/09513599609023605.

[213] de Wilde MA, Veltman-Verhulst SM, Goverde AJ, et al. Preconception predictors of gestational diabetes: a multicentre prospective cohort study on the predominant complication of pregnancy in polycystic ovary syndrome. Hum Reprod 2014;29(6):1327-36. Available from: https://doi.org/10.1093/humrep/deu077.

[214] Gozukara YM, Aytan H, Ertunc D, et al. Role of first trimester total testosterone in prediction of subsequent gestational diabetes mellitus. J Obstet Gynaecol Res 2015;41(2):193-8. Available from: https://doi.org/10.1111/jog.12525.

[215] Powe CE. Early pregnancy biochemical predictors of gestational diabetes mellitus. Curr Diab Rep 2017;17(2):12. Available from: https://doi.org/10.1007/s11892-017-0834-y.

[216] Belkacemi L, Kjos S, Nelson DM, Desai M, Ross MG. Reduced apoptosis in term placentas from gestational diabetic pregnancies. J Dev Orig Health Dis 2013;4(3):256-65. Available from: https://doi.org/10.1017/S2040174413000068.

[217] Madazli R, Tuten A, Calay Z, Uzun H, Uludag S, Ocak V. The incidence of placental abnormalities, maternal and cord plasma malondialdehyde and vascular endothelial growth factor levels in women with gestational diabetes mellitus and nondiabetic controls. Gynecol Obstet Invest 2008;65(4):227-32. Available from: https://doi.org/10.1159/000113045.

[218] Meng Q, Shao L, Luo X, et al. Expressions of VEGF-A and VEGFR-2 in placentae from GDM pregnancies. Reprod Biol Endocrinol 2016;14(1):61. Available from: https://doi.org/10.1186/s12958-016-0191-8.

[219] Wang K, Zheng J. Signaling regulation of fetoplacental angiogenesis. J Endocrinol 2012;212(3):243-55. Available from: https://doi.org/10.1530/JOE-11-0296.

[220] Zhou J, Ni X, Huang X, et al. Potential role of hyperglycemia in fetoplacental endothelial dysfunction in gestational diabetes mellitus. Cell Physiol Biochem 2016;39(4):1317-28. Available from: https://doi.org/10.1159/000447836.

[221] Rudnicka E, Suchta K, Grymowicz M, et al. Chronic low grade inflammation in pathogenesis of PCOS. Int J Mol Sci 2021;22(7):3789.

[222] Boulman N, Levy Y, Leiba R, et al. Increased C-reactive protein levels in the polycystic ovary syndrome: a marker of cardiovascular disease. J Clin Endocrinol Metab 2004;89(5):2160-5. Available from: https://doi.org/10.1210/jc.2003-031096.

[223] Rudnicka E, Kunicki M, Suchta K, Machura P, Grymowicz M, Smolarczyk R. Inflammatory markers in women with polycystic ovary syndrome. Biomed Res Int 2020;2020:4092470. Available from: https://doi.org/10.1155/2020/4092470.

[224] Xiong YL, Liang XY, Yang X, Li Y, Wei LN. Low-grade chronic inflammation in the peripheral blood and ovaries of women with polycystic ovarian syndrome. Eur J Obstet Gynecol Reprod Biol 2011;159(1):148-50. Available from: https://doi.org/10.1016/j.ejogrb.2011.07.012.

[225] Kelly CC, Lyall H, Petrie JR, Gould GW, Connell JM, Sattar N. Low grade chronic inflammation in women with polycystic ovarian syndrome. J Clin Endocrinol Metab 2001;86(6):2453-5. Available from: https://doi.org/10.1210/jcem.86.6.7580.

[226] Orio Jr F, Palomba S, Cascella T, et al. The increase of leukocytes as a new putative marker of low-grade chronic inflammation and early cardiovascular risk in polycystic ovary syndrome. J Clin Endocrinol Metab 2005;90(1):2-5.

[227] Souza dos Santos AC, Soares NP, Costa EC, de Sá JCF, Azevedo GD, Lemos TMAM. The impact of body mass on inflammatory markers and insulin resistance in polycystic ovary syndrome. Gynecol Endocrinol 2015;31(3):225-8.

[228] Tola EN, Yalcin SE, Dugan N. The predictive effect of inflammatory markers and lipid accumulation product index on clinical symptoms associated with polycystic ovary syndrome in nonobese adolescents and younger aged women. Eur J Obstet Gynecol Reprod Biol 2017;214:168-72.

[229] Escobar-Morreale HF, Luque-Ramírez M, González F. Circulating inflammatory markers in polycystic ovary syndrome: a systematic review and metaanalysis. Fertil Steril 2011;95(3):1048-58 e2.

[230] Toulis KA, Goulis DG, Mintziori G, et al. Meta-analysis of cardiovascular disease risk markers in women with polycystic ovary syndrome. Hum Reprod update 2011;17(6):741-60.

[231] Deligeoroglou E, Vrachnis N, Athanasopoulos N, et al. Mediators of chronic inflammation in polycystic ovarian syndrome. Gynecol Endocrinol 2012;28(12):974-8.

[232] Escobar-Morreale HCF, Botella-Carretero JI, Villuendas G, Sancho J, San Millán JL. Serum interleukin-18 concentrations are increased in the polycystic ovary syndrome: relationship to insulin resistance and to obesity. J

Clin Endocrinol Metab 2004;89(2):806-11.
[233] Kaya C, Pabuccu R, Berker B, Satıroglu H. Plasma interleukin-18 levels are increased in the polycystic ovary syndrome: relationship of carotid intima-media wall thickness and cardiovascular risk factors. Fertil Steril 2010; 93(4):1200-7.
[234] Boots CE, Jungheim ES. Inflammation and human ovarian follicular dynamics. Thieme Medical Publishers; 2015, p. 270-5.
[235] Duleba AJ, Dokras A. Is PCOS an inflammatory process? Fertil Steril 2012;97(1):7-12.
[236] González F. Nutrient-induced inflammation in polycystic ovary syndrome: role in the development of meta-bolic aberration and ovarian dysfunction. Thieme Medical Publishers; 2015, p. 276-86.
[237] Spritzer PM, Lecke SB, Satler F, Morsch DM. Adipose tissue dysfunction, adipokines, and low-grade chronic inflammation in polycystic ovary syndrome. Reproduction. 2015;149(5):R219-27.
[238] Shorakae S, Ranasinha S, Abell S, et al. Inter-related effects of insulin resistance, hyperandrogenism, sympathetic dysfunction and chronic inflammation in PCOS. Clin Endocrinol (Oxf) 2018;89(5):628-33. Available from: https://doi.org/10.1111/cen.13808.
[239] González F. Inflammation in polycystic ovary syndrome: underpinning of insulin resistance and ovarian dys-function. Steroids 2012;77(4):300-5. Available from: https://doi.org/10.1016/j.steroids.2011.12.003 2012/03/10/.
[240] Tan AS, Ahmed N, Berridge MV. Acute regulation of glucose transport after activation of human peripheral blood neutrophils by phorbol myristate acetate, fMLP, and granulocyte-macrophage colony-stimulating factor. Blood, J Am Soc Hematol 1998;91(2):649-55.
[241] Chanock SJ, El Benna J, Smith RM, Babior BM. The respiratory burst oxidase. J Biol Chem 1994;269(40):24519-22.
[242] Löms Ziegler-Heitbrock H-W. The biology of the monocyte system. Eur J Cell Biol 1989;49(1):1-12.
[243] Aguirre V, Uchida T, Yenush L, Davis R, White MF. The c-Jun NH(2)-terminal kinase promotes insulin resistance during association with insulin receptor substrate-1 and phosphorylation of Ser(307). J Biol Chem 2000;275(12): 9047-54. Available from: https://doi.org/10.1074/jbc.275.12.9047.
[244] Chen G, Goeddel DV. TNF-R1 signaling: a beautiful pathway. Science 2002;296(5573):1634-5. Available from: https://doi.org/10.1126/science.1071924.
[245] Weisberg SP, McCann D, Desai M, Rosenbaum M, Leibel RL, Ferrante AW. Obesity is associated with macrophage accumulation in adipose tissue. J Clin Investig 2003; 112 (12):1796-808.
[246] Fain J, Bahouth S, Madan A. TNF α release by the nonfat cells of human adipose tissue. Int J Obes 2004; 28(4): 616-22.
[247] Gonzalez F, Nair KS, Daniels JK, Basal E, Schimke JM. Hyperandrogenism sensitizes mononuclear cells to promote glucose-induced inflammation in lean reproductive-age women. Am J Physiol Endocrinol Metab 2012; 302(3): E297-306. Available from: https://doi.org/10.1152/ajpendo.00416.2011.
[248] Gonzalez F, Nair KS, Daniels JK, Basal E, Schimke JM, Blair HE. Hyperandrogenism sensitizes leukocytes to hyperglycemia to promote oxidative stress in lean reproductive-age women. J Clin Endocrinol Metab 2012; 97 (8):2836-43. Available from: https://doi.org/10.1210/jc.2012-1259.
[249] Gonzalez F, Sia CL, Bearson DM, Blair HE. Hyperandrogenism induces a proinflammatory TNFalpha response to glucose ingestion in a receptor-dependent fashion. J Clin Endocrinol Metab 2014;99(5): E848-54. Available from: https://doi.org/10.1210/jc.2013-4109.
[250] Gonzalez F. Nutrient-induced inflammation in polycystic ovary syndrome: role in the development of meta-bolic aberration and ovarian dysfunction. Semin Reprod Med 2015;33(4):276-86. Available from: https://doi.org/10.1055/s-0035-1554918.
[251] Best CL, Pudney J, Welch WR, Burger N, Hill JA. Localization and characterization of white blood cell populations within the human ovary throughout the menstrual cycle and menopause. Hum Reprod 1996;11(4): 790-7. Available from: https://doi.org/10.1093/oxfordjournals.humrep.a019256.
[252] Sancho-Tello M, Perez-Roger I, Imakawa K, Tilzer L, Terranova PF. Expression of tumor necrosis factor-alpha in the rat ovary. Endocrinology 1992;130(3):1359-64. Available from: https://doi.org/10.1210/endo.130.3.1537297.
[253] Spaczynski RZ, Arici A, Duleba AJ. Tumor necrosis factor-alpha stimulates proliferation of rat ovarian theca-interstitial cells. Biol Reprod 1999;61(4):993-8. Available from: https://doi.org/10.1095/biolreprod61.4.993.
[254] Ortega I, Villanueva JA, Wong DH, et al. Resveratrol potentiates effects of simvastatin on inhibition of rat ovarian theca-interstitial cells steroidogenesis. J Ovarian Res 2014;7:21. Available from: https://doi.org/10.1186/1757-2215-7-21.
[255] Carlberg M, Nejaty J, Fröysa B, Guan Y, Söder O, Bergqvist A. Elevated expression of tumour necrosis factor α in cultured granulosa cells from women with endometriosis. Hum Reprod 2000;15(6):1250-5. Available from: https://doi.org/10.1093/humrep/15.6.1250.
[256] Cianci A, Calogero AE, Palumbo MA, et al. Relationship between tumour necrosis factor α and sex steroid concentrations in the follicular fluid of women with immunological infertility. Hum Reprod 1996;11(2):265-8.
[257] Lee KS, Joo BS, Na YJ, Yoon MS, Choi OH, Kim WW. Relationships between concentrations of tumor necrosis factor-α and nitric oxide in follicular fluid and oocyte quality. J Assist Reprod Genet 2000;17(4):222-8.
[258] Amato G, Conte M, Mazziotti G, et al. Serum and follicular fluid cytokines in polycystic ovary syndrome during stimulated cycles. Obstet Gynecol 2003;101(6):1177-82. Available from: https://doi.org/10.1016/S0029-7844(03)00233-3 2003/06/01/.
[259] Adashi EY, Resnick CE, Packman JN, Hurwitz A, Payne DW. Cytokine-mediated regulation of ovarian function: tumor necrosis factor a inhibits gonadotropin-supported progesterone accumulation by differentiating and luteinized murine granulosa cells. Am J Obstet Gynecol 1990;162(4):889-99.
[260] Roby K, Terranova P. Tumor necrosis factor alpha alters follicolar steroidogenesis in vitro. Endocrinology 1988;123 (6):2952-4.
[261] Zolti M, Meirom R, Shemesh M, et al. Granulosa cells as a

[262] Darbon J, Oury F, Laredo J, Bayard F. Tumor necrosis factor-α inhibits follicle-stimulating hormone-induced differentiation in cultured rat granulosa cells. Biochem Biophys Res Commun 1989;163(2):1038-46. source and target organ for tumor necrosis factor-α. FEBS Lett 1990;261(2):253-5.

[263] Wang LJ, Brannstrom M, Pascoe V, Norman RJ. Cellular composition of primary cultures of human granulosa-lutein cells and the effect of cytokines on cell proliferation. Reprod Fertil Dev 1995;7(1):21-6. Available from: https://doi.org/10.1071/rd9950021.

[264] Tal R, Seifer DB, Arici A. The emerging role of angiogenic factor dysregulation in the pathogenesis of polycystic ovarian syndrome. Semin Reprod Med 2015;33(3):195-207. Available from: https://doi.org/10.1055/s-0035-1552582.

[265] Agrawal R, Sladkevicius P, Engmann L, et al. Serum vascular endothelial growth factor concentrations and ovarian stromal blood flow are increased in women with polycystic ovaries. Hum Reprod 1998;13(3):651-5. Available from: https://doi.org/10.1093/humrep/13.3.651.

[266] Artini PG, Monti M, Matteucci C, Valentino V, Cristello F, Genazzani AR. Vascular endothelial growth factor and basic fibroblast growth factor in polycystic ovary syndrome during controlled ovarian hyperstimu-lation. Gynecol Endocrinol 2006;22(8):465-70. Available from: https://doi.org/10.1080/09513590600906607.

[267] Tal R, Seifer DB, Grazi RV, Malter HE. Follicular fluid placental growth factor is increased in polycystic ovarian syndrome: correlation with ovarian stimulation. Reprod Biol Endocrinol 2014;12(1):1-7. Available from: https://doi.org/10.1186/1477-7827-12-82 82.

[268] Tal R, Seifer DB, Grazi RV, Malter HE. Angiopoietin-1 and angiopoietin-2 are altered in polycystic ovarian syndrome (PCOS) during controlled ovarian stimulation. Vasc Cell 2013;5(1):18. Available from: https://doi.org/10.1186/2045-824X-5-18.

[269] Scotti L, Parborell F, Irusta G, et al. Platelet-derived growth factor BB and DD and angiopoietin1 are altered in follicular fluid from polycystic ovary syndrome patients. Mol Reprod Dev 2014;81(8):748-56. Available from: https://doi.org/10.1002/mrd.22343.

[270] Raja-Khan N, Kunselman AR, Demers LM, Ewens KG, Spielman RS, Legro RS. A variant in the fibrillin-3 gene is associated with TGF-β and inhibin B levels in women with polycystic ovary syndrome. Fertil Steril 2010;94(7):2916-19. Available from: https://doi.org/10.1016/j.fertnstert.2010.05.047.

[271] Tal R, Seifer DB, Shohat-Tal A, Grazi RV, Malter HE. Transforming growth factor-β1 and its receptor soluble endoglin are altered in polycystic ovary syndrome during controlled ovarian stimulation. Fertil Steril 2013;100(2):538-43. Available from: https://doi.org/10.1016/j.fertnstert.2013.04.022.

[272] Costa C, Incio J, Soares R. Angiogenesis and chronic inflammation: cause or consequence? Angiogenesis 2007;10(3):149-66. Available from: https://doi.org/10.1007/s10456-007-9074-0.

[273] Wang L, Qi H, Baker PN, et al. Altered circulating inflammatory cytokines are associated with anovulatory polycystic ovary syndrome (PCOS) women resistant to clomiphene citrate treatment. Med Sci Monit 2017;23:1083-9. Available from: https://doi.org/10.12659/msm.901194.

[274] Long X, Li R, Yang Y, Qiao J. Overexpression of IL-18 in the proliferative phase endometrium of patients with polycystic ovary syndrome. Reprod Sci 2017;24(2):252-7. Available from: https://doi.org/10.1177/1933719116653681.

[275] Piltonen TT, Chen JC, Khatun M, et al. Endometrial stromal fibroblasts from women with polycystic ovary syndrome have impaired progesterone-mediated decidualization, aberrant cytokine profiles and promote enhanced immune cell migration in vitro. Hum Reprod 2015;30(5):1203-15. Available from: https://doi.org/10.1093/humrep/dev055.

[276] Fasshauer M, Kralisch S, Klier M, et al. Adiponectin gene expression and secretion is inhibited by interleukin-6 in 3T3-L1 adipocytes. Biochem Biophys Res Commun 2003;301(4):1045-50.

[277] García V, Oróstica L, Poblete C, et al. Endometria from obese PCOS women with hyperinsulinemia exhibit altered adiponectin signaling. Hormone Metab Res 2015;47(12):901-9.

[278] Orostica L, Astorga I, Plaza-Parrochia F, et al. Proinflammatory environment and role of TNF-α in endometrial function of obese women having polycystic ovarian syndrome. Int J Obes 2016;40(11):1715-22.

[279] Oróstica L, García P, Vera C, García V, Romero C, Vega M. Effect of TNF-α on molecules related to the insulin action in endometrial cells exposed to hyperandrogenic and hyperinsulinic conditions characteristics of polycystic ovary syndrome. Reprod Sci 2018;25(7):1000-9.

[280] Jasper MJ, Tremellen KP, Robertson SA. Reduced expression of IL-6 and IL-1α mRNAs in secretory phase endometrium of women with recurrent miscarriage. J Reprod Immunol 2007;73(1):74-84.

[281] Zhao DM, Shan YH, Li FH, Jiang L, Qu QL. Correlation between endometrial receptivity with expressions of IL-1 and VEGF in rats with polycystic ovary syndrome. Eur Rev Med Pharmacol Sci 2019;23(13):5575-80. Available from: https://doi.org/10.26355/eurrev_201907_18291.

[282] Khatun M, Arffman RK, Lavogina D, et al. Women with polycystic ovary syndrome present with altered endometrial expression of stanniocalcin-1. Biol Reprod 2019;102(2):306-15. Available from: https://doi.org/10.1093/biolre/ioz180.

[283] Palomba S, Falbo A, Chiossi G, et al. Low-grade chronic inflammation in pregnant women with polycystic ovary syndrome: a prospective controlled clinical study. J Clin Endocrinol Metab 2014;99(8):2942-51. Available from: https://doi.org/10.1210/jc.2014-1214.

[284] Maliqueo M, Sundstrom Poromaa I, Vanky E, et al. Placental STAT3 signaling is activated in women with polycystic ovary syndrome. Hum Reprod 2015;30(3):692-700. Available from: https://doi.org/10.1093/humrep/deu351.

[285] Aye IL, Lager S, Ramirez VI, et al. Increasing maternal body mass index is associated with systemic inflam-mation in the mother and the activation of distinct placental inflammatory pathways. Biol Reprod 2014;90(6):129. Available from: https://doi.org/10.1095/biolreprod.113.116186.

[286] Roberts KA, Riley SC, Reynolds RM, et al. Placental structure and inflammation in pregnancies associated with obesity. Placenta 2011;32(3):247-54. Available from: https://doi.org/10.1016/j.placenta.2010.12.023.

[287] Du M, Basu A, Fu D, et al. Serum inflammatory markers

and preeclampsia in type 1 diabetes: a prospective study. Diabetes Care 2013;36(7):2054 – 61. Available from: https://doi.org/10.2337/dc12-1934.

[288] Sacks GP, Seyani L, Lavery S, Trew G. Maternal C-reactive protein levels are raised at 4 weeks gestation. Hum Reprod 2004;19(4):1025 – 30. Available from: https://doi.org/10.1093/humrep/deh179.

[289] Wolf M, Sandler L, Hsu K, Vossen-Smirnakis K, Ecker JL, Thadhani R. First-trimester C-reactive protein and subsequent gestational diabetes. Diabetes Care 2003;26(3): 819 – 24. Available from: https://doi.org/10.2337/diacare.26.3.819.

第 24 章

反复妊娠丢失和反复种植失败女性免疫反应的代谢调控

Metabolic control of immune responses in women with recurrent pregnancy loss and recurrent implantation failure

Yiqiu Wei[1,*], Songchen Cai[2,*], Jinli Ding[1], Yong Zeng[2], Tailang Yin[1] and Lianghui Diao[2]

[1] Reproductive Medicine Center, Renmin Hospital of Wuhan University, Wuhan, Hubei, P. R. China
[2] Shenzhen Key Laboratory for Reproductive Immunology of Peri-implantation, Shenzhen Zhongshan Institute for Reproduction and Genetics, Shenzhen Zhongshan Urology Hospital, Shenzhen, P. R. China

1 引言

代谢和免疫是机体维持组织稳态的核心机制。广泛的研究已证实这两个途径在妊娠过程中扮演的角色。在妊娠初期，免疫细胞通过适应性的代谢重编程，赋予胚胎"免疫特权"，以保障胎儿能够正常发育至分娩。由于代谢影响细胞功能，免疫细胞对同种异体移植物的代谢反应不足可能是不利于胎盘形成和妊娠结局的病理条件[1]。反复妊娠丢失（RPL）和反复种植失败（RIF）是患者和医生共同面临的两大挑战。虽然 RIF 和 RPL 发生在生殖过程的不同阶段，但它们的实验室结果往往相似，因此这两种生殖问题通常由同一组医生或在同一科室进行评估和治疗。

RPL 最主要的原因是胚胎染色体异常，其次是神经内分泌、免疫和代谢因素[2]。然而，RIF 的定义、发病率和干预措施仍存在争议[3,4]。在所有病因中，内分泌、代谢和免疫因素被归类为母体因素。以往的研究通常从同种免疫和自身免疫两个角度来解释免疫发病机制。同种异体免疫的发病机制主要基于"胎儿同种异体移植物悖论"的概念。一旦建立妊娠，母体免疫系统会主动适应胎儿抗原的暴露，从而达到免疫内稳态的状态[5]。与妊娠相关的免疫稳态失调包括 Th1/Th2 细胞失衡[6]、Treg/Th17 细胞失衡[7]、自然杀伤（NK）细胞活性增加[8]、M1/M2 细胞失衡[9]、细胞因子及其受体表达异常[10]。自身免疫性疾病通常表现为对自身抗原的过度免疫反应，产生自身抗体或攻击宫内胎儿和胎盘血管，导致胚胎/胎儿丢失。自身抗体包括抗磷脂抗体、抗胰岛素受体抗体、抗甲状腺抗体等。基于生殖免疫学的最新进展，研究人员认识到妊娠更像是癌症，而不是移植[11]。癌症免疫代谢方面的突破也促使人们重新审视妊娠期间的免疫代谢状况以及营养和代谢紊乱对不良妊娠结局的影响[12]。

由于胚胎因素在其他章节有更详细的论述，本章主要从免疫学和代谢的角度讨论 RPL 和 RIF 的病因、机制、评估和治疗。

2 定义和患病率

表 24.1 总结了 RPL 和 RIF 中免疫代谢疾病的患病率。有证据表明，许多免疫代谢疾病与 RPL 和 RIF 的发生有关，如抗磷脂综合征（APS）、胰岛素抵抗（IR）、多囊卵巢综合征（PCOS）、自身免疫性甲状腺疾病（AITD）、高泌乳素血症和其他自身免疫相关疾病。

2.1 抗磷脂综合征与反复妊娠丢失/反复种植失败

APS 也称为 Hughes 综合征，是一种以实验室

表 24.1　与反复妊娠丢失和反复种植失败相关的免疫和代谢疾病患病率

患病率	育龄期女性	不孕女性	RPL	RIF
抗磷脂综合征(APS)	2.7%～7%	20%～25%	5%～15%	9%～20%
胰岛素抵抗(IR)	10%	20%	20%～30%	20%～30%
多囊卵巢综合征(PCOS)	8%～13%	30%～40%	27%～40%	27%～40%
自身免疫性甲状腺疾病(AITD)	6%～20%	15%～30%	17%～33%	15%～30%
高泌乳素血症	0.4%	5%	36%	—

检测抗磷脂抗体(aPL)阳性为特征的免疫性疾病,临床表现为血栓形成风险增加和妊娠丢失[13]。在RPL患者中,符合Sapporo标准的APS患病率为2.5%,而aPL单次阳性率为10.7%,复发阳性率为4.5%[2]。然而,很少发现RIF患者有持续性aPL。在RIF患者中进行aPL检测的价值仍存争议,需要更多的数据以提出明确的建议[14]。

2.2 胰岛素抵抗和多囊卵巢综合征与反复妊娠丢失/反复种植失败

IR是机体对胰岛素反应不良,不能有效摄取葡萄糖进行代谢的一种病理状态。因此,胰岛素的降血糖作用无法发挥。高血糖会刺激机体分泌多量胰岛素,即高胰岛素血症。虽然PCOS的诊断不需要IR,但它似乎会在许多患者中引起或加剧高雄激素血症,而胰岛素增敏剂治疗可以降低雄激素水平。最近的一项研究表明,IR对非PCOS的瘦型患者的体外受精(IVF)结局有不利影响[15]。尽管在非PCOS患者中IR与RPL之间的相关机制仍不确定。然而,目前的研究发现,约70%的PCOS患者存在IR[16]。此外,据报道,27%～40%的RPL女性患有PCOS[16,17]。

2.3 自身免疫性甲状腺疾病与反复妊娠丢失/反复种植失败

AITD是一种常见的器官特异性自身免疫性疾病,包括自身免疫性甲状腺炎和Graves病。在育龄期女性中,甲状腺功能不全和甲状腺自身免疫(TAI)常同时存在,可能与排卵功能障碍和不良妊娠结局有关[18]。在未经选择的女性中,患病率为6%～20%[19,20],RPL女性的患病率更高,为17%～33%[21,22]。然而,导致甲状腺功能亢进的Graves病对RPL或RIF的影响尚未见报道。

2.4 高泌乳素血症与反复妊娠丢失/反复种植失败

高泌乳素血症定义为血清泌乳素(PRL)水平异常升高,通常定义为女性PRL高于25 μg/L(530 mU/L)[23,24]。一些生理状态,包括妊娠、母乳喂养、压力、运动和睡眠,也可导致PRL升高[24]。某些处方药,如钙通道阻滞剂、甲基多巴、三环类药物,以及选择性5-羟色胺再摄取抑制剂、抗抑郁剂、阿片类药物和雌激素,也可增加泌乳素水平[25]。其他原因还包括生殖细胞系功能缺失突变、特发性高泌乳素血症、甲状腺功能减退、胸壁损伤、雌激素治疗、慢性肾功能衰竭、PCOS和大泌乳素瘤[26]。过多的PRL通过反馈作用于下丘脑相应的受体,抑制垂体促性腺激素的分泌,引起无排卵和闭经。临床观察发现,RPL患者的泌乳素水平明显较高,RPL患者的高泌乳素血症发生率约为36%[27],表明高泌乳素血症与流产的发生有因果关系,尤其是在无其他明显原因的RPL患者中[28,29]。

2.5 其他免疫和代谢因素与反复妊娠丢失/反复种植失败

系统性红斑狼疮(SLE)是一种自身免疫性疾病,多见于女性,常与APS相关,可导致流产风险增加[30]。干燥综合征[31]、类风湿关节炎[32]和系统性硬化症[33]也在一定程度上与妊娠并发症的发生相关,但与RPL或RIF的直接联系则相对较少。维生素D(VitD)缺乏被认为是自身免疫性疾病的潜在原因之一,且已在TAI患者中观察到VitD水平降低[34]。反之,VitD缺乏也与不孕和妊娠丢失有关,这表明TAI、VitD与不良妊娠结局之间可能存在相互影响。

3 与反复妊娠丢失和反复种植失败相关的潜在免疫代谢病理学

有充分的证据表明,成功的妊娠取决于滋养细胞对母体免疫系统的有效调节，以及母胎界面的适当交互对话[35]。驻留在子宫内的免疫细胞表现出组织特异性表型和功能，参与人类生殖各个阶段的免疫调节[5]。近年来，免疫细胞如何通过免疫代谢调整自身以适应妊娠的过程逐渐受到关注。细胞代谢是一种维持细胞存活的基本过程，也是对细胞命运具有高度适应性调节作用的力量[36]。介导不同免疫细胞功能的代谢途径可发生重编程，这种可塑性能改变免疫细胞的功能[37]。本部分将主要阐述女性 RPL 和 RIF 的免疫代谢变化及其机制。

3.1 抗磷脂综合征

抗磷脂抗体介导的妊娠丢失与胎盘血管血栓形成、蜕膜血管病变、绒毛间纤维蛋白沉积和胎盘床梗死相关[38-40]。在一项对 RPL 患者的研究中，56% 产科 APS 患者的外周 NK 细胞（pNK）水平较高[41]，表明 NK 细胞可能参与了 APS 诱导的 RPL。pNK 细胞的细胞毒性和百分比在妊娠期间动态变化[42]。根据欧洲人类生殖与胚胎学会（ESHRE）的论证，RPL 与 pNK 数量之间的关联较弱[43]。研究表明 NK 细胞的复杂性和可塑性，使得 NK 细胞亚群的表型定义不一致。$CD56^{dim}CD16^+$ NK 和 $CD56^{bright}CD16^-$ NK 是典型的功能亚群。大多数 pNK 是 $CD56^{dim}CD16^+$ NK，具有更强的细胞毒功能，而许多子宫 NK 是 $CD56^{bright}CD16^-$ NK，具有更强的分泌细胞因子的能力。不同的代谢特征可能是识别 NK 细胞功能命运的可靠标志。例如，葡萄糖驱动的糖酵解和氧化代谢对于细胞毒能力是必需的，而低氧和糖酵解受限的条件则有利于调节功能[44]，这表明在产科 APS 患者中，pNK 细胞的糖酵解和氧化代谢活动较高。

免疫细胞在妊娠期间进行的免疫代谢包括糖酵解增加、氧化磷酸化减少、脂肪酸（FA）合成增加以及能量利用模式的其他转换[45]。这一过程通常通过激活哺乳动物雷帕霉素靶蛋白（mTOR）来增强糖酵解和线粒体功能[46,47]。APS 相关血管病变已被证实与异常 mTOR 信号有关[48]。mTOR 还参与调节 aPL 诱导的单核细胞组织因子（TF）和 IL-8 的表达以及血小板的活化/聚集[49,50]。此外，TF/FⅦa/PAR2 信号转导介导 APS 的中性粒细胞活化和胎儿死亡。因此，作为肝脏胆固醇合成的限速酶抑制剂，他汀类药物可能是治疗 aPL 诱导的妊娠并发症的最佳候选药物[51]，因为这一过程的免疫病理学被认为是通过抑制胆固醇合成来调节的。

3.2 胰岛素抵抗

IR 的发生可能与产生针对胰岛素受体自身抗原的自身抗体有关，导致胰岛素不能与其受体结合而发挥调节血糖的作用。NK 细胞是肥胖诱导应激时脂肪细胞上关键的巨噬细胞极化和 IR 调节因子[52]。代谢激活对于 NK 细胞产生效应蛋白（包括 IFN-γ 和颗粒酶 B）以及与靶细胞形成正确的免疫突触至关重要[53]。在 NK 细胞激活过程中，通过激活 mTOR，糖酵解和线粒体功能增强[46]。FA 和过氧化物酶体增殖激活受体激动剂抑制 mTOR 介导的糖酵解、效应器功能和 NK 细胞的代谢[53]。

脂肪组织炎症与肥胖及其多种并发症相关[54]。在肥胖人群中观察到的 Treg 细胞数量减少会导致全身性 IR，因为 Treg 细胞通常可以改善糖耐量和胰岛素敏感性[55]。短链脂肪酸可影响 Th17 和 Treg 的稳态，从而导致意外的妊娠丢失[56]。此外，$CD4^+/CD8^+$ 的增加与肿瘤坏死因子-α（TNF-α）水平呈正相关[57]。值得注意的是，甘油三酯（TG）能通过增加极低密度脂蛋白颗粒的产生而诱导血浆 TNF-α 水平升高[58]。TNF-α 的表达增加有助于全身性 IR，其通常能改善糖耐量和胰岛素敏感性[55]。此外，外周血单个核细胞和脂肪组织中 CC 趋化因子配体 5（CCL5）和 CC 趋化因子受体 5（CCR5）水平升高与 PCOS 患者高雄激素血症和 IR 相关[59]。相反，脂肪组织中的 B 细胞可能通过激活促炎性巨噬细胞和 T 细胞并释放抵抗素来促进 IR[60,61]。

除脂质代谢外，PCOS 患者的糖代谢也存在紊乱[62]。据报道，有 6 种蛋白质组学生物标志物可预测 PCOS 患者早产的风险，其中丙酮酸激酶同工酶 M1/M2（PKM1/PKM2）升高与糖代谢缺陷密切相关[63]。PCOS 患者的激活和终末补体途径组分增加，尤其是在 IR 和肥胖的情况下[64]。一项研究表明，2 型糖尿病患者 $CD8^+PD-1^+$ T 细胞的代谢-免疫轴发生紊乱，而二甲双胍治疗可通过增加有氧糖酵解活性来挽救抗原特异性信号转导和细胞因子的产生[65]。此外，胰岛素受体缺陷的 T 细胞表现出炎症潜能降低和保护性免疫功能低下，这表明胰岛素受体通过控制细胞代谢直接调节 T 细胞功能[66]。IR 引起的代谢紊乱破坏了与 RPL 和 RIF 密切相关的各种免疫细胞的平衡，值得进一步研究。

3.3 自身免疫性甲状腺疾病

TAI 是导致甲状腺功能减退的主要原因。即使在甲状腺功能正常的女性中，也有研究发现甲状腺自身抗体，尤其是甲状腺过氧化物酶抗体（TPOAb）与不良妊娠结局之间存在联系[67]。在许多不明原因 RPL 女性中，TPOAb 阳性预示活产率降低[68]。据报道，在 22.5% 有 RPL 病史的女性和 14.5% 的健康对照者中检测到甲状腺自身抗体，两者间存在显著差异[69]。目前，甲状腺自身抗体引起 RPL 的机制尚不清楚。已提出了三个假说[70,71]：第一个是自身抗体可能损害甲状腺功能，导致妊娠期代谢异常。第二个是甲状腺抗体破坏胎盘屏障，导致胎盘和胎儿的异常排斥反应。第三个是甲状腺自身抗体引起母体自身免疫系统异常，通过细胞和体液免疫激活对胎儿产生类似的"排斥"。事实上，TAI 受损女性的外周血固有免疫发生了 Th1 改变，表明异常 T 细胞可能是 TAI 和不孕症的基础[71]。在患有 AITD 的女性中，有多达 40% 的细胞毒性 NK 细胞过度活跃和迁移，从而改变子宫免疫和激素反应[71]。NK 细胞增多和过度活跃也与不孕症相关，在 TAI 中更为常见。在 TAI 患者中，NK 细胞和 NKT 样细胞的百分比增加，NK 细胞的细胞毒性增加，表明免疫状态发生了改变，可能影响妊娠结局[72]。

3.4 其他免疫因素

关于其他免疫代谢因子如何影响 RPL 和 RIF 的研究很少。以 SLE 为代表的自身免疫性疾病导致流产的原因与 APS 相似。除 aCL 和抗 β2 GP1 外，SLE 患者的抗 PT 抗体和抗 Anx V 抗体可能在 RPL 中发挥重要作用[73]。维生素 D 的免疫调节特性归因于其对固有和适应性免疫细胞的影响，包括巨噬细胞、树突状细胞[74]，以及 T 淋巴细胞和 B 淋巴细胞[75]，所有这些细胞都含有维生素 D_3 受体。体外研究表明，在表达维生素 D 的 T 细胞中，CD4 激活促进 Th2 表型（产生 IL-4 和 IL-5），抑制 Th1 活性（产生干扰素-γ 和 IL-2）[75]。

4 评估

对于有关免疫和代谢紊乱的 RPL 和 RIF 诊断，应首先考虑是否存在上述临床症状，然后根据临床症状进一步分析实验室检查。当患者出现不明原因的反复血栓形成、反复胎儿丢失、子痫、子痫前期、血小板减少、下肢溃疡或网织细胞增多症时，应考虑 APS[76]。建议进行抗磷脂抗体检测，如 aCL、抗 β2 GP1 或 LA。中高滴度的抗磷脂抗体提示可能存在 APS[76]。

肥胖、血脂异常、动脉粥样硬化、凝血功能障碍、高血压、糖尿病、高尿酸血症、餐前低血糖症状和黑棘皮病提示需要进行 IR 评估。高胰岛素正葡萄糖钳夹被广泛认为是检测外周胰岛素敏感性的"金标准"。然而，这种方法成本高、耗时长、且有创，在临床上并不实用。口服糖耐量试验和空腹替代试验，以及定量胰岛素敏感性检查指数，可作为大规模临床研究的替代方案[77]。此外，高甘油三酯血症和高游离 FA 可进一步加重 IR，应引起重视。对于月经稀少、闭经和多毛症的女性应评估 PCOS。高雄激素血症是诊断 PCOS 的一个关键指标，而先天性肾上腺增生、库欣综合征和雄激素分泌肿瘤等疾病需在诊断 PCOS 时予以排除[78]。

当出现甲状腺肿大、畏寒、便秘、皮肤干燥和黏液性水肿等甲状腺功能减退症相关症状时，需要进行甲状腺功能检查。甲状腺功能检查的结果可能因疾病的不同阶段而异。早期阶段，三碘甲状腺原氨酸（T_3）和甲状腺素（T_4）升高，促甲状腺激素（TSH）降低。到了后期，可能会出现相反的情况。自身免疫性甲状腺炎患者血清中可能存在 TPOAb 或甲状腺球蛋白抗体（TgAb）。此外，值得注意的是，甲状腺功能减退症通常与高胆固醇血症和高甘油三酯血症并存[79]。

5 治疗和生殖结局

针对代谢途径中关键酶或关键分子的干预措施可有效管理人类自身免疫和代谢疾病[36]。多种针对代谢和免疫的药物已获得美国食品药品管理局的批准（表 24.2，图 24.1）。

迄今为止，多种免疫代谢调节药物已被使用或有望用于治疗与不良妊娠结局相关的代谢紊乱疾病。然而，免疫代谢靶向药物的安全性和有效性仍然存在许多谜团（图 24.2）。在临床实践中，需要更多的证据来应用免疫抑制剂和代谢药物以帮助获得妊娠。

5.1 抗磷脂综合征的治疗

阿司匹林联合低分子肝素（LMWH）是 APS 的标准治疗方法。研究表明，静脉注射免疫球蛋白

表 24.2　目前美国食品药品管理局批准的针对代谢和免疫反应的药物

药物	靶点	机制	FDA 妊娠药物分级
二甲双胍	AMPK	增加 FAO；抑制复合物 I；降低线粒体 ROS	B
奥利司他	胃肠道脂肪酶	抑制脂肪水解	B
西罗莫司	mTOR	抑制淋巴因子驱动的 T 细胞增殖	C
他克莫司	mTOR（FKBP12）	抑制 T 细胞活化	C
羟氯喹	未知	抑制炎症、抗凝血、降低胆固醇和 LDL	C
免疫球蛋白	免疫球蛋白受体	诱导抗炎细胞因子，抑制单核细胞和巨噬细胞活化，抑制 B 细胞增殖并调节抗体产生，抑制自身反应性 B 细胞及中和细胞因子，扩增 T 调节细胞诱导 DC、Th1 和 Th17 细胞凋亡，抑制 NK 细胞水平和细胞毒性，抑制 DC 成熟和分化	C
普伐他汀 辛伐他汀 阿托伐他汀	HMG-CoA 还原酶	抑制胆固醇合成	X

注：AMPK，AMP 活化蛋白激酶；FAO，脂肪酸氧化；ROS，活性氧；mTOR，哺乳动物雷帕霉素靶蛋白；FKBP12，FK506 结合蛋白 12；LDL，低密度脂蛋白；HMG-CoA，3-羟基-3-甲基戊二酰辅酶 A。

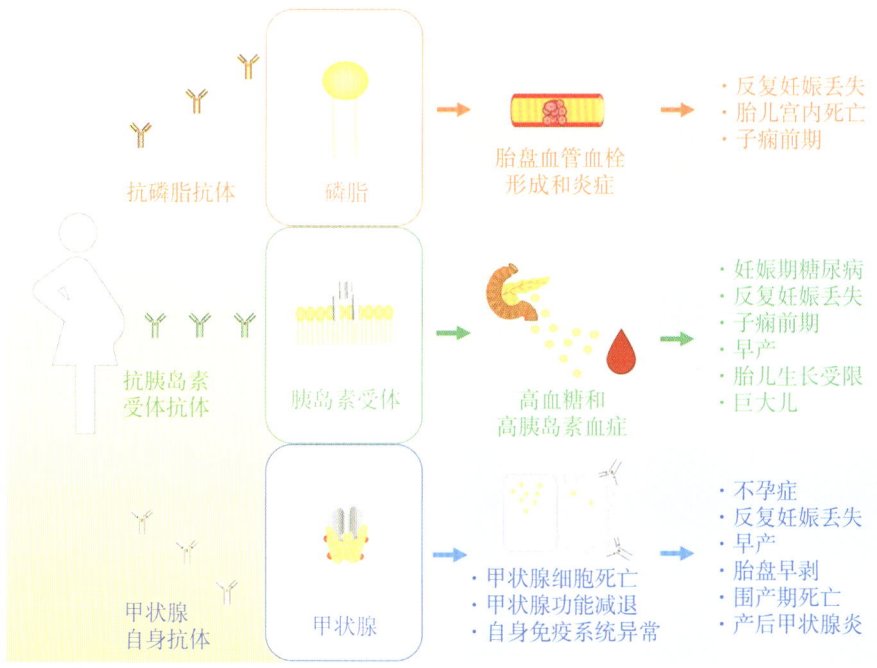

图 24.1　与生殖相关的免疫代谢病理示意图。

该图展示了导致不良妊娠结局的三种典型免疫代谢紊乱的潜在病理机制。上半部分：抗磷脂抗体通过磷脂结合蛋白与磷脂间接结合，损伤血管上皮，诱发血栓形成。当胎盘血栓形成时，胎盘血管循环减少，导致胎儿丢失或死亡。中间部分：抗胰岛素受体抗体与细胞膜上的胰岛素受体结合，降低其胰岛素敏感性，从而使胰腺分泌的胰岛素无法正常发挥作用，导致高血糖和高胰岛素血症，引起一系列代谢紊乱和不良妊娠结局。下半部分：自身抗体与甲状腺细胞结合，破坏甲状腺的正常功能。因此，甲状腺功能减退和母体自身免疫系统异常会导致不良妊娠结局。

240 免疫性反复妊娠丢失和反复种植失败

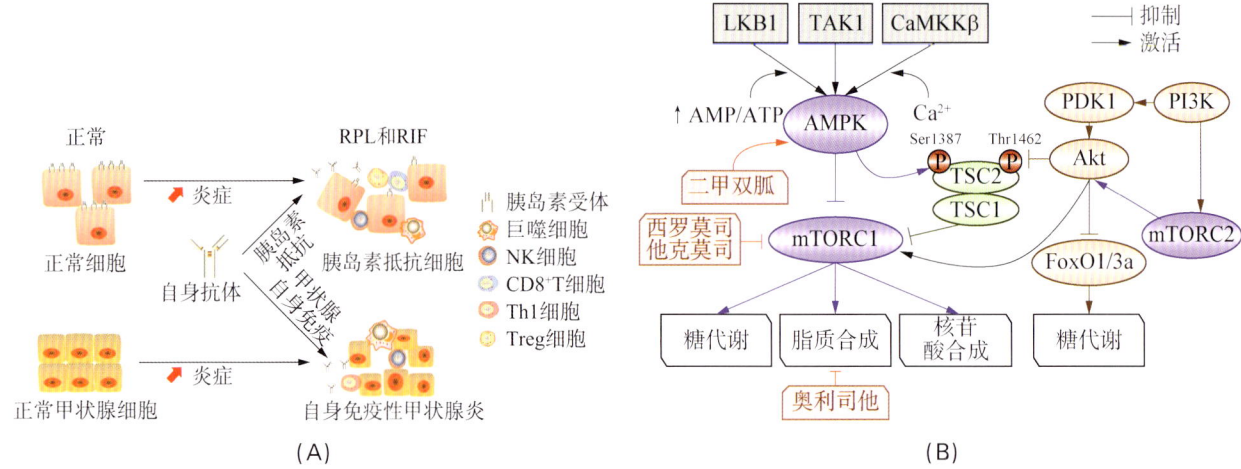

图 24.2 反复妊娠丢失（RPL）和反复种植失败（RIF）的免疫和代谢病因评估及治疗目标。
(A)正常孕妇和 RPL/RIF 患者细胞水平的免疫和代谢变化。(B)相关代谢途径和可能的治疗靶点。mTOR,哺乳动物雷帕霉素靶蛋白；AMPK,5′-磷酸腺苷活化蛋白激酶；LKB1,肝激酶 B1；TAK1,转化生长因子 β 活化激酶 1；CaMKKb,Ca²⁺/钙调蛋白依赖性蛋白激酶 β；TSC,结节性硬化症；PI3K,磷脂酰肌醇 3-激酶；Akt,丝氨酸苏氨酸激酶；PDK1,磷酸肌醇依赖性激酶-1；FoxO1/3a,叉头盒蛋白 O1/3a。

（IVIG）可降低 APS 患者的胎儿丢失率[80,81]。阿司匹林和低分子肝素通过抑制炎症因子、结合整合素和参与补体反应来调节 RPL 和 RIF 患者的免疫应答。不幸的是，20%～30%的 APS 女性仍无法通过标准治疗分娩活产儿。这些病例被定义为"难治性产科 APS"，需要考虑其他新方法，如 IVIG 或羟氯喹。羟氯喹具有免疫调节和抗凝特性，可促进滋养细胞迁移并减少 aPL 与滋养细胞的结合[82]。

他汀类药物对 aPL 阳性患者具有抗炎和抗血栓作用。尽管临床数据仍然不足，他汀类药物可能在抗凝治疗无效的 APS 患者中发挥辅助作用[82]。他汀类药物对孕妇有一定的不良反应。然而，他汀类药物对孕妇的潜在益处促使人们对妊娠期使用他汀类药物的风险/收益比进行新的评估[83]。

西罗莫司，亦称为雷帕霉素，抑制 mTOR 复合物（mTORC），可能是对标准治疗方案耐药的 aPL 阳性微血管病变患者的一种选择[50]。妊娠期间，蜕膜 CD8⁺T 细胞表现出短暂的功能障碍，IFN-γ 高表达，穿孔素和颗粒酶 B 低表达[84]。雷帕霉素可抑制 mTORC1 和 mTORC2，抑制 T 细胞增殖，这似乎有些自相矛盾。然而，它以 T 细胞记忆的形式促进免疫。雷帕霉素可以促进记忆性 CD8⁺T 细胞和记忆性 Treg 细胞的分化，可能有助于维持妊娠[85,86]。然而，其在妊娠期的治疗效果和安全性尚未确定。

IVIG 可能通过调节 Th1/Th2 细胞平衡和 Treg/Th17 细胞平衡，降低 NK 细胞毒性，从而改善妊娠结局。IVIG 的副作用少见，大多是轻微和短暂的。对于细胞免疫标志物阳性的女性，如 NK 细胞毒性增加、NK 细胞计数增加或 Th1/Th2 增加，应在孕前给予 IVIG 治疗[87]。

总之，早期识别与不良妊娠结局相关的风险因素可能是制订治疗标准的最佳策略，如免疫抑制剂、IVIG 和血浆置换[88]。

5.2 胰岛素抵抗和多囊卵巢综合征的治疗

代谢异常在 PCOS 患者胰岛素抵抗的发生、发展中起重要作用。二甲双胍联合克罗米芬可诱导 PCOS 患者排卵，提高临床妊娠率[89]。此外，二甲双胍可改善 PCOS 患者的血管内皮功能，降低流产率[90,91]。随机对照试验（RCT）发现，二甲双胍能显著减少 PCOS 患者的晚期流产和早产[92]。奥利司他是一种胰脂肪酶抑制剂，可负性调节 FA 合成，有效调节 PCOS 患者的代谢。二甲双胍和奥利司他均能改善肥胖无排卵 PCOS 患者的体重、排卵率和雄激素水平[93]。

在免疫代谢中，二甲双胍参与 T 细胞分化，诱导 T 细胞分化为 Treg 细胞和记忆性 T 细胞[94]。此外，二甲双胍可通过调节各种细胞因子的分泌，抑制 MMP-2 和 MMP-9 的表达，激活 p38 MAPK 信号转导，降低孕激素受体（PGR）的表达，减少雌、孕激素诱导的子宫内膜基质细胞蜕膜化[95]。作为一种代谢应激因子，二甲双胍还可激活 AMPK 能量传感器，增强 CD8⁺T 细胞的产生[96]。奥利司他可减弱 FA 代谢重编程，抑制 FABP5 诱导的宫颈癌淋巴结转移[97]。在啮齿动物模型中,通过激活 Nrf2 信号通路,可能对代谢功能障碍相关的脂肪肝具有保护和治疗作用[98]。然而,二甲双胍和奥利司他能否通过调节免疫代谢影响妊娠尚不清楚。

5.3 自身免疫性甲状腺疾病的治疗

一项荟萃分析研究表明,患有 RPL 的女性应筛查/治疗主要的甲状腺疾病,而不仅仅是 TAI[99]。据报道,补充左旋甲状腺素和 IVIG 治疗可预防 AITD 女性的流产。外源性补充合成甲状腺激素类似物以降低 AITD 女性的流产风险是基于考虑 AITD 与妊娠期甲状腺功能减退之间的关系。然而,一项 RCT 的荟萃分析报告,在 TPOAb 阳性的女性中,左甲状腺素与临床妊娠结局改善无关[100],提示存在其他机制,而不是激素缺乏导致流产。根据目前的证据,建议在妊娠期检测 AITD 女性的血清 TSH。此外,对于甲状腺功能减退的女性(TSH≥2.5 和<4.3),应评估 ATA。

6 总结和建议

- RIF 和 RPL 的病因是多样化的,免疫和代谢紊乱在其发病机制中占相当大的比例。
- 生活方式的改变,社会支持和药物控制可以改善这些女性的妊娠结局。
- 值得注意的是,靶向免疫细胞的代谢调节是改善 RPL 和 RIF 妊娠结局的有效手段之一,但需要在准确诊断后进行。
- 对于在其他领域已被证明有效的新型免疫调节和代谢治疗方法,应特别注意对母婴的安全性,包括长期影响。

资助:本章的编写得到深圳市自然科学基金会(JCYJ20190813161801676)的资助。

参考文献

[1] Cha J, Sun X, Dey SK. Mechanisms of implantation: strategies for successful pregnancy. Nat Med 2012;18(12):1754-67.

[2] Sugiura-Ogasawara M, Ozaki Y, Katano K, Suzumori N, Kitaori T, Mizutani E. Abnormal embryonic karyotype is the most frequent cause of recurrent miscarriage. Hum Reprod 2012;27(8):2297-303.

[3] Shaulov T, Sierra S, Sylvestre C. Recurrent implantation failure in IVF: a canadian fertility and andrology society clinical practice guideline. Reprod Biomed Online 2020;41(5):819-33.

[4] Garneau AS, Young SL. Defining recurrent implantation failure: a profusion of confusion or simply an illusion? Fertil Steril 2021;116(6):1432-5.

[5] Schumacher A, Sharkey DJ, Robertson SA, Zenclussen AC. Immune cells at the fetomaternal interface: how the microenvironment modulates immune cells to foster fetal development. JI. 2018;201(2):325-34.

[6] Raghupathy R, Makhseed M, Azizieh F, Hassan N, Al-Azemi M, Al-Shamali E. Maternal Th1- and Th2-type reactivity to placental antigens in normal human pregnancy and unexplained recurrent spontaneous abortions. Cell Immunol 1999;196(2):122-30.

[7] Qian J, Zhang N, Lin J, et al. Distinct pattern of Th17/Treg cells in pregnant women with a history of unexplained recurrent spontaneous abortion. Biosci Trends 2018;12(2):157-67.

[8] King K, Smith S, Chapman M, Sacks G. Detailed analysis of peripheral blood natural killer (NK) cells in women with recurrent miscarriage. Hum Reprod 2010;25(1):52-8.

[9] Tsao FY, Wu MY, Chang YL, Wu CT, Ho HN. M1 macrophages decrease in the deciduae from normal pregnancies but not from spontaneous abortions or unexplained recurrent spontaneous abortions. J Formos Med Assoc 2018;117(3):204-11.

[10] Jasper MJ, Tremellen KP, Robertson SA. Reduced expression of IL-6 and IL-1alpha mRNAs in secretory phase endometrium of women with recurrent miscarriage. J Reprod Immunol 2007;73(1):74-84.

[11] Patil R, Patil SA, Beaman KD, Patil SA. Indole molecules as inhibitors of tubulin polymerization: potential new anticancer agents, an update (2013-2015). Future Med Chem 2016;8(11):1291-316.

[12] Thiele K, Diao L, Arck PC. Immunometabolism, pregnancy, and nutrition. Semin Immunopathol 2018;40(2):157-74.

[13] Garcia D, Erkan D. Diagnosis and management of the antiphospholipid syndrome Longo DL, (ed.) N Engl J Med 2018;378(21):2010-21.

[14] Mascarenhas M, Jeve Y, Polanski L, et al. Management of recurrent implantation failure: British Fertility Society policy and practice guideline. Hum Fertil 2021;1-25.

[15] Wang H, Zhang Y, Fang X, Kwak-Kim J, Wu L. Insulin resistance adversely affect IVF outcomes in lean women without PCOS. Front Endocrinol (Lausanne) 2021;12:734638.

[16] Goodarzi MO, Korenman SG. The importance of insulin resistance in polycystic ovary syndrome. Fertil Steril 2003;80(2):255-8.

[17] Rai R, Backos M, Rushworth F, Regan L. Polycystic ovaries and recurrent miscarriage — a reappraisal. Hum Reprod 2000;15(3):612-5.

[18] Thangaratinam S, Tan A, Knox E, Kilby MD, Franklyn J, Coomarasamy A. Association between thyroid auto-antibodies and miscarriage and preterm birth: meta-analysis of evidence.

BMJ. 2011;342(may09 1):d2616.

[19] Stagnaro-Green A, Glinoer D. Thyroid autoimmunity and the risk of miscarriage. Best Pract Res Clin Endocrinol Metab 2004;18(2):167-81.

[20] Poppe K, Velkeniers B, Glinoer D. The role of thyroid autoimmunity in fertility and pregnancy. Nat Clin Pract Endocrinol Metab 2008;4(7):394-405.

[21] Ticconi C, Giuliani E, Veglia M, Pietropolli A, Piccione E, Di Simone N. Thyroid autoimmunity and recurrent miscarriage. Am J Reprod Immunol 2011;66(6):452-9.

[22] Sarkar D. Recurrent pregnancy loss in patients with thyroid dysfunction. Indian J Endocrinol Metab 2012;16 (Suppl 2): S350-1.

[23] Chahal J, Schlechte J. Hyperprolactinemia. Pituitary. 2008; 11(2):141-6.

[24] Melmed S, Casanueva FF, Hoffman AR, et al. Diagnosis and treatment of hyperprolactinemia: an endocrine society clinical practice guideline. J Clin Endocrinol & Metab 2011;96(2): 273-88.

[25] Molitch ME. Drugs and prolactin. Pituitary. 2008;11(2): 209-18.

[26] Prabhakar VKB, Davis JRE. Hyperprolactinaemia. Best Pract & Res Clin Obstet & Gynaecol 2008;22(2):341-53.

[27] Bussen S, Sütterlin M, Steck T. Endocrine abnormalities during the follicular phase in women with recurrent spontaneous abortion. Hum Reprod 1999;14(1):18-20.

[28] Ando N, Gorai I, Hirabuki T, Onose R, Hirahara F, Minaguchi H. [Prolactin disorders in patients with habitual abortion]. Nihon Sanka Fujinka Gakkai Zasshi 1992;44(6): 650-6.

[29] Hirahara F, Andoh N, Sawai K, Hirabuki T, Uemura T, Minaguchi H. Hyperprolactinemic recurrent miscarriage and results of randomized bromocriptine treatment trials. Fertil Steril 1998;70(2):246-52.

[30] Chen D, Lao M, Zhang J, et al. Fetal and maternal outcomes of planned pregnancy in patients with systemic lupus erythematosus: a retrospective multicenter study. J Immunol Res 2018;2018:2413637.

[31] De Carolis S, Salvi S, Botta A, et al. The impact of primary Sjogren's syndrome on pregnancy outcome: our series and review of the literature. Autoimmun Rev 2014; 13 (2): 103-7.

[32] Ota K, Dambaeva S, Lee J, Gilman-Sachs A, Beaman K, Kwak-Kim J. Persistent high levels of IgM anti-phospholipid antibodies in a patient with recurrent pregnancy losses and rheumatoid arthritis. Am J Reprod Immunol 2014;71(3): 286-92.

[33] Blagojevic J, AlOdhaibi KA, Aly AM, et al. Pregnancy in systemic sclerosis: results of a systematic review and meta-analysis. J Rheumatol 2020;47(6):881-7.

[34] Twig G, Shina A, Amital H, Shoenfeld Y. Pathogenesis of infertility and recurrent pregnancy loss in thyroid autoimmunity. J Autoimmun 2012;38(2-3):J275-81.

[35] Gellersen B, Brosens JJ. Cyclic decidualization of the human endometrium in reproductive health and failure. Endocr Rev 2014;35(6):851-905.

[36] Jung J, Zeng H, Horng T. Metabolism as a guiding force for immunity. Nat Cell Biol 2019;21(1):85-93.

[37] Pearce EL, Pearce EJ. Metabolic pathways in immune cell activation and quiescence. Immunity. 2013;38(4):633-43.

[38] Rand JH, Wu XX, Andree HA, et al. Pregnancy loss in the antiphospholipid-antibody syndrome — a possible thrombogenic mechanism. N Engl J Med 1997;337(3):154-60.

[39] Kwak-Kim J, Agcaoili MSL, Aleta L, et al. Management of women with recurrent pregnancy losses and anti-phospholipid antibody syndrome. Am J Reprod Immunol 2013; Published online March.

[40] Pantham P, Abrahams VM, Chamley LW. The role of anti-phospholipid antibodies in autoimmune reproductive failure. Reproduction. 2016;151(5):R79-90.

[41] Perricone C, De Carolis C, Giacomelli R, et al. High levels of NK cells in the peripheral blood of patients affected with anti-phospholipid syndrome and recurrent spontaneous abortion: a potential new hypothesis. Rheumatol (Oxf) 2007; 46(10):1574-8.

[42] Gabrilovac J, Zadjelović J, Osmak M, Suchanek E, Zupanović Z, Boranić M. NK cell activity and estrogen hormone levels during normal human pregnancy. Gynecol Obstet Invest 1988;25(3):165-72.

[43] The ESHRE Guideline Group on RPL, Bender Atik R, Christiansen OB, et al. ESHRE guideline: recurrent pregnancy loss. Hum Reprod Open 2018;2018(2):hoy004.

[44] Poznanski SM, Ashkar AA. What defines NK cell functional fate: phenotype or metabolism? Front Immunol 2019; 10:1414.

[45] Loftus RM, Finlay DK. Immunometabolism: cellular metabolism turns immune regulator. J Biol Chem 2016; 291 (1):1-10.

[46] Donnelly RP, Loftus RM, Keating SE, et al. mTORC1-dependent metabolic reprogramming is a prerequisite for NK cell effector function. J Immunol 2014;193(9):4477-84.

[47] Chi H. Regulation and function of mTOR signalling in T cell fate decisions. Nat Rev Immunol 2012;12(5):325-38.

[48] Canaud G, Bienaimé F, Tabarin F, et al. Inhibition of the mtorc pathway in the antiphospholipid syndrome. N Engl J Med 2014;371(4):303-12.

[49] Xia L, Zhou H, Wang T, et al. activation of mTOR is involved in anti-β2GPI/β2GPI-induced expression of tissue factor and IL-8 in monocytes. Thromb Res 2017; 157: 103-10.

[50] Hollerbach A, Müller-Calleja N, Ritter S, et al. Platelet activation by antiphospholipid antibodies depends on epitope specificity and is prevented by mTOR inhibitors. Thromb Haemost 2019;119(7):1147-53.

[51] Redecha P, Franzke CW, Ruf W, Mackman N, Girardi G. Neutrophil activation by the tissue factor/Factor VIIa/PAR2 axis mediates fetal death in a mouse model of anti-phospholipid syndrome. J Clin Invest 2008;118(10):3453-61.

[52] Wensveen FM, Jelenčić V, Valentić S, et al. NK cells link obesity-induced adipose stress to inflammation and insulin resistance. Nat Immunol 2015;16(4):376-85.

[53] Michelet X, Dyck L, Hogan A, et al. Metabolic reprogramming of natural killer cells in obesity limits antitumor responses. Nat Immunol 2018;19(12):1330-40.

[54] Zeng Q, Sun X, Xiao L, Xie Z, Bettini M, Deng T. A unique population: adipose-resident regulatory T cells. Front Immunol 2018;9:2075.

[55] Bapat SP, Myoung Suh J, Fang S, et al. Depletion of fat-resident Treg cells prevents age-associated insulin resistance. Nature. 2015;528(7580):137-41.

[56] Smith PM, Howitt MR, Panikov N, et al. The microbial metabolites, short-chain fatty acids, regulate colonic treg cell homeostasis. Science. 2013;341(6145):569-73.

[57] Wang K, Wang DC, Feng YQ, Xiang-Feng L. Changes in cytokine levels and CD4+/CD8+ T cells ratio in draining lymph node of burn wound. J Burn Care Res 2007;28(5): 747-53.

[58] Deng Y, Scherer PE. Adipokines as novel biomarkers and regulators of the metabolic syndrome. Ann N Y Acad Sci 2010;1212:E1-19.

[59] Juan CC, Chen KH, Chen CW, et al. Increased regulated on activation, normal T-cell expressed and secreted levels and cysteine-cysteine chemokine receptor 5 upregulation in omental adipose tissue and peripheral blood mononuclear cells are associated with testosterone level and insulin resistance in polycystic ovary syndrome. Fertil Steril 2021; 116 (4): 1139-46.

[60] Nishimura S, Manabe I, Nagasaki M, et al. CD8+ effector T cells contribute to macrophage recruitment and adipose tissue inflammation in obesity. Nat Med 2009;15(8):914-20.

[61] Lauterbach MAR, Wunderlich FT. Macrophage function in obesity-induced inflammation and insulin resistance. Pflug Arch-Eur J Physiol 2017;469(3-4):385-96.

[62] Kim JY, Song H, Kim H, et al. Transcriptional profiling with a pathway-oriented analysis identifies dysregulated molecular phenotypes in the endometrium of patients with polycystic ovary syndrome. J Clin Endocrinol & Metab 2009; 94(4):1416-26.

[63] Galazis N, Docheva N, Nicolaides KH, Atiomo W. Proteomic biomarkers of preterm birth risk in women with polycystic ovary syndrome (PCOS): a systematic review and biomarker database integration. PLoS One 2013; 8 (1): e53801.

[64] Lewis RD, Narayanaswamy AK, Farewell D, Rees DA. Complement activation in polycystic ovary syndrome occurs in the postprandial and fasted state and is influenced by obesity and insulin sensitivity. Clin Endocrinol (Oxf) 2021;94(1): 74-84.

[65] Nojima I, Eikawa S, Tomonobu N, et al. Dysfunction of CD8+ PD-1+ T cells in type 2 diabetes caused by the impairment of metabolism-immune axis. Sci Rep 2020;10(1): 14928.

[66] Tsai S, Clemente-Casares X, Zhou AC, et al. Insulin receptor-mediated stimulation boosts T cell immunity during inflammation and infection. Cell Metab 2018;28(6):922-34 e4.

[67] Bussen S, Steck T. Thyroid autoantibodies in euthyroid non-pregnant women with recurrent spontaneous abortions. Hum Reprod 1995;10(11):2938-40.

[68] Bliddal S, Feldt-Rasmussen U, Rasmussen ÁK, et al. Thyroid peroxidase antibodies and prospective live birth rate: a cohort study of women with recurrent pregnancy loss. Thyroid. 2019;29(10):1465-74.

[69] Muller AF, Verhoeff A, Mantel MJ, De Jong FH, Berghout A. Decrease of free thyroxine levels after controlled ovarian hyperstimulation. J Clin Endocrinol Metab 2000; 85 (2): 545-8.

[70] Cavagna M, Mantese JC. Biomarkers of endometrial receptivity — a review. placenta. 2003;24(suppl b):s39-47.

[71] kim ny, cho hj, kim hy, et al. thyroid autoimmunity and its association with cellular and humoral immunity in women with reproductive failures: thyroid autoimmunity and reproductive failures. Am J Reprod Immunol 2011;65(1):78-87.

[72] Miko E, Meggyes M, Doba K, et al. Characteristics of peripheral blood NK and NKT-like cells in euthyroid and subclinical hypothyroid women with thyroid autoimmunity experiencing reproductive failure. J Reprod Immunol 2017; 124:62-70.

[73] Bizzaro N, Tonutti E, Villalta D, Tampoia M, Tozzoli R. Prevalence and clinical correlation of anti-phospholipid-binding protein antibodies in anticardiolipin-negative patients with systemic lupus erythematosus and women with unexplained recurrent miscarriages. Arch Pathol Lab Med 2005;129(1):61-8.

[74] Penna G, Adorini L. 1α,25-dihydroxyvitamin D 3 inhibits differentiation, maturation, activation, and survival of dendritic cells leading to impaired alloreactive T cell activation. J Immunol 2000;164(5):2405-11.

[75] Boonstra A, Barrat FJ, Crain C, Heath VL, Savelkoul HFJ, O'Garra A. 1α,25-dihydroxyvitamin D3 has a direct effect on naive CD4− T cells to enhance the development of Th2 cells. J Immunol 2001;167(9):4974-80.

[76] Sammaritano LR. Anti-phospholipid syndrome. Best Pract & Res Clin Rheumatol 2020;34(1):101463.

[77] Otten J, Ahrén B, Olsson T. Surrogate measures of insulin sensitivity vs the hyperinsulinaemic-euglycaemic clamp: a meta-analysis. Diabetologia. 2014;57(9):1781-8.

[78] Fauser BCJM, Tarlatzis BC, Rebar RW, et al. Consensus on women's health aspects of polycystic ovary syndrome (PCOS): the Amsterdam ESHRE/ASRM-sponsored 3rd PCOS consensus workshop group. Fertil Steril 2012;97(1): 28-38 e25.

[79] Alexander EK, Pearce EN, Brent GA, et al. Guidelines of the American thyroid association for the diagnosis and management of thyroid disease during pregnancy and the postpartum. Thyroid 2017;27(3):315-89 2017.

[80] Heilmann L, von Tempelhoff GF, Pollow K. Antiphospholipid syndrome in obstetrics. Clin Appl Thromb Hemost 2003; 9 (2):143-50.

[81] Ziakas PD, Pavlou M, Voulgarelis M. Heparin treatment in antiphospholipid syndrome with recurrent pregnancy loss: a systematic review and meta-analysis. Obstet & Gynecol 2010; 115(6):1256-62.

[82] Sevim E, Willis R, Erkan D. Is there a role for immunosuppression in anti-phospholipid syndrome? Hematol Am Soc Hematol Educ Program 2019;2019(1):426-32.

[83] Vahedian-Azimi A, Makvandi S, Banach M, Reiner Ž, Sahebkar A. Fetal toxicity associated with statins: a systematic review and meta-analysis. Atherosclerosis. 2021; 327:59-67.

[84] Liu L, Huang X, Xu C, et al. Decidual CD8+ T cells exhibit both residency and tolerance signatures modulated by decidual stromal cells. J Transl Med 2020;18(1):221.

[85] Powell JD, Delgoffe GM. The mammalian target of rapamycin: linking T cell differentiation, function, and metabolism. Immunity. 2010;33(3):301-11.

[86] Araki K, Turner AP, Shaffer VO, et al. mTOR regulates memory CD8 T-cell differentiation. Nature. 2009; 460 (7251):108-12.

[87] Yang X, Meng T. Is there a role of intravenous immunoglobulin in immunologic recurrent pregnancy loss? Bayry J. (ed.) J Immunol Res 2020;2020:1-14.

[88] De Carolis S, Tabacco S, Rizzo F, et al. Anti-phospholipid syndrome: an update on risk factors for pregnancy outcome. Autoimmun Rev 2018;17(10):956-66.

[89] Practice Committee of the American Society for Reproductive Medicine. Electronic address: ASRM@asrm.org, practice

committee of the American society for reproductive medicine. Role of metformin for ovulation induction in infertile patients with polycystic ovary syndrome (PCOS): a guideline. Fertil Steril 2017;108(3):426-41.

[90] Attia GR, Rainey WE, Carr BR. Metformin directly inhibits androgen production in human thecal cells. Fertil Steril 2001;76(3):517-24.

[91] Jakubowicz DJ, Iuorno MJ, Jakubowicz S, Roberts KA, Nestler JE. Effects of metformin on early pregnancy loss in the polycystic ovary syndrome. J Clin Endocrinol Metab 2002;87(2):524-9.

[92] Løvvik TS, Carlsen SM, Salvesen Ø, et al. Use of metformin to treat pregnant women with polycystic ovary syndrome (PregMet2): a randomised, double-blind, placebo-controlled trial. Lancet Diabetes Endocrinol 2019;7(4):256-66.

[93] Metwally M, Amer S, Li TC, Ledger WL. An RCT of metformin vs orlistat for the management of obese anovulatory women. Hum Reprod 2009;24(4):966-75.

[94] Pereira FV, Melo ACL, Low JS, et al. metformin exerts antitumor activity via induction of multiple death pathways in tumor cells and activation of a protective immune response. Oncotarget. 2018;9(40):25808-25.

[95] Xiong F, Xiao J, Bai Y, Zhang Y, Li Q, Lishuang X. Metformin inhibits estradiol and progesterone-induced decidualization of endometrial stromal cells by regulating expression of progesterone receptor, cytokines and matrix metalloproteinases. Biomed Pharmacother 2019;109:1578-85.

[96] Pearce EL, Walsh MC, Cejas PJ, et al. Enhancing CD8 T-cell memory by modulating fatty acid metabolism. Nature. 2009;460(7251):103-7.

[97] Zhang C, Liao Y, Liu P, et al. FABP5 promotes lymph node metastasis in cervical cancer by reprogramming fatty acid metabolism. Theranostics. 2020;10(15):6561-80.

[98] Zakaria Z, Othman ZA, Bagi Suleiman J, Jalil NAC, Ghazali WSW, Mohamed M. Protective and therapeutic effects of orlistat on metabolic syndrome and oxidative stress in high-fat diet-induced metabolic dysfunction-associated fatty liver disease (MAFLD) in rats: role on Nrf2 activation. Vet Sci 2021;8(11):274.

[99] Dong AC, Morgan J, Kane M, Stagnaro-Green A, Stephenson MD. Subclinical hypothyroidism and thyroid autoimmunity in recurrent pregnancy loss: a systematic review and meta-analysis. Fertil Steril 2020;113(3):587-600 e1.

[100] Wang X, Zhang Y, Tan H, et al. Effect of levothyroxine on pregnancy outcomes in women with thyroid autoimmunity: a systematic review with meta-analysis of randomized controlled trials. Fertil Steril 2020;114(6):1306-14.

第 25 章

子宫内膜异位症与生殖障碍

Endometriosis and reproductive failures

Gentaro Izumi, Kaori Koga and Yutaka Osuga

Department of Obstetrics and Gynecology, Graduate School of Medicine, The University of Tokyo, Tokyo, Japan

1 引言

子宫内膜异位症的特征是子宫内膜组织在子宫外的种植和生长,如卵巢、输卵管以及包括腹膜壁在内的其他盆腔腹膜器官,是育龄期女性常见的妇科疾病,可引起痛经和慢性盆腔疼痛。众所周知,子宫内膜异位症会导致不孕症,大规模研究表明,该类不孕症的患病率为25%～40%[1]。

子宫内膜异位症与生殖障碍之间的关系仍在讨论中。一些研究表明,子宫内膜异位症可损害子宫内膜功能,导致反复妊娠丢失和种植失败。对体外受精(IVF)结果的荟萃分析显示,子宫内膜异位症患者的胚胎种植率低于对照组[2]。子宫内膜异位症不影响胚胎非整倍体率,但影响种植率,因此人们认为子宫内膜异位症患者会出现种植失败。然而,最近的一项研究表明,子宫内膜异位症患者的整倍体囊胚冷冻移植后的活产率与对照组相似[3]。Senapati等[4]利用辅助生殖技术学会数据库分析了IVF结局数据,得出结论:孤立性子宫内膜异位症不是早期妊娠丢失的危险因素,但伴有输卵管因素的子宫内膜异位症与早期妊娠丢失的风险增加相关。与无子宫内膜异位症的不孕症女性相比,患有子宫内膜异位症并伴有不孕症的患者,如输卵管性不孕、不明原因不孕及所有其他诊断,活产率显著降低[4]。这些近期的研究表明,当子宫内膜异位症合并其他生殖道改变时,活产的机会降低。因此,子宫内膜异位症相关不孕症的治疗可提高种植失败或反复妊娠丢失患者的妊娠和活产机会。本章将讨论子宫内膜异位症相关不孕症的有效治疗方案。

2 子宫内膜异位症相关生殖功能障碍的机制

许多研究报道了子宫内膜异位症导致不孕的机制。其中一个主要机制是输卵管纤维化、粘连和慢性炎症引起输卵管拾卵和运送胚胎的功能障碍。子宫内膜异位症还被认为会改变子宫内膜容受性,进而导致生殖功能障碍。

与子宫内膜异位症相关子宫内膜功能障碍的机制尚不清楚。然而,一些研究提出了假设(图25.1)。已有研究报道了子宫内膜异位症患者子宫内膜中对胚胎种植起重要作用的基因表达异常[5]。此外,子宫内膜异位症患者子宫内膜中的孕酮抵抗会导致雌激素无拮抗状态,不适宜胚胎种植[6]。这些异常的分子和激素功能障碍被认为损害子宫内膜异位症患者的子宫内膜容受性。

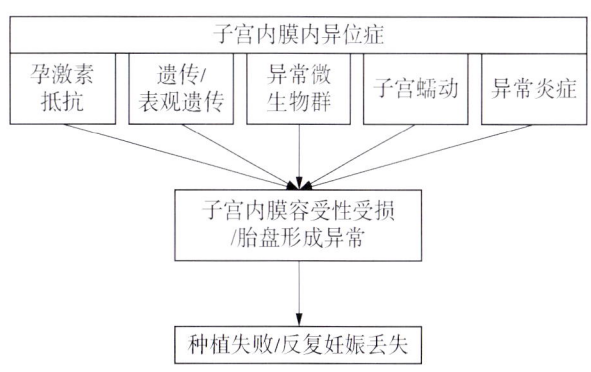

图25.1 子宫内膜异位症相关种植失败和反复妊娠丢失的机制。

3 子宫内膜异位症相关妊娠失败的免疫因素

3.1 慢性子宫内膜炎

近期有研究报道,慢性子宫内膜炎与子宫内膜异位症之间存在密切联系[7]。慢性子宫内膜炎是子宫内膜的一种持续性炎症,通常由子宫内膜微生物群改变诱发。由于慢性子宫内膜炎在种植失败和反复妊娠丢失患者中的发病率较高[8,9],过去报道的一些与子宫内膜异位症相关的生殖障碍可能与同时存在的慢性子宫内膜炎有关。

3.2 细胞因子

子宫内膜异位症患者存在异常炎症状态或免疫细胞功能异常。在子宫内膜异位症患者的腹腔液中,各种细胞因子水平均高于对照组,包括白细胞介素(IL)-1、IL-6、IL-8、IL-10和肿瘤坏死因子(TNF)-α[10]。免疫细胞功能障碍可能是这些细胞因子失调的原因之一。子宫内膜异位症患者的巨噬细胞具有较高的活化状态[11],分泌的促炎细胞因子增多[12]。肥大细胞、中性粒细胞和树突状细胞也可分泌多种促炎细胞因子,参与子宫内膜异位症的病理过程[13,14]。这些促炎细胞因子是生殖所必需的;而其异常分泌则被认为对生殖有害。例如,IL-6在滋养细胞黏附和胚胎种植过程中起重要作用;然而,必须对其活性进行适当调节,以避免种植失败或反复流产[15]。

3.3 对经血逆流的免疫细胞监视

子宫内膜异位症发生发展的一个重要机制是对经血逆流所产生的不恰当免疫反应。Sampson提出子宫内膜异位症是由经血逆流引起的子宫内膜组织植入所致[16],这一理论已被广泛接受。然而,大多数育龄期女性都存在经血逆流。对于子宫内膜异位病灶的形成,免疫细胞在增强子宫内膜细胞存活、促进其种植并诱导子宫内膜异位病灶血管生成方面发挥重要作用[17]。自然杀伤(NK)细胞的细胞毒性[18,19]和巨噬细胞的吞噬活性[20,21]在子宫内膜异位症患者中降低,这有助于子宫内膜细胞的存活。巨噬细胞是血管内皮生长因子(VEGF)的关键来源[22],促进子宫内膜异位病灶血管的生长。然而,子宫内膜异位症的发病步骤与滋养细胞植入相似。因此,子宫内膜异位症患者免疫细胞功能异常的治疗可能会抑制胚胎种植,从而使子宫内膜异位症相关不孕症的免疫治疗变得困难。

4 治疗方案

4.1 激素治疗

由于激素治疗常用于缓解子宫内膜异位症的疼痛症状,Cochrane综述报道,抑制卵巢功能的激素治疗,如促性腺激素释放激素(GnRH)激动剂、口服避孕药和达那唑,对改善患有子宫内膜异位症的不孕女性的生育能力无效[23]。因此,不应向计划妊娠的子宫内膜异位症患者提供激素治疗,因为这些治疗会推迟妊娠时间并产生副作用。

4.2 子宫输卵管造影

子宫输卵管造影是一种用于评估输卵管通畅性的诊断性检查,也是一些不孕症病例评估的一部分。此外,有研究表明,使用油性造影剂冲洗输卵管可直接提高子宫输卵管造影术后数月内的妊娠率[24]。Johnson等[25]报道,油性造影剂对子宫内膜异位症患者的生育力提高效果高于非子宫内膜异位症患者。油性造影剂提高生育力的作用机制尚不清楚。已提出的潜在机制包括:①冲洗输卵管中的碎片。②调节腹腔免疫的特征,如巨噬细胞、树突状细胞和调节性T细胞[26-28]。③调节子宫内膜容受性[29]。事实上,据报道,在没有油性造影剂从输卵管溢出的患者中观察到了生育能力提高的效果,这支持了油性造影剂对种植失败的治疗效果[30]。相反,一项随机对照试验表明,IVF周期前子宫输卵管造影并不能提高子宫内膜异位症或反复种植失败患者的活产率[31]。

4.3 免疫治疗

目前已尝试了多种免疫疗法,但仍没有足够的证据推荐将免疫疗法作为子宫内膜异位症标准疗法。有两项研究表明,在IVF周期中使用皮质类固醇可能对自身抗体阳性的子宫内膜异位症患者有效[32,33]。Onalan等[34]报道了一项对IVF周期中TNF-α拮抗剂治疗的回顾性分析,结果显示TNF-α拮抗剂治疗组的妊娠率和活产率均高于对照组。然而,目前尚无随机对照试验证实这些药物的益处,仍需进一步研究。

4.4 腹腔镜手术

腹腔镜手术对子宫内膜异位症既有诊断作用,

又有治疗作用。然而,子宫内膜异位症相关不孕症的手术治疗对子宫内膜异位症相关妊娠失败的影响有限。一项荟萃分析表明,腹腔镜下子宫内膜异位病灶切除术和消融术可减轻总体疼痛,提高妊娠率[35]。然而,支持改善妊娠结局的证据有限。一项随机对照研究(RCT)显示,腹腔镜手术治疗轻微或轻度子宫内膜异位症不会影响胎儿丢失[36]。此外,在接受 IVF 治疗的患者中,手术组和期待治疗组的妊娠率和流产率没有差异[37]。有很多证据表明,手术通常是首选治疗方法。然而,很少有证据支持手术治疗的生殖结局优于辅助生殖技术。

4.5 体外受精方案的选择

IVF 是子宫内膜异位症相关不孕症的最重要且有效的治疗方法。

然而,目前尚无针对子宫内膜异位症患者的 IVF 方案。非随机研究报道,使用 GnRH 激动剂和拮抗剂进行控制性卵巢刺激的方案对子宫内膜异位症患者的 IVF 结局有相似的影响[38,39]。

多项研究评估了在卵巢刺激前进行药物治疗对提高活产率的影响。2002 年,Surrey 等报道,GnRH 激动剂(醋酸亮丙瑞林 3.75 mg,每 28 天一次,共三次)治疗 3 个月能提高持续妊娠率[40]。值得注意的是,他们还报道了 GnRH 激动剂能改善种植率。已经发表了几项类似的研究,2006 年的一项荟萃分析表明,子宫内膜异位症患者在 IVF 周期前 3 个月或更长时间的垂体下调可增加活产率[41]。然而,最近的研究表明,GnRH 激动剂预处理组和对照组之间的妊娠率没有显著差异[42]。2019 年发表的一项荟萃分析发现,与未进行预处理相比,子宫内膜异位症患者 IVF/卵胞浆内单精子注射(ICSI)前的长期 GnRH 激动剂治疗会影响活产率和总体并发症的发生率[43]。由于这些随机对照试验的标准(如子宫内膜异位症的诊断、子宫内膜异位症的分期及合并子宫内膜异位症)不同,这些结果被认为是非常低质量的证据。一些研究对孕激素预处理也提出了质疑,就像 GnRH 激动剂一样,这些结果都存在争议。Tamura 等[44]报道,第四代孕激素地诺孕素预处理不会影响接受 IVF 周期的子宫内膜异位症患者的活产率。相比之下,Barra 等[45]发现,地诺孕素预处理可改善 IVF 结局。有趣的是,以前研究中使用的所有胚胎都是冷冻的[44],而在后者中则移植了新鲜胚胎[45]。根据这些数据,推测在胚胎移植前立即使用 GnRH 激动剂或孕激素预处理可能有助于提高子宫内膜异位症患者的生育能力。未来需要设计良好的临床试验以证实上述发现。

4.6 新鲜与冷冻胚胎移植

一些研究还比较了子宫内膜异位症患者行新鲜胚胎移植和冷冻胚胎移植的 IVF 结局。Wu 等[16]回顾性比较了匹配队列的活产率和种植率,发现冷冻胚胎移植组的活产率和种植率均高于新鲜胚胎移植组。Bourdon 等[47]也报道,在子宫内膜异位症患者中,冷冻胚胎移植组的活产率和种植率高于新鲜胚胎移植组。而另一项研究表明,冷冻胚胎移植策略对子宫内膜异位症患者没有益处。两项研究均为回顾性配对队列研究。在这方面还需要进一步的探索,尤其是设计良好的 RCT。使用 GnRH 激动剂或孕激素预处理后进行冷冻胚胎移植可能是子宫内膜异位症患者的一种治疗选择。

5 总结和建议

- 子宫内膜异位症是否为种植失败和反复妊娠丢失的原因仍存争议。然而,一些研究表明,子宫内膜异位症降低了子宫内膜容受性。
- 对于子宫内膜异位症患者的种植失败或反复妊娠丢失,目前尚无特异性的治疗方法。然而,子宫内膜异位症相关不孕症的治疗对这些患者也是有效的。
- 体外受精是治疗子宫内膜异位症最有效的方法。冷冻胚胎移植和促性腺激素释放激素激动剂或孕激素预处理可提高生育能力。

参考文献

[1] Ozkan S, Murk W, Arici A. Endometriosis and infertility: epidemiology and evidence-based treatments. Ann N Y Acad Sci 2008;1127:92-100.

[2] Barnhart K, Dunsmoor-Su R, Coutifaris C. Effect of endometriosis on in vitro fertilization. Fertil Steril 2002;77(6):1148-55.

[3] Bishop LA, et al. Endometriosis does not impact live-birth rates in frozen embryo transfers of euploid blastocysts. Fertil Steril 2021;115(2):416-22.

[4] Senapati S, et al. Impact of endometriosis on in vitro fertilization outcomes: an evaluation of the Society for assisted reproductive technologies database. Fertil Steril 2016;106(1):164-71 e1.

[5] Macer ML, Taylor HS. Endometriosis and infertility: a review of the pathogenesis and treatment of endometriosis-associated infertility. Obstet Gynecol Clin North Am 2012;39(4):535-49.

[6] Lessey BA, Kim JJ. Endometrial receptivity in the eutopic endometrium of women with endometriosis: it is affected, and let me show you why. Fertil Steril 2017;108(1):19-27.

[7] Takebayashi A, et al. The association between endometriosis and chronic endometritis. PLoS One 2014;9(2):e88354.

[8] Kimura F, et al. Review: chronic endometritis and its effect on reproduction. J Obstet Gynaecol Res 2019;45(5):951-60.

[9] McQueen DB, Bernardi LA, Stephenson MD. Chronic endometritis in women with recurrent early pregnancy loss and/or fetal demise. Fertil Steril 2014;101(4):1026-30.

[10] Wu MY, Ho HN. The role of cytokines in endometriosis. Am J Reprod Immunol 2003;49(5):285-96.

[11] Lousse JC, et al. Increased activation of nuclear factor-kappa B (NF-kappaB) in isolated peritoneal macrophages of patients with endometriosis. Fertil Steril 2008;90(1):217-20.

[12] Montagna P, et al. Peritoneal fluid macrophages in endometriosis: correlation between the expression of estrogen receptors and inflammation. Fertil Steril 2008;90(1):156-64.

[13] Binda MM, Donnez J, Dolmans MM. Targeting mast cells: a new way to treat endometriosis. Expert Opin Ther Targets 2017;21(1):67-75.

[14] Izumi G, et al. Involvement of immune cells in the pathogenesis of endometriosis. J Obstet Gynaecol Res 2018;44(2):191-8.

[15] Prins JR, Gomez-Lopez N, Robertson SA. Interleukin-6 in pregnancy and gestational disorders. J Reprod Immunol 2012;95(1-2):1-14.

[16] Sampson JA. Metastatic or embolic endometriosis, due to the menstrual dissemination of endometrial tissue into the venous circulation. Am J Pathol 1927;3(2):93-110 43.

[17] Giudice LC, Kao LC. Endometriosis. Lancet 2004;364(9447):1789-99.

[18] Thiruchelvam U, Wingfield M, O'Farrelly C. Natural killer cells: key players in endometriosis. Am J Reprod Immunol 2015;74(4):291-301.

[19] Kang YJ. An increased level of IL-6 suppresses NK cell activity in peritoneal fluid of patients with endometriosis via regulation of SHP-2 expression. Hum Reprod 2014;29(10):2176-89.

[20] Chuang PC, et al. Inhibition of CD36-dependent phagocytosis by prostaglandin E2 contributes to the development of endometriosis. Am J Pathol 2010;176(2):850-60.

[21] Wu MH, et al. Suppression of annexin A2 by prostaglandin E(2) impairs phagocytic ability of peritoneal macrophages in women with endometriosis. Hum Reprod 2013;28(4):1045-53.

[22] McLaren J, et al. Vascular endothelial growth factor is produced by peritoneal fluid macrophages in endometriosis and is regulated by ovarian steroids. J Clin Invest 1996;98(2):482-9.

[23] Hughes E, et al. Ovulation suppression for endometriosis. Cochrane Database Syst Rev 2007;(3):CD000155.

[24] Wang R, et al. Tubal flushing for subfertility. Cochrane Database Syst Rev 2020;10:CD003718.

[25] Johnson NP, et al. The FLUSH trial-flushing with lipiodol for unexplained (and endometriosis-related) subfertility by hysterosalpingography: a randomized trial. Hum Reprod 2004;19(9):2043-51.

[26] Johnson JV, Montoya IA, Olive DL. Ethiodol oil contrast medium inhibits macrophage phagocytosis and adherence by altering membrane electronegativity and microviscosity. Fertil Steril 1992;58(3):511-17.

[27] Sawatari Y, Horii T, Hoshiai H. Oily contrast medium as a therapeutic agent for infertility because of mild endometriosis. Fertil Steril 1993;59(4):907-11.

[28] Izumi G, et al. Oil-soluble contrast medium (OSCM) for hysterosalpingography modulates dendritic cell and regulatory T cell profiles in the peritoneal cavity: a possible mechanism by which OSCM enhances fertility. J Immunol 2017;198(11):4277-84.

[29] Johnson NP, et al. Lipiodol alters murine uterine dendritic cell populations: a potential mechanism for the fertility-enhancing effect of lipiodol. Fertil Steril 2005;83(6):1814-21.

[30] Court KA, et al. Establishment of lipiodol as a fertility treatment — prospective study of the complete innovative treatment data set. Aust N Z J Obstet Gynaecol 2014;54(1):13-19.

[31] Reilly SJ, et al. The IVF-LUBE trial — a randomized trial to assess lipiodol (R) uterine bathing effect in women with endometriosis or repeat implantation failure undergoing IVF. Reprod Biomed Online 2019;38(3):380-6.

[32] Kim CH, et al. The immunotherapy during in vitro fertilization and embryo transfer cycles in infertile patients with endometriosis. J Obstet Gynaecol Res 1997;23(5):463-70.

[33] Dmowski WP, et al. The effect of endometriosis, its stage and activity, and of autoantibodies on in vitro fertilization and embryo transfer success rates. Fertil Steril 1995;63(3):555-62.

[34] Onalan G, Tohma YA, Zeyneloglu HB. Effect of etanercept on the success of assisted reproductive technology in patients with endometrioma. Gynecol Obstet Invest 2018;83(4):358-64.

[35] Bafort C, et al. Laparoscopic surgery for endometriosis. Cochrane Database Syst Rev 2020;10:CD011031.

[36] Marcoux S, Maheux R, Berube S. Laparoscopic surgery in infertile women with minimal or mild endometriosis. Canadian collaborative group on endometriosis. N Engl J Med 1997;337(4):217-22.

[37] Benschop L, et al. Interventions for women with endometrioma prior to assisted reproductive technology. Cochrane Database Syst Rev 2010;(11):CD008571.

[38] Drakopoulos P, et al. Does the type of GnRH analogue used, affect live birth rates in women with endometriosis undergoing IVF/ICSI treatment, according to the rAFS stage? Gynecol Endocrinol 2018;34(10):884-9.

[39] Rodriguez-Purata J, et al. Endometriosis and IVF: are agonists really better? Analysis of 1180 cycles with the propensity score matching. Gynecol Endocrinol 2013;29(9):859-62.

[40] Surrey ES, et al. Effect of prolonged gonadotropin-releasing hormone agonist therapy on the outcome of in vitro fertilization-embryo transfer in patients with endometriosis. Fertil Steril 2002;78(4):699-704.

[41] Sallam HN, et al. Long-term pituitary down-regulation before in vitro fertilization (IVF) for women with endometriosis. Cochrane Database Syst Rev 2006;(1):CD004635.

[42] Decleer W, et al. RCT to evaluate the influence of adjuvant medical treatment of peritoneal endometriosis on the outcome of IVF. Hum Reprod 2016;31(9):2017-23.

[43] Georgiou EX, et al. Long-term GnRH agonist therapy before in vitro fertilisation (IVF) for improving fertility outcomes in women with endometriosis. Cochrane Database Syst Rev 2019;2019(11).

[44] Tamura H, et al. The clinical outcome of dienogest treatment followed by in vitro fertilization and embryo transfer in infertile women with endometriosis. J Ovarian Res 2019;12(1):123.

[45] Barra F, et al. Pretreatment with dienogest in women with endometriosis undergoing IVF after a previous failed cycle. Reprod Biomed Online 2020;41(5):859-68.

[46] Wu J, et al. Fertility and neonatal outcomes of freeze-all vs. fresh embryo transfer in women with advanced endometriosis. Front Endocrinol (Lausanne) 2019;10:770.

[47] Bourdon M, et al. The deferred embryo transfer strategy improves cumulative pregnancy rates in endometriosis-related infertility: a retrospective matched cohort study. PLoS One 2018;13(4):e0194800.

第 26 章

生殖障碍的实验室检查:生殖障碍的免疫学生物标志物

Laboratory approaches for reproductive failure: immunological biomarkers for reproductive failures

Katharine Wolf, Kenneth Beaman, Svetlana Dambaeva and Alice Gilman-Sachs

Clinical Immunology Laboratory, Faculty of Microbiology and Immunology, Center for Cancer Biology, Infection and Immunology, The Chicago Medical School, Rosalind Franklin University of Medicine and Science, Chicago, IL, United States

1 基因组评估

1.1 人白细胞抗原-C和自然杀伤细胞

妊娠的关键问题是为什么胎儿不会被母亲的免疫系统排斥。人白细胞抗原(HLA)基因在主要组织相容性复合体Ⅰ类(MHC-Ⅰ)蛋白中的表达,调节移植器官的接受或排斥,在妊娠中亦发挥作用。然而,早期数据表明,关键的移植抗原 HLA-A 和 HLA-B 并不参与正常妊娠期间母体对胎儿的免疫反应[1-3]。然而,MHC Ⅰ类基因座与生殖之间存在关系。在妊娠期,HLA-C、HLA-G 和 HLA-E 分子调节母胎免疫反应[4,5]。

虽然传统的移植反应并不像预期那样适用于胎儿-胎盘单位,但自然杀伤(NK)细胞似乎是一个不同的问题。子宫 NK 细胞活性的变化已成为我们对胎儿-胎盘单位最感兴趣的问题,并且在正常月经周期中观察到子宫周期性变化[6,7]。HLA 序列数据库中记录了 6 800 多个 HLA-C 等位基因[8]。这些等位基因可根据氨基酸 80 位点残基的序列分为 C1 和 C2 两组。C1 组编码精氨酸,C2 组编码赖氨酸[4]。由于 HLA-C 具有多态性,对母系和父系的 HLA-C 等位基因进行基因分型可提供胎儿可能的 HLA-C 组别/组合信息,从而有助于评估反复妊娠丢失(RPL)。

胎儿 HLA-C 结合 NK 细胞上发现的一组被称为杀伤免疫球蛋白样受体(KIR)的配体(图 26.1)。与 HLA 的其他配体一样,KIR 基因在遗传上相互关联,可以激活或抑制 NK 细胞的活性。NK 细胞活性的激活或抑制取决于胎儿 HLA-C 等位基因和母体 KIR 等位基因的组合。简便起见,KIR 基因型可分为 AA 型和 Bx 型两组。AA 基因型由抑制性 KIR 等位基因组成,Bx 基因型由一个或多个激活性 KIR 等位基因组成。KIR 和 HLA-C 基因型在妊娠期调节 NK 细胞活化。当 HLA-C2 与 AA 基因型相互作用时,会出现活化不足以及随后缺乏对胎盘形成的支持。其他 HLA-C 和 AA 组合对妊娠结局的影响较小。因此,AA/HLA-C C2 基因型的阴性预测值是评估 RPL 的重要临床指示[9]。

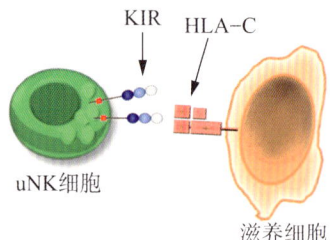

图 26.1 胎盘滋养层细胞的识别是通过人白细胞抗原 (HLA)-C 和杀伤免疫球蛋白样受体完成的。它也可能与 HLA-E 有关。自然杀伤细胞的识别和激活是胎盘的血管化和生长所必需的。

因此，KIR/HLA－C 组合的 NK 细胞活性变化是由于其激活类型的不同，而不是激活或抑制。子宫 NK 细胞虽然名为 NK，但并不具有普遍的破坏性，在妊娠的情况下，它们可以促进滋养细胞的免疫耐受，诱导血管生成，并分泌支持胚胎生长的生长因子[10-12]。对 NK/HLA 相互作用的研究有两个重要的发现：①子宫 NK 细胞活化对于支持妊娠是有益的，而不是有害的。②基于这些机制发现，对 RPL 的治疗干预是有可能的[13,14]。因此，基因组评估应重点关注母系和父系的 HLA－C 等位基因以及母体的 KIR 等位基因。HLA 配体和受体的基因分型对 RPL 的诊断具有重要价值。尽管移植所需的标准 HLA 分型可能仅为评估 RPL 提供有限的信息，但 HLA－C 和 KIR 基因型的分析则可提供有用的诊断信息。

1.2 基因组检测异常的发生率

图 26.2 显示了 KIR 的抑制或激活等位基因，以及 AA 和 3 个 Bx 基因型的代表图。Dambaeva 等[15]进行了一项研究，将患有 RPL 的北美女性与对应的北美人群进行了比较，其中 AA 基因型是最常见的基因型，频率为 32.7%。其余女性分布在 27 个 Bx 基因型中，没有一个基因型频率高于 13%。RPL 患者与参考人群的 KIR 基因型差异无统计学意义。与 KIR 的频率相似，RPL 患者、其配偶或参考人群之间 HLA－C C1 或 C2 等位基因频率没有显著差异。同样，RPL 女性与参考人群之间 HLA－C 等位基因组合频率无显著差异：C1 纯合、C2 纯合或 C1/C2 杂合频率在两组人群中相似。

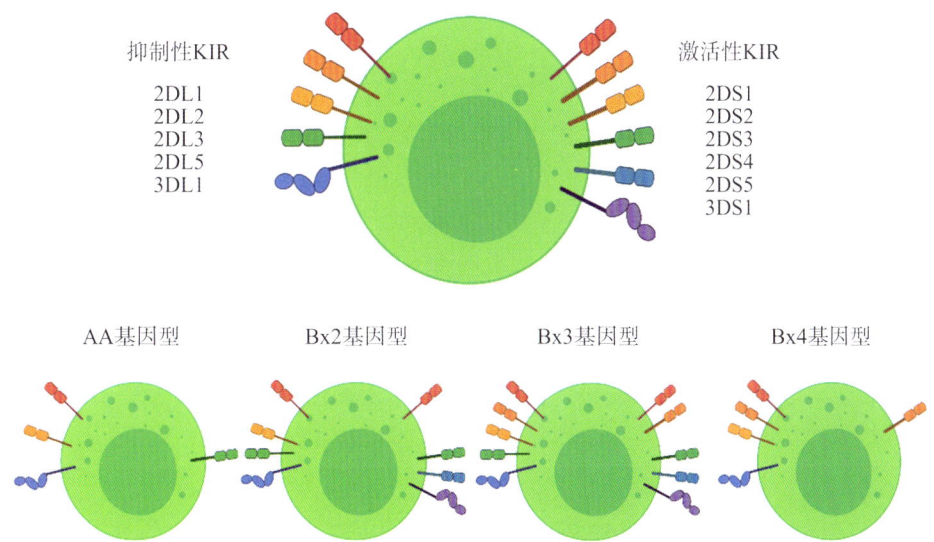

图 26.2 杀伤免疫球蛋白样受体的 AA 基因型或 27 种 Bx 基因型中的任何一种都取决于抑制型或激活型等位基因的数量。

上图展示了部分抑制性或激活性 KIR。下图展示了 AA 基因型和三种 Bx 基因型的代表性图像。

当检测特定 KIR 与 HLA－C 等位基因的遗传组合时，可观察到显著差异[9,15,16]。表达活化 Bx 受体 KIR2DS1 的 RPL 患者更可能携带 HLA－C2 等位基因（图 26.3）。这种组合（KIR2DS1 和同源 HLA－C2）参与 NK 细胞的驯化/许可，并导致携带这两个基因的个体普遍存在功能低下的 NK 细胞[17]。在 RPL 女性的配偶中也观察到 HLA－C2 的频率增加。最后，如上所述，在 RPL 患者中，抑制性 KIR（AA 基因型）与 HLA－C2 组合的频率较高[18-21]。

2 蜕膜化检测

2.1 子宫内膜免疫谱检测

2.1.1 程序

子宫内膜免疫谱（EIP）可利用在冷冻胚胎移植准备的激素替代治疗周期（HRT）或自然周期中所获得的子宫内膜活检样本进行检测。子宫内膜活检按照标准程序进行，约 30 mg 的子宫内膜组织就足以进行分析。

（1）激素替代治疗周期：开始 HRT 周期后，在

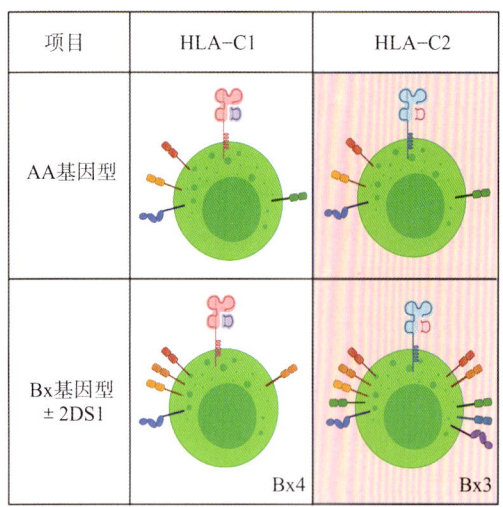

图 26.3 与参考人群相比,某些基因型(红色突出显示)在反复妊娠丢失(RPL)女性中显著富集。

具有 AA 基因型的 RPL 女性同时具有人白细胞抗原(HLA)-C2 的可能性明显更高。具有活化受体 2DS1 的 RPL 女性(例如具有 Bx3 基因型的女性)具有 HLA-C2 的可能性要高得多。

孕酮治疗 5 天后或在预期的冷冻胚胎移植日进行活检[3,22,23]。首次摄入孕酮的日期视为孕酮治疗第 0 天;活检日为孕酮治疗日+5 天。因此,如果首次摄入孕酮日视为孕酮治疗第 1 天,那么活检日为孕酮治疗日+6 天。

(2) 自然周期:黄体生成素达到峰值后的 7~9 天活检,黄体生成素峰值日视为黄体生成素+0 天,则 LH+7~9 天活检。因此,确定黄体生成素峰值的最佳方法是尿黄体生成素检测。

2.1.2 分析

组织学检查受切片数和结果定量的限制。虽然它可以考虑细胞之间的空间关系,但其定量因人而异,不同研究者的定量结果也不尽相同。因此,更好的定量技术是分子检测[24-27]。cDNA 和 mRNA 测序都消除了人为差异和测量因子数量的限制。全序列方法是首先被推广的方法。虽然这种方法成本高、耗时长,它已被报道具有良好的预测结果。

EIP 是一种评估子宫内膜分子免疫表达的检测方法,以确定子宫内膜是否为促进成功妊娠做好了适当准备。这是一种简单、成本较低的方法。为了妊娠成功,子宫内膜必须经历两个过程:蜕膜化和胎盘形成。蜕膜化伴随着母体免疫细胞向蜕膜的大量募集,在妊娠早期,约 70% 的蜕膜淋巴细胞是 NK 细胞。在 EIP 中,检测了 CD56 mRNA 的表达,它与样本中 CD56 NK 细胞的数量相关[6,28,29]。在胎盘形成过程中,胚胎绒毛外滋养层细胞侵入蜕膜,并积极参与螺旋动脉重塑,从而增加了对发育中胚胎/胎儿的血液供应。

研究表明,反复种植失败(RIF)的女性存在子宫 NK 细胞数量过多或减少。与育龄期女性相比,RIF 女性的子宫内膜白细胞介素(IL)-15 和 IL-18,以及肿瘤坏死因子样细胞凋亡弱诱导因子(TWEAK)及其受体 Fn-14(成纤维细胞生长因子诱导分子)水平常发生异常变化。IL-15 和 IL-18 是参与子宫 NK 细胞活化的细胞因子。TWEAK 是一种促血管生成和抗炎的细胞因子,通过 Fn14 发挥作用[13,20,21]。激活信号与控制信号之间的平衡可用 IL-18/TWEAK 和 IL-15/Fn14 比值来测量。通过 CD56 mRNA 转录本定量评估子宫 NK 细胞的丰度。这些比值以及子宫 NK 细胞的评估,已被证明是帮助确定子宫内膜是否能接受胚胎种植和形成胎盘的分子工具。

2.1.3 评价

有 RPL 或 RIF 病史的女性,以及有薄型子宫内膜(厚度≤6 mm)病史的女性可进行该项检查。虽然尚未进行评价,但理论上有理由相信,在开始辅助生殖周期前用 EIP 检测并进行适当治疗的女性,将比未进行筛查和治疗的女性具有更高的活产率[14,20,21,28]。

2.2 子宫内膜蜕膜化评分

Dambaeva 等[27]对多种生长因子和细胞因子进行了研究并发现,与正常生育对照组相比,在生育失败的女性中,观察到有 6 种因子常发生异常。他们确定了可通过医疗干预改变的预测因子,以提高成功妊娠的可能性。利用 ROC 曲线对所有因素综合分析后发现,子宫内膜蜕膜化评分(EDS)的预测性能提高。转录因子 FOXO1、血清和糖皮质激素诱导激酶 1(SGK1)、钠离子通道 SCNN1A 等三个分子均能随孕酮水平的升高而增加。同样,已知葡萄糖转运蛋白溶质载体家族 2 成员 1(SLC2A1)在蜕膜化子宫内膜中上调[30]。与 Ledee 的研究一样,在 IVF 失败和早期妊娠丢失的女性子宫内膜中,NK 细胞标志物颗粒酶 B(GZMB)和细胞因子 IL-15 的 mRNA 表达也发生了改变。在 EDS 中,将这些标志物结合起来,对妊娠结局具有很好的预测价值。如同 HLA-C 和 KIR 分型一样,这些发现可以被纳入干预和预防妊娠丢失的治疗中。

3 外周血细胞分析

虽然通过检测血液中的免疫参数来发现妊娠子宫的变化并不理想，但这往往是我们能做的最好的办法。有人曾经说过：这就像看到消防车在路上开着红灯、鸣着警笛。这可能是紧急情况，也可能是游行。不过，它可以为确定妊娠的成败提供重要信息。20多年来，生殖免疫学家通过检查T细胞和B细胞来评估妊娠，并对NK细胞群进行了近20年的研究[24,25,31]。

3.1 辅助性T细胞(Th)1/Th2细胞比值

最初对RPL的评估是对接受父系淋巴细胞免疫治疗的女性进行免疫反应测试。这种治疗的目的是通过使女性对父系抗原脱敏来改善妊娠结局；然而，由于对干细胞调控的担忧，它在美国已不再使用。尽管如此，这引发了对既往研究结果的回顾，这表明免疫球蛋白或非细胞毒性免疫反应可能对成功妊娠很重要。随后的研究开始揭示，外周血中以细胞毒性或Th1型细胞因子为主的免疫反应不利于成功妊娠。一些研究表明，Th1和Th2产生之间的最佳平衡是妊娠期间适当免疫反应的关键，而Th1/Th2的增加与生殖障碍有关[32]。因此，外周血Th1/Th2检测是诊断RPL的有用指标[28]。

虽然Th1细胞因子(TNF-α和IFN-γ)的增加会导致妊娠丢失，但在适当的时间和浓度下，这些细胞因子在局部子宫胎盘免疫反应中显得又很重要[32]。然而，它们在妊娠早期大量外周血单核细胞中的表达并不表明成功的妊娠结局[28]。在检测妊娠期PD1表达并将RPL与正常妊娠进行比较的研究中，发现Th1/Th2范式与其他标志物如Th17和T调节细胞相对应。虽然这些标志物缺乏统计学上的相关属性，无法在临床环境中成为有用的预后标志物，但它们确实有力支持了Th1/Th2范式[33]。

3.2 自然杀伤细胞水平和细胞毒性

外周血和胎盘界面的另一个重要标志物是NK细胞。NK细胞的检测已经从早期的外周血细胞计数发展到功能活性分析，即细胞毒性的检测。总之，这种评估在检测胎盘生长异常方面具有很高的参考价值。适用于早期妊娠、胚胎种植前和种植期间以及胎儿生长的前3个月。

最初，NK细胞被认为是一种单核细胞，可对缺乏MHC Ⅰ类或Ⅱ类分子的细胞进行细胞溶解。目前已知，它们还能调节免疫系统，介导对肿瘤细胞的自然抵抗，并产生细胞因子。在细胞毒性试验中，单核细胞(包含自然杀伤细胞)与预先用PKH-2(一种结合到细胞膜并发出绿色荧光的亲脂性染料)染色的靶K562细胞孵育2小时[34]。如果绿色的K562被NK细胞杀死，它们的通透性增加，碘化丙啶染料可通过细胞溶解产生的孔隙进入细胞，K562靶细胞会发出明亮的红色/橙色和绿色荧光。然后便可利用流式细胞术测定含有碘化丙啶的被杀靶细胞的百分比。当淋巴细胞与靶细胞以及IgG、脂肪乳剂或强的松一起孵育时，可能会出现细胞毒性抑制。

4 自身抗体在反复妊娠丢失中的作用

4.1 抗磷脂抗体

自身抗体(如抗磷脂抗体、抗甲状腺抗体或抗核抗体)与RPL相关，且易于检测和测量[18,35,36]。抗磷脂综合征(APS)是一种血栓栓塞性疾病，表现为抗磷脂抗体，尤其是抗心磷脂抗体阳性，是这些自身抗体中与RPL最相关的一种。随着各种抗磷脂抗体(其中抗心磷脂抗体是最常见的抗体)检测方法的发展，这些抗体与血栓栓塞性疾病、血小板减少症、系统性红斑狼疮(SLE)、RPL和产科并发症的临床相关性已变得显而易见。梅毒、狼疮抗凝物和抗心磷脂抗体的生物假阳性检测在SLE和RPL患者中得到证实。已建立了针对抗心磷脂抗体和其他抗磷脂抗体的固相ELISA检测方法，该方法具有灵敏和半定量的特点。

抗磷脂抗体的特点是与至少6种不同的磷脂(即心磷脂、磷脂酰丝氨酸、磷脂酰乙醇胺、磷脂酸、磷脂酰甘油、磷脂酰肌醇等)发生交叉反应的异质性自身抗体亚群。2006年，这些抗体被证明与磷脂载体蛋白β-2-糖蛋白Ⅰ(GPI)结合。它们还能与磷脂和这种蛋白质的复合物结合。目前已设计出检测这些单个自身抗体和该复合物特异性自身抗体的检测方法。这些检测方法已经标准化，并按照CLIA 1988的规定进行检测。在孕妇体内已发现了所有这些抗体的IgM、IgG和IgA类抗体。

抗磷脂抗体的检测使用一种具有良好特性的ELISA法。纯化的β2GPI抗原结合在聚苯乙烯微孔板的孔上，将抗原保持在其天然状态。预先稀释的对照组和稀释的患者血清分别加入不同的孔中，使存在的β2GPI IgG 抗体与固定的抗原结合。洗去未结合的样品，并在每个孔中加入酶标记的抗人 IgG 偶联物。第二次孵育使酶标记的抗人 IgG 与附着在微孔上的患者抗体结合。洗去未结合的酶标记抗人类 IgG 后，加入显色底物，测量显色强度以测定剩余的酶活性。利用分光光度计测量患者孔中显影的颜色强度并与五点校准曲线的颜色强度进行比较。

RPL 患者的实验室检查结果和病理表现与经典 APS 综合征患者有所不同，即自身抗体水平较低，很少出现明显的血栓形成。这些自身抗体之间的关系被认为是通过影响抗凝血/凝血复合体来实现的。抗磷脂抗体可与滋养细胞和内皮细胞表面的 GPI 结合，诱导促炎和抗迁移反应，从而阻止胚胎种植和胎盘生长[36]。此外，抗磷脂抗体可结合并激活补体，随后通过与蜕膜结合并抑制滋养细胞的侵袭干扰胎盘的生长。补体激活也可能招募中性粒细胞，从而导致胎盘功能不全、宫内生长受限和胎儿死亡。因此，除了最初推测的血栓形成是这些抗体在妊娠丢失中的作用外，上述其他因素也被推测并证明会导致妊娠丢失。在妊娠早期使用抗凝剂（如肝素、阿司匹林）可防止妊娠丢失，而在妊娠后期则不一定有效。

4.2 抗核抗体

RPL 患者还应检测抗核抗体（ANA），如果发现抗体滴度升高，应进一步区分抗体，以排除干燥综合征（SS-a/RO 和 SS-B/La）或红斑狼疮。高滴度 ANA 阳性结果通常发生在许多自身免疫性疾病中，如系统性红斑狼疮（SLE）、混合性结缔组织病（MCTD）、类风湿关节炎（RA）、干燥综合征（SS）和进行性系统性硬化（PSS）。

每一种不同的风湿性疾病通常表现出特定的 ANA 特征。因此，识别患者 ANA 的特异性对于鉴别诊断这些疾病非常有用。抗 Sm 是一种高度特异性的血清学标志物，在 20%～30% 的 SLE 患者中发现。在多种风湿性疾病中常检测到 RNP 抗体；然而，对该抗原的高滴度反应通常被认为是混合性结缔组织病的诊断。SS-A/Ro 和 SS-B/La 抗体在 SS 中出现的频率最高，尽管在 SLE 患者中也发现了这些抗原特异性。此外，SS-A/Ro 抗体与先天性胎儿心脏传导阻滞之间存在关联。所有这些自身抗体（RNP、Sm、SSA/Ro 和 SS-B/La）均可采用 ELISA 进行检测。

抗 DNA 抗体对妊娠结局产生负面影响并导致 RPL 的机制可能是通过其他致病抗体来实现的。这些抗体可与胎盘细胞或其他组织结合并激活补体，表现为免疫复合物，将中性粒细胞或单核细胞吸引到母胎界面的某个区域，或吸引淋巴或浆细胞样树突状细胞，从而激活其他细胞分泌促炎细胞因子[23]。这些过程可能影响和抑制胎盘或胚胎的生长。

4.3 其他自身抗体

其他多种自身抗体也与 RPL 有关。对于有食物过敏史的女性，可考虑检测抗组织谷氨酰胺转氨酶 IgA 抗体（tTG-IgA 试验），若为阳性，则进行活组织检查，以排除乳糜泻。

5 内分泌检查

建议对患有 RPL 的女性进行内分泌检查，以确定促甲状腺激素（TSH）水平[23,35]。如果发现 TSH 水平异常，则必须检测 T_3、T_4 和甲状腺自身抗体浓度。循环中的甲状腺自身抗体被广泛认为与自身免疫性甲状腺疾病的病因有关，甲状腺球蛋白和甲状腺过氧化物酶自身抗体在临床实践中都是常规检测项目。甲状腺微粒体抗原的血清自身抗体是甲状腺自身免疫性疾病患者常见的抗体。此外，甲状腺疾病与早产和妊娠丢失有关。最近的一篇综述指出，抗 TPO 抗体可能与活产率降低有关。因此，对于患有自身免疫性甲状腺疾病的女性，建议进行甲状腺水平和自身抗体的检测[23]。

6 其他检测

还有许多其他检测方法可用于管理 RPL，例如对各种遗传性血栓性疾病基因（FV Leiden、MTHFR 或 PAI-1）进行基因分型，对其他 Th 亚群（如 T 调节细胞或 Th17 细胞）进行量化，在使用 TNF 抑制剂后确定 TNFα 水平，以及测量细胞外囊泡以监测 RPL[37]。

7 总结和建议

妊娠丢失是一个复杂的免疫、遗传和生理过程，对于具有这种不良结局的女性，应更好了解各种检测结果，以便知道如何治疗 RPL。
- 在目前推荐的 RPL 和 RIF 检测后，仍有超过 50% 的患者可能无法解释原因。
- 相当一部分患有 RPL 和 RIF 的女性存在免疫异常。
- KIR 和 HLA－C 基因分型可提供有关 NK 细胞对妊娠支持作用的信息。
- 外周血 NK 细胞水平、细胞毒性和 Th1/Th2 检测有助于确定具有免疫病因 RPL 和 RIF 的女性。
- APA、ANA、ATA 和抗卵巢抗体等自身抗体的筛查通常有助于研究 RPL 和 RIF 的潜在自身免疫病因。

参考文献

[1] Beaman KD, Dambaeva S, Katara GK, Kulshrestha A, Gilman-Sachs A. The immune response in pregnancy and in cancer is active and supportive of placental and tumor cell growth not their destruction. Gynecol Oncol 2017;145(3):476–80. Available from: https://doi.org/10.1016/j.ygyno.2017.04.019.

[2] Beaman KD, Jaiswal MK, Katara GK, et al. Pregnancy is a model for tumors, not transplantation. Am J Reprod Immunol N Y N 1989 2016;76(1):3–7. Available from: https://doi.org/10.1111/aji.12524.

[3] Moffett A, Chazara O, Colucci F. Maternal allo-recognition of the fetus. Fertil Steril 2017;107(6):1269–72. Available from: https://doi.org/10.1016/j.fertnstert.2017.05.001.

[4] Felker AM, Croy BA. Uterine natural killer cell partnerships in early mouse decidua basalis. J Leukoc Biol 2016;100(4):645–55. Available from: https://doi.org/10.1189/jlb.1HI0515-226R.

[5] Croy BA, Zhang J, Tayade C, Colucci F, Yadi H, Yamada AT. Analysis of uterine natural killer cells in mice. Meth Mol Biol Clifton NJ 2010;612:465–503. Available from: https://doi.org/10.1007/978-1-60761-362-6_31.

[6] Trundley A, Moffett A. Human uterine leukocytes and pregnancy. Tissue Antigens 2004;63(1):1–12. Available from: https://doi.org/10.1111/j.1399-0039.2004.00170.x.

[7] Tukwasibwe S, Nakimuli A, Traherne J, et al. Variations in killer-cell immunoglobulin-like receptor and human leukocyte antigen genes and immunity to malaria. Cell Mol Immunol 2020;17(8):799–806. Available from: https://doi.org/10.1038/s41423-020-0482-z.

[8] Robinson J, Barker DJ, Georgiou X, Cooper MA, Flicek P, Marsh SGE. IPD-IMGT/HLA database. Nucleic Acids Res 2020;48(D1):D948–55. Available from: https://doi.org/10.1093/nar/gkz950.

[9] Hiby SE, Walker JJ, O'Shaughnessy KM, et al. Combinations of maternal KIR and fetal HLA-C genes influence the risk of preeclampsia and reproductive success. J Exp Med 2004;200(8):957–65. Available from: https://doi.org/10.1084/jem.20041214.

[10] Fu B, Zhou Y, Ni X, et al. Natural killer cells promote fetal development through the secretion of growth-promoting factors. Immunity 2017;47(6):1100–13. Available from: https://doi.org/10.1016/j.immuni.2017.11.018 e6.

[11] Lima PDA, Tu MM, Rahim MMA, Peng AR, Croy BA, Makrigiannis AP. Ly49 receptors activate angiogenic mouse DBA$^-$ uterine natural killer cells. Cell Mol Immunol 2014;11(5):467–76. Available from: https://doi.org/10.1038/cmi.2014.44.

[12] Sojka DK, Yang L, Yokoyama WM. Uterine natural killer cells. Front Immunol 2019;10:960. Available from: https://doi.org/10.3389/fimmu.2019.00960.

[13] Petitbarat M, Rahmati M, Sérazin V, et al. TWEAK appears as a modulator of endometrial IL－18 related cytotoxic activity of uterine natural killers. PLoS ONE 2011;6(1):e14497. Available from: https://doi.org/10.1371/journal.pone.0014497.

[14] Lédée N, Gridelet V, Ravet S, et al. Impact of follicular G-CSF quantification on subsequent embryo transfer decisions: a proof of concept study. Hum Reprod Oxf Engl 2013;28(2):406–13. Available from: https://doi.org/10.1093/humrep/des354.

[15] Dambaeva SV, Lee DH, Sung N, et al. Recurrent pregnancy loss in women with killer cell immunoglobulin-like receptor KIR2DS1 is associated with an increased HLA-C2 allelic frequency. Am J Reprod Immunol 2016;75(2):94–103. Available from: https://doi.org/10.1111/aji.12453.

[16] Yang X, Yang E, Wang WJ, et al. Decreased HLA-C1 alleles in couples of KIR2DL2 positive women with recurrent pregnancy loss. J Reprod Immunol 2020;142:103186. Available from: https://doi.org/10.1016/j.jri.2020.103186.

[17] Pittari G, Liu XR, Selvakumar A, et al. NK cell tolerance of self-specific activating receptor KIR2DS1 in individuals with cognate HLA-C2 ligand. J Immunol Baltim Md 1950 2013;190(9):4650–60. Available from: https://doi.org/10.4049/jimmunol.1202120.

[18] Kwak-Kim J, Agcaoili MSL, Aleta L, et al. Management of women with recurrent pregnancy losses and anti-phospholipid antibody syndrome. Am J Reprod Immunol N Y N 1989 2013;69(6):596–607. Available from: https://doi.org/10.1111/aji.12114.

[19] Huhn O, Ivarsson MA, Gardner L, et al. Distinctive phenotypes and functions of innate lymphoid cells in human decidua during early pregnancy. Nat Commun 2020;11(1):381. Available from: https://doi.org/10.1038/s41467-019-14123-z.

[20] Lédée N, Petitbarat M, Chevrier L, et al. The uterine immune profile may help women with repeated unexplained embryo implantation failure after in vitro fertilization. Am J Reprod Immunol N Y N 1989 2016;75(3):388–401. Available from: https://doi.org/10.1111/aji.12483.

[21] Lédée N, Prat-Ellenberg L, Chevrier L, et al. Uterine immune profiling for increasing live birth rate: a one-to-one matched cohort study. J Reprod Immunol 2017;119:23–30.

Available from: https://doi.org/10.1016/j.jri.2016.11.007.

[22] El-Azzamy H, Dambaeva SV, Katukurundage D, et al. Dysregulated uterine natural killer cells and vascular remodeling in women with recurrent pregnancy losses. Am J Reprod Immunol N Y N 1989 2018;80(4):e13024. Available from: https://doi.org/10.1111/aji.13024.

[23] Vomstein K, Feil K, Strobel L, et al. Immunological risk factors in recurrent pregnancy loss: guidelines vs current state of the art. J Clin Med 2021;10(4):869. Available from: https://doi.org/10.3390/jcm10040869.

[24] Beaman KD, Ntrivalas E, Mallers TM, Jaiswal MK, Kwak-Kim J, Gilman-Sachs A. Immune etiology of recurrent pregnancy loss and its diagnosis. Am J Reprod Immunol N Y N 1989 2012;67(4):319–25. Available from: https://doi.org/10.1111/j.1600-0897.2012.01118.x.

[25] Davies ML, Dambaeva SV, Katukurundage D, et al. Predicting NK cell subsets using gene expression levels in peripheral blood and endometrial biopsy specimens. Am J Reprod Immunol N Y N 1989 2017;78(3). Available from: https://doi.org/10.1111/aji.12730.

[26] Shreeve N, Depierreux D, Hawkes D, et al. The CD94/NKG2A inhibitory receptor educates uterine NK cells to optimize pregnancy outcomes in humans and mice. Immunity 2021;54(6):1231–44. Available from: https://doi.org/10.1016/j.immuni.2021.03.021 e4.

[27] Dambaeva S, Bilal M, Schneiderman S, et al. Decidualization score identifies an endometrial dysregulation in samples from women with recurrent pregnancy losses and unexplained infertility. FS Rep 2021;2(1):95–103. Available from: https://doi.org/10.1016/j.xfre.2020.12.004.

[28] Sojka DK, Yang L, Plougastel-Douglas B, Higuchi DA, Croy BA, Yokoyama WM. Cutting edge: local proliferation of uterine tissue-resident NK cells during decidualization in mice. J Immunol Baltim Md 1950 2018;201(9):2551–6. Available from: https://doi.org/10.4049/jimmunol.1800651.

[29] Turco MY, Moffett A. Development of the human placenta. Dev Camb Engl 2019;146(22):dev163428. Available from: https://doi.org/10.1242/dev.163428.

[30] von Wolff M, Ursel S, Hahn U, Steldinger R, Strowitzki T. Glucose transporter proteins (GLUT) in human endometrium: expression, regulation, and function throughout the menstrual cycle and in early pregnancy. J Clin Endocrinol Metab 2003;88(8):3885–92. Available from: https://doi.org/10.1210/jc.2002-021890.

[31] Kwak-Kim JYH, Chung-Bang HS, Ng SC, et al. Increased T helper 1 cytokine responses by circulating T cells are present in women with recurrent pregnancy losses and in infertile women with multiple implantation failures after IVF. Hum Reprod Oxf Engl 2003;18(4):767–73. Available from: https://doi.org/10.1093/humrep/deg156.

[32] Wang W, Sung N, Gilman-Sachs A, Kwak-Kim JT. Helper (Th) cell profiles in pregnancy and recurrent pregnancy losses: Th1/Th2/Th9/Th17/Th22/Tfh cells. Front Immunol 2020;11:2025. Available from: https://doi.org/10.3389/fimmu.2020.02025.

[33] Wang WJ, Salazar Garcia MD, Deutsch G, et al. PD-1 and PD-L1 expression on T-cell subsets in women with unexplained recurrent pregnancy losses. Am J Reprod Immunol N Y N 1989 2020;83(5):e13230. Available from: https://doi.org/10.1111/aji.13230.

[34] Salazar MD, Wang WJ, Skariah A, et al. Post-hoc evaluation of peripheral blood natural killer cell cytotoxicity in predicting the risk of recurrent pregnancy losses and repeated implantation failures. J Reprod Immunol 2022;150:103487. Available from: https://doi.org/10.1016/j.jri.2022.103487.

[35] He Q, Zhang Y, Qiu W, Fan J, Zhang C, Kwak-Kim J. Does thyroid autoimmunity affect the reproductive outcome in women with thyroid autoimmunity undergoing assisted reproductive technology. Am J Reprod Immunol N Y N 1989 2020;84(6):e13321. Available from: https://doi.org/10.1111/aji.13321.

[36] Pantham P, Abrahams VM, Chamley LW. The role of anti-phospholipid antibodies in autoimmune reproductive failure. Reprod Camb Engl 2016;151(5):R79–90. Available from: https://doi.org/10.1530/REP-15-0545.

[37] Rajaratnam N, Ditlevsen NE, Sloth JK, Bæk R, Jørgensen MM, Christiansen OB. Extracellular vesicles: an important biomarker in recurrent pregnancy loss? J Clin Med 2021;10(12):2549. Available from: https://doi.org/10.3390/jcm10122549.

推荐阅读

Bilal MY, Katara G, Dambaeva S, Kwak-Kim J, Gilman-Sachs A, Beaman KD. Clinical molecular genetics evaluation in women with reproductive failures. Am J Reprod Immunol N Y N 1989 2021;85(4):e13313. Available from: https://doi.org/10.1111/aji.13313.